Part 1

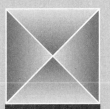

Chemotherapy Principles and Practice

■

Managing Hazardous Drugs

CHEMOTHERAPY PRINCIPLES AND PRACTICE

THE GOAL OF CANCER TREATMENT is to completely destroy or control the growth of neoplastic cells without significantly affecting the viability and function of host cells. Treatments have produced a high rate of tumor regression, enhancing survival or providing palliation for many patients. Today, achieving either complete remission (no evidence of tumor or associated physical, chemical, or symptomatic abnormalities) or partial remission (at least 50% regression in tumor size and only mild symptomatic or performance abnormalities) is an attainable goal for many patients.

Each treatment modality—chemotherapy (cytotoxic drugs and hormonal therapy), biologic response modifiers, targeted therapies, immunotherapy, surgery, and radiation—has specific indications. Depending on various factors, one or more modalities may be used.

Chemotherapy is the primary modality for patients with leukemia or choriocarcinoma. However, virtually all cancer patients receive cytotoxic drugs at one point or another.

• In neoadjunctive chemotherapy, cytotoxic drugs are given before surgery (along with radiation) to reduce or limit the extent of surgical excision.

• In adjuvant chemotherapy, cytotoxic drugs are given after surgery to help prevent cancer recurrence and metastasis.

• Concurrent chemotherapy is commonly given simultaneously with radiation or other modalities.

• Palliative chemotherapy is used to relieve symptoms.

Origins of chemotherapy

German scientist Paul Ehrlich launched the science of chemotherapy in 1910 when he used chemical synthesis to develop Salvarsan, the first syphilis cure. However, cytotoxic drugs were not used successfully against cancer until the 1940s, when the first clinical trial of nitrogen mustard was conducted in lymphoma patients.

Since then, advancements in cancer chemotherapy have hinged on drug discovery. Although the pharmacology of cytotoxic drugs is complex, generally these drugs kill cancer cells by affecting DNA synthesis or function. The prevailing opinion is that cytotoxic drugs cause unbalanced growth of cancer cells, initiating an execution phase in which proteases, nucleases, and endogenous regulators of the cell death pathway are activated and, ultimately, apoptosis (cell death) occurs.

Chemotherapy drug classifications

Nearly all cytotoxic drugs affect DNA synthesis or function—a process that occurs during the cell cycle. The cell cycle has four phases:

• M—mitosis, during which cell division occurs

• G_1—the first gap (postmitotic or presynthetic) phase, during which the cell makes the enzymes necessary for DNA synthesis

• S—characterized by DNA synthesis

• G_2—the second gap (premitotic or postsynthetic) phase, during which RNA and other proteins are synthesized for the M phase.

Cells that complete the M phase either repeat the cell cycle, differentiate and mature into specialized cells and eventually die, or go into the resting phase (G_0). Many chemotherapy drugs appear to act on enzymes involved in DNA synthesis or function; consequently, proliferating cells in the M phase are most susceptible to drug effects.

Most antineoplastic drugs are cytotoxic rather than tumoricidal, acting on biochemical pathways of both normal and neoplastic cells. Although their action is somewhat specific for malignant cells, antineoplastic agents also may affect other rapidly proliferating cells or tissues—most notably, bone marrow, GI epithelium, skin, hair follicles, and embryonic structures.

Based on their effects during the cell-cycle phase, most cytotoxic drugs fall into one of two categories:
• phase-specific drugs, which exert their lethal effects only (or primarily) during a specific phase of the cell cycle (usually the M or S phase)
• phase-nonspecific drugs, which are lethal to cells during multiple phases.

However, some cytotoxic drugs have more than one specificity, or their exact mechanism of action is unknown.

Phase-specific drugs

Cytotoxic drugs that act selectively during certain cell-cycle phases include antimetabolites, vinca alkaloids, taxanes, and type I topoisomerase inhibitors.

Antimetabolites

Antimetabolites are structural analogues of normally occurring metabolites. They interfere with normal nucleic acid biosynthesis by competing with purines and pyrimidines in important metabolic pathways. They can damage DNA indirectly through misincorporation into DNA, by causing abnormal timing or progression through DNA synthesis, or by altering the function of pyrimidine and purine biosynthetic enzymes.

Most antimetabolites exert their action and are most toxic to cells in the S phase, with the degree of toxicity increasing with duration of exposure. Antimetabolites slow the entry of some cells into the S phase, sparing these cells from the drug's effects during a given exposure. Therefore, their cytotoxic effects may be limited.

Antimetabolites are subdivided into three categories.
• **Folic acid antagonists** (such as methotrexate) prevent reduction of folic acid to tetrahydrofolic acid by inhibiting the enzyme dihydrofolic acid reductase. Used with leucovorin as an adjuvant treatment for osteosarcomas, they also are commonly given to children and adults with hematopoietic neoplasms.
• **Purine analogues** (such as azathioprine, cladribine, fludarabine, mercaptopurine, pentostatin, and thioguanine) interfere with nucleic acid synthesis and interconversion of biological purines. Typically, they are used to treat acute lymphoid leukemias and lymphoma.
• **Pyrimidine analogues** (including capecitabine, cytarabine, floxuridine, fluorouracil, and gemcitabine) interfere with uridine and thymine biosynthesis and halt production of cytosine and thymine, preventing new DNA production. They are useful against various solid tumors, such as those of the breast and colon.

Vinca alkaloids

Vinca alkaloids (including vinblastine, vincristine, and vinorelbine) act against cancer through a mechanism that is not fully understood. They are thought to exert cytotoxic effects by binding to tubulin, the protein subunit of the microtubules that forms cellular mitotic spindles or "scaffolding." Formation of vinca alkaloid–tubulin complexes prevents polymerization of the tubulin subunits into microtubules and induces depolymerization of microtubules—ultimately inhibiting microtubule assembly and arresting mitosis in metaphase. Vinca alkaloids are used to treat

Hodgkin's disease, non-Hodgkin's lymphoma, some leukemias, and breast cancer.

Taxanes

Taxanes (docetaxel and paclitaxel) affect the cytoplasmic protein tubulin. They are thought to disrupt the dynamic equilibrium of the microtubule system and block cells in the late G_2 phase and M phase, thereby inhibiting cell replication. Taxanes are used to treat breast and lung cancers.

Type I topoisomerase inhibitors

Type I topoisomerase inhibitors (irinotecan and topotecan) exert their cytotoxic effects during the S phase through an interaction with the DNA-DNA topoisomerase cleavable complex. These agents are used to treat colorectal and ovarian cancers.

Phase-nonspecific drugs

Phase-nonspecific cytotoxic drugs act against both proliferating and resting cells. This category includes alkylating agents, platinum agents, and antitumor antibiotics.

Alkylating agents

The oldest class of antineoplastics, alkylating agents are highly reactive carbonium ions that alter normal biological function by reacting with essential cellular components. Attaching easily to DNA, they react with phosphate, amino, sulfhydryl, hydroxyl, carboxyl, and imidazole groups, causing multiple lesions in both dividing and nondividing cells. Alkylation leads to depurination, cellular miscoding, and crosslinking of DNA strands; these effects in turn interfere with DNA replication and RNA transcription and disrupt nucleic acid function. Crosslinking appears to contribute more to the drugs' cytotoxic effects, whereas depurination and chain scission cause permanent structural modifications resulting in mutagenesis or carcinogenesis. Intracellular enzymes can modify initial DNA damage; however, DNA crosslinking is difficult to repair, especially after high doses of alkylating agents.

Chemically, alkylating agents fall into six groups:
- nitrogen mustards, such as chlorambucil, cyclophosphamide, ifosfamide, mechlorethamine, and melphalan
- estrogen/nitrogen mustard, such as estramustine phosphate sodium
- alkylsulfonates, such as busulfan
- ethylenimines, such as altretamine and thiotepa
- triazenes, such as dacarbazine and temozolomide
- nitrosoureas, such as carmustine, lomustine, and streptozocin.

Platinum agents

Platinums (including carboplatin, cisplatin, and oxaliplatin) are natural metal derivatives that work by crosslinking DNA subunits. This effect causes inhibition of DNA synthesis, transcription, and function.

Antitumor antibiotics

Antitumor antibiotics (such as dactinomycin, daunorubicin, doxorubicin, epirubicin, and possibly mitomycin) are phase-nonspecific. (It is not known whether bleomycin and plicamycin are phase-specific or nonspecific.). Unlike anti-infective antibiotics, they disrupt cellular function by binding to or complexing with DNA. Ultimately, they inhibit protein synthesis by inhibiting DNA-dependent RNA synthesis, directly inhibiting RNA synthesis, altering DNA and subsequently inhibiting RNA synthesis, or reacting with DNA to produce strand scission.

Unclassified chemotherapy drugs

Some drugs used to treat cancer cannot be classified by their effect on the cell cycle because they are not cytotoxic, their action is unknown, their precise mechanism of action is multifaceted, or site of action has not been determined precisely. These drugs include biological response modifiers, targeted therapies, hormonal antineoplastics (used in breast and prostate cancer), some retinoids, and certain other miscellaneous drugs.

Biological response modifiers

Biological response modifiers enhance the host's innate antitumor defense mechanisms. Denileukin diftitox is a recombinant DNA-derived cytotoxic protein designed to direct the cytocidal activity of diphtheria toxin to malignant cells of cutaneous T-cell lymphoma. Studies suggest it interacts with interleukin-2 receptors on the cell surface and inhibits cellular protein synthesis, causing cell death within hours.

Targeted cancer therapies

Targeted cancer therapies (such as monoclonal antibodies; small-molecule inhibitors of the epidermal growth factor receptor [EGFR]–pathway in lung, breast, and colorectal cancers; and proapoptotic and proteasome inhibitors) use drugs that block the growth and spread of cancer by interfering with specific molecules in carcinogenesis and tumor growth. Many targeted cancer therapies are in preclinical testing.

Monoclonal antibodies

Monoclonal antibodies identify and bind to specific antigens on cancer cells, inducing an immunologic response against the target cell. Trastuzumab, a recombinant DNA-derived humanized murine monoclonal antibody, binds specifically to human EGFR 2—a transmembrane receptor protein that is overexpressed in selected cancer cells, such as those found in breast cancer. This binding inhibits tumor cell proliferation.

Rituximab, a chimeric human-murine monoclonal antibody, binds specifically to antigen CD20, a hydrophobic transmembrane protein located on normal pre-B and mature B lymphocytes. A host immune response ensues, resulting in lysis of normal and malignant B cells.

Like rituximab, ibritumomab binds specifically to antigen CD20 on normal and malig-

nant B cells, inducing cellular damage by forming free radicals in target and neighboring cells.

Alemtuzumab, a recombinant DNA-derived humanized anti-CD52 monoclonal antibody, binds specifically to antigen CD52, triggering a host immune response that causes lysis of normal and leukemic cells.

Gemtuzumab ozogamicin, a recombinant humanized monoclonal antibody, binds specifically to antigen CD33—an adhesion protein expressed on leukemic blasts in more than 80% of patients with acute myeloid leukemia. This binding triggers release of calicheamicin, a potent antitumor antibiotic. Calicheamicin binds to the minor groove of DNA, causing doublestrand breaks and cell death.

Small-molecule inhibitors

Small-molecule inhibitors, also called signal-transduction inhibitors, target and block specific enzymes and EGFRs in cancer cell growth. Imatinib mesylate, for example, is a protein-tyrosine inhibitor that competitively inhibits tyrosine phosphorylation of proteins involved in signal transduction and consequently proliferation. It induces apoptosis of Bcr-Abl-positive cells as well as fresh leukemic cells in Philadelphia chromosome–positive chronic myeloid leukemia.and is also used to treat GI stromal tumors.

Apoptosis-inducing drugs

Apoptosis-inducing drugs, such as Velcade and Genasense, cause cancer cells to undergo apoptosis by interfering with proteins necessary for the process. Velcade is used to treat multiple myeloma not responsive to other treatment. Genasense, presently available only in clinical trials, is used to treat leukemia, non-Hodgkin's lymphoma, and solid tumors.

Hormonal antineoplastics

Hormonal antineoplastics decrease the levels of hormones thought to contribute to the growth of certain cancers, such as breast and prostate cancer. Goserelin acetate, leuprolide acetate, and triptorelin pamoate are gonadotropin-releasing hormone (GnRH) analogues that suppress gonadotropin secretion and androgen and estrogen synthesis, inhibiting the growth of hormone-dependent tumors.

Megestrol acetate, a synthetic progestin, may work by inhibiting pituitary function, which causes suppression of luteinizing hormone. Nonsteroidal antiandrogens (including bicalutamide, flutamide, and nilutamide) inhibit the action of androgens by competitively blocking nuclear androgen receptors in such target tissues as the prostate, seminal vesicles, and adrenal cortex.

Tamoxifen and toremifene are estrogen agonist-antagonists (previously called antiestrogens) that compete with estrogen for binding to cytoplasmic estrogen receptors, thereby blocking tumor growth stimulated by estrogen. Fulvestrant—a steroidal estrogen antagonist—competitively binds to, inhibits, and down-regulates estrogen receptors in breast cancer cells. Testolactone (an antiandrogen) and the aromatase inhibitors anastrozole, exemestane, and letrozole inhibit conversion of adrenal androgens to estrogens, thus inhibiting the growth of hormone-dependent tumors.

Retinoids

Alitretinoin (9-*cis*-retinoic acid) and tretinoin (all-*trans* retinoic acid) are endogenous retinoids that increase cellular differentiation, reduce cellular proliferation, and increase apoptosis in both normal cells and cancer cells.

Miscellaneous agents

Arsenic trioxide appears to cause morphologic changes and DNA fragmentation typical of programmed cell death. It also damages or degrades a fusion gene characteristic of acute promyelocytic leukemia.

Asparaginase and pegaspargase interfere with the growth of some leukemic cells by depleting asparaginase, an amino acid required for synthesis of DNA and essential proteins.

Chemotherapy protocols

Antineoplastic drugs usually are given in combinations (also called regimens or protocols) that may include several different drugs. The goal of administering combination chemotherapy in cycles or specific sequences is to produce additive or synergistic therapeutic effects while delaying the emergence of drug resistance and minimizing overwhelming toxicities.

In single-drug therapy, some tumor cells resist the drug; even cells that responded to the drug at first eventually grow resistant. In contrast, combination chemotherapy enhances tumor cell destruction while minimizing drug resistance and toxicities by allowing administration of several drugs with different mechanisms of action and with different toxicities. If a specific overlapping toxicity cannot be avoided, the drugs involved should differ in the onset of that toxicity.

Each drug in the regimen should be effective alone against the specific neoplasm and should potentiate the effects of the other drugs. In some protocols, a cell-cycle phase-nonspecific drug is given first, followed by a phase-specific drug to provoke any cells that survived the first drug into mitosis and thus make them more susceptible to the second drug.

Some drugs are more effective in inducing than maintaining remission. To maximize the benefit of chemotherapy, some sequential regimens consist of drugs that periodically reinduce or reinforce induction, thereby prolonging remission.

Choice of an appropriate protocol centers on patient factors, tumor type, and tumor grade or degree of malignancy. Clinician preferences also play a role. Whichever protocol is used, the clinician must have a thorough understanding of the pharmacology and toxicities of each drug.

Managing chemotherapy

Most antineoplastic drugs have a narrow therapeutic index. Thus, their effective use hinges on balancing their cytotoxic effects against their inherent toxicity to host cells.

The outcome of chemotherapy depends on the interaction among drug, tumor, and patient. Specific drugs, dosages, and administration routes must be chosen on the basis of their relative efficacy and toxicity, tumor growth characteristics, drug effect during the cell cycle, and drug pharmacokinetics. The clinician must carefully consider the patient's clinical and histologic diagnosis, clinical status, age, sex, and previous treatment. Chemotherapy should be given only if expected therapeutic benefits clearly outweigh the hazards.

Dosage calculation

In both children and adults, dosages are more accurately calculated by using body surface area (BSA)— a mathematical function of height and weight—rather than weight alone. Originally, BSA was intended to provide cross-species dosage conversion to determine dosages for patients in phase I chemotherapy trials. Now, it is the standard for determining dosages of chemotherapeutic agents. Dosage calculation must take into accouont such factors as the patient's renal function.

Patient management

Because most antineoplastics are highly toxic, patient management must address complications of the treatment as well as the disease. Toxicity—especially delayed toxicity caused by damage to regenerating tissues—is a common limiting factor for chemotherapy drugs. The risk of toxicity increases in patients who have received previous treatment with antineoplastics or radiation therapy.

During a chemotherapy treatment course, the patient's functional status may decline. Most often, treatment-induced toxicity affects rapidly proliferating tissues, causing varying degrees of myelosuppression and related hematologic toxicities as well as nausea and vomiting. Less common adverse effects include alopecia, diarrhea, and mucositis. More than ever, oncology clinicians are focusing on reducing unfavorable side effects of chemotherapy and improving pain control.

Myelosuppression

Most antineoplastics affect the normal immune response, causing suppression of antibody production with delayed hypersensitivity reactions, reduced cellular immunity, or both. Some drugs also affect the inflammatory reaction and alter the function and number of phagocytes. Immunosuppression may make the patient more susceptible to opportunistic infections and cause febrile neutropenia, anemia, and thrombocytopenia.

Managing neutropenia

Neutropenia peaks 6 to 14 days after conventional doses of anthracyclines, antifolates, and antimetabolites; with alkylating agents, its onset varies. In patients with a nadir neutrophil count above $1,000/mm^3$, the risk of mortality is minimal; when the nadir neutrophil count is below $500/mm^3$, the risk of mortality increases.

Treatment of febrile neutropenia includes antibiotic or antifungal therapy given for the duration of neutropenia symptoms. Antibiotic or antifungal agent selection is based on the suspected organism; careful physical examination of catheter sites, dentition, mucosal surfaces, and perirectal and genital orifices; chest X-ray findings; and urine, blood, and sputum culture results. In some cases, granulocyte colony-stimulating factors may be given to reduce the incidence of febrile neutropenia.

Managing anemia

Typically, if hemoglobin is below 8 g/dl or if compromising conditions (such as pulmonary or cardiac disease) warrant maintaining hemoglobin above 9 g/dl, packed red blood cell transfusions are given. Patients who receive chemotherapy for more than 2 months or who have underlying complications may be candidates for erythropoietin therapy.

Managing thrombocytopenia

Thrombocytopenia rarely complicates chemotherapy for solid tumors but is common in patients with certain hematologic malignancies that have infiltrated the bone marrow. Bleeding related to thrombocytopenia may occur when the platelet count drops below 20,000/mm³ and is common when the platelet count is below 5,000/mm³. In leukemia patients, prophylactic transfusions are warranted to keep the platelet count above 20,000/mm³; in patients with solid tumors, the threshold for transfusions is 10,000/mm³. In clinical investigation, certain cytokines have shown promise in increasing platelet counts.

Nausea and vomiting

Nausea with or without vomiting is the most common chemotherapy adverse effect. Antineoplastic agents vary in emetogenic potential. Actinomycin, cisplatin, dacarbazine, mechlorethamine, and the nitrosoureas are highly emetogenic and cause vomiting in nearly all patients. Other drugs are moderately emetogenic, and a few—for instance, melphalan and chlorambucil—rarely cause emesis when given in standard dosages. With still other antineoplastics, such as antimetabolites, emetogenicity varies with the dosage and dosing schedule.

Successful management of chemotherapy-induced nausea and vomiting centers on giving combinations of antiemetic drugs from different classes based on the drugs' emetogenic potential and the type of emesis (acute, delayed, breakthrough, or anticipatory) the drugs typically cause. Psychological techniques, such as relaxation, also are useful. (For more information on the emetogenicity of chemotherapy drugs and emesis treatment, see the inside front cover and Appendix F.)

Alopecia

Some chemotherapy drugs, such as alkylating agents and anthracyclines, cause nearly total alopecia at recommended dosages. Others—for instance, antimetabolites—cause little, if any, hair loss. To help patients cope with this side effect, provide psychological support and information about cosmetic resources.

Reproductive effects

Alkylating agents and topoisomerase poison-containing regimens cause ovulation cessation and azoospermia. Duration of these effects varies with age and sex. For example, males who receive mechlorethamine and procarbazine for Hodgkin's disease are effectively sterile; on the other hand, fertility usually returns after treatment with cisplatin, etoposide, or vinblastine. Females experience anovulation after receiving alkylating agents; females younger than age 30 at the time of treatment are likely to recover normal menses; those older than age 35 are unlikely to recover normal menses.

Other chemotherapy side effects

Some antineoplastics cause transient diarrhea, constipation, mucositis, stomatitis, esophagitis, fever, pain, body aches, malaise, or anorexia. When appropriate, medications should be prescribed to treat these complaints (as discussed in Appendix F). Nonpharmacologic interventions, such as relaxation, physical therapy, and counseling, may be valuable for many patients.

Chemotherapy of the future

New compounds and new chemical pathways uncovered within the last few decades—and new principles based on these discoveries—have led to entirely new categories of cancer-fighting drugs. Examples include antiangiogenic drugs, which starve the tumor's blood supply; antisense agents, which attach microscopic pieces of DNA or RNA to a tumor, interfering with cancer cell replication; and photodynamic therapy, which uses drugs to debulk tumor size.

The chemotherapy drugs of the future will emerge from a continuous process of discovery and development. Recent advances in nanotechnology, proteomics, genomics, and other fields are likely to lead to the development of drugs that use such novel approaches as:

• affecting a tumor cell's ability to die
• counteracting activated oncogenes
• infecting cancer cells with viruses while leaving normal cells intact
• restoring lost function of tumor-suppressor genes
• preventing normal chromosomal end-replication.

Treatments will become increasingly streamlined, tailored to specific characteristics of a patient's cancer while sparing healthy tissues. Gentler and more effective cancer treatments provide the hope that more cancers can be cured and many others managed as chronic diseases while allowing patients to live normal lives with normal life expectancies.

References

Mosby's Drug Consult. Elsevier. Available online at: http://www.mosbysdrugconsult.com.

Abeloff MD (ed), Armitage JO, Niederhuber JE, et al. *Clinical Oncology.* 3rd ed. New York, NY: Elsevier Churchill Livingstone; 2004.

Kasper DL, Braunwald E, Fauci AS (eds). *Harrison's Principles of Internal Medicine.* 16th ed. New York, NY: McGraw Hill Publishing Co; 2005.

McEvoy GK, Miller J, Litvak K (eds). *AHFS Drug Information 2005.* Bethesda, Md: American Society of Health-System Pharmacists, Americal Hospital Formulary Service; 2005.

National Cancer Institute. Cancer Trends Progress Report, 2005 Update. Available online at: http://progressreport.cancer.gov/introduction.asp.

National Cancer Institute. National Cancer Institute Fact Sheet, Targeted Cancer Therapies: Questions and Answers. Available online at: http://www.cancer.gov/cancertopics/factsheet/Therapy/targeted.

Ross JS, Schenkein DP, Pietrusko R, et al. Targeted therapies for cancer 2004. *Am J Clin Pathol.* 122(4):598-609;2004.

MANAGING
HAZARDOUS DRUGS

FOR THE PAST DECADE, concern about the safety of health care workers who handle hazardous drugs has been growing. Up to 5.5 million health care workers have the potential to be exposed to hazardous drugs. Anyone involved in caring for patients receiving such drugs may be vulnerable. Generally, the activities that pose the greatest risk to health care workers are preparing and administering cancer chemotherapy agents, cleaning up chemotherapy spills, and handling patient excreta.

Several organizations have published guidelines on safe handling of hazardous drugs, including the Occupational Safety & Health Administration (OSHA), National Institute for Occupational Safety and Health (NIOSH), American Society of Health-System Pharmacists, and Oncology Nursing Society.

OSHA published the first national guidelines on safe handling of chemotherapeutic drugs in 1986—yet these recommendations are still not in universal use. In 2004, NIOSH issued an alert on preventing occupational exposure to hazardous drugs in health care settings. (See *NIOSH warning*.) The alert and other information on preventing occupational exposure to hazardous drugs is available on the NIOSH website (www.cdc.gov/niosh/docs/2004-165/).

The guidelines presented in this section reflect the recommendations of the organizations mentioned above. When applied consistently, current recommendations for safe handling can limit workers' exposure—and its

---

NIOSH warning

Warning! Working with or near hazardous drugs in health care settings may cause rashes, infertility, miscarriage, birth defects, and possibly leukemia or other cancers.

This warning comes from "Preventing Occupational Exposure to Antineoplastic and Other Hazardous Drugs in Health Care Settings"—an alert published in 2004 by the National Institute for Occupational Safety and Health. The purpose of the alert is to inform health care workers of the potential risks of handling chemotherapy and other hazardous drugs. Drugs that meet one or more of the following criteria should be considered hazardous and handled appropriately:

- carcinogenic
- genotoxic (mutagenic)
- teratogenic (developmentally toxic)
- toxic to human reproductive capacity
- organotoxic at low doses
- similar in structure or toxicity to drugs that meet the above criteria.

---

effects. However, no single set of guidelines can address all the needs of every health care facility or worker. Health care professionals must rely on their professional judgment, experience, and common sense in applying these recommendations to their unique circumstances. They must also stay abreast of evolving federal, state, and local regulations and the requirements of appropriate accrediting institutions.

Defining hazardous drugs

Hazardous drugs are toxic compounds that meet one or more of the following criteria:
• carcinogenic
• genotoxic (mutagenic)
• teratogenic (developmentally toxic)
• toxic to human reproductive capability
• organotoxic in humans or animals when given in low doses
• new drugs that mimic existing hazardous drugs in structure or toxicity.

Also, on direct contact, these agents may irritate the skin, eyes, and mucous membranes and cause ulceration and tissue necrosis.

Many hazardous drugs used in the treatment of cancer bind to or damage DNA. Other antineoplastics, some antivirals, antibiotics, and bioengineered drugs interfere with cell growth or proliferation or with DNA synthesis. In some cases, these drugs have nonselective actions that disrupt the growth and function of both healthy and diseased cells. Besides causing toxic side effects in patients, these nonselective actions can cause adverse effects in health care workers inadvertently exposed to the drug. (See *Hazardous oncology drugs*.)

As the use and number of cytotoxic drugs increases, so does the number of potentially exposed health care workers. For example, antineoplastics such as cyclophosphamide have immunosuppressant effects that prove beneficial in treating nonmalignant diseases, such as rheumatoid arthritis and multiple sclerosis. Consequently, health care workers in fields other than oncology may be responsible for handling these drugs or caring for patients who have received them.

NIOSH and other organizations continue to gather data on the potential toxicity and health effects of highly potent drugs and bioengineered agents. Health care professionals who work with or around hazardous drugs should use a standard precautions approach and follow the recommendations in the drug manufacturer's Material Safety Data Sheet (MSDS).

Potential effects of exposure

Exposure to hazardous drugs can cause health effects ranging from acute symptoms to late-onset and long-term effects.

Acute symptoms

The most common acute symptoms of hazardous drug exposure are nausea, vomiting, headache, dizziness, hair loss, and hepatic damage. These symptoms correlate with the number of doses handled and the use of personal protective equipment (PPE). Duration of work exposure and volume of drug handling also may play a role; one study found hepatocellular damage in nurses working in an oncology unit.

Reproductive effects

Exposure to chemotherapeutic agents poses a significant risk to reproductive health. Infertility, spontaneous abortions, fetal abnormalities, and menstrual-cycle abnormalities have been reported. Nurses and pharmacists who have had occupational chemotherapy exposure have an increased prevalence of infertility.

Some studies have found that pregnant women exposed to antineoplastics during the first trimester were more than twice as likely to experience fetal loss as pregnant women who were not exposed and carried their pregnancies to full term. One study showed a relative risk for fetal loss of 1.7 (interval of 1.0 to 2.8) among nurses who prepared and administered 18 chemotherapy infusions per week (on average) without PPE. Another study found a link between spontaneous abortions and chemotherapy handling during pregnancy. Several additional adverse reproductive outcomes after cytotoxic drug exposure have been reported, including a higher risk of preterm delivery and small-for-gestational-age

Hazardous oncology drugs

The oncology drugs listed below have been designated as hazardous by the National Institutes of Health and Centers for Disease Control and Prevention. All personnel who handle, prepare, or administer these drugs must follow appropriate guidelines and precautions. This list is intended only as a guide for health care providers in diverse practice settings. It does not include all hazardous drugs in use or reflect an exhaustive review of all approved medications that may be considered hazardous. Drug names followed by an asterisk (*) are carcinogens according to the International Agency for Research on Cancer.

Aldesleukin
Alemtuzumab
Altretamine
Amifostine
Anastrozole
Arsenic trioxide
Asparaginase
Azacitidine*
Azathioprine*
Bacillus Calmette-Guerin vaccine
Bexarotene
Bicalutamide
Bleomycin*
Bortezomib
Busulfan*
Capecitabine
Carboplatin
Carmustine*
Chlorambucil*
Cisplatin*
Cladribine
Clofarabine
Cyclophosphamide*
Cytarabine
Dacarbazine*
Dactinomycin
Daunorubicin hydrochloride*
Denileukin
Docetaxel
Doxorubicin*

Epirubicin
Estrogens
Estramustine phosphate sodium
Estrogens, conjugated
Etoposide*
Exemestane
Floxuridine
Fludarabine
Fluorouracil
Flutamide
Fulvestrant
Gemcitabine
Gemtuzumab ozogamicin
Goserelin
Hydroxyurea
Ibritumomab tiuxetan
Idarubicin
Ifosfamide
Imatinib mesylate
Interferon alfa-2a
Interferon alfa-2b
Interferon alfa-n1
Interferon alfa-n3
Irinotecan hydrochloride
Letrozole
Leuprolide acetate
Lomustine*
Mechlorethamine*
Megestrol
Melphalan*
Mercaptopurine

Methotrexate
Mitomycin*
Mitotane
Mitoxantrone hydrochloride*
Nilutamide
Oxaliplatin
Paclitaxel
Pegaspargase
Pentostatin
Plicamycin
Procarbazine*
Raloxifene
Rituximab
Streptozocin*
Tamoxifen*
Temozolomide
Teniposide*
Testolactone
Thalidomide
Thioguanine
Thiotepa*
Topotecan
Toremifene citrate
Tositumomab
Tretinoin
Triptorelin
Valrubicin
Vinblastine sulfate
Vincristine sulfate
Vinorelbine tartrate

neonates and an increased incidence of miscarriages and malformed offspring.

Some authorities recommend that women who are pregnant, trying to conceive, or breastfeeding avoid exposure to chemotherapy drugs. According to OSHA, health care facilities should inform employees of the potential risks of handling hazardous drugs before or during pregnancy and should offer alternative duty, if requested, to employees who are pregnant or trying to conceive.

Genotoxic effects

The genetic effects of exposure to a broad spectrum of antineoplastics have been studied extensively. Genotoxic activity has occurred both in patients who received antineoplastics and health care workers who administered them. The incidence of DNA single-strand breaks in peripheral mononuclear blood cells was 50% higher in nurses who did not use recommended safety precautions when administering these drugs. This finding is significant because other major carcinogens (such as environmental smoke) cause identical DNA strand breaks. Chromosomal aberrations also occurred in nurses and physicians who handled antineoplastics. The length of handling exposure was the main factor correlating with the degree of chromosomal damage.

Carcinogenic effects

Health care workers generally have an increased risk of cancer (predominately leukemia). One study found that hospital workers were almost three times more likely than nonhospital workers to develop acute myelogenous leukemia.

Research on cancer occurrence among health care personnel who handle antineoplastics is limited and has focused predominantly on leukemia. Nonetheless, a wealth of information exists in the literature regarding occupational chemotherapy exposure and elevated levels of nonspecific markers for carcinogen exposure.

Occupational exposure routes

Exposure to hazardous drugs most likely results from dermal absorption (via direct skin contact with the drugs or handling of contaminated material), ingestion, injection, and inhalation. In some cases, hazardous drugs or their metabolites also are present in patients' excreta, making it an exposure source for health care workers who handle excreta.

During drug preparation or administration, the primary exposure routes to hazardous drugs are inhalation of aerosolized drugs and direct skin contact. A drug may become aerosolized or may spray or splatter when a needle is withdrawn from the drug vial, when syringes and needles or filter straws are used for drug transfer, when ampules are opened, and when air is expelled from a syringe during measurement of precise drug volumes.

Ingestion can result from consuming drug-contaminated foods or beverages and from other hand-to-mouth contact. Accidental injection may result from needlesticks or other injuries from contaminated sharps.

Preparation of parenteral hazardous drugs requires the use of aseptic techniques and a sterile environment. Many pharmacies provide a horizontal laminar-flow work bench for drug preparation. Although these units protect the drug product, they may expose the operator and other room occupants to aerosols generated during drug preparation. For this reason, hazardous drugs should be prepared in a biological safety cabinet (BSC) that filters incoming air through a high-efficiency particulate air filter.

During drug administration, health care workers should avoid clearing air from a syringe or infusion line and should take measures to avoid leakage at tubing, syringe, or stopcock connections to reduce opportunities for accidental skin contact and aerosal generation. Syringes and needles should be disposed of intact—and without recapping—into a leakproof, puncture-resistant container.

Disposal of cytotoxic drugs and trace-contaminated materials (such as gloves, gowns, needles, syringes, and vials) also may expose pharmacists, nurses, physicians, and ancillary personnel (including housekeeping staff) to hazardous drugs. Also, excreta from patients receiving cytotoxic drugs may contain high drug concentrations. All personnel should be aware of these potential exposure sources and take appropriate precautions to avoid accidental contact.

Components of a safe drug handling program

Health care facilities should have a well-designed program that addresses all aspects of safe handling of hazardous drugs. The program should address the following:
• identification of specific hazardous drugs
• proper procedures for drug preparation and administration, spill management, and waste management
• which personnel are permitted to handle hazardous drugs
• educational and competency requirements for personnel who handle hazardous drugs
• required training for all employees who work with or around hazardous drugs, including appropriate use of established precautions and required PPE
• policy on hazardous drug handling by female employees who are pregnant, actively trying to conceive, or breastfeeding and by male employees attempting to father a child.

The safe drug handling program should address all situations in which hazardous drugs are used, including preparation and administration. The program should be a collaborative effort, with input from all affected departments, such as pharmacy, nursing, medical staff, housekeeping, transportation, maintenance, employee health, risk management, industrial hygiene, clinical laboratories, and safety officers.

Employers are required by law to have an MSDS available for all hazardous agents in the workplace. The facility's safety program must include a process for monitoring and updating

the MSDS database. When a hazardous drug is purchased for the first time, the MSDS must be received from the manufacturer or distributor. The MSDS defines appropriate handling precautions for the drug, including protective equipment, controls, and spill management. In many cases, the MSDS is available online through the drug manufacturer or safety information services.

Labeling, packaging, and storage of hazardous drugs

Drugs that require safe handling precautions must be clearly labeled at all times during transport and use. Drug packages and bins, shelves, and storage areas used for hazardous drugs must have distinctive labels identifying those drugs as requiring special handling precautions (for example, "Caution: Cytotoxic agent"). Segregating hazardous drugs from other drug inventory improves control, reduces the number of staff members potentially exposed, and decreases opportunities for drug errors (such as pulling a look-alike vial from an adjacent drug bin).

Hazardous drugs should be stored in areas with general exhaust ventilation sufficient to dilute and remove airborne contaminants. To prevent potential breakage, hazardous drug products placed in inventory should be stored in bins with high fronts and on shelves that have guards to prevent accidental falls.

Several studies have documented contamination on the outside of drug vials when delivered by the manufacturer. To protect against this exposure source, workers must wear a double set of gloves when stocking, performing inventory control, or selecting hazardous drug packages for further handling.

Hazardous drug packages must be placed in sealed containers and labeled with a unique identifier. Staff members who handle hazardous drugs or clean areas where hazardous drugs are stored or handled must be trained to recognize the unique identifying labels used to distinguish these drugs and areas.

Warning labels and signs must be clear to non-English readers.

Transport of hazardous drug packages

Hazardous drug packages must be transported in a manner that reduces environmental contamination in the event of accidental dropping. All persons transporting hazardous drugs must receive safety training that includes spill control. Spill kits must be immediately accessible.

Compounding and preparation environment

Hazardous drugs should be compounded in a controlled area where access is limited to authorized personnel with special training in handling requirements. Preferably, this area should be either a contained environment with negative air pressure or an area protected by an airlock or anteroom. If a positive-pressure environment is unavoidable, it should be augmented with an appropriately designed antechamber to avoid potential spread of airborne hazardous drug contamination from packaging contamination, poor handling technique, and spills.

Ventilation and engineering controls

Ventilation or engineering controls should be used to control emission of airborne contaminants. Depending on the design, ventilated cabinets also may be used to provide the critical environment necessary to compound sterile preparations.

When asepsis is not required, a Class I BSC or a containment isolator may be used to prepare hazardous drugs. Compounding of sterile hazardous drugs requires a Class II or Class III BSC or an isolator intended for asepsis and containment. Adding a closed-system drug transfer device to the drug preparation process in a class II BSC prevents escape of hazardous drug solution or vapor and guards against entry of environmental contaminants. Several closed-system drug transfer devices are available to reduce drug leakage during preparation and handling. However, these devices are not a substitute for a ventilated cabinet.

Commercial air-venting devices can be used to avoid overpressurizing vials during reconstitution, which can cause aerosolization and leakage. Devices known as chemo adjuncts also are available. Some use a filtered, vented spike to aid reconstitution and removal of hazardous drugs during compounding. However, chemo adjuncts are not considered closed-system transfer devices.

Drug administration area

Access to the drug administration area should be limited to essential personnel and patients receiving therapy. Food or beverage consumption by employees should not be permitted and food should not be stored in this area. In inpatient therapy areas where lengthy administration techniques may be required, hazardous drugs should be hung or removed in a manner that minimizes exposure of family members and ancillary staff and avoids potential contamination of personnel and food trays.

The facility's safe handling program should describe required measures to minimize environmental contamination and maximize cleaning and decontamination efficacy in all settings where hazardous drugs are administered. In these areas, surfaces should be made of materials that can be easily cleaned and decontaminated. Upholstered and carpeted surfaces should be avoided.

In some cases, hazardous drugs must be administered in nontraditional locations (such as operating rooms) or through unusual routes. This poses a challenge to training and containment. For instance, intracavitary administration of a hazardous drug (such as into the bladder, peritoneal cavity, or chest cavity) frequently requires equipment for which locking connections may not be readily available. When hazardous drugs are given by unusual routes or in nontraditional locations, techniques and ancillary devices that minimize the risks of open systems should be used.

Personal protective equipment

Workers must wear appropriate PPE when handling hazardous drug packages, cartons, and drug vials; performing inventory control procedures; and gathering hazardous drugs and supplies for drug compounding. Types of PPE include gloves, gown, eye and face protection, shoe covers, and respiratory devices. During compounding, workers must wear gloves and gowns to prevent skin surfaces from coming in contact with the drug.

Gloves

Many latex and nonlatex materials provide effective protection against penetration and permeation by most hazardous drugs. Gloves made of nitrile or neoprene rubber and polyurethane have been successfully tested against various antineoplastics. The American Society for Testing and Materials (ASTM) has developed testing standards for assessing the resistance of medical gloves to permeation by chemotherapy drugs. Gloves that meet this testing standard earn the designation of "chemotherapy gloves." All gloves used with hazardous drugs should meet this standard. Powder-free gloves are preferred because they avoid contamination of the sterile processing area with powder particulates. Powdered gloves, in contrast, may absorb hazardous drug contaminants, increasing the risk of skin contact.

Recommendations for the use of gloves when preparing and administering hazardous drugs include the following:
- Select high-quality, powder-free gloves made of latex, nitrile, polyurethane, neoprene, or other materials that meet the ASTM standards for chemotherapy gloves.
- Inspect gloves for visible defects before donning them.
- Sanitize gloves with 70% alcohol or other appropriate disinfectant before performing an aseptic activity.
- Wash hands thoroughly before donning gloves and after removing them.

- Wear a double pair of gloves for all activities involving hazardous drugs, including handling of drug shipping cartons or drug vials, compounding and administering hazardous drugs, handling drug waste or waste from patients recently treated with hazardous drugs, and cleaning up spills. Wear the inner (first) pair of gloves under the cuff of the gown and the second (outer) pair over the cuff.
- Change gloves every 30 minutes during compounding.
- Change gloves immediately if they become damaged or contaminated.
- Remove the outer gloves after wiping down the final drug preparation but before labeling or removing the preparation from the BSC. Place these gloves in an appropriate containment bag.
- Wear the clean inner pair of gloves to surface-clean the final preparation, attach the label, and remove the product from the BSC.
- Place the prepared product in a clean transport bag.
- Remove gloves with care to avoid contamination. Follow your facility's specific procedures for glove removal.
- Remove and discard gloves into an appropriate cytotoxic waste container.
- Change gloves after administering a hazardous drug dose or when leaving the immediate drug administration area.

Gowns

Commercially available materials vary in their ability to resist penetration by hazardous drugs. Only gowns with polyethylene or vinyl coatings provide adequate splash protection and prevent penetration by the drug. Selection of gowning material depends on the situation. Use disposable chemotherapy gowns. Never reuse gowns.

Current recommendations for the use of gowns include the following:
- Wear a gown or coverall when compounding a sterile preparation, compounding or administering a hazardous drug, cleaning up a

hazardous drug spill, or handling waste from a patient recently treated with a hazardous drug.

• Select a disposable gown of a material with proven efficacy against the specific hazardous drug.

• When compounding, do not wear a coated gown for more than 3 hours.

• Change the gown immediately if it becomes damaged or contaminated.

• Remove the gown with care to avoid contamination of clothing. Follow your facility's procedures for gown removal.

• Immediately after removing the gown, dispose of it as hazardous waste.

• Wash your hands after removing and disposing of the gown.

Eye and face protection

Use eye and face protection whenever exposure from splashing or uncontrolled aerosolization of hazardous drugs is possible, such as when containing a spill or handling a damaged drug shipping carton. In these situations, a face shield (rather than safety glasses or goggles) is recommended because it provides improved skin protection.

NIOSH-approved respiratory protection should be worn when the possibility of exposure to hazardous drug aerosols exists. Activities that require respirator use include administering drugs by inhalation and cleaning up spills. All workers who may use a respirator must be fit-tested and trained to use the appropriate respirator according to the OSHA Respirator Standard. Be aware that surgical masks do not provide respiratory protection.

Proper sequence for donning PPE

After washing your hands, don the first (inner) pair of gloves. Then don the gown and face shield. Next, don the second (outer) pair of gloves. Make sure these gloves extend beyond the elastic or knit cuff of the gown.

Other PPE

Workers who perform sterile compounding should wear shoe and hair coverings to minimize particulate contamination of the critical work zone and the drug preparation. When removing shoe and hair coverings, wear gloves and use caution to prevent contamination from spreading to clean areas. Be sure to place hair and shoe coverings in appropriate containers and discard them (along with used gloves) as hazardous waste.

Managing spills

Hazardous drug spills must be contained and cleaned up immediately by trained workers. Facilities must have policies and procedures that address spill prevention and clean-up. Written procedures must specify who is responsible for spill management based on the size and scope of the spill.

Spill kits containing all materials needed to clean up hazardous drug spills should be readily available in all areas where hazardous drugs are routinely handled. A spill kit should accompany injectable hazardous drugs delivered to patient care areas (even though the drugs are transported in a sealable plastic bag or container). If hazardous drugs will be prepared or administered in a nonroutine area (such as a patient's home or an unusual patient care area), the drug handler must obtain a spill kit and respirator.

Other recommendations for managing hazardous drug spills include the following:

• Obtain a spill kit and respirator.

• Don appropriate PPE, including inner and outer gloves and a respirator.

• Assess the size and scope of the spill. Call for additional trained help if necessary. Spills that cannot be contained by two spill kits may require outside assistance.

• Post signs to limit access to the spill area.

• Carefully remove any broken glass fragments and place them in a puncture-resistant container.

• Absorb hazardous liquids with spill pads.

Absorb hazardous powders with damp, disposable pads or soft towels.

• Clean in a systematic manner, proceeding from areas of lesser to greater contamination.

• Completely remove and place all contaminated material in disposal bags.

• Rinse the spill area with water and then clean it with detergent, sodium hypochlorite solution, and neutralizer.

• Rinse the area several times and place all materials used for containment and clean-up in disposal bags. Seal the bags and place them in the appropriate final container for disposal as hazardous waste.

• Carefully remove all PPE while still wearing the inner gloves. Place all disposable PPE in an appropriate disposal bag; seal the bag and place it in an appropriate final container.

• Remove the inner gloves and place them in a small, sealable bag. Then place that bag in the appropriate final container for disposal as hazardous waste. Do not push or force contaminated materials into the container.

• Wash your hands thoroughly with soap and water.

• After the initial clean-up, the area should be recleaned by housekeeping, janitorial, or environmental services.

Waste management and disposal

The Resource Conservation and Recovery Act (RCRA) gives the Environmental Protection Agency responsibility for tracking hazardous waste from its generation to disposal. For regulatory purposes, materials are defined as hazardous waste when discarded if they possess certain characteristics (acute toxicity, reactivity, ignitability, or corrosivity) or are "listed" as a particular type of waste.

The RCRA applies to some drugs, as well as chemicals discarded by pharmacies, hospitals, clinics, and other commercial entities. Covered drugs include epinephrine, mercury (thimerosal), nicotine, nitroglycerin, and physostigmine.

In addition, eight chemotherapy drugs (arsenic trioxide, chlorambucil, cyclophospha-

mide, daunomycin [daunorubicin], melphalan, mitomycin C, streptozotocin [streptozocin], and uracil mustard) appear on the "U list" of commercial chemicals (named for their hazardous waste identification numbers, which begin with the letter "U"). These drugs must be disposed of as RCRA hazardous waste and placed in containers that will be incinerated in a regulated medical waste incinerator.

Not all chemotherapy drugs are considered hazardous waste by the EPA, even though many have similar characteristics to the eight drugs listed above. The EPA list has not been updated in 30 years.

Handling unlisted hazardous drug waste

Hazardous drugs not listed as hazardous waste should be handled as described below:

• Handle hazardous drug waste and contaminated materials separately from other trash.

• Place drug-contaminated syringes and needles in chemotherapy sharps containers for disposal.

• Discard contaminated needles, syringes, I.V. tubing, butterfly clips, and similiar materials intact to prevent aerosol generation and injury. *Do not recap needles.* Place all contaminated items in a puncture-resistant disposal container labeled "Cytotoxic waste only" (or similar wording).

• Do not place sharps used for hazardous drug preparation in red sharps containers or needle boxes. (These containers typically are disinfected by autoclaving or microwaving, which has no effect on chemical residue.)

• Clean and decontaminate work areas before and after each activity involving hazardous drugs, and at the end of each shift.

• Wear PPE when handling linen contaminated with drugs or patient excreta or body fluids.

• Discard cytotoxic drugs (which are considered regulated wastes) in cytotoxic waste containers. These containers should be sealed and disposed of according to federal, state, and local requirements.

Preparing and administering parenteral drugs

Wear gloves, a gown, and a face shield (if necessary) when preparing, handling, and administering hazardous parenteral drugs. Use stringent aseptic technique during any procedure in which sterile dosage forms are manipulated with needles and syringes. Using needleless devices reduces the risk of blood-borne pathogen exposure and accidental exposure to hazardous drugs caused by needlesticks.

Drug reconstitution, withdrawal, and transfer

When reconstituting a hazardous drug in a vial, avoid pressurizing the vial contents, which may cause the drug to spray out around the needle or through a needle hole or a loose seal. To avoid pressurization, create a *slight* negative pressure in the vial. After drawing up the diluent, insert the needle into the vial and pull back the plunger; this action creates a slight negative pressure inside the vial, which draws air into the syringe. Transfer small amounts of diluent slowly as equal volumes of air are removed.

Keeping the needle in the vial, swirl the contents carefully until they dissolve. With the vial inverted, gradually withdraw the proper amount of drug solution while equal volumes of air are exchanged for solution. Measure the exact volume needed while the needle is in the vial; any excess drug should remain in the vial. With the vial upright, withdraw the plunger past the original starting point to create a slight negative pressure before removing the needle. Make sure the needle hub is clear before you remove the needle.

To withdraw a hazardous drug from an ampule, gently tap the neck or top portion of the ampule. Then wipe the neck with alcohol and attach a 5-micron filter needle or straw to a syringe large enough so that it is no more than three-quarters full when holding the drug. Next, draw the fluid through the filter needle or straw and clear it from the needle and hub. Exchange the needle or straw for a needle of similar gauge and length; eject any air and excess drug into a sterile vial (leaving the desired volume in the syringe), taking care to avoid aerosolization.

If the dose will be dispensed in the syringe, draw back the plunger to clear fluid from the needle and hub. Replace the needle with a locking cap, and surface-decontaminate and label the syringe. Use a syringe that is no more than three-quarters full when filled with the solution; this reduces the risk of the plunger separating from the syringe barrel.

When transferring a hazardous drug to an I.V. bag, take care to puncture only the septum of the injection port; avoid puncturing the sides of the port or the bag. After the drug solution has been injected into the I.V. bag, surface-decontaminate the I.V. port, container, and set. Label the final preparation (including an auxiliary warning, such as "Caution: Cytotoxic agent") and cover the injection port with a protective shield.

General recommendations

General recommendations for administering hazardous parenteral drugs include the following:

- Always work below eye level.
- Visually examine the drug dose while it is still in the transport bag. If the dose appears to be intact, remove it from the transport bag.
- Place a plastic-backed absorbent pad under the drug administration area to absorb leaks and prevent drug contact with the patient's skin.
- Whenever possible, use a needleless system to administer a hazardous I.V. drug. Use Luer-Lok fittings for all needleless systems, syringes, needles, infusion tubing, and pumps. However, such systems may result in leakage of droplets at connection points; therefore, place gauze pads under the connection at injection ports to catch leaks and have a spill kit and hazardous drug waste container readily available.
- If the administration site must be primed, prime the I.V. tubing with a solution that does

not contain hazardous drugs, or use the back-flow method.

• When administering hazardous I.M. or sub-cutaneous drugs, use Luer-Lok safety needles or retracting needles or shields. Make sure syringes have Luer-locking connections and are less than three-quarters full. Have a spill kit and hazardous drug waste container readily available. Remove the syringe cap and connect the appropriate safety needle. Do not expel air from the syringe or prime the safety needle. After administration, discard the syringe, with safety needle attached, directly into a hazardous drug waste container.

• Discard hazardous drug containers with the administration sets attached; do not remove the sets.

• Use a transport bag as a containment bag for materials contaminated with hazardous drugs, drug containers, and sets.

• Use detergent, sodium hypochlorite solution, and neutralizer (if appropriate) to wash surfaces that may have come in contact with hazardous drugs.

• Wearing gloves, contain and dispose of materials contaminated with hazardous drugs and remaining PPE as hazardous waste. Make sure the hazardous drug waste container is large enough to hold all the discarded material and PPE. Do not push or force contaminated materials into the container.

• After disposing of materials, carefully remove, contain, and discard your gloves. Then wash your hands thoroughly.

Preparing and administering oral and noninjectable drugs

Oral forms of certain hazardous drugs may be prescribed for small children or for adults with feeding tubes. Recipes for extemporaneously compounded oral liquids may start with the parenteral form or may require crushing of tablets or opening of capsules, which may cause fine dust formation and local environmental contamination. Also, tablets or capsules may be coated with a dust of residual hazardous drug that could be inhaled, ab-sorbed through the skin, or ingested or could spread to other locations. In addition, liquid formulations may be aerosolized or spilled. Never crush or compound a hazardous oral drug in an unprotected environment.

To avoid release of aerosolized powder or liquid into the environment during hazardous drug manipulation, facilities must develop procedures for preparation and use of such equipment as filtered hoods.

Recommendations for preparing and administering hazardous oral or noninjectable drugs include the following:

• Work below eye level during drug preparation.

• Visually examine the drug dose while it is still in the transport bag. If the dose appears to be intact, remove it from the transport bag.

• Keep a spill kit and hazardous drug waste container readily available.

• Wash hands and don double gloves. Wear a face shield if the potential for sprays, aerosols, or splashing exists.

• Place a plastic-backed absorbent pad on the work area, if necessary, to contain spills.

• After administering the drug, contain and dispose of materials contaminated with the hazardous drug into a hazardous drug waste container. Do not push or force contaminated materials into the container.

• Carefully remove, contain, and discard your gloves. Then wash your hands thoroughly.

Dealing with accidental exposure

Facilities should ensure that emergency treatment supplies (such as soap, eyewash, and sterile saline solution for eye irrigation) are readily available in areas where hazardous drugs are compounded or administered.

In case of skin contact with a cytotoxic drug, immediately remove contaminated clothing and wash the affected area thoroughly with soap and water. (Do not use a scrub brush because this could abrade the skin.) Rinse the area thoroughly. Call for help, if needed. Then obtain medical attention.

In case of eye contact, flush the affected eye (while holding back the eyelid) with copious amounts of water or normal saline solution for at least 15 minutes. Call for help, if needed. Then obtain medical attention.

Employee monitoring and medical surveillance

A facility's safety program for controlling workplace exposure to hazardous drugs should identify workers with potential exposure and those who might be at higher risk for adverse health effects from such exposure. All incidents of employee exposure to hazardous drugs should be documented in the employee's medical record and medical surveillance log.

The facility's medical surveillance program should include assessment and documentation of symptom complaints, physical findings, and laboratory values (such as blood counts) to identify deviations from expected norms. The program should routinely monitor all workers who handle hazardous drugs.

In facilities without medical surveillance programs, NIOSH encourages workers who handle hazardous drugs to inform their personal health care providers of their occupation and possible hazardous drug exposure when obtaining routine medical care.

Martha Polovich, RN, MN, AOCN
Oncology Clinical Nurse Specialist
Southern Regional Health System
Riverdale, Georgia

References

American Society of Health-System Pharmacists. ASHP guidelines on handling hazardous drugs. *Am J Health Syst Pharm.* 2006;63(12): in press.

Environmental Protection Agency. Introduction to containers (40 CFR Parts 264/265, Subpart I; §261.7). Available online at: http://www.epa.gov/epaoswer/hotline/training/cont05.pdf. Accessed March 23, 2006.

Environmental Protection Agency. Introduction to hazardous waste identification (40 CFR Part 261). Available online at: http://www.epa.gov/epaoswer/hotline/training/hwid05.pdf . Accessed March 23, 2006.

Martin S. The adverse health effects of occupational exposure to hazardous drugs. *Community Oncology.* 2005;2(5):397-400.

National Institute for Occupational Safety and Health. Preventing occupational exposure to antineoplastic and other hazardous drugs in health care settings. Available online at: http://www.cdc.gov/niosh/docs/2004-165/. Accessed January 8, 2006.

Occupational Safety and Health Administration. Technical Manual, TED 1-0.15A, Section VI, Chapter 2. Available online at: http://www.osha.gov/dts/osta/otm/otm_vi/otm_vi_2.html. Accessed January 8, 2006.

Polovich M. Developing a hazardous drug safe-handling program. *Community Oncology.* 2005;2(5):403-405.

Polovich M. Safe handling of hazardous drugs. Available online at: http://www.nursingworld.org/ojin/topic25/tpc25_5.html.

Part 2

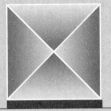

Drugs A to Z

abarelix
Plenaxis

Classification: Antineoplastic, hormone/ hormone modifier, gonadotropin-releasing hormone analogue
Pregnancy risk category X

Pharmacology
Abarelix suppresses luteinizing hormone (LH) and follicle-stimulating hormone secretion, reducing testosterone secretion. No initial increase in serum testosterone level occurs.

Pharmacokinetics
Drug is absorbed slowly, peaking 3 days after injection. It is widely distributed; half-life is approximately 13 days. It is metabolized in liver and excreted in urine.

How supplied
Powder for injectable solution: 113-mg single-dose vial

Indications and dosages

FDA-APPROVED

➡ Palliative treatment of advanced symptomatic prostate cancer when LH–releasing hormone agonist therapy is inappropriate or surgical castration has been refused and one or more of the following exists: risk of neurologic compromise due to metastases, ureteral or bladder outlet obstruction due to local encroachment or metastatic disease, or severe bone pain from skeletal metastases persisting despite opioid analgesia
Adults: 100 mg I.M. into gluteal muscle on days 1, 15, and 29, and every 4 weeks thereafter

⊠ WARNINGS

• Immediate-onset systemic allergic reactions (some resulting in hypotension and syncope) have occurred, including after initial dose. Cumulative risk of allergic reaction increases with treatment duration.
• Only physicians enrolled in Plenaxis PLUS (Plenaxis User Safety) Program may prescribe drug.
• Efficacy in suppressing serum testosterone to castration levels may decrease with continued use. Efficacy beyond 12 months has not been established.
• Treatment failure can be detected by measuring serum total testosterone before administration on day 29 and every 8 weeks thereafter.

Contraindications and precautions
Contraindicated in hypersensitivity to drug or its components and in women and *children.*

Use cautiously with other drugs that may cause QTc prolongation (for example, amiodarone, quinidine, and sotalol), and in patients weighing more than 225 lb (102 kg).

Preparation and administration
• Obtain serum transaminase levels before starting drug and periodically thereafter.
• Before reconstituting, gently shake vial. Hold at 45-degree angle and tap lightly on table to break up caking.
• Reconstitute one vial (113 mg) with 2.2 ml normal saline injection to provide 100-mg dose (50 mg/ml) for single I.M. injection.
• Withdraw 2.2 ml normal saline injection using enclosed 18G × 1.5" needle and 3-ml syringe. Inject diluent quickly. Discard remaining diluent.
• Shake immediately for 15 seconds. Allow vial to stand for 2 minutes. Tap vial to reduce foaming, and swirl vial occasionally. Repeat.
• Invert vial and draw up some suspension into syringe. Without removing needle from vial, reinject it at remaining solids in vial. Repeat until all solids are dispersed.
• Swirl vial before withdrawal; withdraw entire contents (at least 2 ml).
• Use separate needles for reconstitution and injection by exchanging 18G × 1.5" needle

with enclosed 22G × 1.5" Safety Glide injection needle.
• Give entire reconstituted suspension I.M. immediately, and observe for allergic response.
• For at least 30 minutes after each injection, watch for allergic reaction. If reaction includes hypotension or syncope, use supportive measures, such as leg elevation, oxygen, I.V. fluids, antihistamines, corticosteroids, and epinephrine alone (or in combination). Observe patient until event resolves.
• Monitor patient response by measuring total serum testosterone level before administration on day 29 and every 8 weeks thereafter.
• Store unreconstituted drug at 77° F (25° C).

Adverse reactions

CNS: pain, sleep disturbance, dizziness, headache, fatigue
CV: QTc prolongation, peripheral edema
EENT: eye or eyelid swelling
GI: constipation, nausea, diarrhea
GU: breast enlargement, breast pain, nipple tenderness, dysuria, frequent voiding, urinary retention, urinary tract infection
Musculoskeletal: back pain
Respiratory: upper respiratory tract infection, wheezing, rapid or irregular respiratory rate, dyspnea, chest tightness
Skin: pruritus, urticaria
Other: hot flushes, severe allergic reaction with fainting or loss of consciousness

Interactions

Drug-drug. *Drugs that may cause QTc prolongation (such as amiodarone, quinidine, sotalol):* possible risk of increased QTc prolongation
Drug-diagnostic tests. *Hemoglobin:* slightly decreased
Serum transaminases, triglycerides: increased

Toxicity and overdose

• Maximum tolerated dosage has not been determined. Although no accidental overdoses have been reported, expect such episodes to cause pronounced manifestations of adverse effects.

• If overdose occurs, treatment is supportive and symptomatic. No antidote exists.

Special considerations

• Periodic serum prostate-specific antigen measurement may also be considered. Maintain strict monitoring of serum testosterone level in obese patients and patients weighing more than 225 lb (102 kg).
• Extended treatment may decrease bone mineral density.

Patient education

• Instruct patient to visit physician regularly to receive injection.
• Advise patient to have periodic blood tests to ensure drug efficacy.

acetaminophen and codeine phosphate

Capital with Codeine Suspension, EZ III, Phenaphen with Codeine No. 2, Phenaphen with Codeine No. 3, Phenaphen with Codeine No. 4, Tylenol with Codeine, Tylenol with Codeine #2, Tylenol with Codeine #3, Tylenol with Codeine #4

Classification: Opioid analgesic, antipyretic
Controlled substance schedule III
Pregnancy risk category C

Pharmacology

Acetaminophen is a nonopioid, nonsalicylate analgesic and antipyretic whose specific mechanism of analgesic action is unknown. Antipyretic properties result from inhibition of hypothalamic heat-regulating center. Codeine binds to opiate receptors in CNS and inhibits ascending pain pathways.

Pharmacokinetics

Both ingredients are well absorbed orally. Plasma half-life is 1 to 4 hours, but may increase in liver damage or overdose. About 85% of oral dose appears in urine within 24 hours.

After absorption, codeine is metabolized in liver. It retains at least half its analgesic activity when given orally. About 10% is demethylated to morphine (which may explain drug's analgesic activity). Half-life is 2.5 to 3 hours. Metabolic products are excreted in urine.

How supplied
Elixir: 120 mg acetaminophen and 12 mg codeine/5 ml
*Suspension:*120 mg acetaminophen and 12 mg codeine/5 ml
Tablets: 300 mg acetaminophen and 15 mg codeine, 300 mg acetaminophen and 30 mg codeine, 300 mg acetaminophen and 60 mg codeine

Indications and dosages

FDA-APPROVED

➥ Mild to moderately severe pain
Adults: 1 or 2 tablets containing acetaminophen with 15 or 30 mg codeine P.O. or 1 tablet containing acetaminophen with 60 mg codeine P.O. every 4 hours as needed; for oral solution or suspension, 1 tbs (3 tsp) P.O. every 4 hours p.r.n.
Children ages 7 to 12: 10 ml (2 tsp) oral solution or suspension P.O. three or four times daily
Children ages 3 to 6: 5 ml (1 tsp) oral solution or suspension P.O. three or four times daily

DOSAGE MODIFICATIONS

• Adjust dosage according to pain severity and patient response.
• For patients with hepatic impairment, usual maximum acetaminophen dosage is 2,000 mg daily.

Contraindications and precautions
Contraindicated in hypersensitivity to drug or its components.

Use cautiously in sulfite sensitivity, head injury, intracranial lesions, preexisting intracranial pressure increase, acute abdominal conditions, severe hepatic or renal impairment, hypothyroidism, Addison's disease, prostatic hypertrophy, urethral stricture, pregnancy or breastfeeding, and in debilitated or *elderly patients*. Safety and efficacy have not been established for *children younger than age 3.*

Preparation and administration
• Store in tight, light-resistant container with child-resistant closure at controlled temperature of 59° to 86° F (15° to 30° C). Protect from light. Do not refrigerate or freeze elixir.

Adverse reactions
CNS: drowsiness, sedation, dizziness, agitation, lethargy, restlessness, euphoria, seizures
CV: bradycardia, palpitations, orthostatic hypotension, tachycardia, circulatory collapse
GI: nausea, vomiting, anorexia, constipation
GU: urinary retention
Respiratory: respiratory depression, respiratory paralysis
Skin: rash, urticaria, pruritus
Other: flushing, dependency, anaphylaxis

Interactions
Drug-drug. *Antianxiety agents, antipsychotics, other CNS depressants and opioid analgesics:* additive CNS depression
Anticholinergics: increased risk of paralytic ileus
Drug-diagnostic tests. *Urinary 5-hydroxyindoleacetic acid:* false-positive (acetaminophen)
Drug-food. *Cabbage:* increased acetaminophen metabolism
Drug-herb. *Black cohosh:* increased risk of hepatotoxicity
Dandelion, milk thistle: possible increased acetaminophen clearance
Ginkgo: increased acetaminophen level
Ginseng (Panax and Siberian), goldenseal, kava, pomegranate: increased codeine level
St. John's wort: increased sedation, increased analgesia

Toxicity and overdose

Acetaminophen

• Fatal hepatic necrosis is most serious overdose effect. Renal tubular necrosis, hypoglycemic coma, and thrombocytopenia may also occur. Signs and symptoms of hepatotoxicity may not appear for 48 to 72 hours after ingestion; these may include nausea, vomiting, diaphoresis, and general malaise.

• Empty stomach promptly by lavage or emesis induction. Obtain serum acetaminophen assay as soon as possible, but no sooner than 4 hours after ingestion. Obtain liver function studies initially; repeat at 24-hour intervals. Give N-acetylcysteine (antidote), preferably within 16 hours.

Codeine

• Opioid triad of pinpoint pupils, respiratory depression, and loss of consciousness indicates toxicity. Seizures may occur.

• Serious effects of overdose include respiratory depression, extreme somnolence progressing to stupor or coma, skeletal muscle flaccidity, cold and clammy skin, and sometimes bradycardia and hypotension that may progress to apnea, circulatory collapse, cardiac arrest, and death in severe overdose.

• Gastric emptying may help remove unabsorbed drug. Establish adequate respiratory exchange through patent airway and assisted or controlled ventilation. In severe cases, consider hemodialysis (preferred) or peritoneal dialysis. Administer appropriate naloxone dose (preferably I.V.) simultaneously with respiratory resuscitation efforts. Because codeine's duration of action may exceed that of antagonist, continually monitor patient.

• Do not give antagonist if significant respiratory or cardiovascular depression is absent. Use oxygen, I.V. fluids, vasopressors, and other supportive measures as indicated.

Special considerations

• Tablets contain sodium metabisulfite, which may cause allergy-type reactions (including anaphylaxis and life-threatening or less severe asthmatic episodes) in susceptible patients.

Sulfite sensitivity occurs more often in asthmatic patients.

• Tolerance may develop with continued use; incidence of untoward effects is dose-related.

Patient education

• Instruct patient to shake liquid form (suspension) well before using and measure with measuring spoon or dropper (not kitchen spoon).

• Tell patient to seek immediate medical attention for yellowing of eyes or skin, wheezing, trouble swallowing or breathing, lightheadedness or fainting, or dizziness when standing or sitting up.

• Warn patient not to drink alcohol before or after taking drug.

• Caution patient not to take more than one dose at a time.

• Tell patient to use extra caution when driving or operating machinery on days when he takes drug.

acetaminophen and hydrocodone bitartrate

Anexsia, Anolor DH5, Bancap HC, Ceta Plus, Co-Gesic, Dolacet, Hy-Phen, Stagesic, Stagesic-10, T-Gesic, Vanacet, Vicodin, Vicodin ES, Vicodin HP, Zydone

Classification: Opioid analgesic, antipyretic
Controlled substance schedule III
Pregnancy risk category C

Pharmacology

Acetaminophen is a nonopiate, nonsalicylate analgesic and antipyretic whose specific mechanism of analgesic action is unknown. Antipyretic properties result from inhibition of hypothalamic heat-regulating center. Hydrocodone is a semisynthetic opioid analgesic and antitussive, with multiple actions qualitatively similar to those of codeine. Precise mechanism of action is unknown, but it may be related to opiate receptors in CNS.

Pharmacokinetics
Acetaminophen is metabolized by liver. Plasma half-life is 1 to 4 hours, but may increase in liver damage or overdose. About 85% of oral dose appears in urine within 24 hours. Hydrocodone is metabolized in liver. It has elimination half-life of 3.5 to 4.1. hours and is excreted primarily in urine.

How supplied
Capsules: 500 mg/5 mg
Elixir: 500 mg/5 mg/15 ml, 500 mg/7.5 mg/ 15 ml
Tablets: 325 mg/5 mg, 325 mg/7.5 mg, 325 mg/10 mg, 400 mg/5 mg, 400 mg/ 7.5 mg, 400 mg/10 mg, 500 mg/2.5 mg, 500 mg/5 mg, 500 mg/7.5 mg, 500 mg/10 mg, 650 mg/7.5 mg, 650 mg/10 mg, 660 mg/ 10 mg, 750 mg/7.5 mg, 750 mg/10 mg

Indications and dosages

FDA-APPROVED

➥ Moderate to moderately severe pain
Adults: 325 mg/5 mg, 400 mg/5 mg, 500 mg/2.5 mg tablets; 500 mg/5 mg capsules or tablets—1 to 2 tablets P.O. every 4 to 6 hours as needed. Do not exceed 8 capsules or tablets daily.
Adults: 325 mg/7.5 mg, 325 mg/10 mg, 400 mg/ 7.5 mg, 400 mg/10 mg, 500 mg/7.5 mg, 500 mg/ 10 mg, 650 mg/7.5 mg, 650 mg/10 mg, 660 mg/ 10 mg tablets—1 tablet P.O. every 4 to 6 hours as needed. Do not exceed 6 tablets daily.
Adults: 750 mg/7.5 mg, 750 mg/10 mg tablets— 1 tablet P.O. every 4 to 6 hours as needed. Do not exceed 5 tablets daily.
Adults: 500 mg/5 mg/15 ml or 500 mg/7.5 mg/ 15 ml elixir—15 ml P.O. every 4 to 6 hours as needed. Do not exceed 90 ml daily.

DOSAGE MODIFICATIONS
• Adjust dosage according to pain severity and response.

• For patients with hepatic impairment, usual maximum acetaminophen dosage is 2,000 mg daily.

Contraindications and precautions
Contraindicated in hypersensitivity to drug or its components.
  Use cautiously in head injury, intracranial lesions, preexisting intracranial pressure increase, acute abdominal conditions, severe hepatic or renal impairment, hypothyroidism, Addison's disease, prostatic hypertrophy, urethral stricture, pulmonary disease, high doses, postoperative or debilitated patients, pregnancy or breastfeeding, and *elderly patients.* Safety and efficacy in *children* have not been established.

Preparation and administration
• Store at controlled temperature of 59° to 86° F (15° to 30° C).
• Keep in tight, light-resistant container with child-resistant closure.

Adverse reactions
CNS: drowsiness, dizziness, light-headedness, confusion, headache, sedation, euphoria, dysphoria, weakness, hallucinations, disorientation, mood changes, seizures
CV: palpitations, tachycardia, bradycardia, change in blood pressure, circulatory depression, syncope
EENT: blurred vision, miosis, diplopia, tinnitus
GI: nausea, vomiting, anorexia, constipation, cramps, dry mouth
GU: increased urine output, dysuria, urinary retention
Respiratory: respiratory depression
Skin: rash, urticaria, pruritus
Other: dependence, allergic reactions

Interactions
Drug-drug. *Antianxiety agents, antihistamines, antipsychotics, opioids, other CNS depressants:* additive CNS depression

Anticholinergics: increased risk of paralytic ileus

MAO inhibitors, tricyclic antidepressants: increased effect of either drug

Drug-diagnostic tests. *Urinary 5-hydroxyindoleacetic acid:* false-positive (acetaminophen)

Drug-food. *Cabbage:* increased acetaminophen metabolism

Drug-herb. *Black cohosh:* increased risk of hepatotoxicity

Dandelion, milk thistle: possible increased acetaminophen clearance

Ginkgo: increased acetaminophen level

Ginseng (Panax *and Siberian*), *goldenseal, kava, pomegranate:* increased codeine level

Jamaican dogwood, lavender, mistletoe, nettle, pokeweed, poppy, senega, valerian: increased sedation

St. John's wort: increased sedation, increased analgesia

Toxicity and overdose

Acetaminophen

• Fatal hepatic necrosis is most serious overdose effect. Renal tubular necrosis, hypoglycemic coma, and thrombocytopenia may also occur. Signs and symptoms of hepatotoxicity may not appear for 48 to 72 hours after ingestion and may include nausea, vomiting, diaphoresis, and general malaise.

• Empty stomach promptly by lavage or emesis induction. Obtain serum acetaminophen assay as soon as possible, but no sooner than 4 hours after ingestion. Obtain liver function studies initially and repeat at 24-hour intervals. Give N-acetylcysteine (antidote), preferably within 16 hours of overdose.

Hydrocodone

• Opioid triad of pinpoint pupils, respiratory depression, and loss of consciousness indicates toxicity. Seizures may occur.

• Serious signs and symptoms of overdose include respiratory depression, extreme somnolence progressing to stupor or coma, skeletal muscle flaccidity, cold and clammy skin, and sometimes bradycardia and hypotension that

may progress to apnea, circulatory collapse, cardiac arrest, and death in severe overdose.

• Gastric emptying may help remove unabsorbed drug. Establish adequate respiratory exchange through patent airway and assisted or controlled ventilation. In severe cases, consider hemodialysis (preferred) or peritoneal dialysis. Administer appropriate dose of naloxone (preferably I.V.) simultaneously with respiratory resuscitation efforts. Because duration of hydrocodone's action may exceed that of antagonist, continually monitor patient; give repeated antagonist doses as needed to maintain adequate respiration.

• Do not administer antagonist if significant respiratory or cardiovascular depression is absent. Use oxygen, I.V. fluids, vasopressors, and other supportive measures as indicated.

Special considerations

• Tolerance may develop with continued use; incidence of untoward effects is dose-related.

Patient education

• Instruct patient to seek immediate medical attention for yellowing of eyes or skin, wheezing, trouble swallowing or breathing, lightheadedness or fainting, or dizziness when standing or sitting up.

• Caution patient not to drink alcohol before or after taking drug.

• Tell patient not to take drug during labor.

• Caution patient not to take more than one dose at a time.

• Advise patient to use extra caution when driving or operating machinery on days when he takes drug.

Only common or life-threatening adverse reactions are listed.

acetaminophen and oxycodone hydrochloride

Endocet, Percocet-2.5/325, Percocet-5/325, Percocet-7.5/325, Percocet-7.5/500, Percocet-10/325, Percocet-10/650, Roxicet, Roxilox, Tylox

Classification: Opioid analgesic, antipyretic
Controlled substance schedule II
Pregnancy risk category C

Pharmacology

Acetaminophen is a nonopiate, nonsalicylate analgesic and antipyretic whose specific mechanism of analgesic action is unknown. Antipyretic properties result from inhibition of hypothalamic heat-regulating center. Oxycodone is a semisynthetic opioid analgesic and antitussive with multiple actions qualitatively similar to those of morphine. Precise mechanism of action is unknown but it may be related to opiate receptors in CNS.

Pharmacokinetics

Acetaminophen is metabolized by liver. Plasma half-life is 1 to 4 hours, but may increase in liver damage or overdose. About 85% of oral dose appears in urine within 24 hours. Oxycodone has onset of action of 15 to 30 minutes. Level peaks in 1 hour; duration of action is 4 to 6 hours. Drug is metabolized by liver and kidneys and excreted primarily in urine.

How supplied

Tablets: 2.5 mg/325 mg, 5 mg/325 mg, 7.5 mg/325 mg, 10 mg/325 mg, 7.5 mg/500 mg, 10 mg/650 mg

Indications and dosages

> **FDA-APPROVED**

➠ Moderate to moderately severe pain
Adults: 325 mg/7.5 mg and 325 mg/10 mg tablets—1 tablet P.O. every 6 hours as needed.

Adults: 325 mg/5 mg, 500 mg/7.5 mg, and 650 mg/10 mg tablets—1 tablet P.O. every 6 hours as needed. Maximum daily dosage is 4 g.
Adults: 325 mg/2.5 mg tablet—1 or 2 tablets P.O. every 6 hours as needed.

> **DOSAGE MODIFICATIONS**

• Adjust dosage according to pain severity and response.
• For patients with hepatic impairment, usual maximum acetaminophen dosage is 2,000 mg/day.

Contraindications and precautions

Contraindicated in hypersensitivity to drug or its components.

Use cautiously in head injury, intracranial lesions, preexisting intracranial pressure increase, acute abdominal conditions, severe hepatic or renal impairment, hypothyroidism, Addison's disease, prostatic hypertrophy or urethral stricture, and in pregnancy or breast-feeding. Also use cautiously in debilitated or *elderly patients.* Safety and efficacy in *children* have not been established.

Preparation and administration

• Store at controlled temperature of 59° to 86° F (15° to 30° C).
• Keep in tight, light-resistant container with child-resistant closure.

Adverse reactions

CNS: drowsiness, dizziness, confusion, headache, sedation, euphoria
CV: palpitations, bradycardia, blood pressure changes
EENT: blurred vision, miosis, diplopia, tinnitus
GI: nausea, vomiting, anorexia, constipation, cramps
GU: increased urine output, dysuria, urinary retention
Respiratory: respiratory depression
Skin: rash, urticaria, bruising, diaphoresis, pruritus
Other: dependency, flushing

Interactions

Drug-drug. *Antipsychotics, other opioids, seda-tive-hypnotics, skeletal muscle relaxants:* additive CNS depression

Drug-diagnostic tests. *Amylase:* increased

Drug-food. *Cabbage:* increased acetamino-phen metabolism

Drug-herb. *Black cohosh:* increased risk of he-patotoxicity

Dandelion, milk thistle: possible increased acet-aminophen clearance

Ginkgo: increased acetaminophen level

Ginseng (Panax *and Siberian), goldenseal, kava, pomegranate:* increased codeine level

Jamaican dogwood, lavender, mistletoe, nettle, pokeweed, poppy, senega, valerian: increased se-dation

St. John's wort: increased sedation, increased analgesia

Toxicity and overdose

Acetaminophen

• Fatal hepatic necrosis is most serious over-dose effect. Renal tubular necrosis, hypo-glycemic coma, and thrombocytopenia may also occur. Signs and symptoms of hepatotox-icity may not appear for 48 to 72 hours after ingestion and may include nausea, vomiting, diaphoresis, and general malaise.

• Empty stomach promptly by lavage or eme-sis induction. Obtain serum acetaminophen assay as soon as possible, but no sooner than 4 hours after ingestion. Obtain liver function studies initially and repeat at 24-hour inter-vals. Give *N*-acetylcysteine (antidote), prefer-ably within 16 hours of overdose.

Oxycodone

• Serious signs and symptoms of overdose in-clude respiratory depression, extreme somno-lence progressing to stupor or coma, skeletal muscle flaccidity, cold and clammy skin, and sometimes bradycardia and hypotension that may progress to apnea, circulatory collapse, cardiac arrest, and death in severe overdose.

• Establish adequate respiratory exchange through patent airway and assisted or con-trolled ventilation. In severe cases, consider

hemodialysis (preferred) or peritoneal dialysis. Give appropriate naloxone dose (preferably I.V.) simultaneously with respiratory resuscita-tion efforts. Because duration of drug's action may exceed that of antagonist, continuously monitor patient; give repeated antagonist dos-es as needed to maintain adequate respiration.

• Do not administer antagonist if significant respiratory or cardiovascular depression is ab-sent. Use oxygen, I.V. fluids, vasopressors, and other supportive measures as indicated.

• Gastric emptying may help remove unab-sorbed drug.

Special considerations

• Tolerance may develop with continued use; incidence of untoward effects is dose-related.

Patient education

• Instruct patient to shake liquid form well and measure dose with measuring spoon or dropper (not kitchen spoon).

• Advise patient to seek immediate medical attention for yellowing of eyes or skin, wheez-ing, difficulty swallowing or breathing, light-headedness or fainting, or dizziness when standing or sitting up.

• Caution patient not to drink alcohol before or after taking drug and not to take more than one dose at a time.

• Instruct patient to use extra caution when driving or performing other hazardous activi-ties on days when he takes drug.

aldesleukin
Proleukin

Classification: Antineoplastic, biological response modifier (recombinant DNA origin)
Pregnancy risk category C

Pharmacology

Aldesleukin is a synthetic interleukin (IL)-2 agent that activates cellular immunity through profound lymphocytosis, eosinophilia, and thrombocytopenia and cytokine production (including tumor necrosis factor, IL-1, and gamma interferon). Drug inhibits tumor growth.

Pharmacokinetics
Drug attains high plasma concentration. Onset is 5 minutes, peak is 13 minutes, and half-life is about 8 minutes. It is eliminated by kidneys with little or no bioactive protein excreted in urine.

How supplied
Solution for infusion: 22 million international units in single-use vial

Indications and dosages

FDA-APPROVED

➡ Metastatic renal cell carcinoma
Adults: 600,000 international units/kg by I.V. infusion over 15 minutes every 8 hours for maximum of 14 doses. After 9-day rest, repeat schedule for another 14 doses, to maximum of 28 doses per course, as tolerated.
➡ Metastatic melanoma
Adults: 600,000 international units/kg by I.V. infusion over 15 minutes every 8 hours for maximum of 14 doses. After 9-day rest, repeat schedule for another 14 doses, to maximum of 28 doses per course, as tolerated.

OFF-LABEL USES (SELECTED)

➡ Malignant melanoma
Adults: Variable dosing schedule
➡ Non-Hodgkin's lymphoma
Adults: Variable dosing schedule

DOSAGE MODIFICATIONS

• Withhold drug (rather than reduce dosage) if adverse events requiring dosage modification occur.
• Withhold drug in patients with reduced organ perfusion (as shown by altered mental status, reduced urine output, significant hypotension, or arrhythmia). Recovery from

capillary leak syndrome (CLS) begins shortly after drug is discontinued.
• Discontinue drug if moderate to severe lethargy or somnolence develops.

⊠ WARNINGS

• Restrict therapy to patients with normal cardiac and pulmonary function. Use cautiously in patients with normal thallium stress tests and pulmonary function tests with history of cardiac or pulmonary disease.
• Use cautiously in patients with fixed requirements for large fluid volume, such as those with hypercalcemia.
• Drug may cause CLS, resulting in hypotension and reduced organ perfusion (which may be severe and fatal), arrhythmias (supraventricular and ventricular), angina, myocardial infarction, respiratory insufficiency requiring intubation, GI bleeding or infarction, renal insufficiency, edema, and mental status changes.
• Impaired neutrophil function and increased risk of disseminated infection (including sepsis and bacterial endocarditis) may occur. Bacterial infections should be adequately treated before therapy. Patients with indwelling central lines have a high risk of infection with gram-positive microorganisms. Antibiotic prophylaxis with oxacillin, nafcillin, ciprofloxacin, or vancomycin has been linked to reduced incidence of staphylococcal infections.
• Withhold drug in patients developing moderate to severe lethargy or somnolence; continued use may result in coma.

Contraindications and precautions
Contraindicated in hypersensitivity to IL-2 or its components, abnormal thallium stress test or pulmonary function tests, organ allografts, or drug-related toxicities with previous therapy.
Use cautiously in abnormal cardiac, pulmonary, hepatic, or CNS function at start of therapy; CLS; and hepatic or renal impair-

ment. Safety and efficacy in *children* have not been established.

Preparation and administration
• Follow hazardous drug guidelines for handling, preparation, and administration. (See "Managing hazardous drugs," page 11.)
• Reconstitute with 1.2 ml sterile water for injection. Avoid excess foaming by directing diluent at side of vial and gently swirling contents. Swirl but do not shake vial. After reconstitution, each ml contains 18 million units (1.1 mg/ml).
• Dilute reconstituted drug in 50 ml D_5W and infuse over 15 minutes.
• Reconstituted or diluted solutions are stable for up to 48 hours if refrigerated.
• Do not administer with in-line filters because filter may absorb drug.
• Store vials at 36° to 46° F (2° to 8° C).

Adverse reactions
CNS: confusion, stupor, coma, psychosis, transient ischemic attacks, meningitis, cerebral edema, somnolence, anxiety, dizziness, malaise, asthenia
CV: hypotension, supraventricular tachycardia, blood pressure fluctuations, myocardial infarction (MI), ventricular tachycardia, cardiac arrest, myocarditis, pericarditis, vasodilation, arrhythmia, asymptomatic ECG changes, heart failure
EENT: permanent or transient blindness secondary to optic neuritis, rhinitis
GI: duodenal ulcers, bowel necrosis, tracheoesophageal fistula, diarrhea, vomiting, nausea, stomatitis, anorexia, abdominal pain, enlarged abdomen
GU: oliguria, anuria, acute renal failure, allergic interstitial nephritis
Hematologic: thrombocytopenia, anemia, leukopenia, intravascular coagulopathy
Metabolic: acidosis, hypomagnesemia, hypocalcemia
Respiratory: dyspnea, apnea, adult respiratory distress syndrome, respiratory failure,

worsened cough, pulmonary congestion, crackles, rhonchi, pulmonary infiltrates, unspecified pulmonary changes
Skin: rash, pruritus, exfoliative dermatitis
Other: fever, infection, sepsis, edema, peripheral edema, weight gain, chills, pain

Interactions
Drug-drug. *Analgesics, antiemetics, opioids, other CNS agents, sedatives, tranquilizers:* increased severity of CNS adverse reactions
Beta blockers, other antihypertensives: increased risk of hypotension
Cardiotoxic, hepatotoxic, myelotoxic, and nephrotoxic agents: increased organ toxicity
Cisplatin, dacarbazine, interferon alfa, tamoxifen: increased risk of hypersensitivity reactions
Glucocorticoids: possible reduction in aldesleukin antitumor efficacy
Interferon alfa: increased risk of MI, myocarditis, ventricular hypokinesia, severe rhabdomyolysis, crescentic IgA glomerulonephritis, oculobulbar myasthenia gravis, inflammatory arthritis, thyroiditis, bullous pemphigoid, and Stevens-Johnson syndrome
Iodinated contrast media: delayed (1 to 4 hours) adverse reactions to drug, including fever, chills, nausea, vomiting, pruritus, rash, diarrhea, hypotension, edema, and oliguria
Other antineoplastics: safety not established
Drug-diagnostic tests. *BUN; ALP, ALT, bilirubin; creatine kinase; creatinine; lactate dehydrogenase; serum and urinary uric acid; urinary albumin and protein:* increased
ECG: reduced QRS voltage, ST segment and T-wave changes
Left ventricular ejection fraction, left ventricular stroke work index: decreased
Prothrombin time: prolonged
Serum albumin, bicarbonate, calcium, magnesium, phosphate, potassium, protein, sodium: decreased

Toxicity and overdose

• Adverse reactions are dose-related and reflect cardiac, renal, and hepatic toxicity.
• Symptoms persisting after therapy ends should be treated supportively. Life-threatening toxicities warrant I.V. dexamethasone, which may cancel out drug's therapeutic effect.

Special considerations

• Evaluate patient's response 4 weeks after course ends and immediately before scheduled start of next course. Patient should receive additional course only if tumor has shrunk since previous course and retreatment is not contraindicated. Separate treatment courses by rest period of at least 7 weeks from discharge.
• Patients sensitive to *Escherichia coli*–derived proteins may be sensitive to drug.
• Watch for delayed adverse reactions, which may occur 4 weeks to several months after drug therapy.
• Monitor patient for irritability, confusion, and depression, which may indicate bacteremia or early bacterial sepsis, hypoperfusion, occult CNS cancer, or direct drug-induced CNS toxicity. Drug-induced mental status changes may progress for several days before recovery begins.
• Drug may exacerbate preexisting autoimmune disease or initial presentation of autoimmune and inflammatory disorders.
• Decreased neutrophil function may lead to infection, delayed healing, and gingival bleeding.
• Watch for unexplained weight changes, hypotension, chest pain, heart murmurs, palpitations, irregular pulse, dyspnea or other respiratory impairment, and abnormal bleeding.
• Concomitant use of nephrotoxic or hepatotoxic drugs may worsen renal or hepatic toxicity. Monitor kidney and liver function test results frequently.
• Stomatitis may be severe enough to require a liquid diet.

• Monitor patient for pulmonary infiltration, which may appear by day 4 of therapy and usually resolves within a few weeks after drug is stopped. Intubation may be needed for respiratory failure.
• Evaluate patient for vision problems shortly after start of therapy.
• Monitor patient for macular erythema 2 to 3 days after start of therapy. Condition begins to resolve 2 to 3 days after drug is stopped. Monitor palms and soles for skin peeling; skin appears normal within 2 to 3 weeks after drug withdrawal.
• Watch for other dermatologic effects, including angioedema, urticaria, and erythema nodosum.

Patient education

• Instruct patient to immediately report fever or chills, cough or hoarseness, lower back or side pain, painful or difficult urination, unusual bleeding or bruising, blood in urine or stool, black tarry stools, or pinpoint red spots on skin.
• Inform patient that nausea and vomiting are expected.
• Advise patient to practice proper oral hygiene during treatment, including cautious use of regular toothbrushes, dental floss, and toothpicks. Tell patient to check with prescriber before dental work.
• Tell patient that drug may cause weight gain of more than 10% of pretreatment weight; reversal of gain may take up to 2 weeks after therapy ends.
• Caution patient to avoid persons with infections, especially during periods of low blood cell counts.

alemtuzumab

Campath

Classification: Antineoplastic, monoclonal antibody
Pregnancy risk category C

Pharmacology

Alemtuzumab binds to antigen CD52 on cell surface of normal and malignant B and T lymphocytes. Proposed mechanism of action is antibody-dependent lysis of leukemic cells after cell surface binding.

Pharmacokinetics

Peak and trough levels rise during first few weeks and reach maintenance levels by about week 6. Serum level rise corresponds with malignant lymphocytosis reduction. Average half-life is 12 days.

How supplied

Solution for injection: 30 mg/3 ml in single-use ampule

Indications and dosages

FDA-APPROVED

➡ B-cell chronic lymphocytic leukemia in patients treated with alkylating agents who failed fludarabine therapy
Adults: 3 mg subcutaneously (commonly used but not FDA-approved route) daily or as 2-hour I.V. infusion daily. When tolerated, increase to 10 mg. When tolerated, initiate maintenance dosage of 30 mg/day three times a week on alternate days for up to 12 weeks. Dosage escalation takes 1 to 2 weeks.

DOSAGE MODIFICATIONS

• Dosage increase to 30 mg may be accomplished in 3 to 7 days in most patients.
• Stop therapy during serious infection, serious hematologic toxicity, or other serious toxicity until event resolves.

• Stop therapy permanently if autoimmune anemia or thrombocytopenia occurs. (See table below.)

Adjusting dosage when hematologic toxicity occurs

Hematologic toxicity	Dosage modification and therapy reinitiation
First occurrence of absolute neutrophil count (ANC) below 250/mm³ and/or platelet count of 25,000/mm³ or less	Withhold drug. When ANC is 500/mm³ or more and platelet count is 50,000/mm³ or more, resume drug at same dose. If delay between dosing is 7 days or more, start drug at 3 mg and escalate to 10 mg and then to 30 mg as tolerated.
Second occurrence of ANC below 250/mm³ and/or platelet count of 25,000/mm³ or less	Withhold drug. When ANC is 500/mm³ or more and platelet count is 50,000/mm³ or more, resume drug at 10 mg. If delay between dosing is 7 days or more, start drug at 3 mg and escalate to 10 mg only.
Third occurrence of ANC below 250/mm³ and/or platelet count of 25,000/mm³ or less	Discontinue drug permanently.
Decrease of ANC and/or platelet count to 50% or less of baseline value in patients starting drug with baseline ANC of 500/mm³ or less and/or baseline platelet count of 25,000/mm³ or less	Withhold drug. When ANC and/or platelet count returns to baseline, resume drug. If delay between dosing is 7 days or more, start drug at 3 mg and escalate to 10 mg and then to 30 mg as tolerated.

⚠ WARNINGS

• Serious and, in rare cases, fatal pancytopenia, bone marrow hypoplasia, autoimmune idiopathic thrombocytopenia, and autoimmune hemolytic anemia have occurred. Single doses above 30 mg or cumulative doses above

90 mg/week should not be given because of their link to higher pancytopenia incidence.
• Serious infusion reactions may occur. Carefully monitor patient during infusions; discontinue drug if indicated. Gradual escalation to maintenance dosage is required at initiation and after therapy interruption of 7 or more days.
• Serious, and sometimes fatal bacterial, viral, fungal, and protozoan infections have occurred. Obtain weekly CBC and platelet counts during therapy or more frequently if anemia, neutropenia, or thrombocytopenia worsens. Prophylaxis for *Pneumocystis carinii* pneumonia and herpesvirus infections has decreased incidence of (but not eliminated) these infections.

Contraindications and precautions
Contraindicated in type I hypersensitivity or anaphylactic reaction to drug or its components, active systemic infections, and immunodeficiency.

Use cautiously in bone marrow depression, existing or recent chickenpox, herpes zoster, ischemic heart disease, previous cytotoxic drug or radiation therapy, and pregnancy or breastfeeding. Safety and efficacy in *elderly patients* and *children* have not been established.

Preparation and administration
• Follow hazardous drug guidelines for handling, preparation, and administration. (See "Managing hazardous drugs," page 11.)
• Obtain baseline CBC with differential and platelet count.
• Do not administer by I.V. bolus or push. I.V. infusion has caused severe adverse reactions; this route has been replaced almost completely by subcutaneous injection.
• For I.V. infusion, dilute in 100 ml normal saline solution or D_5W and infuse over 2 hours. Administer diphenhydramine and acetaminophen, as indicated, 30 minutes before

infusion to decrease risk of serious adverse reactions.
• Prescribe anti-infective prophylaxis to minimize risk of opportunistic infections.
• Store drug in refrigerator at 36° to 46° F (2° to 8° C). Do not freeze. Discard if ampule has been frozen. Protect from direct sunlight.

Adverse reactions
CNS: asthenia, dysesthesia, dizziness, fatigue, headache, insomnia
CV: chest pain, edema, hypertension, hypotension, tachycardia, supraventricular tachycardia
EENT: pharyngitis
GI: abdominal pain, anorexia, diarrhea, dyspepsia, nausea, vomiting
Hematologic: bone marrow depression, anemia, neutropenia, thrombocytopenia, pancytopenia, purpura
Musculoskeletal: skeletal pain, myalgia
Respiratory: bronchitis, bronchospasm, cough, dyspnea, pneumonitis
Skin: herpes simplex infection, pruritus, rash, urticaria
Other: infusion-related reactions, sepsis, allergic reactions, anaphylactoid reaction

Interactions
Drug-drug. *Antihypertensives:* hypotension
Blood dyscrasia–causing drugs: increased anemia, leukopenia, and thrombocytopenia
Bone marrow depressants: additive bone marrow depression
Drug-diagnostic tests. *Antibody tests:* possible interference with subsequent diagnostic serum tests that use antibodies

Toxicity and overdose
• Overdose is associated with higher pancytopenia incidence.
• No specific antidote is known; discontinue drug and use supportive treatments. Blood products or modifiers may be used to treat bone marrow toxicity.

Special considerations

- Evaluate for hypotension during infusion.
- Monitor patient for signs and symptoms of infection; therapy may be stopped if severe infection occurs.
- Monitor patient weekly for anemia, neutropenia, and thrombocytopenia (platelet count below 50,000/mm³) and more frequently if these worsen during therapy.
- Evaluate CD4+ count after treatment until it recovers to 200 cells/mm³ or more.
- Take precautions against excessive bleeding and use extreme caution during invasive procedures.
- Inspect and test secretions for blood.

Patient education

- Instruct patient to report signs and symptoms of infection immediately.
- Urge patient to maintain follow-up appointments, especially for weekly CBC and platelet counts, during therapy. Failure to do so may lead to serious adverse reactions.
- Advise breastfeeding patient to stop breastfeeding during therapy and for 3 months afterward.

altretamine
Hexalen

Classification: Antineoplastic, alkylating agent
Pregnancy risk category D

Pharmacology

Altretamine appears to be activated by liver to metabolites (pentemethlymelamine and tetramethlymelamine) that bind with nucleic acids, preventing cell uptake and inhibiting DNA and RNA synthesis.

Pharmacokinetics

Drug is well absorbed. It undergoes rapid and extensive demethylation in liver, causing plasma levels to vary. It peaks in 30 minutes to 3 hours. Elimination half-life is 4 to 13 hours. It is excreted in urine.

How supplied

Capsules: 50 mg

Indications and dosages

FDA-APPROVED

⊖ Palliative treatment of persistent or recurrent ovarian cancer after cisplatin or alkylating agent–based combination therapy
Adults: 260 mg/m² P.O. daily in four divided doses for either 14 or 21 consecutive days in 28-day cycle

OFF-LABEL USES (SELECTED)

➥ Small-cell lung carcinoma
Adults: 60 to 400 mg/m² P.O. daily for 5 to 21 days; used only with other drugs proven to be effective in small-cell lung carcinoma

DOSAGE MODIFICATIONS

- Temporarily discontinue (for 14 days or longer) and subsequently restart at 200 mg/m² daily if GI intolerance does not improve with symptomatic measures, WBC count is below 2,000/mm³, granulocyte count is below 1,000/mm³, platelet count is below 75,000/mm³, or progressive neurotoxicity occurs.
- If neurologic symptoms fail to stabilize on reduced dosage schedule, discontinue drug indefinitely.
- Dosage is usually decreased to 150 mg/m² daily for 14 days when drug is combined with other bone marrow depressants.
- Dosage may be decreased if nausea and vomiting persist despite supportive antiemetic therapy.

⊠ WARNINGS

- Monitor peripheral blood counts at least monthly, before each course begins, and as clinically indicated.

Only common or life-threatening adverse reactions are listed.

A

• Drug causes mild to moderate bone marrow depression and neurotoxicity. Blood counts and neurologic examination should be performed before each course and dosage adjusted as clinically indicated.

Contraindications and precautions

Contraindicated in hypersensitivity to drug or its components, preexisting severe bone marrow depression, and severe neurologic toxicity.

Use cautiously in preexisting cisplatin neuropathies, bone marrow depression, concurrent radiation therapy, concurrent MAO inhibitor therapy, pregnancy or breastfeeding, and in *elderly patients*. Safety and efficacy in *children* have not been established.

Preparation and administration

• Follow hazardous drug guidelines for handling, preparation, and administration. (See "Managing hazardous drugs," page 11.)
• Evaluate peripheral blood counts before each course.
• Give an antiemetic before administration to help control nausea and vomiting.
• Give after meals or at bedtime to help prevent adverse reactions.
• Store at controlled temperature of 59° to 86° F (15° to 30° C).

Adverse reactions

CNS: peripheral neuropathy
GI: nausea, vomiting
Hematologic: anemia, leukopenia, thrombocytopenia
Hepatic: hepatotoxicity

Interactions

Drug-drug. *Blood dyscrasia–causing drugs:* increased anemia, leukopenia, and thrombocytopenia
Cimetidine: increased altretamine serum level
MAO inhibitors (including furazolidone, procarbazine, and selegiline): severe orthostatic hypotension

Drug-diagnostic tests. *ALP, BUN, creatinine:* increased
Renal function tests: altered

Toxicity and overdose

• Although no known acute overdose cases have occurred, anticipated signs and symptoms include nausea, vomiting, peripheral neuropathy, and severe bone marrow depression.
• Treatment is supportive. Pyridoxine may significantly reduce neurotoxicity but adversely affect response duration, suggesting it should not be given with altretamine or cisplatin.

Special considerations

• Monitor neurologic function, especially in patients with preexisting cisplatin neuropathies.
• Monitor hematocrit, hemoglobin, platelet count, and WBC count with differential at least monthly, before each course, and as clinically indicated.

Patient education

• Instruct patient to take drug at same time every day, preferably with meals and at bedtime.
• Caution patient not to take more than one dose at a time. If he forgets dose, advise him to skip that dose and take next dose at regular time.
• Advise patient to seek immediate medical attention for yellowing of eyes or skin or dizziness when standing or sitting up.
• Counsel women with childbearing potential to avoid pregnancy.
• Instruct breastfeeding patient to stop breastfeeding during therapy.

amifostine
Ethyol

Classification: Cytoprotective
Pregnancy risk category C

Pharmacology
Amifostine reduces cytotoxicity of radiation and alkylating agents such as cisplatin by detoxifying reactive metabolites. It protects normal tissues through higher capillary alkaline phosphatase activity, higher pH, and better vascularity, which increases thiol metabolite concentration in normal tissues.

Pharmacokinetics
Drug is rapidly metabolized and cleared from plasma. Distribution half-life is less than 1 minute; elimination half-life is about 8 minutes. Metabolites are excreted mainly in urine.

How supplied
Powder for injection: 500 mg in 10-ml vial

Indications and dosages

FDA-APPROVED

➲ Reduction of incidence of moderate to severe xerostomia in patients undergoing postoperative radiation treatment for head and neck cancer
Adults: 200 mg/m² I.V. once daily, infused over 3 minutes, starting 15 to 30 minutes before standard fraction radiation therapy (1.8 to 2 Gy)
➲ Reduction of cumulative renal toxicity caused by repeated cisplatin administration in patients with advanced ovarian cancer or non-small-cell lung cancer
Adults: 910 mg/m² I.V. once daily infused over 15 minutes, starting 30 minutes before chemotherapy. If full dose cannot be given, subsequent cycles should be administered at 740 mg/m².

OFF-LABEL USES (SELECTED)

➡ Myelodysplastic syndromes
Adults: Commonly used dosage schedule is either three times a week or once weekly. Three-times-a-week dosages include 100 mg/m², 200 mg/m², and 400 mg/m² I.V. infusion. Once-weekly dose of 740 mg/m² I.V. infusion has been studied.
➡ Protection against cisplatin- and paclitaxel-induced neurotoxicity
Adults: Commonly used dosages include 500 mg I.V. infusion 20 minutes before chemotherapy or 740 mg/m² I.V. infusion 15 minutes before chemotherapy.
➡ Protection against salivary secretion disturbance by radioiodine; protection against cyclophosphamide-induced granulocytopenia and thrombocytopenia, cisplatin-induced thrombocytopenia, and carboplatin-induced generalized bone marrow depression
Adults: Commonly used dosages range from 740 mg/m² to 910 mg/m² as I.V. infusion about 15 minutes before chemotherapy.
➡ Reduction of mucositis in patients receiving radiation therapy or radiation combined with chemotherapy
Adults: Commonly used dosages include 200 mg/m², 740 mg/m², and 910 mg/m² as I.V. infusion 15 to 30 minutes before therapy.

DOSAGE MODIFICATIONS

• Temporarily discontinue infusion if systolic blood pressure decreases. Restart if baseline blood pressure returns within 5 minutes; otherwise, reduce dosage.

Contraindications and precautions
Contraindicated in sensitivity to aminothiol compounds.

Use cautiously in preexisting cardiovascular or cerebrovascular conditions, cutaneous reactions, hypotension, dehydration, concurrent antihypertensive therapy or chemotherapy for other cancers, definitive radiation therapy, risk of hypocalcemia, and pregnancy or breastfeeding. Safety and efficacy in *elderly*

Only common or life-threatening adverse reactions are listed.

patients (*older than age 70*) and *children* have not been established.

Preparation and administration
- Give antiemetics, including I.V. dexamethasone and serotonin 5-HT$_3$ receptor antagonist, before and during amifostine administration.
- Interrupt antihypertensive therapy for 24 hours before amifostine administration. Do not use drug in patients whose antihypertensive therapy cannot be interrupted for 24 hours.
- Ensure adequate hydration before infusion.
- Dilute with normal saline solution.
- Administer as short-term I.V. infusion over 15 minutes; prolonged infusions increase risk of hypotension and vomiting.
- Keep patient supine during infusion.
- Monitor blood pressure every 5 minutes during infusion and thereafter as indicated. If hypotension occurs, place patient in Trendelenburg position. Start normal saline infusion using separate I.V. line.
- Immediately and permanently discontinue drug if patient develops acute allergic reaction, such as serious or severe cutaneous reaction, cutaneous reaction associated with fever, or other symptoms of unknown etiology.
- Store at controlled temperature of 68° to 77° F (20° to 25°C).

Adverse reactions
CNS: dizziness, somnolence
CV: hypotension, syncope
EENT: sneezing
GI: nausea, vomiting, hiccups
Metabolic: hypocalcemia, hypomagnesemia
Skin: rash, Stevens-Johnson syndrome
Other: flushing, feeling of warmth, chills

Interactions
Drug-drug. *Antihypertensives:* worsened hypotension
Drug-diagnostic tests. *Calcium, magnesium:* decreased

Toxicity and overdose
- Signs and symptoms include hypotension. Anxiety and reversible urinary retention may occur at high doses.
- Manage with infusions of normal saline solution and other supportive measures as indicated.

Special considerations
- Monitor hydration status carefully, especially when giving drug with chemotherapy agents with high emetic risk, such as cisplatin.
- Monitor serum calcium levels in patients at risk for hypocalcemia, such as those with nephrotic syndrome or those receiving multiple doses. If necessary, give calcium supplements.
- Continue to monitor blood pressure and hydration throughout therapy.

Patient education
- Tell patient he will be kept in supine position and blood pressure will be monitored frequently during infusion.
- Instruct patient to report dizziness, rash, pruritus, or other adverse reactions.
- Inform women of childbearing potential that drug may harm fetus if used during pregnancy.
- Tell breastfeeding patient to discontinue breastfeeding during therapy.

aminoglutethimide
Cytadren

Classification: Adrenal steroid inhibitor, antineoplastic, aromatase inhibitor
Pregnancy risk category D

Pharmacology
Aminoglutethimide inhibits aromatase enzymes needed to convert androgens to estrogens and inhibits desmolase, an enzyme needed for steroid production. It also blocks adre-

nal steroid biosynthesis by interfering with enzymatic conversion of cholesterol to delta-5 pregnenolone, and decreases production of glucocorticoids, mineralocorticoids, estrogens, and androgens.

Pharmacokinetics

Drug is well absorbed and metabolized in liver. It is 25% plasma protein–bound; elimination half-life is 7 to 9 hours. It is excreted as unchanged drug and metabolites in urine.

How supplied

Tablets: 250 mg

Indications and dosages

OFF-LABEL USES (SELECTED)

➡ Metastatic prostate cancer
Adults: Commonly prescribed dosage is 500 to 1,000 mg P.O. daily in divided doses.
➡ Breast and prostatic carcinoma
Adults: Initially, 125 mg P.O. twice daily for several days to 1 week, then two or three times a day for approximately 2 weeks in combination with hydrocortisone 100 mg P.O. daily in three divided doses for 1 to 2 weeks, then hydrocortisone 40 mg P.O. daily (10 mg in morning and at 5 P.M. and 20 mg at bedtime). For maintenance, 250 mg P.O. four times daily, preferably every 6 hours in combination with hydrocortisone 40 mg P.O. daily (10 mg in morning and at 5 P.M. and 20 mg at bedtime).

DOSAGE MODIFICATIONS

• Severe or significant adverse effects may necessitate dosage reduction or temporary discontinuation.
• If rash persists beyond 8 days or becomes severe, discontinue drug. Restart at lower dosage after mild or moderate rash disappears. Mineralocorticoid replacement, such as fludrocortisone, may be necessary. If glucocorticoid replacement is needed, 20 to 30 mg hydrocortisone P.O. in morning replaces endogenous secretion.

Contraindications and precautions

Contraindicated in severe hypersensitivity to glutethimide or aminoglutethimide.

Use cautiously in abnormal thyroid or hepatic function; stressful conditions, such as surgery, trauma, or acute illness; pregnancy or breastfeeding; and in *elderly patients.* Safety and efficacy in *children* have not been established.

Preparation and administration

• Institute treatment in hospital until patient achieves stable dosage regimen.
• Store in tight, light-resistant container.
• Do not store above 86° F (30° C).

Adverse reactions

CNS: ataxia, dizziness, drowsiness, headache
CV: hypotension
GI: anorexia, nausea, vomiting
Metabolic: adrenocortical hypofunction, hypothyroidism
Musculoskeletal: myalgia
Skin: maculopapular eruptions
Other: fever

Interactions

Drug-drug. *Coumarin, warfarin:* reduced anticoagulant effect
Dexamethasone: increased dexamethasone metabolism
Sedative-hypnotics, tranquilizers, tricyclic antidepressants: aggravated aminoglutethimide signs and symptoms
Drug-diagnostic tests. *ALP, AST, bilirubin:* increased
Thyroid function tests: decreased
Drug-herb. *Ginseng (Siberian), L-tryptophan, stinging nettle, valerian:* increased sedation

Toxicity and overdose

• Common overdose signs and symptoms include respiratory depression, hyperventilation, hypotension, hypovolemic shock, somnolence, lethargy, coma, ataxia, dizziness, fatigue, nausea, vomiting, sodium and water

---

Only common or life-threatening adverse reactions are listed.

loss, hyponatremia, hypochloremia, hyperkalemia, and hypoglycemia.
• Treat overdose with gastric lavage and supportive measures. If circulating glucocorticoid deficiency develops, give I.V. infusion of hydrocortisone (100 mg hydrocortisone sodium succinate in 500 ml normal saline solution) and 50 ml 40% glucose solution within 3 hours. After initial infusion, continue I.V. hydrocortisone at 10 mg/hour until patient can take oral cortisone. If hypovolemia or hypotension occurs, give I.V. norepinephrine, according to patient need and response. After rehydration, patient may require plasma or blood to maintain sufficient circulatory volume. In severe toxicity, consider dialysis.

Special considerations
• Monitor serum electrolyte levels periodically.
• Monitor liver function test results.
• Observe adrenocortical response by carefully monitoring plasma cortisol level until desired suppression level occurs.
• Observe patient for signs and symptoms of hypothyroidism and monitor thyroid function studies as indicated.
• Adrenocortical hypofunction may occur, especially with stressful conditions. Monitor patient and give hydrocortisone and mineralocorticoid supplements as indicated. Do not use dexamethasone.
• Drug may suppress adrenal aldosterone production and may cause orthostatic or persistent hypotension. Monitor blood pressure at appropriate intervals.

Patient education
• Instruct patient to take drug at same time every day, and not to take more than one dose at a time.
• Caution patient not to consume alcohol before or after taking drug.
• Inform patient that drug may cause hypotension; describe symptoms.
• Caution patient to avoid driving and other potentially hazardous activities; drug may cause drowsiness.

• Counsel female patient not to use drug if she is pregnant, expects to become pregnant, or is breastfeeding.

anastrozole
Arimidex

Classification: Antineoplastic, aromatase inhibitor, hormone/hormone modifier
Pregnancy risk category D

Pharmacology
Anastrozole significantly decreases serum estradiol levels by selectively inhibiting conversion of androgen to estrogen. This leads to decreased tumor mass or delayed growth.

Pharmacokinetics
Drug is well absorbed from GI tract; food may decrease absorption. It is metabolized in liver. Maximum plasma levels occur within 2 hours. Half-life is 50 hours. Drug is eliminated in urine.

How supplied
Tablets: 1 mg

Indications and dosages

FDA-APPROVED

➡ Hormone-receptor-positive or hormone-receptor unknown locally advanced or metastatic breast cancer in postmenopausal women; advanced breast cancer in postmenopausal women with disease progression after tamoxifen therapy
Adults: 1 mg P.O. daily continued until tumor progression

Contraindications and precautions
Contraindicated in hypersensitivity to drug or its components.
Use cautiously in history of thromboembolism, hepatic impairment, or hypercholes-

terolemia. Drug should not be used in pre-menopausal, pregnant, or breastfeeding women. Safety and efficacy in *children* have not been established.

Preparation and administration

• Follow hazardous drug guidelines for handling, preparation, and administration. (See "Managing hazardous drugs," page 11.)
• Exclude pregnancy before starting treatment.
• Administer with food.
• Store at 68° to 77° F (20° to 25° C).

Adverse reactions

CNS: headache, lethargy, depression, dizziness, confusion, insomnia, anxiety
CV: chest pain, hypertension, thrombophlebitis, thromboembolism
EENT: rhinitis, sinusitis, pharyngitis
GI: nausea, vomiting, diarrhea, constipation, abdominal pain, dry mouth, altered taste leading to anorexia
GU: breast pain, vaginal bleeding, vaginal dryness, pruritus vulvae, urinary tract infection
Hematologic: leukopenia, anemia
Metabolic: hypercholesterolemia
Musculoskeletal: bone pain, neck pain, myalgia, asthenia, bone fractures, pelvic pain
Respiratory: cough, dyspnea, bronchitis
Skin: rash, alopecia
Other: edema, hot flashes, weight gain or loss, tumor flare, flulike syndrome, sweating, accidental injury, infection

Interactions

Drug-drug. *Estrogen therapies:* reduced anastrozole efficacy
Tamoxifen: reduced anastrozole plasma level
Drug-diagnostic tests. *ALP, ALT, AST, GGT, low-density lipoproteins, total serum cholesterol:* increased
Bone mineral density: reduced
Drug-herb. *Dehydroepiandrosterone:* possible interference with drug's antiestrogen effects
Glutamine: enhanced tumor growth

Toxicity and overdose

• Maximum dosage has not been established. Expected overdose symptoms may include severe gastric irritation (necrosis, gastritis, ulceration, and hemorrhage).
• No specific antidote exists. Consider that patient may have taken multiple agents. Induce vomiting if patient is alert. Dialysis may prove helpful (drug is not highly protein-bound). Treat symptomatically and provide general supportive care, including frequent vital sign monitoring and close observation.

Special considerations

• Monitor CBC count, blood chemistry and liver function test results, and serum lipid levels.
• Evaluate patient regularly for chest pain and dyspnea (symptoms of thromboembolism).
• Monitor patient for changes in tumor size.
• Therapy should continue even if nausea, vomiting, or diarrhea occurs.
• Patients with estrogen receptor-negative disease or who failed to respond to previous tamoxifen therapy rarely respond to anastrozole.

Patient education

• Educate patient about signs and symptoms of serious adverse reactions, and tell him to report these.
• Instruct patient to keep taking drug even if nausea, vomiting, or diarrhea occurs.
• Inform patient that drug may cause hair loss and that after therapy ends, new hair growth may differ in color or texture.
• Advise patient that tumor flare (increased tumor size and bone pain) may occur, but will subside rapidly. Recommend analgesics.
• Instruct women with childbearing potential about pregnancy testing before treatment starts.
• Tell patient to inform prescriber if she is breastfeeding or plans to breastfeed.

Only common or life-threatening adverse reactions are listed.

aprepitant
Emend, Emend 3-Day

Classification: Antiemetic, antivertigo agent, substance P antagonist
Pregnancy risk category B

Pharmacology
Aprepitant inhibits emesis induced by cytotoxic chemotherapeutic agents such as cisplatin in both acute and delayed emesis phases. It also augments antiemetic activity of dexamethasone and the 5-HT$_3$ receptor antagonist ondansetron.

Pharmacokinetics
Drug is metabolized in liver. It is well distributed and more than 95% bound to plasma protein. It peaks in about 4 hours, has a terminal half-life of 9 to 13 hours, and is excreted in urine and feces.

How supplied
Capsules: 80 mg, 125 mg

Indications and dosages

FDA-APPROVED

➡ Prevention of acute and delayed nausea and vomiting associated with initial and repeat courses of highly or moderately emetogenic cancer chemotherapy, including high-dose cisplatin
Adults: 125 mg P.O. 1 hour before treatment (day 1) and 80 mg once daily in morning on days 2 and 3

DOSAGE MODIFICATIONS

• Patients with mild to moderate hepatic insufficiency (Child-Pugh score of 5 to 9) do not require dosage adjustment. No clinical data exist for patients with severe hepatic insufficiency (Child-Pugh score above 9).

Contraindications and precautions
Contraindicated in hypersensitivity to drug or its components and concurrent pimozide, terfenadine, astemizole, or cisapride therapy.
   Use cautiously in concurrent chemotherapy (primarily agents metabolized through CYP3A4); therapy with docetaxel, paclitaxel, etoposide, irinotecan, ifosfamide, imatinib, vinorelbine, vinblastine, or vincristine; and in pregnancy or breastfeeding. *Elderly patients.* may be more sensitive to drug effects. Safety and efficacy in *children* have not been established.

Preparation and administration
• Administer with corticosteroid and 5-HT$_3$ antagonist.
• Give with or without food.
• Store at 68° to 77° F (20° to 25° C). Keep desiccant in original bottle.

Adverse reactions
CNS: fatigue, headache, somnolence, dizziness
GI: anorexia, constipation, diarrhea, nausea, heartburn
Hematologic: neutropenia
Respiratory: hiccups
Skin: Stevens-Johnson syndrome
Other: dehydration, angioedema

Interactions
Drug-drug. *Astemizole, cisapride, clarithromycin, dexamethasone, docetaxel, etoposide, ifosfamide, imitinib, irinotecan, itraconazole, ketoconazole, methylprednisolone, midazolam, nefazodone, nelfinavir, paclitaxel, pimozide, ritonavir, terfenadine, troleandomycin, vinorelbine, vincristine:* increased serum levels of these drugs
Carbamazepine, phenytoin, rifampin: reduced aprepitant efficacy
Hormonal contraceptives: reduced contraceptive efficacy
Phenytoin, tolbutamide, warfarin: decreased serum levels of these drugs
Drug-diagnostic tests. *ALP, ALT, AST, BUN, serum creatinine, urine protein, WBCs:* increased

Drug-food. *Grapefruit juice:* increased aprepitant level

Drug-herb. *Butterbur, comfrey:* increased toxic metabolites of these herbs

Cat's claw, echinacea, eucalyptus, feverfew, kava, licorice, peppermint oil, pomegranate, valerian: increased aprepitant level

Toxicity and overdose

• Single doses up to 600 mg have been well tolerated in healthy patients. Signs and symptoms of overdose include drowsiness and headache.

• If overdose occurs, discontinue drug and provide general supportive treatment. Because of drug's antiemetic activity, drug-induced emesis may not be effective. Hemodialysis does not remove drug.

Special considerations

• Long-term, continuous therapy is not recommended because drug interaction profile may change with such use.

• Administration with warfarin may significantly increase INR or prothrombin time. For patients on long-term warfarin therapy, closely monitor INR in 2-week period (particularly at 7 to 10 days) after starting 3-day regimen with each chemotherapy cycle.

Patient education

• Instruct patient to take initial dose 1 hour before chemotherapy.

• Advise patient that he may take drug with or without food.

• Urge patient to seek immediate medical attention for leg pain and swelling, fever, chills, sore throat, or other infection symptoms.

• Caution patient to take drug only as prescribed and never to take more than one dose at a time.

• Recommend alternative or back-up contraceptive methods to patients with childbearing potential.

• Provide guidance to help breastfeeding patient decide whether to discontinue breastfeeding or stop drug.

arsenic trioxide
Trisenox

Classification: Antineoplastic, miscellaneous
Pregnancy risk category D

Pharmacology

Arsenic trioxide has an unclear mechanism of action. It causes morphologic changes and DNA fragmentation in NB4 human promyelocytic leukemia cells, resulting in cell death. It also degrades fusion protein PML/RAR alpha.

Pharmacokinetics

Drug is methylated and metabolized in liver. Distribution half-life is approximately 1 hour; elimination half-life is 12 hours. Drug is eliminated extensively in bile and minimally in urine.

How supplied

Solution for injection: 1 mg/ml in 10-ml ampule

Indications and dosages

FDA-APPROVED

◉ Induction of remission and consolidation of acute promyelocytic leukemia (APL) in patients who are refractory to, or have relapsed from, retinoid and anthracycline chemotherapy and whose APL is characterized by presence of t(15;17) translocation or PML/RAR-alpha gene expression

Adults: For induction, 0.15 mg/kg I.V. daily until bone marrow remission. Total induction dosage should not exceed 60 doses. For consolidation, begin 3 to 6 weeks after induction therapy ends and give 0.15 mg/kg I.V. daily for 25 doses over 5 weeks.

➡ Relapsed or refractory multiple myeloma
Adults: 0.25 mg/kg I.V. daily for 5 days for first 2 weeks of 28-day cycle

➡ Chronic myeloid leukemia (CML) in chronic, accelerated, and blast crisis
Adults: Up to 6 mg I.V. three times daily

Only common or life-threatening adverse reactions are listed.

➥ Myelodysplastic syndromes
Adults: Commonly used dosages range from
0.15 mg/kg to 0.25 mg/kg I.V. daily for 2
weeks.

DOSAGE MODIFICATIONS

• Safety and efficacy of drug in patients with
renal and hepatic impairment have not been
studied. However, particular caution is needed in patients with renal failure because renal
excretion is main elimination route.

⊠ WARNINGS

• Some patients with APL who receive drug
experience symptoms similar to those of
retinoic acid–acute promyelocytic leukemia or
APL differentiation syndrome, which can be
fatal.
• At first indication of APL differentiation
syndrome (abnormal chest auscultatory findings, radiographic abnormalities, or unexplained fever, dyspnea, or weight gain), high-
dose steroid therapy should begin immediately, irrespective of WBC count, and continue
for at least 3 days until signs and symptoms
have abated. Usually, arsenic trioxide need not
be discontinued during treatment of syndrome.
• Drug may cause complete AV block and QT
interval prolongation, which can lead to potentially fatal torsades de pointes–type ventricular arrhythmia.
• Before therapy, 12-lead ECG should be performed and serum electrolyte and creatinine
levels should be evaluated; preexisting electrolyte abnormalities should be corrected and,
if possible, drugs known to prolong QT interval should be discontinued.

Contraindications and precautions
Contraindicated in hypersensitivity to drug or
its components.

Use cautiously in heart failure, renal insufficiency, hypokalemia, hypomagnesemia, prolonged QT intervals, history of torsades de
pointes, pregnancy or breastfeeding, and *elderly patients* with renal impairment. Safety
and efficacy in *children* have not been established.

Preparation and administration
• Follow hazardous drug guidelines for handling, preparation, and administration. (See
"Managing hazardous drugs," page 11.)
• Obtain baseline 12-lead ECG, creatinine
level, and serum potassium, calcium, and
magnesium levels before start of therapy.
• Dilute with 100 to 250 ml D_5W or normal
saline injection immediately after withdrawing
from ampule.
• Do not mix with other drugs.
• Administer I.V. over 1 to 2 hours. Infusion
may last up to 4 hours if acute vasomotor reactions occur.
• Store undiluted drug at 77° F (25° C). Do
not freeze. After dilution, drug is chemically
and physically stable when stored for 24 hours
at room temperature and for 48 hours when
refrigerated.

Adverse reactions
CNS: anxiety, confusion, insomnia, somnolence, headache, paresthesia, depression,
dizziness, tremor, seizures, agitation, coma,
weakness, fatigue, rigors, pain
CV: hypotension, hypertension, atrial arrhythmias, prolonged QT interval, other ECG
changes, chest pain, tachycardia, torsades de
pointes
EENT: epistaxis, postnasal drip, sinusitis, sore
throat
GI: abdominal pain, abdominal distention,
oral candidiasis, oral blistering, constipation,
diarrhea, dyspepsia, fecal incontinence, GI
hemorrhage, dry mouth, nausea, vomiting,
anorexia
GU: vaginal hemorrhage, intermenstrual
bleeding, renal failure, renal impairment, oliguria, urinary incontinence

Hematologic: leukocytosis, anemia, thrombocytopenia, neutropenia, disseminated intravascular coagulation

Metabolic: hyperkalemia, hypokalemia, hypomagnesemia, hyperglycemia, acidosis

Respiratory: pleural effusion, dyspnea, cough, wheezing, crackles, tachypnea, rhonchi, crepitation

Skin: rash, pruritus, ecchymosis, hyperpigmentation, nonspecific skin lesions, local exfoliation, herpes simplex, herpes zoster, dry skin

Other: weight gain or loss, severe edema, sweating, injection site reactions, bacterial infection (nonspecific), sepsis

Interactions

Drug-drug. *Amphotericin B, diuretics:* electrolyte abnormalities
Antiarrhythmics, other drugs that can prolong QT interval, thioridazine: prolonged QT interval
Drug-diagnostic tests. *ALT, AST, serum glucose:* increased
ECG: prolonged QT interval (may be fatal), complete AV block
Serum magnesium: decreased
Serum potassium: increased or decreased
Drug-herb. *Alpha-lipoic acid, coenzyme Q10:* decreased chemotherapy efficacy
Glutamine: possible enhanced tumor growth

Toxicity and overdose

• Signs and symptoms of overdose include seizures, muscle weakness, and confusion. If these occur, stop therapy immediately.
• Consider chelation therapy. Conventional therapy for acute arsenic intoxication includes 3 mg/kg dimercaprol I.M. every 4 hours until immediate life-threatening toxicity subsides. Thereafter, 250 mg penicillamine P.O. may be given up to four times daily.

Special considerations

• Monitor electrolyte, hematologic, and coagulation profiles at least twice weekly. Monitor clinically unstable patients more often during induction and at least weekly during consolidation.
• Maintain potassium level above 4 mEq/dl and magnesium level above 1.8 mg/dl. If absolute QT interval value exceeds 500 msec, reevaluate patient and take immediate steps to correct concomitant risk factors (if any). Also weigh risks and benefits of continuing therapy.
• Obtain weekly ECG to check for prolonged QT interval. Evaluate clinically unstable patients more frequently during induction and consolidation.
• Initiate corrective measures for QT interval greater than 500 msec.

Patient education

• Inform patient that he may need to undergo blood testing before starting therapy, twice weekly during induction, and at least weekly during consolidation.
• Tell patient ECGs may be obtained frequently during therapy.
• Instruct patient to report adverse reactions (including fainting and rapid pulse).
• Advise women with childbearing potential to avoid pregnancy.
• Instruct breastfeeding patient to discontinue either drug or breastfeeding. (Drug appears in breast milk and may cause serious adverse reactions in breastfeeding infant.)

asparaginase
Elspar

Classification: Antineoplastic, enzyme
Pregnancy risk category C

Pharmacology

Asparaginase inhibits protein synthesis, and ultimately DNA and RNA synthesis, by rapidly depleting cellular asparagine (which tumor cells need for protein synthesis). Cell death results from cell fragmentation into membrane-bound particles, which are then eliminated through phagocytosis.

Pharmacokinetics

Drug is metabolized intravascularly by proteolysis. With I.V. use, it peaks immediately and has an immediate onset. Elimination half-life is 8 to 30 hours, with little excretion required. Trace amounts are excreted in urine.

How supplied

*Powder for injection:*10,000 international units in 10-ml vial

Indications and dosages

FDA-approved

➥ Acute lymphocytic leukemia in combination with other antineoplastics
Adults: 200 international units/kg I.V. daily for 28 days, usually combined with other agents in specific regimens. Typical combination dosage is 500 mg/kg, but some regimens call for 200 mg/kg on specific days of cycle (for example, days 8, 15, 22).
Children: 6,000 international units/m² I.V. on treatment days 4, 7, 10, 13, 16, 19, 22, 25, and 28 in combination with vincristine and prednisone. Or 1,000 international units/kg daily for 10 days beginning on treatment day 22 in combination with vincristine and prednisone. When used as sole induction agent, give 200 international units/kg I.V. daily for 28 days.

Dosage modifications

• Stop therapy permanently in patients who develop pancreatitis.

☒ WARNINGS

• For each patient, physician must carefully weigh possibility of achieving therapeutic benefit versus risk of toxicity. All data should be thoroughly reviewed before administration.

Contraindications and precautions

Contraindicated in previous anaphylactic reaction to drug (unless desensitized) and in pancreatitis or history of pancreatitis.

Use cautiously in hepatic impairment, secondary malignancy, infection, concurrent radiation therapy, patients who have had previous course of therapy or previous anaphylactoid reaction to drug, and pregnancy or breastfeeding.

Preparation and administration

• Follow hazardous drug guidelines for handling, preparation, and administration. (See "Managing hazardous drugs," page 11.)
• I.V. asparaginase administration with or immediately before a course of vincristine and prednisone may be linked to increased toxicity.
• Perform intradermal skin test before initial administration and when drug has not been given for at least 1 week. Observe skin test site for at least 1 hour. Wheal or erythema indicates positive reaction, although negative reaction does not rule out allergic reaction.
• For I.V. use with 10,000 international unit–vials, reconstitute powder with 5 ml sterile water for injection or sodium chloride injection. Solution may be used for direct I.V. administration within 8 hours.
• Reconstituted drug should be clear and colorless. Discard if cloudy.
• Before infusion, dilute with normal saline solution or D_5W. Infuse within 8 hours if clear.
• Use 5-micron filter during administration.
• If administering I.M., reconstitute with 2 ml sodium chloride injection in 10,000 international unit–vial. Use within 8 hours if clear.
• Refrigerate dry and reconstituted solution at 36° to 46° F (2° to 8° C).

Adverse reactions

CNS: irritability, headache, coma, depression, fatigue, confusion, hallucinations, lethargy, drowsiness, agitation, Parkinson-like syndrome

GI: nausea, vomiting, anorexia, diarrhea, cramps, pancreatitis
GU: urinary retention, renal failure, glycosuria, polyuria, azotemia, uric acid neuropathy, proteinuria
Hematologic: thrombocytopenia, leukopenia, bone marrow depression, anemia, decreased clotting factors (V, VII, VIII, IX), decreased fibrinogen, increased INR
Hepatic: hepatotoxicity
Metabolic: hyperglycemia, hypoglycemia
Musculoskeletal: arthralgia
Respiratory: fibrosis
Skin: rash, urticaria
Other: chills, fever, hyperthermia, anaphylaxis, weight loss

Interactions

Drug-drug. *Antidiabetic agents, such as sulfonylurea and insulin:* altered blood glucose level
Corticosteroids, glucocorticoids (especially prednisone), vincristine: enhanced hyperglycemic effect of asparaginase, increased risk of neuropathy, disturbed erythropoiesis
Immunosuppressants (such as azathioprine, chlorambucil, cyclophosphamide, cyclosporine, mercaptopurine, and muromonab-CD): increased immunosuppressive effects
Methotrexate: decreased methotrexate effect on cancer cells
Prednisone, vincristine: increased asparaginase toxicity
Drug-diagnostic tests. *ALP, ALT, AST, bilirubin, blood ammonia, serum amylase:* increased
Blood glucose: increased or decreased
Serum albumin: decreased
Thyroid function tests: rapid, marked reduction in serum thyroxine–binding globulin within 2 days of first dose, normaling within 4 weeks of last dose
WBCs: significantly decreased lymphoblast count, often accompanied by marked serum uric acid rise
Drug-herb. *Alpha-lipoic acid, coenzyme Q10:* decreased chemotherapy efficacy
Glutamine: enhanced tumor growth

Toxicity and overdose

• Overdose signs and symptoms include nausea and diarrhea. Toxicity is less common in children.
• Treatment is supportive.

Special considerations

• Use as sole induction agent only when combined regimen is inappropriate because of toxicity or other specific patient-related factors, or in cases refractory to other therapy.
• Allergic reactions occur frequently, especially during retreatment. Reactions cannot be accurately predicted through intradermal skin tests. Anaphylaxis and death have occurred in hospital settings with experienced observers.
• Drug adversely affects liver in most patients and may increase preexisting hepatic impairment caused by previous therapy or underlying disease.
• Monitor patient for decreased urine output, which may result from uric acid nephropathy. To prevent nephropathy, allopurinol may be prescribed. Encourage increased fluid intake.
• Obtain frequent serum amylase levels to detect early evidence of pancreatitis. Watch for signs and symptoms of pancreatitis, allergic reaction, and cyanosis. Stop therapy permanently if pancreatitis occurs.
• Monitor blood glucose level; fatal hyperglycemia may occur.
• Monitor temperature frequently; elevated temperature may indicate early infection.

Patient education

• Tell patient to report breathing changes or coughing and to perform deep-breathing exercises three or four times daily in semi-Fowler's position.
• Instruct patient to drink 2 to 3 L daily to prevent urate deposits and calculi.
• If stomatitis develops, advise patient to brush teeth two or three times daily with soft brush or cotton-tipped applicator, and to use unwaxed dental floss.
• Advise females of childbearing potential to

use contraception because drug can harm fetus.
- Provide guidance to help breastfeeding patient decide whether to discontinue breastfeeding or stop drug.

azacitidine
Vidaza

Classification: Antineoplastic, antimetabolite
Pregnancy risk category D

Pharmacology
Azacitidine may exert its antineoplastic effects by causing DNA hypomethylation and direct cytotoxicity of abnormal hematopoietic bone marrow cells. Cytotoxic effects cause death of rapidly dividing cells, including cancer cells no longer responsive to normal growth control mechanisms.

Pharmacokinetics
Drug is deaminated in liver. It has an elimination half-life of 3 to 6 hours and is excreted in urine in 24 hours.

How supplied
Powder for injection: 100 mg

Indications and dosages

FDA-APPROVED
➡ Myelodysplastic syndrome with the following subtypes: refractory anemia, refractory anemia with ringed sideroblasts (if accompanied by neutropenia or thrombocytopenia or requiring transfusions), refractory anemia with excess blasts, refractory anemia with excess blasts in transformation, and chronic myelomonocytic leukemia
Adults: 75 mg/m^2 subcutaneously daily for 7 days every 4 weeks; may increase to 100 mg/m^2 if no beneficial effect after two treatment cycles and if no toxicity other than nausea and vomiting occurs.

OFF-LABEL USES (SELECTED)
➡ Acute myeloid leukemia
Adults: Commonly used dosage is 50 to 300 mg/m^2 I.V. by continuous infusion daily for 5 days, or 150 to 200 mg/m^2 I.V. two times a week for 2 to 8 weeks

DOSAGE MODIFICATIONS
- Dosage adjustment is based on hematologic laboratory values, including WBC, absolute neutrophil, and platelet counts. After giving recommended dosage for first cycle, reduce dosage or delay for subsequent cycles based on nadir counts and hematologic response.
- If unexplained serum bicarbonate reduction to below 20 mEq/L occurs, reduce dosage by 50% for next course. If unexplained BUN or serum creatinine elevations occur, delay next cycle until values return to normal or baseline, and reduce dosage by 50% for next treatment course.

Contraindications and precautions
Contraindicated in hypersensitivity to drug or mannitol and in patients with advanced, malignant hepatic tumors.

Use cautiously in hepatic or renal impairment and in pregnancy or breastfeeding. Risk of renal toxicity increases in *elderly patients* with renal impairment. Safety and efficacy in *children* have not been established.

Preparation and administration
≫ Follow hazardous drug guidelines for handling, preparation, and administration. (See "Managing hazardous drugs," page 11.)
- Obtain liver function test results and serum creatinine level before therapy begins.
- Premedicate patient for nausea and vomiting.
- Divide doses above 4 ml equally in two syringes and inject subcutaneously in two separate sites.
- Rotate sites for each injection; never inject in tender, bruised, red, or hard area.

• Invert syringe two or three times and gently roll between palms for 30 seconds immediately before administration.
• Store unreconstituted vials at 77° F (25° C).

Adverse reactions

CNS: confusion, lethargy, malaise, fatigue, restlessness, insomnia, headache, dizziness, anxiety, depression, hypoesthesia, rigors
CV: chest pain, pallor, heart murmur, tachycardia, hypotension, syncope
EENT: sinusitis, epistaxis, rhinorrhea, postnasal drip, pharyngitis
GI: nausea, vomiting, anorexia, constipation, diarrhea, abdominal pain and tenderness, abdominal distention, gingival bleeding, oral mucosal petechiae, tongue ulceration, stomatitis, dyspepsia, dysphagia, hemorrhoids
GU: dysuria, urinary tract infection
Hematologic: neutropenia, leukopenia, thrombocytopenia, anemia, hematoma
Metabolic: hypokalemia
Musculoskeletal: myalgia, arthralgia, limb pain, back pain, muscle weakness and cramps
Respiratory: cough, dyspnea, upper respiratory tract infection, pneumonia, rhonchi, crackles, crackles, wheezing, decreased breath sounds, pleural effusion, atelectasis
Skin: dry skin, pruritus, urticaria, ecchymosis, petechiae, skin lesions, herpes simplex, cellulitis, injection site reactions
Other: peripheral edema, pitting edema, weight loss, decreased appetite, pyrexia, pain, increased sweating, night sweats, lymphadenopathy, postprocedural hemorrhage

Interactions

Drug-herb. *Alpha-lipoic acid, coenzyme Q10:* decreased chemotherapy efficacy

Toxicity and overdose

• Signs and symptoms of toxicity (diarrhea, nausea, vomiting) have appeared after single I.V. dose of about 290 mg/m^2.
• For overdose, monitor appropriate blood counts and provide supportive treatment, as necessary. No specific antidote exists.

Special considerations

• Monitor CBCs before each dosing cycle and as often as necessary between cycles to evaluate for hematologic adverse reactions (for example, neutropenia, leukopenia, anemia, and thrombocytopenia).
• Azacitidine metabolites are primarily excreted by kidneys; evaluate for renal toxicity in patients with existing renal impairment.

Patient education

• Caution patient not to miss or double a dose. Tell him to consult prescriber if he misses dose.
• Urge patient to keep follow-up health care appointments, especially for periodic blood tests.
• Inform female of childbearing potential that drug may harm fetus and that she should avoid pregnancy during therapy.
• Advise males not to father a child while taking drug.
• Instruct women not to breastfeed during therapy.

BCG live, intravesical
TheraCys, Tice BCG

Classification: Antineoplastic, biological response modifier
Pregnancy risk category C

Pharmacology

BCG live, a freeze-dried suspension of attenuated strain of *Mycobacterium bovis* (Bacillus Calmette and Guerin [BCG]), promotes local inflammatory reaction, which leads to sloughing of bladder wall epithelium and cancer cell destruction in superficial bladder cancer. Exact mechanism of action is unknown, but antitumor effect seems to be T lymphocyte–dependent.

Pharmacokinetics

Viability and immunogenicity may vary among strains.

How supplied

Powder for suspension, lyophilized (TheraCys): 81-mg vial containing $10.5 \pm 8.7 \times 10^8$ colony-forming units (CFU), equivalent to roughly 81 mg dry weight

Powder for suspension, lyophilized (Tice BCG): vial containing 1 to 8×10^8 CFU, equivalent to roughly 50 mg wet weight

Indications and dosages

FDA-APPROVED

➥ Prophylaxis and treatment of urinary bladder carcinoma in situ; prophylaxis of primary or recurrent stage Ta and/or T1 papillary bladder tumors after transurethral resection (TUR)
Adults: One dose (TheraCys) of 81 mg (dry weight) in 3 ml diluent provided, suspended in 50 ml preservative-free normal saline solution given intravesically once weekly for 6 weeks, then one treatment 3, 6, 12, 18, and 24 months after initial treatment; begin 7 to 14 days after TUR. Or one dose (Tice BCG) (one vial in 50 ml normal saline solution) given intravesically once weekly for 6 weeks; may repeat once; then continue monthly for 6 to 12 months; begin 7 to 14 days after TUR.

⊠ WARNINGS

• Drug contains live, attenuated mycobacteria. Because of potential transmission risk, it should be handled, prepared, and disposed of as biohazardous material.
• BCG infections have been reported in health care workers—mainly from accidental needle sticks or skin lacerations during drug preparation. Nosocomial infections have occurred in immunosuppressed patients receiving parenteral drugs prepared in same areas as BCG live. Drug may disseminate when given intra-

vesically, and serious infections (some fatal) have occurred.

B

Contraindications and precautions

Contraindicated in immunosuppression or congenital or acquired immunodeficiencies; concurrent febrile illness; urinary tract infection; active tuberculosis (TB); gross hematuria; and within 7 to 14 days after bladder biopsy, TUR, or traumatic bladder catheterization.

Use cautiously in concurrent anti-infective therapy, tuberculin sensitivity, high risk for HIV infection, small bladder capacity, and pregnancy or breastfeeding. Safety and efficacy in *children* have not been established.

Preparation and administration

• Follow hazardous drug guidelines for handling, preparation, and administration. (See "Managing hazardous drugs," page 11.)
TheraCys and Tice BCG
• Products labeled for use only in bladder cancer treatment are not intended for use as TB immunization.
• Before starting intravesical therapy, rule out active TB in PPD-positive patients.
• Do not inject drug subcutaneously or I.V.
• Do not remove rubber stopper from vial.
• Do not give drug within 1 week of TUR because of risk of serious complications (including deaths from disseminated BCG infection).
• If traumatic catheterization occurs (such as one associated with bleeding or false passage), do not give drug, and delay treatment at least 1 week.
• Postpone intravesical instillation if patient has fever or suspected infection or is receiving antimicrobials. (Antimicrobial therapy may interfere with BCG efficacy).
• Patient should not drink fluids for 4 hours before treatment, and should empty bladder before administration.
• Withhold drug if patient has signs and symptoms of systemic infection; treat immediately with antitubercular antibiotics.

• Refrigerate at 35° to 46° F (2° to 8° C) and protect from light.

TheraCys

• Dilute each dose (three reconstituted vials) in 50 ml preservative-free normal saline solution for a total of 53 ml.

• Use immediately after reconstitution; do not use after 2 hours. Do not use reconstituted product with flocculation or clumping that gentle shaking does not disperse.

Tice BCG

• Draw 1 ml of sterile, preservative-free normal solution into syringe and add to one vial to resuspend.

• Draw mixture into syringe and gently expel back into ampule three times to ensure thorough mixing and thus minimize mycobacteria clumping.

• Dispense cloudy suspension into top end of catheter-tip syringe containing 49 ml saline diluent, for total volume of 50 ml. Gently rotate syringe.

• Use suspended drug immediately after preparation. Discard after 2 hours.

• Do not filter vial contents.

TheraCys and TICE BCG

• Instill reconstituted and diluted drug into empty bladder by gravity flow through urethral catheter immediately after preparation. Do not depress plunger to force flow.

• Have patient retain instilled fluid for 1 to 2 hours, depending on irritative symptoms and ability to retain solution.

• During first hour after instillation, instruct patient to alternate between prone and supine positions and from left to right side, with 15 minutes in each position, to maximize bladder surface exposure to drug. Then allow him to be upright but retain suspension for another 60 minutes, for total of 2 hours. If necessary, instruct him to void sooner. After 2 hours, have him void in seated position.

Adverse reactions

CNS: lethargy, malaise

GI: anorexia, diarrhea, nausea, vomiting

GU: dysuria; hematuria; urinary frequency, urgency, and incontinence; urinary tract infection; cystitis; renal toxicity; contracted bladder

Hematologic: anemia, leukopenia, myelosuppression

Skin: rash, skin ulcer

Other: systemic infection, flulike syndrome (malaise, fever, chills)

Interactions

Drug-drug. *Antimicrobials:* impaired drug response

Bone marrow depressants, immunosuppressants: impaired drug response, increased risk of osteomyelitis or disseminated BCG infection

Drug-diagnostic tests. *Liver function tests:* abnormal

Tuberculin skin test (PPD): positive conversion

Urinalysis: microscopic pyuria

Toxicity and overdose

• Traumatic catheterization, too-early instillation after TUR, or administering more than one vial or instillation can lead to BCG toxicity, marked by self-limited cystitis that escalates to systemic infection with subsequent instillations, hematuria, pyuria, fever, chills, malaise, arthralgia, and possibly death.

• If patient develops persistent fever or acute febrile illness consistent with BCG infection, discontinue drug and immediately evaluate and treat for BCG infection. Otherwise, use supportive treatment, including antituberculotics.

Special considerations

• Carefully monitor patients receiving anti-infectives for other infections to evaluate whether such therapy will interfere with effects of BCG live.

• Drug may cause tuberculin sensitivity, which could complicate interpretation of skin test reactions when diagnosing suspected mycobacterial infections.

• Small bladder capacity has been associated with increased risk of severe local reactions.

Only common or life-threatening adverse reactions are listed.

- Local adverse reactions generally follow third intravesical instillation (usually by 2 to 4 hours) and persist for 24 to 72 hours.
- Manage bladder irritation symptomatically with phenazopyridine, propantheline, and acetaminophen.
- Monitor urinary status carefully for BCG live inflammatory response, which manifests as hematuria, urinary frequency, dysuria, and bacterial urinary tract infection.
- Watch for signs and symptoms of systemic BCG infection, such as temperature above 103° F (39° C), persistent temperature above 101° F (38° C) for more than 2 days, and severe malaise.

Patient education

- Instruct patient not to drink fluids for 4 hours before treatment. Have him empty bladder before administration.
- Explain instillation procedure to patient.
- Encourage patient to maintain adequate hydration in hours after treatment, to flush bladder.
- Inform patient that burning may occur with first urination.
- Advise patient to immediately report blood in urine, fever or chills, increased voiding frequency, frequent urge to urinate, painful urination, joint pain, nausea and vomiting, rash, or cough (possible indications of BCG systemic infection).
- For 6 hours after instillation, instruct patient to disinfect voided urine with household bleach, letting urine stand for 15 minutes before flushing.
- Advise female patient to avoid pregnancy and breastfeeding during therapy.

bevacizumab
Avastin

B

Classification: Antineoplastic, monoclonal antibody
Pregnancy risk category C

Pharmacology
Bevacizumab binds vascular endothelial growth factor (VEGF) and prevents it from interacting with endothelial cell-surface receptors. VEGF interaction with these receptors causes proliferation and new blood vessel formation. By binding VEGF, drug prevents this interaction, thus inhibiting development of new blood vessels and metastatic disease progression.

Pharmacokinetics
Clearance varies with weight, gender, and tumor burden. Half-life is about 20 days (range of 11 to 50 days).

How supplied
Solution for infusion: 25 mg/ml in 4-ml (100-mg) and 16-ml (400-mg) single-use vials

Indications and dosages

FDA-APPROVED

➡ Metastatic colon or rectal carcinoma (in combination with I.V. 5-fluorouracil-based chemotherapy)
Adults: 5 mg/kg by I.V. infusion once every 14 days until disease progression occurs. Do not start therapy for at least 28 days after major surgery and until surgical incision is fully healed.

OFF-LABEL USES (SELECTED)

➡ Breast cancer
Adults: Dosages of 3, 10, and 20 mg/kg every 2 weeks as monotherapy have been studied.
➡ Non-small-cell lung cancer, first-line treatment in combination with paclitaxel and car-

boplatin for advanced or metastatic non-squamous-cell disease

Adults: Commonly used dosages are 7.5 and 15 mg/kg every 3 weeks.

DOSAGE MODIFICATIONS

• Discontinue drug permanently in patients with hypertensive crisis and temporarily in those with severe hypertension not controlled by medical management.

• Discontinue drug in patients with nephrotic syndrome.

• Regularly monitor patients with moderate to severe proteinuria based on 24-hour collections until improvement or resolution occurs.

• Temporarily suspend drug in patients with evidence of moderate to severe proteinuria, pending further evaluation.

⊠ WARNINGS

• GI perforation and wound dehiscence, complicated by intra-abdominal abscesses, have occurred increasingly. Perforation with or without abscesses may be fatal. GI perforation typically presents as abdominal pain, constipation, and vomiting. Therapy should be permanently discontinued in patients with GI perforation or wound dehiscence requiring medical intervention.

• Serious and fatal hemoptysis has occurred in patients with non-small-cell lung cancer treated with bevacizumab.

Contraindications and precautions

No known contraindications exist.

Use cautiously in hypersensitivity to drug or its components, significant cardiovascular disease, recent hemoptysis, and pregnancy or breastfeeding. *Elderly patients* are more prone to adverse reactions. Safety and efficacy in *children* have not been established.

Preparation and administration

• Do not give to patients with recent hemoptysis.

• Do not administer or mix infusions with dextrose solutions.

• Do not give as I.V. push or bolus. Deliver initial dose over 90 minutes as I.V. infusion. If first infusion is well tolerated, may administer second infusion over 60 minutes; if well tolerated, may administer all subsequent infusions over 30 minutes.

• Store in original carton until time of use. Do not freeze or shake. Protect vial from light.

• Store diluted solutions for infusion at 36° to 46° F (2° to 8° C) for up to 8 hours.

Adverse reactions

CNS: dizziness, confusion, headache, asthenia
CV: congestive heart failure, hypertension, hypertensive crisis, myocardial infarction, deep vein thrombosis, intra-abdominal thrombosis
EENT: epistaxis
GI: hemorrhage, perforation, abdominal pain, constipation, nausea, vomiting, diarrhea, anorexia, stomatitis, taste disorder, flatulence
GU: proteinuria, nephrotic syndrome
Hematologic: leukopenia, neutropenia, thrombocytopenia, hemorrhage
Metabolic: hypokalemia
Musculoskeletal: myalgia, arthralgia
Respiratory: cough, dyspnea, upper respiratory tract infection
Skin: alopecia, dry skin, exfoliative dermatitis
Other: fever, pain, weight loss

Interactions

Drug-drug. *Irinotecan:* worsened adverse reactions of diarrhea and neutropenia
Drug-diagnostic tests. *Potassium:* decreased
Urinalysis: proteinuria
Drug-herb. *Alpha-lipoic acid, coenzyme Q10:* decreased chemotherapy efficacy

Toxicity and overdose

• Signs and symptoms include headache.
• Treatment is supportive; no known antidote exists.

Only common or life-threatening adverse reactions are listed.

B

Special considerations

• Drug may impair wound healing; suspend therapy before elective surgery. Appropriate interval between last dose and elective surgery is unknown; however, consider drug half-life of about 20 days.
• Other reported serious bleeding events are uncommon and include GI and subarachnoid hemorrhage and hemorrhagic stroke.
• Before each dose, monitor urine protein with serial urinalyses for development or worsening of proteinuria. Patients with 2+ or greater urine dipstick reading should undergo further assessment, such as 24-hour urine collection.
• Monitor blood pressure throughout therapy and frequently thereafter in patients with hypertension.

Patient education

• Inform patient that infusion initially takes 90 minutes but is later reduced to 60 minutes, then 30 minutes if tolerated.
• Instruct patient to report bleeding.
• Caution female patient not to get pregnant during therapy because drug may harm fetus and cause pregnancy loss. Explain that drug effects linger even after therapy ends, possibly harming fetus.
• Counsel breastfeeding patient to stop breastfeeding during and for prolonged time after therapy because of drug's long half-life.

bexarotene
Targretin

Classification: Antineoplastic, retinoid
Pregnancy risk category X

Pharmacology

Bexarotene regulates expression of genes that control cellular differentiation and proliferation. It may inhibit growth of some hematopoietic and squamous tumor cell lines. Exact mechanism of action is unknown but may relate to selective binding to some retinoid X receptors as well as apoptosis induction.

Pharmacokinetics

Drug has good oral bioavailability, which increases with high-fat meal. (Topical drug is absorbed sporadically.) It is metabolized in liver by CYP450 3A4 to oxidative metabolites (which are glucuronidated). Drug is more than 99% protein-bound. It peaks in 2 to 4 hours.

How supplied

Capsules (soft gelatin): 75 mg
Gel 1%: 60 g (600 mg active bexarotene)/tube

Indications and dosages

FDA-APPROVED

➡ Cutaneous manifestations of cutaneous T-cell lymphoma in patients refractory to at least one previous systemic therapy
Adults: 300 mg/m² P.O.daily.
➡ Treatment of cutaneous lesions in patients with cutaneous T-cell lymphoma (stage IA and IB) who have refractory or persistent disease after other therapies or who have not tolerated other therapies
Adults: Gel applied topically once every other day for first week, increased at weekly intervals up to four times daily, according to individual lesion tolerance

DOSAGE MODIFICATIONS

• Oral dosage may be adjusted to 200 mg/m² daily and then 100 mg/m² daily, or drug may be temporarily suspended if necessitated by toxicity or increased liver function test values. When toxicity is controlled, oral dosage may be carefully readjusted upward.
• If no tumor response occurs after 8 weeks of treatment and initial dose of 300 mg/m² daily is well tolerated, dosage may be increased to 400 mg/m² daily with careful monitoring.

• Generally, patients can maintain oral dosing frequency of two to four times a day. Most responses occur at dosing frequencies of two times a day or more.

• If severe local irritation occurs with topical application, dosage can be reduced or drug temporarily discontinued for a few days until symptoms subside.

⊠ WARNINGS

• Capsules are a member of retinoid class associated with birth defects and must not be given to pregnant women.

Contraindications and precautions

Contraindicated in hypersensitivity to drug or its components and in pregnancy.

Use cautiously in hepatic and renal insufficiency, diabetes mellitus, uncontrolled hyperlipidemia, concurrent vitamin A supplementation, concurrent tamoxifen use, sunburn, and breastfeeding. Safety and efficacy in *children* have not been established.

Preparation and administration

• Follow hazardous drug guidelines for handling, preparation, and administration. (See "Managing hazardous drugs," page 11.)

• Obtain baseline liver function test results before administering drug.

• Measure blood lipid levels before administering. Fasting triglyceride levels should be normal or normalized with appropriate interventions before therapy starts.

• Apply sufficient gel to cover lesion generously. Allow gel to dry before covering with clothing. Unaffected skin may become irritated, so avoid applying to normal skin surrounding lesion. Do not apply near mucosal surfaces. Do not use occlusive dressings with gel.

• Store capsules at 36° to 77° F (2° to 25° C) and gel at 77° F. Avoid exposing to high temperatures and humidity after opening. Protect from light.

Adverse reactions

CNS: headache, fatigue, lethargy, asthenia
CV: peripheral edema, thrombophlebitis
GI: nausea, abdominal pain, diarrhea, acute pancreatitis
Hematologic: leukopenia, neutropenia, anemia
Hepatic: hepatic failure
Metabolic: hypothyroidism, hypercalcemia, hyperlipidemia
Skin: rash, contact dermatitis, pruritus, dry skin, photosensitivity
Other: infection, chills

Interactions

Drug-drug. *Erythromycin, gemfibrozil, itraconazole, ketoconazole, other CYP450 3A4 inhibitors:* enhanced bexarotene efficacy
Hormonal contraceptives: reduced efficacy of oral and other systemic contraceptives
Insulin, sulfonylureas, troglitazone, other antidiabetic agents: enhanced action, resulting in hypoglycemia
Phenobarbital, phenytoin, rifampin, other CYP450 3A4 inducers: reduced bexarotene efficacy
Vitamin A: increased risk of retinoid toxicity
Drug-diagnostic tests. *Blood lipids, CA125 assay values in patients with ovarian cancer, hepatic enzymes:* increased
Thyroid-stimulating hormone, total thyroxine: decreased
Drug-food. *Grapefruit juice:* possible altered levels of drugs cleared by CYP450 3A4 enzyme
High-fat meal: enhanced drug efficacy
Drug-herb. *American elder, cat's claw, echinacea, eucalyptus, feverfew, kava, licorice, milk thistle, peppermint oil, pomegranate, St. John's wort:* possible altered levels of drugs cleared by CYP450 3A4 enzyme

Toxicity and overdose

• Dosages up to 30 times greater than recommended on mg/m² basis have been tolerated without acute toxicity. Anticipated signs and symptoms of toxicity are those of most com-

---

Only common or life-threatening adverse reactions are listed.

mon adverse reactions, such as rash, contact dermatitis, and pruritus.
- Treat with supportive care.

Special considerations
- Obtain baseline WBC count with differential and periodically during treatment. Leukopenia and neutropenia rarely are associated with severe sequelae.
- Carefully monitor liver function tests after 1, 2, and 4 weeks of treatment; if stable, monitor at least every 8 weeks thereafter. Consider suspending or stopping capsules if levels exceed 3 × ULN for AST, ALT, or bilirubin.
- Consider thyroid hormone supplements for patients with laboratory evidence of hypothyroidism. Obtain baseline thyroid function tests and monitor patient during treatment.
- Monitor for and treat major lipid abnormalities that occur during long-term therapy.
- Response to gel may occur as soon as 4 weeks after first application, although most patients take longer to respond.

Patient education
- Advise patient to take capsules with food.
- Instruct patient using capsules to minimize exposure to sunlight and artificial ultraviolet light.
- Advise patient using gel to avoid strong sunlight on gel application days.
- If patient applies gel only once daily and forgets a dose, instruct him to apply dose as soon as he remembers and then apply next day's dose at regular time.
- Inform patient using gel not to use insect repellents containing DEET.
- Urge patient to seek immediate medical attention for severe stomach pain or yellowing of eyes or skin.
- Inform patient he may need to undergo periodical laboratory tests during therapy.
- Tell patient to consult health care professional before taking vitamin A or multiple vitamin supplement.
- Urge patient with vision problems to have regular eye examinations.

- Advise patients with childbearing potential to use effective contraception for 1 month before starting therapy, during therapy, and at least 1 month afterward. Tell them to use two reliable contraceptive methods simultaneously (unless they are abstinent).
- Tell male patient to use condoms during intercourse (to avoid pregnancy) during therapy and for at least 1 month after last dose.

bicalutamide
Casodex

Classification: Antineoplastic, nonsteroidal antiandrogen, hormone/hormone modifier
Pregnancy risk category X

Pharmacology
Bicalutamide competitively inhibits action of androgens by binding to cytosol androgen receptors in target tissue. Drug also may inhibit androgen uptake in pituitary gland.

Pharmacokinetics
Drug is well absorbed and converted to inactivated metabolites in liver. It is highly proteinbound, and peaks in 30 hours. Terminal half-life is several days. Parent drug and metabolites are excreted in urine and feces.

How supplied
Tablets: 50 mg

Indications and dosages

FDA-approved

➡ Stage D_2 metastatic carcinoma of prostate (in combination with luteinizing hormone–releasing hormone [LH-RH] analogue)
Adults: One 50-mg tablet P.O. once daily

Contraindications and precautions
Contraindicated in hypersensitivity to drug or its components, in women, and in pregnancy.

Use cautiously in moderate to severe hepatic impairment and in renal impairment. Safety and efficacy in **children** have not been established.

Preparation and administration

• Follow hazardous drug guidelines for handling, preparation, and administration. (See "Managing hazardous drugs," page 11.)
• Measure serum transaminase levels before treatment, at regular intervals for first 4 months of treatment, and periodically thereafter.
• Drug is given with LH-RH analogue, starting at same time
• Drug should be given at same time each day, with or without food.
• Store at controlled temperature of 68° to 77° F (20° to 25° C).

Adverse reactions

CNS: dizziness, paresthesia, insomnia, anxiety, neuropathy, headache, asthenia
CV: hypertension, chest pain, heart failure, edema
EENT: dry mouth
GI: diarrhea, constipation, nausea, vomiting, anorexia, melena, abdominal pain
GU: erectile dysfunction; decreased libido; gynecomastia; breast tenderness; nocturia; hematuria; urinary tract infection; dysuria; urinary incontinence, frequency, retention, and urgency
Hematologic: anemia
Musculoskeletal: bone pain, back pain
Respiratory: dyspnea
Skin: rash, sweating, dry skin, pruritus, alopecia
Other: hot flashes, infection, flulike symptoms, weight loss

Interactions

Drug-drug. *Activated charcoal:* decreased bicalutamide absorption
Coumarin-derived anticoagulants such as warfarin: reduced warfarin efficacy
Drug-diagnostic tests. *ALP, ALT, AST, bilirubin, blood glucose, BUN, creatinine, estradiol, testosterone:* increased
Hemoglobin, WBCs: decreased
Drug-herb. *Aloe, cascara, pomegranate, rhubarb, tannic acid:* decreased drug absorption

Toxicity and overdose

• Signs and symptoms of overdose may include nausea, vomiting, and hepatotoxicity.
• No specific antidote for overdose exists. Provide general supportive care, including frequent monitoring of vital signs and close observation. Induce vomiting if patient is alert. Dialysis rarely is helpful.

Special considerations

• Evaluate serum prostate specific antigen (PSA) regularly to help monitor patient's response. If PSA level rises during therapy, evaluate for clinical progression.
• If patient develops signs or symptoms of hepatic dysfunction, measure serum transaminase levels (especially ALT) immediately. If jaundice occurs or ALT level rises above 2 × ULN, discontinue drug immediately and monitor hepatic function closely.
• Drug can displace coumarin anticoagulants such as warfarin from protein-binding sites. If patient is receiving coumarin anticoagulant, closely monitor prothrombin time; adjust anticoagulant dosage if needed.

Patient education

• Inform patient that drug and LH-RH analogue therapy should begin at same time. Caution him not to interrupt or stop therapy without consulting prescriber.
• Instruct patient to take drug one dose at a time and at same time daily, with or without food.
• Tell patient to immediately report nausea, vomiting, abdominal pain, fatigue, anorexia, flulike symptoms, dark urine, jaundice and right upper quadrant tenderness.
• Advise patient to seek medical attention for chest pain, heart failure, fainting, or bloody urine.

Only common or life-threatening adverse reactions are listed.

bleomycin sulfate

Blenoxane

Classification: Antineoplastic, antitumor antibiotic

Pregnancy risk category D

Pharmacology

Bleomycin sulfate binds to, splits, and fragments double-stranded DNA, resulting in single-strand breaks. This effect inhibits DNA synthesis and, to a lesser degree, RNA and protein synthesis.

Pharmacokinetics

After I.V. infusion, drug is incompletely metabolized by intracellular aminopeptidases and widely distributed in skin, lungs, kidney, peritoneum, and lymphatics. Onset is immediate (onset for I.M. route is unknown); drug peaks in 20 to 60 minutes. Elimination half-life is 3 to 5 hours. Kidneys excrete about 50% as unchanged drug and metabolites.

How supplied

Powder for injection: 15-unit and 30-unit vials

Indications and dosages

FDA-APPROVED

➡ Squamous-cell carcinoma, non-Hodgkin's lymphoma

Adults and adolescents: 0.25 to 0.5 unit/kg (10 to 20 units/m^2) I.V., I.M., or subcutaneously weekly or twice weekly

➡ Testicular carcinoma

Adults: 0.25 to 0.5 unit/kg (10 to 20 units/m^2) I.V., I.M., or subcutaneously weekly or twice weekly. In BEP regimen, bleomycin 30 units I.V. on days 2, 9, and 16, with etoposide 100 mg/m^2 on days 1 to 5, and cisplatin 20 mg/m^2 on days 1 to 5; repeated every 21 days

➡ Hodgkin's disease

Adults and adolescents: 0.25 to 0.5 unit/kg (10 to 20 units/m^2) I.V., I.M., or subcutaneously weekly or twice weekly; then, after 50% response, maintenance dosage of 1 unit daily or 5 units weekly I.V. or I.M. In ABVD regimen, doxorubicin 25 mg/m^2, bleomycin 10 units/m^2, vinblastine 6 mg/m^2, and dacarbazine 375 mg/m^2 I.V. on days 1 and 15; repeated every 28 days.

⊖ Malignant pleural effusion

Adults and adolescents: 60 units in 50 to 100 ml normal saline solution given as a single-dose bolus intrapleural injection

OFF-LABEL USES (SELECTED)

➡ Cutaneous malignancies (basal-cell carcinoma, squamous-cell carcinoma, advanced metastatic melanoma, Kaposi's sarcoma)

Adults: Commonly used intralesional bleomycin dosages combined with electric pulses (electrochemotherapy), 0.5 unit for tumors measuring up to 100 mm^3, 0.75 unit for tumors 100 to 150 mm^3, 1 unit for tumors 150 to 500 mm^3, 1.5 units for tumors 500 to 1,000 mm^3, 2 units for tumors 1,000 to 2,000 mm^3, 2.5 units for tumors 2,000 to 3,000 mm^3, 3 units for tumors 3,000 to 4,000 mm^3, 3.5 units for tumors 4,000 to 5,000 mm^3, and 4 units for tumors larger than 5,000 mm^3

DOSAGE MODIFICATIONS

- If no acute reaction occurs, follow regular dosage schedule.
- Some practitioners limit total lifetime dose to 300 to 400 units because of risk of pulmonary toxicity.
- Patients with moderate renal failure (glomerular filtration rate [GFR] of 10 to 50 ml/minute) should receive 75% of usual dose at normal dosage interval; patients with severe renal failure (GFR below 10 ml/minute) should receive 50% of usual dose at normal dosage interval. No dosage adjustment is necessary for patients with GFR above 50 ml/minute.

⊠ WARNINGS

- Pulmonary fibrosis (frequently presenting as pneumonitis) is most severe toxicity. It occurs more frequently in elderly patients, in patients who received previous pulmonary radiation, in those who received high oxygen levels after treatment, and in those receiving more than 400 units as a total dose or more than 25 units/m²/dose.
- Severe idiosyncratic reaction—consisting of hypotension, mental confusion, fever, chills, and wheezing—may occur after first or second dose. Careful monitoring is required. Recommended test dose for high-risk patients receiving first dose is 2 units subcutaneously or I.V. 2 hours before dose is given.

Contraindications and precautions

Contraindicated in hypersensitivity or idiosyncratic reaction to drug.

Use with extreme caution in significant renal impairment or compromised pulmonary function. Use cautiously in concurrent radiation therapy, pregnancy or breastfeeding, and *elderly patients*. Safety and efficacy in *children* have not been established.

Preparation and administration

≫ Follow hazardous drug guidelines for handling, preparation, and administration. (See "Managing hazardous drugs," page 11.)

- Premedicate with acetaminophen, corticosteroids, and diphenhydramine to prevent fever and decrease risk of anaphylaxis.
- Before first treatment, 2-unit test dose is recommended for lymphoma patients to decrease risk of anaphylactoid reaction.
- Carefully monitor patient for severe idiosyncratic reaction (similar to anaphylaxis), signs of which include hypotension, mental confusion, fever, chills, and wheezing that usually occur after first dose.
- Reconstitute 15-unit vial with 1 to 5 ml sterile water for injection, normal saline solution for injection, or sterile bacteriostatic wa-

ter for injection. Reconstitute 30-unit vial with 2 to 10 ml of above diluents. Discard drug reconstituted in normal saline solution after 24 hours.

- For I.V. injection, dissolve contents of 15- or 30-unit vial in 5 ml or 10 ml, respectively, of normal saline solution for injection. Administer slowly over 10 minutes.
- For intermittent infusion, dilute further and infuse over 15 minutes or longer (typically diluted in 50 to 100 ml D₅W or normal saline solution for injection and infused over 15 to 30 minutes or 1 unit/minute).
- Keep prolonged infusions in glass containers.
- For intrapleural use, dissolve 60 units in 50 to 100 ml normal saline injection, and administer through thoracostomy tube after drainage of excess pleural fluid and confirmation of complete lung expansion.
- Clamp thoracostomy tube after instillation. Move patient from supine to left and right lateral positions several times over next 4 hours. Remove clamp and reestablish suction. Length of time chest tube remains in place after sclerosis depends on clinical situation.
- Sterile powder is stable at 36° to 46° F (2° to 8° C) for 24 months.

Adverse reactions

CNS: headache, confusion
CV: hypotension
GI: nausea, vomiting, anorexia, stomatitis, mouth or lip ulcers
Respiratory: fibrosis, pneumonitis, wheezing, pulmonary toxicity
Skin: rash, hyperkeratosis, "radiation recall," nail changes, alopecia, pruritus, acne, striae, peeling
Other: weight loss, fever, chills, anaphylaxis, Raynaud's phenomenon, pain at tumor site

Interactions

Drug-drug. *Cisplatin:* delayed drug clearance and toxicity, even with low doses
General anesthetics: rapid pulmonary deterioration

Only common or life-threatening adverse reactions are listed.

Other antineoplastics: increased drug toxicity, including bone marrow depression (rarely caused by bleomycin alone), mucosal and pulmonary toxicity
Phenytoin: decreased phenytoin level
Drug-herb. *Alpha-lipoic acid, coenzyme Q10:* decreased chemotherapy efficacy
Glutamine: possible enhanced tumor growth

Toxicity and overdose

• Signs and symptoms of overdose include fever, chills, pulmonary fibrosis, hyperpigmentation, and pneumonitis. Pulmonary toxicity is dose-related; give total doses of more than 400 units with great caution. When drug is used with other antineoplastics, pulmonary toxicity may occur at lower dosages.
• No specific antidote exists. Treatment is supportive.

Special considerations

• Evaluate respiratory status regularly. Obtain baseline chest X-ray and repeat every 1 to 2 weeks to detect pulmonary changes.
• Pulmonary toxicity may be more common in patients older than age 70.
• Monitor renal function, chest X-ray, and pulmonary status throughout therapy.

Patient education

• Inform patient that most serious side effect is a condition that impedes lung function. Urge him to seek immediate medical attention for breathing or swallowing difficulty; wheezing; light-headedness or fainting; sudden swelling of face, lips, tongue, legs, or arms; dizziness when standing or sitting up; confusion; or sudden high fever.
• Inform patient that prescriber may need to adjust dosage several times for best effect.
• Caution women with childbearing potential to avoid becoming pregnant during therapy.
• Advise breastfeeding patient not to breastfeed during therapy.

bortezomib
Velcade

Classification: Antineoplastic, proteasome inhibitor
Pregnancy risk category D

Pharmacology

Bortezomib reversibly inhibits chymotrypsin-like activity of 26S proteasome, a large protein complex that regulates normal protein homeostatic mechanisms, inducing cell apoptosis. It also has antiangiogenic properties and inhibits interleukin 6–mediated cell growth and cellular adhesion molecules.

Pharmacokinetics

Drug is metabolized in liver and distributed to most body tissues, including myocardium. More than 80% is bound to protein. Duration is 72 hours; median response time is 30 to 127 days. After first dose, mean elimination half-life ranges from 9 to 15 hours.

How supplied

Powder for injection: 3.5 mg in 10-ml vial

Indications and dosages

FDA-APPROVED

➡ Multiple myeloma in patients who have received at least one previous therapy
Adults: Standard schedule is 1.3 mg/m^2 as bolus I.V. injection over 3 to 5 seconds twice weekly for 2 weeks (days 1, 4, 8, and 11), followed by 10-day rest period (days 12 to 21); repeated every 21 days as tolerated. For therapy of more than 8 weeks, give on standard schedule or maintenance schedule of once weekly for 4 weeks (days 1, 8, 15, and 22) followed by 13-day rest period (days 23 to 35). Allow at least 72 hours between consecutive doses.

➡ Relapsed, refractory non-Hodgkin's lymphoma (primarily mantle-cell lymphoma)
Adults: Commonly used dosage is 1.3 to 1.5 mg/m² as bolus I.V. injection over 3 to 5 seconds twice weekly for 2 weeks (days 1, 4, 8, and 11) followed by 10-day rest period (days 12 to 21); repeated every 21 days as tolerated.

DOSAGE MODIFICATIONS

• Discontinue temporarily if patient experiences Grade 4 thrombocytopenia. Drug may be reinitiated at reduced dosage after thrombocytopenia resolves.
• Withhold drug at onset of Grade 3 nonhematologic or Grade 4 hematologic toxicities, excluding neuropathy. Once toxicity symptoms resolve, may reinitiate at 25% reduced dosage.
• Patients with preexisting severe neuropathy should receive drug only after careful consideration. If patient develops neuropathic pain or peripheral sensory neuropathy while receiving drug, manage according to the following guidelines:
Grade 1 with pain or Grade 2: Decrease to 1 mg/m².
Grade 2 with pain or Grade 3: Withhold drug until toxicity resolves; reinstitute at 0.7 mg/m²/week.
Grade 4: Discontinue drug.

Contraindications and precautions

Contraindicated in hypersensitivity to bortezomib, boron, or mannitol.
Use cautiously in peripheral neuropathy, history of syncope, hypotension or administration of agents linked to hypotension, cardiovascular disorders, GI disorders that may lead to dehydration, hepatic or renal impairment, long-term therapy, women of childbearing potential, and breastfeeding. Safety and efficacy in *children* have not been established.

Preparation and administration

• Administer fluid and electrolyte replacement to prevent dehydration caused by drug-induced nausea, diarrhea, constipation, and vomiting.
• Reconstitute each vial with 3.5 ml normal saline injection for a concentration of 1 mg/ml. Solution should be clear and colorless. Give within 8 hours of reconstitution.
• Administer by I.V. bolus over 3 to 5 seconds.
• Allow 72 hours between consecutive doses.
• Store unopened vials at 77° F (25° C); excursions are permitted from 59° to 86° F (15° to 30° C). Keep in original package to protect from light.

Adverse reactions

CNS: dizziness, headache, fatigue, asthenia, syncope
CV: orthostatic hypotension, edema
EENT: blurred vision, diplopia
GI: constipation, diarrhea, anorexia, nausea, vomiting
Hematologic: anemia, neutropenia, thrombocytopenia
Musculoskeletal: arthralgia, back pain, bone pain, muscle cramps, myalgia
Respiratory: pneumonia, dyspnea, cough
Skin: rash, pruritus
Other: dehydration, peripheral neuropathy

Interactions

Drug-drug. *CYP450 3A4 inhibitors or inducers:* drug toxicity or reduced efficacy
Oral antidiabetic drugs: hypoglycemia, hyperglycemia
Drug-food. *Grapefruit juice:* increased drug blood level, increased risk of toxicity
Drug-herb. *Alpha-lipoic acid, coenzyme Q10:* decreased chemotherapy efficacy
Glutamine: Possible enhanced tumor growth
Herbs undergoing metabolism by CYP450 isoenzyme system: increased risk of drug toxicity or reduced efficacy

Toxicity and overdose

• Toxicity is associated with decreased blood pressure, increased heart rate and contractility and, ultimately, terminal hypotension.

Only common or life-threatening adverse reactions are listed.

• No specific antidote exists. If overdose occurs, monitor vital signs and provide appropriate supportive care to maintain blood pressure and body temperature.

Special considerations

• Because thrombocytopenia has occurred in approximately 40% of patients throughout therapy (maximal at day 11, usually recovered by next cycle), monitor CBCs (including platelet counts) frequently.
• Drug causes peripheral neuropathy that is predominantly sensory but may be mixed sensorimotor. Closely monitor patients with preexisting numbness, pain, or burning in feet or hands or with signs and symptoms of peripheral neuropathy. Patients experiencing new or worsening peripheral neuropathy may require dosage and schedule change.

Patient education

• Advise patient to seek immediate medical attention for fever, pneumonia, diarrhea, vomiting, dehydration, nausea, or fainting.
• Inform patient that he may need to undergo laboratory tests during therapy.
• Caution patient that drug may impair ability to drive or perform other hazardous activities.
• Advise patient to not take drugs that may cause peripheral neuropathy or decrease blood pressure.
• Instruct patient to report symptoms of peripheral neuropathy, including burning sensation, hyperesthesia, hypoesthesia, paresthesia, discomfort, or neuropathic pain.
• Advise women with childbearing potential to avoid pregnancy during therapy.
• Caution breastfeeding patient not to breastfeed during therapy.

busulfan

B

Busulfex, Myleran

Classification: Antineoplastic, alkylating agent
Pregnancy risk category D

Pharmacology

Busulfan hydrolyzes to release methanesulfonate groups, producing reactive carbonium ions. These ions can alkylate DNA and disrupt RNA transcription, causing cell rupture and death. DNA damage may account for much of drug's cytotoxicity. Activity is cell cycle phase-nonspecific.

Pharmacokinetics

Drug is metabolized extensively in liver. With oral use, onset of initial response is 10 to 15 days; peak response is 12 to 20 weeks. With I.V. use, peak response is 4 days; duration, 13 days. Elimination half-life is 2.5 hours. Parent drug and metabolites are excreted in urine.

How supplied

Solution for injection: 6 mg/ml in 10-ml ampule
Tablets: 2 mg

Indications and dosages

FDA-APPROVED

⊖ Conditioning regimen before allogeneic hematopoietic progenitor cell transplantation for chronic myelogenous leukemia (in combination with cyclophosphamide)
Adults: 0.8 mg/kg of ideal body weight (IBW) or actual weight (whichever is lower) I.V. every 6 hours for 4 days (total of 16 doses) as 2-hour infusion through central venous catheter. Cyclophosphamide 60 mg/kg is given on each of 2 days as 1-hour I.V. infusion, starting 3 days before bone marrow transplant day and no sooner than 6 hours after 16th busulfan dose.

➥ Palliative treatment of chronic myeloge-nous (myeloid, myelocytic, or granulocytic) leukemia

Adults and children: For remission induction, approximately 60 mcg/kg or 1.8 mg/m^2 (for adults, usually 4 to 8 mg) P.O.; reserve dosages above 4 mg daily for patients with most compelling symptoms. With remission of less than 3 months, maintenance therapy of 1 to 3 mg P.O. daily may be advisable to control hematologic status and prevent rapid relapse.

OFF-LABEL USES (SELECTED)

➥ Conditioning regimen before allogeneic hematopoietic progenitor-cell transplantation for various malignant hematologic diseases (in combination with cyclophosphamide)

Children: 1.1 mg/kg I.V. over 2 hours every 6 hours for 4 days (total of 16 doses) or 1 mg/kg P.O. four times a day for 16 doses if patient's actual weight is 12 kg (26 lb) or more; or 0.8 mg/kg I.V. over 2 hours every 6 hours for 4 days (total of 16 doses) if patient's actual weight is less than 12 kg

DOSAGE MODIFICATIONS

• For obese or severely obese patients, administer drug based on adjusted IBW. Calculate IBW (height in cm and weight in kg) as:

IBW (kg; men) = 50 + 0.91 × (height in cm − 152);

IBW (kg; women) = 45 + 0.91 × (height in cm − 152).

Calculate adjusted ideal body weight (AIBW) as:

AIBW = IBW + 0.25 × (actual weight [kg] − IBW).

• With remission of less than 3 months, maintenance dosage of 1 to 3 mg daily may control hematologic status and prevent rapid relapse.

• Drug effects may be delayed. If levels of formed blood elements fall sharply or exceptionally quickly, temporary drug withdrawal may be necessary.

• To measure adequate AUC at dose 1 and adjust subsequent doses to achieve desired target AUC (1,125 μM·min), use this formula:

Adjusted dose (mg) = Actual dose (mg) × target AUC (μM·min)/actual AUC μM·min)

For example, if patient received dosage of 11 mg and corresponding AUC was 800 μM·min, for target AUC of 1,125 μM·min, use this formula to find target mg dose:

11 mg × 1,125 μM·min/800 μM·min =15.5 mg

• WBC count rarely drops during first 10 to 15 days of oral therapy. Instead, it may increase, which does not indicate drug resistance or warrant dosage increase.

• Because WBC count may continue to decrease for more than 1 month after therapy ends, drug must be discontinued before total WBC count falls to normal range. When it declines to roughly 15,000/mm^3, withhold drug.

⊠ WARNINGS

• Drug must be diluted before use.
• Busulfan injection is a potent cytotoxic drug that causes profound bone marrow depression at recommended dosages. It should be administered under supervision of qualified physician experienced in allogeneic hematopoietic stem cell transplantation, use of cancer chemotherapeutic drugs, and management of patients with severe pancytopenia. Appropriate management of therapy and complications is possible only when adequate diagnostic and treatment facilities are readily available.

Contraindications and precautions

Contraindicated in hypersensitivity to drug or its components (oral and I.V forms) and when diagnosis of chronic myelogenous leukemia has not been firmly established (oral form).

Use cautiously in history of seizure disorder, head trauma, concurrent use of other potentially epileptogenic drugs, possible compromised bone marrow reserve due to previous irradiation or chemotherapy, and marrow recovery from previous cytotoxic therapy. Also use cautiously in pregnancy or breastfeeding.

Although drug is used off-label for this age-group, safety and efficacy of I.V. use in *children* have not been established.

Preparation and administration

>> Follow hazardous drug guidelines for handling, preparation, and administration. (See "Managing hazardous drugs," page 11.)

• Always premedicate with phenytoin; busulfan can cross blood-brain barrier and induce seizures (which typically occur on days 3 or 4 of therapy).

• Give antiemetics before initial dose and continue on fixed schedule throughout treatment.

• Use administration set with minimal residual hold-up volume (2 to 5 ml).

• Use only 5-micron nylon filter included in package with each ampule. Do not use polycarbonate syringes.

• Dilute solution with either normal saline solution for injection or D_5W injection to a diluent:drug ratio of 10:1. Final concentration is 0.5 mg/ml.

• Always add busulfan injection to diluent (not diluent to busulfan), and mix thoroughly.

• Give I.V. through central venous catheter as 2-hour infusion.

• Use infusion pump to administer solution. Set flow rate to deliver entire prescribed dose over 2 hours. Flush indwelling catheter line before and after infusion with 5 ml normal saline solution or D_5W. Do not infuse concomitantly with I.V. solutions of unknown compatibility. Rapid infusion is not recommended.

• Infuse solutions in normal saline solution or D_5W within 8 hours when stored at 77° F (25° C). Infuse solutions reconstituted with normal saline solution within 12 hours when refrigerated at 36° to 46° F (2° to 8° C).

• Unopened ampule is stable until expiration date when refrigerated at 36° to 46° F.

• Store tablets in dry place at 59° to 77° F (15° to 25° C).

Adverse reactions

CNS: seizures (high doses), asthenia, unusual fatigue, weakness

CV: chest pain, tachycardia, cardiac tamponade (high doses with cyclophosphamide), pericardial fibrosis

EENT: cataracts

GI: nausea, vomiting, anorexia, dry mouth, stomatitis, mucositis

GU: erectile dysfunction, sterility, amenorrhea, gynecomastia

Hematologic: thrombocytopenia, leukopenia, anemia, pancytopenia, severe bone marrow depression (nadir is 14 to 21 days, with recovery after 28 days)

Hepatic: hepatic veno-occlusive disease with high doses (increased risk with AUC above 1,500 mg/ml/minute)

Metabolic: adrenal insufficiency–like syndrome, hyperuricemia secondary to tumor lysis syndrome

Respiratory: irreversible pulmonary fibrosis ("busulfan lung")

Skin: hyperpigmentation

Other: weight loss, secondary cancers

Interactions

Drug-drug. *Acetaminophen:* decreased busulfan clearance when acetaminophen is given more than 72 hours before or at same time

Blood dyscrasia–causing drugs: increased anemia, leukopenia, or thrombocytopenia

Cyclophosphamide: increased risk of cardiac tamponade in patients with thalassemia

Cytotoxic therapy: additive drug-induced pulmonary toxicity

Itraconazole: decreased busulfan clearance, causing increased drug plasma level and increased risk of toxicity

Metronidazole: increased busulfan trough level, causing increased risk of toxicity

Phenytoin: increased busulfan clearance, causing decreased plasma concentration

Drug-diagnostic tests. *ALP, ALT, AST, bilirubin, BUN, creatinine, glucose, urinary uric acid:* increased

CBC and differential; platelets; serum calcium, magnesium, and potassium: decreased
Cytology studies of lung, bladder, breast, or uterine cervix tissue: interpretation problems due to cytologic dysplasia caused by busulfan
Drug-food. Grapefruit juice: possible altered levels of drugs cleared by CYP450 3A4 enzyme
Drug-herb. American elder, cat's claw, echinacea, eucalyptus, feverfew, kava, licorice, milk thistle, peppermint oil, pomegranate, St. John's wort: possible altered levels of drugs cleared by CYP450 3A4 enzyme

Toxicity and overdose

• Common signs and symptoms of overdose include profound bone marrow hypoplasia or aplasia and pancytopenia. CNS, liver, lungs, and GI tract may also be affected.
• No antidote exists except hematopoietic progenitor cell transplantation. Provide vigorous supportive measures as indicated. Induce vomiting or gastric lavage if ingestion was recent. Consider dialysis.

Special considerations

• Total WBC count declines exponentially with constant busulfan dose. Weekly plotting of WBC count on semilogarithmic graph paper helps predict when therapy should be discontinued. Normal WBC count usually occurs in 12 to 20 weeks with recommended dosage.
• Evaluate hematologic status frequently and monitor patient closely for infection or bleeding. Profound bone marrow depression is universal and may present as neutropenia, thrombocytopenia, or anemia.
• Severe granulocytopenia, thrombocytopenia, anemia, or combination may occur. Monitor CBCs (including WBC differential) and quantitative platelet counts frequently during treatment and until recovery is achieved. Use antibiotic therapy and platelet and RBC support when indicated.
• Ovarian suppression and amenorrhea commonly occur in premenopausal women re-

ceiving long-term, low-dose therapy for chronic myelogenous leukemia. Sterility, azoospermia, and testicular atrophy have been reported in males.
• Drug may cause cellular dysplasia in lungs and other organs. Cytologic abnormalities, characterized by giant, hyperchromatic nuclei, have occurred in lymph nodes, pancreas, thyroid, adrenal glands, liver, and bone marrow.

Patient education

• Instruct patient to take tablets at same time each day, maintain adequate fluid intake (2 to 3 L/day), and have blood counts measured periodically.
• Urge patient to immediately report difficulty swallowing or breathing; light-headedness or fainting; hypersensitivity reactions (including hives, pruritus, and sudden swelling of face, lips, tongue, legs, or arms); nosebleed; unusual bruising; fever, chills, or other infection symptoms; persistent cough; or congestion.
• Inform patient that long-term therapy may cause diffuse pulmonary fibrosis.
• Urge patient to report abrupt weakness, unusual fatigue, anorexia, weight loss, nausea and vomiting, mouth sores, and melanoderma (possibly associated with syndrome resembling adrenal insufficiency).
• Inform patient of drug's other toxic effects, including risk of seizures, infertility, amenorrhea, skin hyperpigmentation, dry mucous membranes, and cataracts (rare).
• Tell patient that prescriber may need to adjust dosage several times for best effect.
• Counsel women with childbearing potential to avoid becoming pregnant during therapy.
• Advise breastfeeding patient to stop breastfeeding during therapy.

Only common or life-threatening adverse reactions are listed.

capecitabine
Xeloda

Classification: Antineoplastic, antimetabolite
Pregnancy risk category D

Pharmacology
Capecitabine converts to 5-fluorouracil (5-FU) in liver and inhibits formation of necessary precursor of thymidine triphosphate (essential for DNA synthesis). It also interferes with RNA processing and protein synthesis. It produces higher fluorouracil levels in tumor tissue than normal tissues. Activity is cell cycle S-phase–specific.

Pharmacokinetics
Drug is readily absorbed in GI tract and metabolized to fluorouracil in liver, peripheral tissues, and tumor tissue by thymidine phosphorylase. It peaks in about 2 hours. Elimination half-life is 38 to 45 minutes. Drug is excreted by kidneys.

How supplied
Tablets: 150 mg, 500 mg

Indications and dosages

FDA-APPROVED
➡ Metastatic colorectal carcinoma when treatment with a fluoropyrimidine such as capecitabine alone is preferred
Adults: 1,250 mg/m² P.O. twice daily (morning and evening; 2,500 mg/m² total daily dose) for 2 weeks followed by 1-week rest, given as 3-week cycles
➡ Metastatic breast cancer resistant to both paclitaxel and anthracycline-containing chemotherapy regimen or resistant to paclitaxel and when further anthracycline therapy is not indicated (monotherapy) or after failure of previous anthracycline-containing chemotherapy (combination therapy with docetaxel)
Adults: As single agent, 1,250 mg/m² P.O. twice daily (morning and evening) for 2 weeks followed by 1-week rest, given as 3-week cycles. Alternatively, 1,250 mg/m² P.O. twice daily for 2 weeks followed by 1-week rest, in combination with docetaxel 75 mg/m² as 1-hour I.V. infusion every 3 weeks

OFF-LABEL USES (SELECTED)
➡ Colorectal cancer
Adults: Actively being investigated to replace 5-FU in many combination regimens, such as CAPOX (capecitabine 1,000 mg/m² P.O. twice daily for 14 days + oxaliplatin 130 mg/m² I.V. on day 1, repeated every 21 days) and CAPIRI (capecitabine 1,000 mg/m² twice daily for 14 days + irinotecan 100 mg/m² on days 1 and 8, repeated every 22 days)
➡ Renal cell carcinoma
Adults: Being studied for use as single agent; 2,500 mg/m² divided into two doses for 14 days and then 7 days off; also being investigated in combination with gemcitabine or immunotherapy

DOSAGE MODIFICATIONS
• For patients with moderate renal impairment (baseline creatinine clearance of 30 to 50 ml/minute), reduce dosage to 75% of starting dose when used as monotherapy or in combination with docetaxel.
• If Grade 2 or 3 hand-and-foot syndrome occurs (characterized by numbness, dysesthesia or paresthesia, tingling, painless swelling or erythema of hands or feet, or discomfort disrupting normal activities), interrupt therapy until event resolves or decreases to Grade 1. After Grade 3 hand-and-foot syndrome, decrease subsequent dosages.
• If drug-related Grade 2 to 4 elevations in bilirubin occur, interrupt therapy until hyperbilirubinemia resolves or decreases to Grade 1. NCIC Grade 2 hyperbilirubinemia is defined as 1.5 × normal, Grade 3 as 1.5 to 3 × normal, and Grade 4 as more than 3 × normal.

• Carefully monitor phenytoin level in patients receiving capecitabine and phenytoin; phenytoin dosage may need to be reduced.

⊠ WARNINGS

• Altered coagulation parameters, bleeding, and death have occurred in patients taking drug concomitantly with coumarin-derivative anticoagulants, such as warfarin and phenprocoumon. INR or prothrombin time (PT) should be monitored frequently so anticoagulant dosage can be adjusted accordingly.
• Significant PT and INR increases have occurred in patients stabilized on anticoagulants when capecitabine was introduced. Increases occurred in patients with and without liver metastases within several days to several months after starting capecitabine and, in a few cases, within 1 month after stopping. Patients older than age 60 are at increased risk for coagulopathy.

Contraindications and precautions

Contraindicated in hypersensitivity to drug or its components or to 5-FU, dihydropyrimidine dehydrogenase deficiency, and severe renal impairment.

Use cautiously in renal or hepatic disease, concurrent use of CYP2C9 substrates, concurrent radiation therapy, and in pregnancy or breastfeeding. **Elderly patients** may be more sensitive to toxic effects. Risk of severe GI effects (diarrhea, nausea, and vomiting) may increase in patients ages 80 and older. Safety and efficacy in **children** have not been established.

Preparation and administration

• Follow hazardous drug guidelines for handling, preparation, and administration. (See "Managing hazardous drugs," page 11.)
• Premedicate according to product label before giving to patients receiving capecitabine-docetaxel combination.

• Give with water within 30 minutes after meals.
• Store at 77° F (25° C) in tightly closed container.

Adverse reactions

CNS: dizziness, headache, paresthesia, fatigue, insomnia
EENT: eye irritation
GI: nausea, vomiting, diarrhea (dose-limiting toxicity), anorexia, stomatitis, abdominal pain, constipation, dyspepsia
Hematologic: neutropenia, lymphopenia, thrombocytopenia, bone marrow depression, anemia, leukopenia (dose-limiting toxicity)
Musculoskeletal: myalgia, limb pain
Skin: hand-and-foot syndrome, dermatitis, nail disorder
Other: fever, edema, dehydration

Interactions

Drug-drug. *Antacids containing aluminum hydroxide and magnesium hydroxide:* increased capecitabine plasma level
Blood dyscrasia–causing drugs: increased leukopenia or thrombocytopenia
Bone marrow depressants: additive bone marrow depression
Fosphenytoin, phenytoin: elevated phenytoin level
Leucovorin: increased 5-FU concentration and toxicity
Oral coumarin-derivative anticoagulants: altered coagulation or bleeding
Drug-diagnostic tests. *ALP, ALT, AST, bilirubin:* increased, especially in patients with hepatic metastases
INR, PT, triglycerides: increased
Magnesium, potassium: decreased

Toxicity and overdose

• Common signs and symptoms of acute overdose include nausea, vomiting, diarrhea, GI irritation and bleeding, hand-and-foot syndrome, and bone marrow depression. Cardiotoxicity has occurred and may present as

---

Only common or life-threatening adverse reactions are listed.

myocardial infarction, angina, arrhythmias, cardiac arrest, ECG changes, and cardiomyopathy. Cardiotoxicity is more common in patients with history of coronary artery disease.
• Treatment should include supportive medical interventions. Dialysis may help to reduce circulating concentrations of 5'-deoxy-5'-fluorouridine (5'-DFUR).

Special considerations
• Monitor patient closely for toxicity.
• Evaluate patient for diarrhea. If severe, therapy may need to be interrupted.

Patient education
• Tell patient to take tablets with water within 30 minutes after meals (breakfast and dinner) at same time every day.
• Advise patient he may need to take two different-strength tablets simultaneously.
• Instruct patient to seek medical attention for swelling, redness, or sores in throat or mouth; pain, swelling, or redness of hands or feet; temperature above 100.5° (38° C); or bloody bowel movements.
• Urge patient to contact prescriber right away if he has more than four bowel movements daily, if diarrhea occurs during sleep, if he vomits more than once in a 24-hour period, or if his appetite decreases.

carboplatin
Paraplatin

Classification: Antineoplastic, platinum agent
Pregnancy risk category D

Pharmacology
Carboplatin inhibits DNA synthesis, replication, and transcription by inducing equal numbers of drug-DNA cross-links. This effect causes growth imbalance and cell death. Activity is cell cycle phase-nonspecific.

Pharmacokinetics
Drug is not bound to plasma protein, but platinum from carboplatin becomes irreversibly bound to plasma protein and is slowly eliminated, with minimum half-life of 5 days. When creatinine level is 60 ml/minute or more, 65% of dose is excreted in urine within 12 hours and 71% within 24 hours.

How supplied
Carboplatin aqueous solution injection: 50-mg/5-ml, 150-mg/15-ml, 450-mg/45-ml, and 600-mg/60-ml multidose vials
Powder for injection: 50-mg, 150-mg, and 450-mg vials

Indications and dosages

FDA-APPROVED

➡ Advanced ovarian cancer (combined with cyclophosphamide)
Adults: 300 mg/m² I.V. (with 600 mg/m² cyclophosphamide) I.V. on day 1 every 4 weeks for six cycles
➡ Ovarian cancer recurring after chemotherapy
Adults: 360 mg/m² I.V. on day 1 every 4 weeks

OFF-LABEL USES (SELECTED)

➡ Bladder cancer
Adults: Carboplatin adequate AUC 5 mg/ml/minute and paclitaxel 175 to 200 mg/m² I.V. every 21 days is being investigated.
➡ Non-small-cell lung cancer
Adults: Commonly used dosages are carboplatin (AUC 5 to 7 mg/ml/minute) and paclitaxel 175 mg/m² I.V. over 3 hours every 21 days
➡ Small-cell lung cancer
Adults: Commonly used dosages are carboplatin 450 mg/m² I.V. on day 1 and etoposide 100 mg/m² on days 1 to 3 every 28 days

DOSAGE MODIFICATIONS

• Adjust dosage according to platelet and neutrophil counts. For platelet count above

100,000/mm³ and neutrophil count above 2,000/mm³, adjust to 125% of previous course. For platelet count of 50,000 to 100,000/mm³ and neutrophil count of 500 to 2,000/mm³, do not adjust. For platelet count below 50,000/mm³ and neutrophil count below 500/mm³, adjust to 75% of previous course. (Percentages apply to carboplatin as single agent or carboplatin and cyclophosphamide in combination.)

• For creatinine clearance of 41 to 59 ml/ minute, adjust day-1 dosage to 250 mg/m². For creatinine clearance of 16 to 40 ml/ minute, adjust day-1 dosage to 200 mg/m².

• Dosage may be calculated mathematically based on preexisting renal function or on renal function and desired platelet nadir. In this case, use Calvert formula for carboplatin dosing:

Total dose (mg) = (target AUC) × (GFR + 25).
(Total dosage is calculated in mg, not mg/m².)

• Use formula dosing based on estimates of glomerular filtration rate in elderly patients to provide predictable plasma carboplatin AUCs and minimize toxicity risk.

• Emesis may be more severe in patients who previously received emetogenic therapy. Antiemetics may help. Extending single I.V. administration to 24 hours or dividing total dose over 5 consecutive daily pulse doses has resulted in reduced emesis.

⊠ WARNINGS

• Bone marrow depression is dose-related and may be severe, resulting in infection or bleeding. Anemia may be cumulative and require transfusions. Vomiting may occur.
• Anaphylactic-like reactions may occur within minutes of administration. Epinephrine, corticosteroids, and antihistamines can relieve symptoms.

Contraindications and precautions
Contraindicated in severe hypersensitivity to mannitol, cisplatin, or other compounds containing platinum; severe bone marrow depression; and significant bleeding.

Use cautiously in patients previously treated with cisplatin, concurrent radiation therapy, pregnancy or breastfeeding, and in *elderly patients*. Safety and efficacy in *children* have not been established.

Preparation and administration
• Follow hazardous drug guidelines for handling, preparation, and administration. (See "Managing hazardous drugs," page 11.)
• Dilute each 10 mg with 1 ml sterile water for injection, D_5W, or normal saline solution. Further dilute with normal saline solution or D_5W to 1 to 4 mg/ml.
• Infuse for 15 minutes or longer. No pre- or posttreatment hydration or forced diuresis is required. Discard solution after 8 hours.
• Injection site reactions, including redness, swelling, pain, and necrosis associated with extravasation, have been reported.
• Multidose vials for injection maintain microbial, chemical, and physical stability for up to 14 days at 77° F (25° C) after multiple needle entries.
• Protect unopened vials from light, and store at 77° F.

Adverse reactions
CNS: seizures, central neurotoxicity, dizziness, confusion
CV: cardiac abnormalities
EENT: visual changes, tinnitus, hearing loss, vestibular toxicity
GI: severe nausea, vomiting, diarrhea, mucositis, anorexia, constipation, taste changes
GU: renal tubular damage, renal insufficiency, erectile dysfunction, sterility, amenorrhea, gynecomastia
Hematologic: thrombocytopenia (dose-limiting, with nadir within 2 to 3 weeks and recovery 1 to 2 weeks later), leukopenia, pancytopenia, neutropenia, anemia, bleeding
Metabolic: hypomagnesemia, hypocalcemia, hypokalemia, hyponatremia, hyperuremia

---

Only common or life-threatening adverse reactions are listed.

Skin: alopecia, dermatitis, rash, erythema, pruritus, urticaria
Other: weight loss, anaphylaxis, peripheral neuropathy

Interactions

Drug-drug. *Blood dyscrasia–causing drugs:* increased leukopenia and thrombocytopenia
Bone marrow depressants: additive bone marrow depression
Cisplatin: increased risk of neurotoxicity or ototoxicity
Nephrotoxic compounds: worsened renal effects
Nephrotoxic or ototoxic agents: increased risk of ototoxicity and nephrotoxicity
Drug-diagnostic tests. *ALP, AST, bilirubin, BUN, creatinine:* increased
Serum calcium, magnesium, potassium, sodium: decreased
Drug-herb. *Alpha-lipoic acid, coenzyme Q10:* possible enhanced tumor growth

Toxicity and overdose

• Signs and symptoms of overdose include bone marrow depression and hepatotoxicity.
• No antidote exists.

Special considerations

• Bone marrow depression (leukopenia, neutropenia, and thrombocytopenia) is a dose-dependent and dose-limiting toxicity. Monitor peripheral blood counts during therapy and, when appropriate, until recovery occurs. Median nadir occurs at day 21 in patients receiving single-agent carboplatin. In general, single intermittent courses should not be repeated until WBC, neutrophil, and platelet counts recover.
• Bone marrow depression is increased in patients who have received previous therapy (especially regimens including cisplatin) and in patients with impaired renal function. Reduce initial dosages in these patients appropriately and monitor blood counts carefully between courses. Combination therapy with other bone marrow depressants must be carefully

managed with respect to dosage and timing to minimize additive effects.
• Some patients may need transfusions during treatment, particularly those receiving prolonged therapy.
• Peripheral neurotoxicity is infrequent but increased in patients older than age 65 and in those previously treated with cisplatin.
• Vision loss has been reported with doses higher than those recommended in package insert. Significant hearing loss has occurred in children who received higher-than-recommended doses combined with other ototoxic agents.
• Manage allergic reactions (which may occur within minutes of administration) with appropriate supportive therapy. Patients previously exposed to platinum therapy are at increased risk for allergic reactions, including anaphylaxis.
• High doses (more than four times recommended dose) have caused severe liver function abnormalities.
• Creatinine clearance is most sensitive measure of renal function in patients receiving drug, and is most useful test for correlating drug clearance with bone marrow depression.

Patient education

• Inform patient that vomiting is a common side effect.
• Advise patient to seek immediate medical attention for unusual bleeding or bruising; sudden fever; yellowing of eyes or skin; fever, chills, sore throat, or other infection symptoms; trouble swallowing or breathing; wheezing; light-headedness or fainting; or sudden swelling of face, lips, tongue, legs, or arms.
• Urge patient to keep all appointments with health care professional to monitor progress.
• Inform patient that prescriber may need to change dosage several times for best effect.
• Caution women with childbearing potential to avoid pregnancy because drug can harm fetus.

carmustine (BCNU)
BiCNU, Gliadel

Classification: Antineoplastic, alkylating agent, nitrosourea
Pregnancy risk category D

Pharmacology
Carmustine inhibits DNA and RNA synthesis by cross-linking with DNA and RNA strands. This effect prevents cellular division and interferes with protein synthesis, causing cell death. Activity is cell cycle phase-nonspecific.

Pharmacokinetics
After I.V. dose, drug is metabolized to active compounds in liver and is rapidly distributed into tissues, with significant amounts into cerebrospinal fluid. It peaks in 15 minutes. Duration is 6 weeks; half-life is 15 to 20 minutes. Drug is excreted by kidneys.

How supplied
Powder for injection (BiCNU): 100-mg vials
Wafer implant (Gliadel): 7.7 mg

Indications and dosages

FDA-APPROVED

➥ Palliative therapy (as single agent or in combination) for glioblastoma, brainstem glioma, medulloblastoma, astrocytoma, ependymoma, metastatic brain tumors, and multiple myeloma (in combination with prednisone); secondary palliative therapy in Hodgkin's disease and non-Hodgkin's lymphoma (in combination with other approved drugs) in patients who relapse during or fail to respond to primary therapy
Adults: 150 to 200 mg/m² I.V. infusion over 1 to 2 hours every 6 weeks (as single agent in previously untreated patients) as single dose or divided into daily injections, such as 75 to 100 mg/m² on 2 successive days

➔ Newly diagnosed high-grade malignant glioma as adjunct to surgery and radiation, or recurrent glioblastoma multiforme as adjunct to surgery
Adults: 61.6 mg (eight wafers) by implantation into resection cavity, if size and shape allow

OFF-LABEL USES (SELECTED)

➥ Disseminated malignant melanoma
Adults: 150 mg/m² I.V. infusion as single dose every 4 to 6 weeks; as part of Dartmouth regimen (carmustine 150 mg/m² daily on day 1 every 6 weeks, cisplatin 25 mg/m² daily on days 1 to 3 every 3 weeks, dacarbazine 220 mg/m² daily on days 1 to 3 every 3 weeks, and tamoxifen 20 mg P.O. daily)

DOSAGE MODIFICATIONS

• Adjust dosage when drug is combined with other myelosuppressants and in patients with depleted bone marrow reserve.
• Schedule below is suggested as a guide to dosage adjustment.

Nadir after previous dose

Leukocytes/mm³	Platelets/mm³	Percentage of previous dose to be given
Above 4,000	Above 100,000	100%
3,000-3,999	75,000-99,999	100%
2,000-2,999	25,000-74,999	70%
Below 2,000	Below 25,000	50%

• Do not give repeat carmustine course until circulating blood elements have returned to acceptable levels (platelets above 100,000/mm³ and WBCs above 4,000/mm³), which usually occurs in 6 weeks.
• Bone marrow toxicity is cumulative, and adjustment must be considered on basis of nadir blood counts with previous dose.
• If resection cavity does not accommodate eight wafers, maximum allowable number of wafers should be placed. No more than eight should be used per surgical procedure.

Only common or life-threatening adverse reactions are listed.

WARNINGS

Powder for injection

• Most common and severe toxic effect is bone marrow depression—notably thrombocytopenia and leukopenia—which may contribute to bleeding and overwhelming infections in already compromised patient.

• Blood counts should be monitored weekly for at least 6 weeks after dose. At recommended dosage, courses should not be given more frequently than every 6 weeks.

• Because bone marrow toxicity is cumulative, dosage adjustment must be considered on basis of nadir blood counts with previous dose.

• Patients receiving more than 1,400 mg/m^2 cumulative dose are at significantly higher risk for pulmonary toxicity. Such toxicity can occur years after treatment and may cause death, particularly in patients treated in childhood.

Contraindications and precautions

Contraindicated in hypersensitivity to drug or its components.

Administer I.V. injection cautiously in bone marrow depression, concurrent radiation therapy, baseline below 70% of predicted forced vital capacity or carbon monoxide diffusing capacity, hepatic or renal impairment, and pregnancy or breastfeeding. Safety and efficacy in *children* have not been established.

Preparation and administration

≫ Follow hazardous drug guidelines for handling, preparation, and administration. (See "Managing hazardous drugs," page 11.)

Powder for injection

• Administer antiemetic 30 to 60 minutes before drug.

• Dissolve drug with 3 ml supplied sterile diluent (dehydrated alcohol injection). Aseptically add 27 ml sterile water for injection. Each ml of resulting solution contains 3.3 mg of drug in 10% ethanol. Protect solution from light.

• Reconstituted clear, colorless to yellowish solution may be diluted further with 5% dextrose injection. Inspect for particulates and discoloration if solution and container permit.

• Ask patient about alcohol sensitivity or intolerance because I.V. diluent contains alcohol.

• Lyophilized dosage formulation contains no preservatives and is not intended as a multidose vial.

• Use only glass containers for administration.

• Use reconstituted solution I.V. only; administer by I.V. drip.

• Do not administer over less than 1 to 2 hours, to avoid intense pain and burning at injection site (although true thrombosis is rare). Rapid I.V. infusion may produce intensive skin flushing and conjunctiva suffusion within 2 hours, lasting about 4 hours.

• Store vials at room temperature when reconstituted as directed and further diluted to a concentration of 0.2 mg/ml in 5% dextrose injection. Protect from light and use within 8 hours.

• Drug has low melting point; exposure to temperatures of 86.9° to 89.6° F (30.5° to 32° C) or higher causes drug to liquefy and appear as oily film on vials. Discard vial should this occur.

• Refrigerate unopened vials at 36° to 46° F (2° to 8° C) to provide 2-year stability. Reconstituted solution is stable for 8 hours at 77° F (25° C) when protected from light.

Wafer

• Wafers are packaged in two aluminum-foil laminate pouches. Inner pouch is sterile and designed to maintain product sterility and protect against moisture. Outer pouch is peelable overwrap; outside surface is not sterile.

• Pouches containing wafers should remain unopened until implantation.

• Up to eight implants may be placed to cover as much of resection cavity as possible. Slight overlapping is acceptable. Wafers broken in half may be used, but those broken into more than two pieces should be discarded in biohazard container. Oxidized regenerated cellulose (Surgicel) may cover wafers to secure them against cavity surface. After placement, irrigate resection cavity and close dura in watertight fashion.

• Keep unopened foil pouches at ambient room temperature for no longer than 6 hours.
• Store wafers at or below –4° F (–20° C).

Adverse reactions
Powder for injection
GI: nausea, vomiting, anorexia, stomatitis
GU: azotemia, renal failure
Hematologic: bone marrow depression, thrombocytopenia, leukopenia, anemia
Hepatic: hepatotoxicity
Respiratory: fibrosis, pulmonary infiltrates
Skin: burning, hyperpigmentation at injection site
Wafer
CNS: hydrocephalus, depression, abnormal thinking, confusion, ataxia, dizziness, insomnia, monoplegia, coma, amnesia, paranoid reaction, aphasia, brain edema, seizures, headache, hemiplegia, intracranial hypertension, meningitis, abscess, somnolence, stupor, asthenia, deep wound infection of subgaleal space, bone, meninges, or neural parenchyma
CV: hypertension, hypotension, deep vein thrombophlebitis
EENT: diplopia, visual field defects, eye pain
GI: nausea, vomiting, diarrhea, constipation, dysphagia, GI hemorrhage, fecal incontinence, oral candidiasis
GU: urinary incontinence
Metabolic: hyponatremia, hyperglycemia, hypokalemia
Musculoskeletal: neck pain, back pain
Hematologic: thrombocytopenia, leukocytosis, anemia
Respiratory: infection, pneumonia, aspiration pneumonia, pulmonary embolism
Skin: rash
Other: peripheral edema, accidental injury, allergic reaction, chest pain, sepsis, abnormal healing (cerebrospinal fluid leak, subdural fluid collection, subgaleal or wound effusions, wound breakdown)

Interactions
Powder for injection
Drug-drug. *Blood dyscrasia–causing drugs:* increased leukopenia and thrombocytopenia
Bone marrow depressants: additive bone marrow depression
Cimetidine: increased risk of bone marrow depression
Drugs that inhibit aldehyde dehydrogenase-2 or cause disulfiram-like reaction: increased risk of disulfiram-like reaction
Etoposide: increased risk of severe hepatic dysfunction with hyperbilirubinemia, ascites, and thrombocytopenia
Hepatotoxic or nephrotoxic drugs: increased hepatotoxicity or nephrotoxicity
Phenytoin: decreased phenytoin efficacy
Drug-diagnostic tests. *ALP, AST, bilirubin, BUN, blood glucose:* increased
Sodium, potassium: decreased
Drug-herb. *Alpha-lipoic acid, coenzyme Q10:* decreased chemotherapy efficacy
Glutamine: possible enhanced tumor growth

Toxicity and overdose
Powder for injection
• Signs and symptoms of overdose include pulmonary infiltrates or fibrosis, bone marrow depression (thrombocytopenia, leukopenia, anemia), hepatotoxicity (increased ALP and bilirubin levels), and renal abnormalities (azotemia and renal failure).
• No proven antidotes have been identified.
Wafer
• Short-term and long-term toxicity profiles when given with chemotherapy have not been fully explored. When given with radiotherapy, implant does not appear to cause short- or long-term toxicities.

Special considerations
Powder for injection
• Monitor platelet, WBC, and neutrophil counts weekly for acceptable levels.

Only common or life-threatening adverse reactions are listed.

- Do not give repeat course before 6 weeks because hematologic toxicity is delayed and cumulative.
- Long-term use of nitrosoureas has been associated with secondary cancers.
- Monitor liver and kidney function tests periodically.

Wafer

- Avoid communication between surgical resection cavity and ventricular system, to prevent wafer migration into ventricular system (which causes obstructive hydrocephalus). If communication larger than wafer diameter exists, close before wafer implantation.
- CT scans and MRI of head may show enhancement in brain tissue surrounding resection cavity after implantation. This may represent edema and inflammation caused by implant or tumor progression.

Patient education

- Inform patient that blood counts will be measured weekly for first 6 weeks of therapy.
- Advise patient to seek immediate medical attention for chest pain; sudden fever; unusual bleeding or bruising; difficulty swallowing or breathing; wheezing; light-headedness or fainting; sudden swelling of face, lips, tongue, legs, or arms; yellowing of eyes or skin; or fever, chills, sore throat, or other infection symptoms.
- Caution women with childbearing potential to avoid pregnancy because drug can harm fetus.
- Advise breastfeeding patient to stop breastfeeding during therapy.

cetuximab
Erbitux

Classification: Antineoplastic, monoclonal antibody, epidermal growth factor receptor (EGFR) inhibitor
Pregnancy risk category C

Pharmacology

Cetuximab binds specifically to EGFR on both normal and malignant tumor cells. This effect blocks phosphorylation and activation of receptor-associated kinases, inhibiting cell growth, inducing apoptosis, and decreasing matrix metalloproteinase and vascular endothelial growth factor production.

Pharmacokinetics

Steady-state concentration occurs by third weekly infusion. Initial response occurs within 6 weeks. Elimination half-life ranges from 41 to 213 hours, with mean of 97 hours.

How supplied

Solution for injection: 100 mg (2 mg/ml)

Indications and dosages

FDA-APPROVED

➥ EGFR-expressing, metastatic colorectal cancer in patients refractory to irinotecan-based chemotherapy (in combination with irinotecan); EGFR-expressing, metastatic colorectal cancer in patients intolerant of irinotecan-based chemotherapy (single agent)
Adults: 400 mg/m² as initial loading dose by I.V. infusion over 2 hours (maximum infusion rate is 5 ml/minute), and weekly maintenance dose of 250 mg/m² infused over 1 hour (maximum infusion rate is 5 ml/minute)

OFF-LABEL USES (SELECTED)

➥ Relapsed or refractory head and neck cancer
Adults: Commonly used in combination with

platinum-based chemotherapy—400 mg/m^2 loading dose I.V. infusion over 2 hours followed weekly by 250 mg/m^2 infused I.V. over 1 hour, or loading dose of 100 to 500 mg/m^2 I.V. and maintenance dose of 100 to 250 mg/m^2 I.V. weekly for 7 weeks; or 200 to 400 mg/m^2 I.V. weekly with no loading dose

➡ Breast cancer

Adults: Commonly prescribed dosage is 50 to 200 mg/m^2 I.V. weekly for 6 weeks.

➡ Tumors overexpressing EGFR

Adults: Commonly prescribed dosage is 5 to 100 mg/m^2 I.V. weekly or loading dose of 100 to 500 mg/m^2 and maintenance dose of 5 to 400 mg/m^2 weekly.

DOSAGE MODIFICATIONS

• If patient experiences mild or moderate (Grade 1 or 2) infusion reaction, permanently reduce infusion rate by 50%.

• For first occurrence of severe acneiform rash, delay infusion 1 to 2 weeks. If condition improves, continue therapy at 250 mg/m^2; if no improvement, discontinue therapy. For second occurrence, delay infusion 1 to 2 weeks. If condition improves, reduce dosage to 200 mg/m^2; if no improvement, discontinue therapy. For third occurrence, delay infusion for 1 to 2 weeks. If condition improves, reduce dosage to 150 mg/m^2; if no improvement, discontinue therapy. On fourth occurrence, discontinue therapy.

⊠ WARNINGS

• Severe infusion reactions (Grade 3 or 4) occurred in about 3% of patients, rarely with fatal outcome (less than 1 in 1,000). About 90% of severe infusion reactions occurred with initial infusion.

• Severe infusion reactions require immediate interruption of infusion and permanent drug discontinuation.

Contraindications and precautions

No known contraindications exist.

Use cautiously in hypersensitivity to drug, its components, or murine proteins and in concurrent radiation therapy. Safety and efficacy in *children* have not been established.

Preparation and administration

• Premedicate with histamine$_1$ antagonist, such as 50 mg diphenhydramine I.V.

• Do not administer as I.V. push or bolus.

• Administer with low–protein-binding 0.22-micron in-line filter. Piggyback drug to infusion line.

• Do not reconstitute.

• Solution should be clear and colorless but may contain trace amounts of white amorphous particulates. Do not shake or dilute.

• Drug may be given by infusion pump or syringe pump.

• Administer initial dose over 2 hours at rate of 5 ml/minute; give subsequent weekly doses over 1 hour. Maximum infusion rate is 5 ml/minute.

• Observe patient for 1 hour after infusion. Severe, potentially fatal infusion reactions have occurred, including rapid onset of airway obstruction (bronchospasm, stridor, hoarseness), urticaria, and hypotension.

• Discard solution after 12 hours if refrigerated or after 8 hours at room temperature.

• Store unopened vials at 36° to 46° F (2° to 8° C).

Adverse reactions

CNS: malaise, asthenia, headache
CV: peripheral edema
GI: diarrhea, abdominal pain, constipation, nausea and vomiting
GU: renal failure
Musculoskeletal: back pain, weakness
Respiratory: interstitial lung disease, pulmonary embolus, dyspnea
Skin: dermatologic toxicity, acneiform rash
Other: dehydration, fever, sepsis, pain, infusion reactions (anaphylactoid-like)

Only common or life-threatening adverse reactions are listed.

Interactions
Drug-herb. *Alpha-lipoic acid, coenzyme Q10:* decreased chemotherapy efficacy
Glutamine: possible enhanced tumor growth

Toxicity and overdose
• Signs and symptoms of overdose include onset of acute or worsening of existing pulmonary symptoms. Dermatologic toxicity presents as inflammatory or infectious sequelae.
• No specific antidote exists. Treat symptomatically; discontinue drug if necessary. Inflammation or infection due to dermatologic toxicity may require oral antibiotics (topical corticosteroids are not recommended).

Special considerations
• Monitor vital signs frequently.
• Watch for signs and symptoms of interstitial lung disease, which necessitate drug discontinuation.
• Patients treated with cetuximab, cisplatin, and radiation experience 95% incidence of rash. Incidence and severity of cutaneous reactions with combined-modality therapy appears to be additive. Use appropriate caution when adding radiation to cetuximab therapy in patients with colorectal cancer.

Patient education
• Tell patient that sunlight may worsen skin reactions. Advise him to use sunscreen, wear hat, and limit sun exposure.
• Instruct patient to report rash, fever, dehydration, shortness of breath, difficulty breathing, and other new signs and symptoms.
• Caution women with childbearing potential to avoid pregnancy because drug can harm fetus.
• Advise breastfeeding patients to stop breastfeeding during and for 60 days after therapy.

chlorambucil
Leukeran

C

Classification: Antineoplastic, alkylating agent, nitrogen mustard derivative
Pregnancy risk category D

Pharmacology
Chlorambucil alkylates DNA and RNA and inhibits enzymes that allow amino acid synthesis in proteins. This effect disrupts cell function. Activity is cell cycle phase-nonspecific.

Pharmacokinetics
Drug is rapidly and completely absorbed from GI tract. It is metabolized in liver to active compound, phenylacetic acid mustard. About 99% is protein-bound (albumin). Drug peaks within 1 hour; half-life is about 2 hours. Approximately 60% is excreted in urine.

How supplied
Tablets: 2 mg

Indications and dosages

FDA-APPROVED

➥ Chronic lymphocytic leukemia (CLL); malignant lymphomas, including lymphosarcoma, giant follicular lymphoma, and Hodgkin's disease
Adults: 0.1 to 0.2 mg/kg P.O. daily for 3 to 6 weeks to response or bone marrow depression

OFF-LABEL USES (SELECTED)

➥ Combination therapy for Hodgkin's disease
Adults: Commonly used regimen is 6 mg/m² P.O. daily on days 1 to 7 (ChIVPP/ EVA hybrid) every 28 days.

DOSAGE MODIFICATIONS

• Carefully adjust dosage to patient response; reduce as soon as WBC count falls abruptly. Patients with Hodgkin's disease usually require 0.2 mg/kg daily; patients with other lymphomas or CLL usually require 0.1 mg/kg daily.

• Alternative schedules for treating CLL using intermittent, biweekly, or once-monthly pulse doses of chlorambucil have been reported. Intermittent schedules begin with initial single dose of 0.4 mg/kg. Doses are generally increased by 0.1 mg/kg until lymphocytosis or toxicity is controlled. Subsequent doses are modified to produce mild hematologic toxicity. In CLL, response rate to biweekly or once-monthly dosing schedule equals or exceeds that previously reported with daily administration and hematologic toxicity is less than or equal to that in studies using daily chlorambucil.

• Drug should not be given at full dosages before 4 weeks after full course of radiation therapy or chemotherapy because of possible bone marrow vulnerability to damage. If pretherapy WBC or platelet count is depressed from bone marrow disease before therapy starts, institute treatment at reduced dosage.

• If bone marrow infiltration is confirmed or bone marrow is hypoplastic, daily dosage should not exceed 0.1 mg/kg.

• Drug need not be discontinued if neutrophil count falls; however, decrease dosage if WBC or platelet count falls below normal. Discontinue if more severe bone marrow depression occurs.

⊠ WARNINGS

• Chlorambucil can severely suppress bone marrow function. It is a carcinogen and probably mutagenic and teratogenic. Drug also causes infertility.

Contraindications and precautions

Contraindicated in drug resistance and hypersensitivity to drug or other alkylating agents.

Use cautiously in patients receiving other potentially epileptogenic drugs and in neutropenia, history of seizure disorder or head trauma, bone marrow depression, chickenpox (concurrent or recent, including recent exposure), herpes zoster, gout, urate renal calculi, infection, tumor cell infiltration of bone marrow, previous cytotoxic drug or radiation therapy, and pregnancy or breastfeeding. Safety and efficacy in *children* have not been established.

Preparation and administration

≫ Follow hazardous drug guidelines for handling, preparation, and administration. (See "Managing hazardous drugs," page 11.)

• Give only to patients with CLL or malignant lymphomas.

• Entire daily dose may be given at once.

• Drug may be given at bedtime and with antiemetic to limit GI effects.

• Refrigerate at 36° to 46° F (2° to 8°C).

Adverse reactions

CNS: confusion, agitation, seizures
GI: diarrhea
GU: hyperuremia
Hematologic: thrombocytopenia, leukopenia, pancytopenia (with prolonged use), permanent bone marrow depression
Hepatic: hepatotoxicity, jaundice
Respiratory: fibrosis, pneumonitis, pulmonary dysplasia
Skin: Stevens-Johnson syndrome, alopecia, dermatitis, rash
Other: weight loss

Interactions

Drug-drug. *Anticoagulants, salicylates:* increased risk of bleeding
Blood dyscrasia–causing drugs: increased leukopenia and thrombocytopenia
Bupropion, clozapine, haloperidol, loxapine, MAO inhibitors (including furazolidone and procarbazine), maprotiline, molindone, phenothiazines, pimozide, thioxanthenes, tricyclic antidepressants: lowered seizure threshold, increased risk of seizures
Other antineoplastics: increased toxicity
Other immunosuppressants, including azathio-

Only common or life-threatening adverse reactions are listed.

C

prine, glucocorticoids, corticotropin, cyclophos-phamide, cyclosporine, cytarabine, mercapto-purine, muromonab-CD3, and tacrolimus: increased risk of infection and neoplasms
Drug-diagnostic tests. *ALP, AST, uric acid (serum and urine):* increased
Drug-food. *Any food:* slowed absorption, but no effect on extent of absorption
Drug-herb. *Alpha-lipoic acid, coenzyme Q10:* decreased chemotherapy efficacy
Glutamine: possible enhanced tumor growth

Toxicity and overdose

• Common signs and symptoms of overdose include reversible pancytopenia and neurologic toxicity ranging from agitated behavior and ataxia to multiple generalized tonic-clonic seizures.
• No antidote exists. Institute general supportive measures, with appropriate blood transfusions, if necessary. Drug is not dialyzable.

Special considerations

• Seizures, infertility, leukemia, and secondary malignancies have occurred when drug was used to treat malignant and nonmalignant diseases.
• Small doses of palliative radiation over isolated foci remote from bone marrow usually do not depress neutrophil and platelet counts. In these cases, drug may be given in usual dosage.
• Administering drug to prepubertal and pubertal males caused high incidence of sterility. Prolonged or permanent azoospermia has occurred in adult males. Drug may also produce amenorrhea in females.
• Drug causes relatively few GI adverse effects or other evidence of toxicity (apart from bone marrow depression). Single oral doses of 20 mg or more may produce nausea and vomiting.
• Monitor patient carefully to avoid life-threatening bone marrow damage. Test blood weekly for hemoglobin, total and differential WBC counts, and quantitative platelet counts.

During first 3 to 6 weeks of therapy, check WBC count 3 or 4 days after each weekly CBC.
• Slowly progressive lymphopenia develops during treatment. Lymphocyte count usually returns to normal rapidly when therapy ends.
• Neutropenia usually develops after third week of treatment and may last up to 10 days after last dose. Severe neutropenia appears in patients who received 6.5 mg/kg or more total dosage in one course and in those on continuous dosing schedule.

Patient education

• Instruct patient to take drug at same time every day.
• Inform patient that drug may cause hypersensitivity, drug fever, bone marrow depression, liver problems, infertility, seizures, GI problems, and secondary cancers. Tell him to notify prescriber of rash, bleeding, fever, jaundice, persistent cough, seizures, nausea, vomiting, amenorrhea, and unusual lumps or masses.
• Urge patient to seek immediate medical attention for skin blisters, unusual bleeding or bruising, sudden high fever, seizures, or hallucinations (visual or auditory).
• Caution patient to avoid drug if she is pregnant, considering pregnancy, or breastfeeding.

chlorpromazine hydrochloride
Thorazine, Thorazine Spansule

Classification: Antiemetic, antivertigo agent, phenothiazine
Pregnancy risk category C

Pharmacology

Chlorpromazine is thought to block post-synaptic dopamine receptors in brain. It exerts sedative and antiemetic activity, acting at all CNS levels (primarily subcortical) and on multiorgan systems. It also exerts strong anti-adrenergic and weaker peripheral anticholinergic activity. It possesses slight antihistaminic and antiserotonin properties.

Pharmacokinetics

Drug is metabolized in liver. It is distributed widely, with 95% bound to plasma proteins. Elimination half-life is 10 to 30 hours. Drug is excreted in urine as metabolites. Other factors vary with administration route.

With immediate-release oral use, absorption varies, drug is widely distributed, onset is erratic (30 to 60 minutes), and duration is 4 to 6 hours. With extended-release oral use, onset is 30 to 60 minutes and duration is 10 to 12 hours. With I.V. use, onset is 5 minutes and peak is 10 minutes. With I.M. use, drug is well absorbed; it peaks in 15 to 20 minutes and has a duration of 4 to 8 hours. With rectal use, onset is erratic and duration is 3 hours.

How supplied

Oral concentrate: 30 mg/ml, 100 mg/ml
Solution for injection: 25 mg/ml
Suppositories (rectal): 25 mg, 100 mg
Syrup: 10 mg/5 ml
Tablets: 10 mg, 25 mg, 50 mg, 100 mg, 200 mg

Indications and dosages

FDA-APPROVED

➡ Nausea and vomiting
Adults: 10 to 25 mg P.O. every 4 to 6 hours as needed, increased as necessary. Or 25 mg I.M. initially and then, if no hypotension occurs, 25 to 50 mg I.M. every 3 to 4 hours as needed until vomiting stops; then switch to P.O. form. Or one 100-mg suppository P.R. every 6 to 8 hours as needed.
➡ Intractable hiccups
Adults: 25 to 50 mg P.O. three or four times daily. If symptoms persist for 2 to 3 days after initial dose, give 25 to 50 mg I.M. If symptoms still persist, give 25 to 50 mg by slow I.V. infusion.

DOSAGE MODIFICATIONS

• Lower dosages are usually sufficient for most elderly patients, but observe closely for hypotension and neuromuscular reactions. Tailor dosage to patient, carefully monitor response, and adjust accordingly. Increase more gradually in elderly patients.
• Drug prolongs and intensifies action of CNS depressants, such as anesthetics, barbiturates, and opioids. When administered concomitantly, about 25% to 50% of usual dosage of such agents is required. When drug is not given to reduce requirements of CNS depressants, stop depressants before starting chlorpromazine. These agents may be reinstated at low doses and increased as needed.

Contraindications and precautions

Contraindicated in hypersensitivity to phenothiazines, coma, angle-closure glaucoma, high dose of CNS depressants, and bone marrow depression.

Use cautiously in sulfite sensitivity (parenteral form); chronic respiratory disorders and acute respiratory infections (particularly in children); cardiovascular, hepatic, or renal disease; history of glaucoma; concurrent use of CNS depressants, atropine or related drugs, and drugs that may prolong QT interval; anticipated exposure to extreme heat or organophosphorus insecticides; previously diagnosed breast cancer; glaucoma; and pregnancy or breastfeeding. Also use cautiously in *elderly patients* and *children*.

Preparation and administration

• Solution is clear and colorless to pale yellow. Slight yellowish discoloration does not alter potency. Discard if markedly discolored.
• Avoid getting solution on hands or clothing; may cause contact dermatitis.
• For I.V. use in intractable hiccups, give in 500 to 1,000 ml normal saline solution by slow I.V. infusion.
• For I.M. use, inject slowly, deep into upper outer quadrant of gluteal muscle.

Only common or life-threatening adverse reactions are listed.

C

• For concentrate, add desired amount of concentrate to 60 ml (2 fl oz) or more of diluent just before administration for palatability and stability. Dilute with tomato or fruit juice, milk, simple syrup, orange syrup, carbonated beverages, coffee, tea, or water. Semisolid foods, such as soups and puddings, may also be used.

• Because of hypotensive effects, reserve parenteral use for bedfast or acute ambulatory patient, and have patient lie down for at least 30 minutes after injection. If irritation develops, dilute injection with normal saline solution or 2% procaine; avoid mixing with other agents in syringe. Avoid injecting undiluted drug into vein.

• Subcutaneous injection is not advised.

• After abrupt withdrawal of high-dose therapy, patient may have signs and symptoms resembling those of physical dependence (such as gastritis, nausea and vomiting, dizziness, and tremulousness). To avoid or reduce these, gradually reduce dosage or continue concomitant antiparkinsonians for several weeks after chlorpromazine withdrawal.

• Ampules and multidose vials contain sodium bisulfite and sodium sulfite, which may cause allergic reactions that require drug withdrawal and immediate treatment (including anaphylactic symptoms and life-threatening or less severe asthmatic episodes) in susceptible patients—especially asthmatics.

• Store solution (protected from light), suppositories, and tablets between 59° and 86° F (15° and 30° C). Store oral concentrate below 77° F (25° C) and protect from light.

Adverse reactions
CNS: pseudoparkinsonism, akathisia, dystonia, tardive dyskinesia, seizures, headache, neuroleptic malignant syndrome (NMS), dizziness
CV: orthostatic hypotension (especially with I.V. use), hypertension, cardiac arrest, ECG changes, tachycardia
EENT: blurred vision, dry eyes, glaucoma

GI: dry mouth, nausea, vomiting, diarrhea, anorexia, constipation
GU: urinary retention, enuresis, erectile dysfunction, amenorrhea, gynecomastia, breast engorgement
Hematologic: anemia, leukopenia, leukocytosis, agranulocytosis
Hepatic: jaundice
Respiratory: laryngospasm, dyspnea, respiratory depression
Skin: rash, photosensitivity, dermatitis, blue-gray skin discoloration
Other: weight gain

Interactions
Drug-drug. *Guanethidine and related compounds:* reduced antihypertensive effects
Metrizamide: seizures
Oral anticoagulants: reduced anticoagulant efficacy
Other CNS depressants: additive effects
Propranolol: increased propranolol and chlorpromazine levels
Thiazide diuretics: additive orthostatic hypotension
Drug-diagnostic tests. *Phenylketonuria:* false positive
Drug-herb. *Alfalfa, bergamot, St. John's wort:* increased photosensitization potential
Belladonna: increased anticholinergic effects
Ephedra (ma huang): additive QT-interval prolongation
Evening primrose oil: increased seizure risk
Ginkgo, ginseng, (Panax and Siberian), goldenseal, pomegranate: possible increased chlorpromazine level
L-tryptophan, melatonin, valerian: increased sedation
Yohimbe: markedly increased alpha$_2$-adrenergic antagonism

Toxicity and overdose
• Common signs and symptoms of overdose include CNS depression to somnolence or coma, hypotension, extrapyramidal symptoms, agitation and restlessness, seizures,

fever, autonomic reactions (such as dry mouth and ileus), ECG changes, and arrhythmias.
- Treatment is symptomatic and supportive. Early gastric lavage is helpful. Maintain observation and open airway. Do not induce emesis. Treat extrapyramidal symptoms with antiparkinsonians, barbiturates, or diphenhydramine. Avoid increasing respiratory depression. If stimulant therapy is desirable, give amphetamine, dextroamphetamine, or caffeine with sodium benzoate. Avoid stimulants that may cause seizures (such as picrotoxin or pentylenetetrazol). If hypotension occurs, consider giving vasoconstrictor. Epinephrine is not recommended because it may lower blood pressure further.

Special considerations
- Use cautiously in patients with history of glaucoma. Avoid in patients with angle-closure glaucoma.
- Monitor patient for aspiration of vomitus.
- To reduce risk of adverse reactions related to cumulative drug effect, periodically evaluate patients receiving long-term therapy with chlorpromazine or other antipsychotics to determine if maintenance dosage could be reduced or drug discontinued.
- Antiemetic action may mask signs of overdose of other drugs and obscure diagnosis and treatment of other conditions, such as intestinal obstruction, brain tumor, and Reye's syndrome.
- When used with chemotherapy drugs, drug may mask toxicity of these agents.
- If tardive dyskinesia occurs in patient taking antipsychotics, consider discontinuing drug. However, some patients may require treatment despite tardive dyskinesia.
- If NMS occurs, immediately discontinue antipsychotics and other drugs not essential to concurrent therapy. Institute intensive symptomatic treatment and medical monitoring, and treat concomitant serious problems for which specific treatments are available. Experts disagree on specific pharmacologic treatment regimens for uncomplicated NMS.

- Do not give drug to patients with bone marrow depression or hypersensitivity reaction to phenothiazines (such as blood dyscrasias and jaundice) unless potential benefit outweighs risk. In this setting, pancytopenia from concurrent chemotherapy and chlorpromazine is not a contraindication; however, do not give drug rectally.
- Monitor blood pressure closely when giving drug I.V.

Patient education
- Advise patient to seek immediate medical attention for high temperature, rigid muscles, uncontrollable thirst, difficulty swallowing or breathing, wheezing, light-headedness or fainting, or dizziness when standing or sitting up.
- Caution patient to avoid alcohol during therapy.
- Urge patient to use caution when driving and performing other hazardous activities until drug effects are known.
- Advise patient to avoid strong sunlight on days when he takes drug.
- Advise patient on moderate- or high-dose long-term therapy to have periodic eye examinations.
- Caution breastfeeding patient to avoid taking drug.

cisplatin
Platinol-AQ

Classification: Antineoplastic, platinum coordination complex, alkylating agent
Pregnancy risk category D

Pharmacology
Cisplastin alkylates DNA and RNA, inhibiting enzymes that allow DNA, RNA, and protein synthesis. Activity is cell cycle phase-nonspecific.

Only common or life-threatening adverse reactions are listed.

Pharmacokinetics

Drug is metabolized in liver and distributed widely and rapidly. About 90% is protein-bound. It peaks in 18 to 23 days; duration is about 40 days. Half-life is 30 to 100 hours; drug accumulates in body tissues for several months. It is excreted in urine, with about 20% to 40% eliminated unchanged.

How supplied

Solution for injection: 1 mg/ml in 50-mg and 100-mg vials

Indications and dosages

FDA-APPROVED

➡ Metastatic testicular cancer (in combination with other approved chemotherapeutic agents)
Adults: 20 mg/m² I.V. daily for 5 days
➡ Metastatic ovarian cancer (in combination with cyclophosphamide)
Adults: 75 to 100 mg/m² I.V. once every 4 weeks
➡ Metastatic ovarian cancer refractory to standard chemotherapy in patients who have not previously received cisplatin (monotherapy)
Adults: 100 mg/m² I.V. once every 4 weeks
➡ Advanced bladder cancer (monotherapy)
Adults: 50 to 70 mg/m² I.V. once every 3 to 4 weeks depending on extent of previous exposure to radiation or chemotherapy. For heavily pretreated patients, give 50 mg/m² repeated every 4 weeks.

OFF-LABEL USES (SELECTED)

➡ Soft-tissue sarcoma, mesothelioma, melanoma, osteosarcoma of unknown primary origin, salvage treatment of lymphomas, bone marrow transplant conditioning regimens
Adults: Multiple dosing strategies are available. Refer to specific regimen or protocol.

DOSAGE MODIFICATIONS

• Modify dosage based on previous radiation therapy or chemotherapy.

• Do not give initial or repeat doses unless serum creatinine level is below 1.5 mg/100 ml or BUN level is below 25 mg/100 ml, platelet count is at least 100,000/mm³, and WBC count is at least 4,000/mm³.
• Do not give subsequent doses until audiometric analysis shows auditory acuity within normal limits.
• Dosage may need to be reduced in elderly patients and those with cardiac, hepatic, or renal disease.

WARNINGS

• Cumulative renal toxicity associated with drug is severe. Other major dose-related toxicities are bone marrow depression, nausea, and vomiting.
• Drug may cause significant ototoxicity, which may be more pronounced in children and manifests as tinnitus, loss of high frequency hearing, and occasionally deafness.
• Anaphylactic-like reactions have occurred. Facial edema, bronchoconstriction, tachycardia, and hypotension may arise within minutes of administration. Epinephrine, corticosteroids, and antihistamines have relieved symptoms.

Contraindications and precautions

Contraindicated in allergic reactions to drug or other compounds containing platinum, preexisting renal impairment, bone marrow depression, and hearing impairment.

Use cautiously in neuropathy, pneumococcus vaccination, concurrent radiation therapy, pregnancy or breastfeeding, *elderly patients,* and *children.*

Preparation and administration

≫ Follow hazardous drug guidelines for handling, preparation, and administration. (See "Managing hazardous drugs," page 11.)
• Before giving dose, hydrate patient with 1 to 2 L fluid infused over 8 to 12 hours. Maintain

adequate hydration and urine output during next 24 hours.

• Pretreat with antiemetic. Nausea and anorexia may persist up to 1 week after treatment. Delayed nausea and vomiting, beginning or persisting for 24 hours or more after chemotherapy, may occur.

• Do not use needles of I.V. sets containing aluminum parts; aluminum reacts with drug, causing black precipitate and potency loss.

• Platinol AQ is prediluted to 1 mg/ml. Initially, dilute each 50-mg vial with 50 ml sterile water for injection to yield 1 mg/ml. Withdraw desired dose. Immediately before use, further dilute each half of single dose in 1 L 5% dextrose in one-quarter or one-half normal saline solution, or normal saline solution containing 12.5 to 25 g mannitol. Do not use D₅W.

• Infuse each 1 L of solution over 3 to 4 hours. Administer total dose of 2 L over 6 to 8 hours.

• If diluted solution will not be used within 6 hours, protect from light. Give by I.V. infusion only.

• Anaphylactoid-like reactions to cisplatin have occurred within minutes of administration in patients with previous exposure. Epinephrine, corticosteroids, and antihistamines have relieved symptoms.

• Local soft-tissue toxicity rarely follows extravasation. Severity relates to solution concentration. Infusion of solutions with concentration above 0.5 mg/ml may cause tissue cellulitis, fibrosis, and necrosis.

• Drug remaining in amber vial after initial entry is stable for 28 days when protected from light or for 7 days under fluorescent room light.

• Store at 59° to 77° F (15° to 25° C). Do not refrigerate. Protect unopened container from light.

Adverse reactions

CNS: seizures
CV: cardiac abnormalities

EENT: tinnitus, hearing loss, vestibular toxicity
GI: severe nausea and vomiting, anorexia, diarrhea
GU: renal tubular damage, renal insufficiency, erectile dysfunction, sterility, amenorrhea, gynecomastia, hyperuremia
Hematologic: thrombocytopenia, leukopenia, pancytopenia
Metabolic: hypomagnesemia, hypocalcemia, hypokalemia, hypophosphatemia
Respiratory: fibrosis
Skin: alopecia, dermatitis
Other: weight loss, anaphylaxis, peripheral neuropathy

Interactions

Drug-drug. *Antihistamines, buclizine, cyclizine, loxapine, meclizine, phenothiazines, thioxanthenes, trimethobenzamide:* masking of ototoxicity symptoms, such as tinnitus, dizziness, and vertigo
Bleomycin: renal impairment
Blood dyscrasia–causing drugs: increased leukopenia and thrombocytopenia
Bone marrow depressants: additive bone marrow depression
Nephrotoxic or ototoxic agents: increased risk of ototoxicity and nephrotoxicity
Phenytoin: reduced phenytoin plasma level and efficacy
Drug-diagnostic tests. *BUN, serum creatinine, serum uric acid:* increased (indicating nephrotoxicity)
Coombs' test: positive result (associated with hemolytic anemia)
Creatinine clearance, serum calcium, magnesium, phosphate, potassium, and sodium: decreased
Serum AST, bilirubin: increased
Drug-herb. *Alpha-lipoic acid, coenzyme Q10:* decreased chemotherapy efficacy
Glutamine: possible enhanced tumor growth

Toxicity and overdose

• Common signs and symptoms of overdose include renal or hepatic failure, deafness, ocular toxicity (including retinal detachment),

significant bone marrow depression, intractable nausea and vomiting, or neuritis.
• No proven antidote has been established. Use general supportive measures. Hemodialysis has little effect because of drug's rapid and marked protein-binding.

Special considerations
• Severe neuropathies have occurred with dosages and dosing frequencies greater than recommended.
• Monitor kidney function tests frequently and peripheral blood counts weekly. Periodically monitor liver function tests, and regularly perform neurologic examinations.
• Perform audiometric testing before initiating therapy and before each subsequent dose because drug's ototoxicity is cumulative.

Patient education
• Inform patient that drug may cause serious or fatal allergic reactions, may lower blood counts to dangerous levels, and may affect kidneys and hearing.
• Urge patient to seek immediate medical attention for sudden high fever, unusual bleeding or bruising, seizures, vision changes, hearing loss, difficulty swallowing or breathing, wheezing, light-headedness or fainting, urinary changes, numbness or tingling in arms or legs, or sudden swelling of face, lips, tongue, arms, or legs.
• Inform patient that prescriber may need to change dosage several times for best effect.
• Caution patient to avoid drug if she is pregnant, considering pregnancy, or breastfeeding.
• Advise breastfeeding patient to stop breastfeeding during therapy.

cladribine
Cladribine Novaplus, Leustatin

C

Classification: Antineoplastic, antimetabolite, purine nucleoside analogue
Pregnancy risk category D

Pharmacology
Cladribine's mechanism of action in hairy cell leukemia is unknown. Phosphorylated metabolites accumulate in lymphocytes and monocytes, inducing DNA single-strand breaks and blocking RNA synthesis. This effect eventually and selectively kills these cells. Drug also induces apoptosis. Activity is cell cycle phase-nonspecific.

Pharmacokinetics
After I.V. dose, drug is distributed rapidly; about 20% is protein-bound. Distribution half-life is 36 minutes; elimination half-life, 7 hours. Roughly 15% to 44% is eliminated by kidney.

How supplied
Solution for injection: 10-ml vial (1 mg/ml)

Indications and dosages

FDA-APPROVED
⊖ Active hairy cell leukemia
Adults: 0.09 mg/kg continuous I.V. infusion over 24 hours as single course for 7 consecutive days

OFF-LABEL USES (SELECTED)
➡ Active hairy cell leukemia
Adults: 3.4 mg/m² subcutaneously daily for 7 days may be prescribed.
➡ Cutaneous T-cell lymphoma, chronic lymphocytic leukemia (CLL), non-Hodgkin's lymphoma
Adults: 0.1 mg/kg continuous I.V. infusion over 24 hours daily for 5 to 7 days (repeated every 28 to 35 days) for two to four cycles, or

0.12 mg/kg I.V. piggyback over 2 hours daily for 5 days (repeated every 28 to 35 days) for two to four cycles may be prescribed.

➥ Acute myeloid leukemia

Adults: 5 mg/m^2 I.V. piggyback over 2 hours daily for 5 days with cytarabine 2 g/m^2 I.V. piggyback over 4 hours daily for 5 days with granulocyte-colony stimulating factor 300 mcg subcutaneously daily on days 0 to 5 may be prescribed.

Children: 8.9 mg/m^2 continuous I.V. infusion daily for 5 consecutive days as monotherapy may be prescribed.

DOSAGE MODIFICATIONS

• Consider delaying or discontinuing therapy if neurotoxicity or renal toxicity occurs.

• For patients taking blood dyscrasia–causing drugs, base dosage adjustment on hematologic parameters.

• Dosage reduction may be needed when two or more bone marrow depressants (including radiation) are used concurrently or consecutively with cladribine.

⊠ WARNINGS

• Drug is approved for I.V. infusion only.

• Injection should be administered under supervision of qualified physician experienced in antineoplastic therapy.

• Anticipate bone marrow suppression (usually reversible and probably dose-related).

• Serious neurologic toxicity (including irreversible paraparesis and quadraparesis) appears to be dose-related and has been reported in hairy cell leukemia patients who receive continuous infusion at high dosages (four to nine times recommended levels). Severe neurologic toxicity rarely follows treatment with standard dosages.

• Acute nephrotoxicity has occurred in patients with hairy cell leukemia who receive high doses (four to nine times recommended levels)—especially when drug was given with other nephrotoxic agents or therapies.

Contraindications and precautions

Contraindicated in hypersensitivity to drug or its components.

Use cautiously in known or suspected renal or hepatic insufficiency, active infection, concurrent radiation therapy, and pregnancy or breastfeeding. Also use cautiously in *children* because safety and efficacy have not been established. (However, drug has been given off-label to children with acute myeloid leukemia).

Preparation and administration

• Follow hazardous drug guidelines for handling, preparation, and administration. (See "Managing hazardous drugs," page 11.)

• Dilute with designated diluent.

• Solution is incompatible with D$_5$W.

• Precipitate may form at low temperatures. Warm naturally to room temperature and shake vigorously.

• To prepare single daily dose, add calculated dose to infusion bag containing 500 ml normal saline for injection.

• Don't mix solution with other I.V. drugs or additives or infuse simultaneously through common I.V. line.

• Benzyl alcohol (constituent of recommended diluent for 7-day infusion) has been linked to fatal "gasping syndrome" in premature infants.

• To prepare 7-day ambulatory continuous I.V. infusion, use bacteriostatic normal saline solution and sterile 0.22-micron filter. Admixtures for 7-day infusion are stable for at least 7 days.

• Consider prophylactic therapy with sulfamethoxazole-trimethoprim in patients receiving multiple courses because of drug's prolonged effects on lymphocytes.

• Once solution has been diluted, administer promptly or refrigerate at 36° to 46° F (2° to 8° C) for no more than 8 hours.

Adverse reactions

CNS: fatigue, headache, asthenia, weakness
CV: edema, tachycardia

Only common or life-threatening adverse reactions are listed.

GI: anorexia
Hematologic: thrombocytopenia, anemia, neutropenia, lymphopenia
Musculoskeletal: myalgia, arthralgia
Skin: rash
Other: fever, infection, injection site reactions

Interactions

Drug-drug. *Blood dyscrasia–causing drugs:* increased leukopenia and thrombocytopenia
Other bone marrow depressants: additive bone marrow depression
Drug-herb. *Alpha-lipoic acid, coenzyme Q10:* decreased chemotherapy efficacy
Glutamine: possible enhanced tumor growth

Toxicity and overdose

• High doses have been linked to irreversible neurologic toxicity (paraparesis or quadriparesis), acute nephrotoxicity, and severe bone marrow depression.
• No known antidote exists. Treatment includes drug discontinuation, careful observation, and appropriate supportive measures. Experts do not know if dialysis or hemofiltration removes drug.

Special considerations

• Closely monitor patient for signs and symptoms of hematologic and nonhematologic toxicity. Periodically evaluate peripheral blood counts, particularly during first 4 to 8 weeks after treatment, to detect anemia, neutropenia, thrombocytopenia, and other sequelae (such as infection or bleeding).
• Monitor renal and hepatic function, especially in patients with underlying renal or hepatic impairment.
• Febrile episodes are common and can occur anytime but typically appear 3 to 4 days into therapy (possibly from cytokine release). Because most fevers occur in neutropenic patients, closely monitor these patients during first month of therapy, and give empiric antibiotics as indicated.
• Severe neurologic toxicity rarely follows treatment with standard dosing regimens.

Patient education

• Inform patient that drug may cause serious side effects, such as paralysis, kidney damage, and reduced blood cell counts.
• Advise patient to seek immediate medical attention for fever or unusual bleeding or bruising.
• Caution women with childbearing potential to avoid pregnancy because drug can harm fetus.
• Provide guidance to help breastfeeding patient decide whether to discontinue breastfeeding or stop drug.

clofarabine
Clolar

Classification: Antineoplastic, purine nucleoside antimetabolite
Pregnancy risk category D

Pharmacology

Clofarabine is sequentially converted intracellularly to 5'-monophosphate metabolite by doxycytidine kinase and mono- and disphophokinases and then to active 5' triphosphate form. It inhibits DNA synthesis and disrupts integrity of mitochondrial membrane, leading to programmed cell death. Drug is cytotoxic to rapidly proliferating and quiescent cancer cell types in vitro.

Pharmacokinetics

Drug undergoes negligible hepatic metabolism; CYP450 inhibitors are unlikely to affect metabolism. It is 47% bound to plasma proteins (mainly albumin). Parent compound has terminal half-life of about 5 hours; active compound, 24 hours. Most of dose (49% to 60%) is excreted unchanged in urine.

How supplied

Solution for injection: 1 mg/ml (20 mg in 20-ml flint vials)

Indications and dosages

FDA-APPROVED

➠ Relapsed or refractory acute lymphoblastic leukemia after at least two previous regimens
Children ages 1 to adults age 21: 52 mg/m^2 by I.V. infusion over 2 hours daily for 5 consecutive days every 2 to 6 weeks, depending on toxicity and response

OFF-LABEL USES (SELECTED)

➠ Relapsed or refractory acute myeloid leukemia
Children: 52 mg/m^2 by I.V. infusion over 2 hours daily for 5 consecutive days every 2 to 6 weeks, depending on toxicity and response
➠ Relapsed or refractory acute leukemias
Adults: 40 mg/m^2 by I.V. infusion over 2 hours daily for 5 consecutive days every 2 to 6 weeks, depending on toxicity and response (monotherapy)
Elderly patients (newly diagnosed): As combination therapy, 40 mg/m^2 as I.V. infusion over 1 hour daily for 5 days (days 2 to 6), followed 4 hours later by cytarabine (ara-C) 1 g/m^2 as I.V. infusion over 2 hours daily for 5 days (days 1 to 5)

DOSAGE MODIFICATIONS

• Repeat treatment cycles after recovery or return to baseline organ function, about every 2 to 6 weeks. Base dosage on patient's body surface area, calculated using height and weight before start of each cycle.
• Stop drug if hypotension develops during the 5 days of treatment. If hypotension is transient and resolves without drug intervention, reinstitute drug (generally at lower dosage).
• Discontinue drug immediately if patient has significant signs or symptoms (such as hypotension) of systemic inflammatory response syndrome (SIRS) or capillary leak syndrome (CLS). Consider giving steroids, diuretics, and albumin. Drug may be reinstituted when patient is stable (generally at lower dosage).
• If creatinine or bilirubin levels rise significantly, discontinue drug. Reinstitute (possibly at lower dosage) when patient is stable and organ function returns to baseline.

Contraindications and precautions

No known contraindications exist.
  Use cautiously in renal or hepatic impairment, active infection, dehydration, hypotension, risk of tumor lysis syndrome (which may result in SIRS or CLS and organ dysfunction), and pregnancy or breastfeeding. Safety and efficacy in adults have not been established; however, drug has been given to adults with relapsed or refractory acute leukemias.

Preparation and administration

• Evaluate hepatic and renal function before and during treatment. Closely monitor respiratory status and blood pressure during infusion.
• Prophylactic steroids (such as 100 mg/m^2 hydrocortisone on days 1 through 3) may help prevent SIRS or CLS. If early signs or symptoms occur, immediately stop drug and use appropriate supportive measures.
• Filter through sterile 0.22-micron syringe filter; then further dilute with D$_5$W or normal saline for injection before I.V. infusion. Resulting admixture may be stored at room temperature, but must be used within 24 hours.
• To prevent incompatibilities, do not administer other drugs through same I.V. line.
• Give continuous I.V. fluids throughout 5 days of treatment to reduce effects of tumor lysis and other adverse events. Administer allopurinol if hyperuricemia is expected.
• Store vials containing undiluted drug at 77° F (25° C); excursions are permitted to 59° to 86° F (15° to 30° C).

Adverse reactions

CNS: headache, fatigue, dizziness, anxiety, irritability, depression, lethargy, tremor, rigors
CV: hypertension, hypotension, flushing, tachycardia, pericardial effusions, transient left ventricular systolic dysfunction, edema
GI: decreased appetite, constipation, diarrhea, nausea, vomiting, abdominal pain

---

Only common or life-threatening adverse reactions are listed.

Hematologic: anemia, leukopenia, thrombocytopenia, neutropenia (Grade III or IV about 10%)
Hepatic: hepatomegaly, jaundice
Musculoskeletal: arthralgia, back pain, myalgia, limb pain
Respiratory: cough, dyspnea, pleural effusion, respiratory distress
Skin: rash, dermatitis, erythema, dry skin, palmar-plantar erythrodysesthesia syndrome, pruritus
Other: SIRS or CLS, fever of unknown origin, pyrexia, tumor lysis syndrome, injection site pain

Interactions
Drug-diagnostic tests. *ALT, AST, bilirubin:* increased
Drug-herb. *Alpha-lipoic acid, coenzyme Q10:* decreased chemotherapy efficacy
Glutamine: possible enhanced tumor growth

Toxicity and overdose
• Toxicities include hyperbilirubinemia, vomiting, maculopapular rash, cardiotoxicity (tachycardia, peripheral perfusion) and bone marrow depression.
• No specific antidote exists. Treat supportively.

Special considerations
• Avoid concurrent use of drugs that may cause renal or hepatic toxicity during 5 days of therapy. Closely monitor patients receiving drugs that affect blood pressure or cardiac function.
• Monitor patient for signs and symptoms of tumor lysis syndrome or cytokine release (such as tachypnea, tachycardia, hypotension, and pulmonary edema) that could develop into SIRS, CLS, or organ dysfunction.
• Monitor hematologic status closely; drug may cause severe bone marrow depression, including neutropenia, anemia, and thrombocytopenia.
• Closely monitor renal and hepatic function during 5 days of therapy.

• ALT and AST elevations are transient; they typically occur within 1 week of administration and last less than 2 weeks. Increased bilirubin level is less common but more persistent, with median time to recovery from Grade III/IV to Grade II of about 6 days.

Patient education
• Counsel patient about appropriate measures to avoid dehydration caused by diarrhea and vomiting.
• Instruct patient to contact prescriber if dizziness, light-headedness, fainting, or decreased urine output occurs.
• Caution women with childbearing potential to avoid becoming pregnant during therapy.
• Advise breastfeeding patient to stop breastfeeding during therapy.

codeine phosphate
codeine sulfate

Classification: Opioid analgesic, antitussive
Controlled substance schedule II
Pregnancy risk category C

Pharmacology
Codeine is a centrally active analgesic with agonist activity at opiate centers. It also depresses respirations and cough center, initiates antidiuretic hormone release, activates vomiting center, causes pupillary constriction, reduces intestinal motility, increases biliary tract pressure and ureteral contraction amplitude, and decreases gastric, pancreatic, and biliary secretions.

Pharmacokinetics
Drug is metabolized in liver. Onset is 10 to 30 minutes; peak, about 30 minutes to 1 hour. Its duration is 4 to 6 hours; half-life, about 3 hours. Drug crosses placental barrier and appears in breast milk. It is excreted by kidneys.

How supplied

Oral solution: 15 mg/5 ml
Solution for injection (phosphate): 15 mg/ml,
30 mg/ml
Tablets: 30 mg, 60 mg (phosphate); 15 mg, 30
mg, 60 mg (sulfate)

Indications and dosages

FDA-APPROVED

➟ Mild to moderate pain
Adults: 15 to 60 mg P.O. every 4 to 6 hours as
needed, or 15 to 60 mg I.M. or subcutaneously (phosphate) every 4 to 6 hours as needed
Children age 1 and older: 0.5 mg/kg or 15
mg/m^2 P.O. every 4 to 6 hours. Dosages above
1.5 mg/kg are not recommended.
➟ Cough
Adults: 10 to 20 mg P.O. every 4 to 6 hours,
not to exceed 120 mg daily
Children: 1 to 1.5 mg/kg P.O. daily in four divided doses, not to exceed 60 mg daily

OFF-LABEL USES (SELECTED)

➟ Diarrhea
Adults: 30 mg P.O.; may repeat four times daily as needed

DOSAGE MODIFICATIONS

• Adjust dosage according to pain severity
and response.
• When giving with other opioid analgesics,
general anesthetics, phenothiazines, tranquilizers, sedative-hypnotics, or other CNS depressants, reduce dosage of one or both drugs.
• For patients with renal disease and creatinine clearance of 10 to 50 ml/minute, give
75% of dose; if creatinine clearance is less
than 10 ml/minute, give 50%.

Contraindications and precautions

Contraindicated in hypersensitivity to drug or
its components.
   Use cautiously in Addison's disease, hypothyroidism, arrhythmias, head injury and increased intracranial pressure, acute abdominal
conditions, prostatic hypertrophy, urethral
stricture, renal or hepatic dysfunction, debilitated or **elderly patients,** and pregnancy or
breastfeeding.

Preparation and administration

• Prepare solution for injection with sterile
water, and filter through 0.22-micron membrane filter.
• Do not use solution if it is more than slightly discolored or contains precipitate.
• Do not mix with other solutions for injection.

Adverse reactions

CNS: drowsiness, sedation, dizziness, agita-
tion, lethargy, restlessness, euphoria, seizures
CV: bradycardia, palpitations, orthostatic hy-
potension, tachycardia, circulatory collapse
GI: nausea, vomiting, anorexia, constipation
GU: urinary retention
Respiratory: respiratory depression, respira-
tory paralysis
Skin: flushing, rash, urticaria, pruritus
Other: dependency, anaphylaxis

Interactions

Drug-drug. *General anesthetics, other CNS depressants, other opioid analgesics, phenothiazines,
sedative-hypnotics, skeletal muscle relaxants,
tranquilizers:* additive depressant effects
MAO inhibitors: increased toxicity
Drug-diagnostic tests. *Serum amylase, lipase:*
increased
Drug-herb. *Corkwood:* increased anticholinergic effect
Ginseng (Panax *and Siberian*), *goldenseal, kava,
pomegranate:* increased codeine level
*Jamaican dogwood, kava, lavender, mistletoe, net-
tle, pokeweed, poppy, senega, valerian:* increased
CNS depression
St. John's wort: increased sedation and in-
creased analgesia

Toxicity and overdose
- Common signs and symptoms of overdose include respiratory depression, sedation, and miosis. Other symptoms include nausea and vomiting, skeletal muscle flaccidity, bradycardia, hypotension, and cool, clammy skin. Apnea, death, and noncardiac pulmonary edema also may occur.
- Protect airway and support ventilation and perfusion. Meticulously monitor and maintain acceptable vital signs, blood gas values, and serum electrolyte levels. Activated charcoal may decrease drug absorption from GI tract. Charcoal has been more effective than emesis or lavage; consider charcoal instead of or in addition to gastric emptying.

Special considerations
- Drug may prolong labor and produce respiratory depression in newborn. Patient may require resuscitation and, in severe depression, naloxone.
- Drug may have prolonged cumulative effect in patients with renal or hepatic impairment.

Patient education
- Urge patient to seek immediate medical attention for difficulty swallowing or breathing, wheezing, light-headedness or fainting, or dizziness when standing or sitting up.
- Instruct patient to use caution when driving and performing other hazardous activities until drug effects are known.
- Advise patient to avoid taking drug with other opioids, sedative-hypnotics, phenothiazines, or alcohol because of additive depressant effects.

cyclophosphamide
Cytoxan, Cytoxan Lyophilized, Neosar

C

Classification: Antineoplastic, alkylating agent, nitrogen mustard derivative, disease-modifying antirheumatic agent
Pregnancy risk category D

Pharmacology
Cyclophosphamide is converted in liver to active alkylating metabolites, which impede growth of susceptible rapidly proliferating cancer cells. Action is thought to involve cross-linking of tumor cell DNA.

Pharmacokinetics
Drug is well absorbed after oral dose (75% bioavailability) and metabolized to inactive forms in liver. It peaks about 1 hour after oral dose and 2 to 3 hours after I.V. dose. Elimination half-life is 3 to 12 hours. It is excreted in urine.

How supplied
Solution for injection: 75 mg mannitol/100 mg cyclophosphamide in 100-mg, 200-mg, 1-g, and 2-g single-dose vials
Tablets: 25 mg, 50 mg

Indications and dosages

FDA-APPROVED

➥ Malignant lymphomas (Stages III and IV of Ann Arbor system), Hodgkin's disease, lymphocytic lymphoma (nodular or diffuse), mixed-cell type lymphoma, histiocytic lymphoma, Burkitt's lymphoma, multiple myeloma, chronic lymphocytic leukemia, chronic granulocytic leukemia, acute myelogenous and monocytic leukemia, acute lymphoblastic (stem cell) leukemia in children, mycosis fungoides (advanced), neuroblastoma (disseminated), ovarian adenocarcinoma, retinoblastoma, carcinoma of breast

Adults and children: 40 to 50 mg/kg I.V. in divided doses over 2 to 5 days; or 10 to 15 mg/kg I.V. every 7 to 10 days; or 3 to 5 mg/kg I.V. twice weekly; or 1 to 5 mg/kg P.O. daily for initial and maintenance dosing

Off-label uses (selected)

➥ Breast, ovarian, cervical, bladder, head and neck, prostrate, and lung cancer (usually small-cell); Ewing's sarcoma
Adults and children: Multiple dosing strategies exist. See specific protocol or regimen. Typical dosage is 60 to 120 mg/m² P.O. or I.V. daily for up to 14 days every 4 to 6 weeks; or 1 to 2.5 mg/kg P.O. or I.V. daily for up to 14 days every 4 to 6 weeks; or 400 to 1,500 mg/m² I.V. every 21 to 28 days.

Dosage modifications

• Adjust dosage based on antitumor activity or leukopenia. Total WBC count is a good objective guide for regulating dosage. Transient decreases in total WBCs to 2,000/mm³ (after short courses) or more persistent reduction to 3,000/mm³ (with continuing therapy) are tolerated without serious infection risk, except in marked granulocytopenia.
• After adrenalectomy, dosages of both replacement steroids and cyclophosphamide may need adjustment.
• For patients taking blood dyscrasia–causing drugs, cyclophosphamide dosage may need adjustment based on hematologic parameters.
• Dosage reduction may be required for patients receiving two or more bone marrow depressants (including radiation) concurrently or consecutively.
• Other hepatic CYP450 enzyme inducers/inhibitors may affect drug blood levels, requiring dosage adjustments.
• Consider dosage adjustment in patients with renal or hepatic insufficiency.
• Serious and sometimes fatal infections may develop in severely immunosuppressed patients. In patients who have or develop viral, bacterial, fungal, protozoan, or helminthic infections, drug may not be indicated, therapy

should be interrupted, or dosage should be reduced.

Contraindications and precautions

Contraindicated in hypersensitivity to drug and severely depressed bone marrow function.

Use cautiously in leukopenia, thrombocytopenia, tumor cell infiltration of bone marrow, renal or hepatic impairment, previous radiation therapy or therapy with other cytotoxic agents, and concurrent administration of other CYP450 enzyme inducers/inhibitors. Also use cautiously in pregnancy, breastfeeding, *elderly patients,* and *children.*

Preparation and administration

≫ Follow hazardous drug guidelines for handling, preparation, and administration. (See "Managing hazardous drugs," page 11.)
• Dilute each 100 mg with 5 ml sterile water for injection to yield 20 mg/ml. May further dilute with 100 to 250 ml D₅W, normal saline solution, 5% dextrose in normal saline solution, or lactated Ringer's solution.
• Shake solution well and allow to stand until clear.
• Drug may be given by I.V. push (each 100 mg given over 1 minute).
• Intermittent infusion is recommended for doses above 500 mg. Dilute with 100 to 250 ml D₅W, normal saline solution, 5% dextrose in normal saline solution, or lactated Ringer's solution; give over 20 to 60 minutes.
• Store at or below 77° F (25° C). Product withstands brief exposure up to 86° F (30° C) but should be protected from temperatures above 86° F.

Adverse reactions

CNS: headache, dizziness
CV: cardiotoxicity (with high doses)
GI: nausea, vomiting, diarrhea, colitis
GU: gonadal suppression, sterility, hemorrhagic cystitis
Hematologic: thrombocytopenia, leukopenia, pancytopenia, bone marrow depression

---

Only common or life-threatening adverse reactions are listed.

Hepatic: hepatotoxicity
Metabolic: syndrome of inappropriate antidiuretic hormone secretion, hyperuricemia
Respiratory: fibrosis
Skin: alopecia, dermatitis
Other: weight loss, secondary neoplasms, anaphylaxis

Interactions

Drug-drug. *Blood dyscrasia–causing drugs:* increased leukopenia and thrombocytopenia
Cocaine: reduced or slowed cocaine metabolism, increasing or prolonging its effects and increasing risk of toxicity
Cytarabine: increased risk of cardiomyopathy
Daunorubicin, doxorubicin: increased cardiotoxicity
Lovastatin: increased risk of rhabdomyolysis and acute renal failure
Oral anticoagulants: increased or decreased anticoagulant activity
Other bone marrow depressants: additive bone marrow depression
Other CYP450 enzyme inducers/inhibitors: interference with cyclophosphamide conversion to its active moiety, with possible effect on drug blood level
Other immunosuppressants, such as azathioprine, chlorambucil, cyclosporine, glucocorticoids, mercaptopurine, and muromonab-CD3: increased risk of infection and neoplasm development
Phenobarbital: increased metabolism and leukopenic activity of cyclophosphamide
Succinylcholine chloride: increased succinylcholine effect
Drug-diagnostic tests. Candida, *mumps, trichophyton, tuberculin PPD skin tests:* suppressed positive reactions
Papanicolaou test: false-positive
Serum pseudocholinesterase: decreased
Serum and urine uric acid: increased
Drug-food. *Grapefruit juice:* increased drug level
Drug-herb. *Alpha-lipoic acid, coenzyme Q10:* decreased chemotherapy efficacy
Cat's claw, echinacea, eucalyptus, feverfew, kava, licorice, peppermint oil, pomegranate, valerian: increased drug level
Glutamine: possible enhanced tumor growth
Melatonin: stimulated immune fraction

Toxicity and overdose

• Signs and symptoms of overdose include nausea, vomiting, cardiotoxicity, bone marrow depression, infection, anorexia, and alopecia.
• No specific antidote exists. Treatment is supportive and may include transfusions and dialysis (which removes about 30% of drug).

Special considerations

• Monitor hematologic profile (particularly neutrophils and platelets) regularly to determine degree of hematopoietic suppression. Examine urine regularly for RBCs.
• Drug has caused secondary cancers (most commonly urinary bladder, myeloproliferative, or lymphoproliferative).
• Drug interferes with oogenesis and spermatogenesis and may cause sterility in both sexes.
• Hemorrhagic cystitis may occur, which may be severe and even fatal (though rarely). Forcing fluid intake helps ensure ample urine output, necessitates frequent voiding, and reduces time drug stays in bladder. Mesna may also be given by I.V. bolus as prophylaxis.
• Serious and sometimes fatal infections may develop in severely immunosuppressed patients.
• Emetogenic potential depends on dosing; nausea and vomiting are commonly delayed.

Patient education

• Tell patient that if he forgets dose, he should take it as soon as he remembers and then take next dose at regular time.
• Instruct patient to drink 3 to 4 L of fluid over at least 24 hours after receiving dose.
• Advise patient to seek immediate medical attention for fever, tiredness, bladder pain, bloody urine, difficulty swallowing or breathing, wheezing, light-headedness or fainting, or dizziness when standing or sitting up.

• Caution women with childbearing potential to avoid pregnancy during therapy because drug may harm fetus.
• Provide guidance to help breastfeeding patient decide whether to discontinue breastfeeding or stop drug.

cytarabine
Cytosar-U

cytarabine liposome
DepoCyt

Classification: Antineoplastic, antimetabolite
Pregnancy risk category D

Pharmacology
Cytarabine primarily kills cells undergoing DNA synthesis. It inhibits DNA polymerase by competing with deoxycytidine triphosphate, ultimately inhibiting DNA synthesis and under certain conditions, blocking cell progression from G1 phase to S phase. Activity is cell cycle phase-specific.

Pharmacokinetics
Drug is metabolized mainly in liver and rapidly distributed throughout body. Highest concentrations occur in intestines, liver, and kidney. With I.V. or subcutaneous dose, drug peaks within 20 to 60 minutes. Elimination half-life is 7 to 20 minutes; terminal half-life, about 2 hours. About 80% of dose is eliminated in urine as metabolites within 24 to 36 hours.
   Liposomal form is metabolized in liver and peaks within 5 hours. Half-life is 100 to 236 hours. Drug is excreted in urine mainly as inactive metabolite.

How supplied
Powder for injection (conventional form): 100-mg, 500-mg, 1-g, and 2-g vials

Solution for injection (liposomal form): 50 mg in 5-ml, single-use vial

Indications and dosages

FDA-APPROVED

➡ Remission induction in acute nonlymphocytic leukemia (used in combination)
Adults and children: 100 mg/m² daily (conventional form) by continuous I.V. infusion (days 1 to 7) or 100 mg/m² (conventional form) I.V. every 12 hours (days 1 to 7)
➡ Postremission therapy in acute nonlymphocytic leukemia (used in combination)
Adults and children: 1 to 3 g/m² (conventional form) I.V. infusion over 1 to 3 hours every 12 hours for 3 to 6 days. Most common regimen is 3 g/m² daily (conventional form) infused over 3 hours every 12 hours on days 1, 3, and 5 for six doses in patients younger than age 60.
➡ Acute lymphocytic leukemia
Adults and children: For multidose strategies, see specific regimens. High-dose cytarabine (conventional form) is given as 1 to 3 g/m² I.V. piggyback over 1 to 3 hours for 2 to 4 doses. For induction phase, 75 to 150 mg/m² (conventional form) I.V. daily on designated days.
➡ Blast phase of chronic myelocytic leukemia
Adults and children: Treat as for acute leukemia. See specific regimen.
➡ Prophylaxis and treatment of meningeal leukemia
Adults: 5 to 75 mg/m² intrathecally once daily for 4 days or once every 4 days until cerebrospinal fluid (CSF) findings are normal, followed by one additional treatment (conventional form). Alternative treatment schedule is twice weekly (conventional form) until CSF clears, then weekly for 4 weeks. However, multiple strategies exist.
◉ Lymphomatous meningitis
Adults: For induction therapy, 50 mg (liposomal form) intrathecally (intraventricular or lumbar puncture) every 14 days for two doses

---

Only common or life-threatening adverse reactions are listed.

(weeks 1 and 3); for consolidation therapy, 50 mg (liposomal form) intrathecally (intraventricular or lumbar puncture) every 14 days for three doses (weeks 5, 7, and 9), followed by one additional dose at week 13. For maintenance, 50 mg (liposomal form) intrathecally (intraventricular or lumbar puncture) every 28 days for four doses (weeks 17, 21, 25, and 29). Give dexamethasone 4 mg P.O. or I.V. twice daily for 5 days, starting on day of liposome injection, with each treatment.

OFF-LABEL USES (SELECTED)

➥ Hodgkin's and non-Hodgkin's lymphoma
Adults: Combination therapy with cisplatin 100 mg/m² by continuous I.V. over 24 hours on day 1, cytarabine 2 g/m² I.V. over 3 hours every 12 hours on day 2, and dexamethasone 40 mg P.O. or I.V. on days 1 to 4

DOSAGE MODIFICATIONS

• If drug-induced neurotoxicity develops with liposomal form, reduce dosage to 25 mg. If neurotoxicity persists, discontinue drug.
• If given with blood dyscrasia–causing drugs, adjust dosage, if necessary, based on hematologic parameters.
• Dosage reduction may be required when two or more bone marrow depressants (including radiation) are used concurrently or consecutively.
• Consider suspending drug or modifying therapy if drug-induced bone marrow depression results in platelet count below 50,000/mm³ or polymorphonuclear granulocyte count below 1,000/mm³.
• Use caution when giving high doses to patients with impaired hepatic or renal function because of increased risk of neurotoxicity.

⊠ WARNINGS

Cytarabine
• For induction, patients should be treated in facility with laboratory and supportive resources sufficient to monitor drug tolerance

and protect and maintain patient compromised by drug toxicity.
• Physician must judge drug's possible benefit against toxic effects in considering if therapy is advisable.
Cytarabine liposome
• Chemical arachnoiditis (manifested primarily by nausea, vomiting, headache, and fever) is a common adverse event that may be fatal if left untreated. Give drug concurrently with dexamethasone to reduce incidence and mitigate symptoms.

Contraindications and precautions
Contraindicated in hypersensitivity to drug or its components (cytarabine and cytarabine liposome) and in active meningeal infection (cytarabine liposome).

Use cautiously in preexisting bone marrow depression, hepatic or renal impairment, concurrent radiation therapy, pregnancy or breastfeeding, and in **elderly patients,** especially those with renal impairment. Liposomal form is not recommended in breastfeeding women. Safety and efficacy of liposomal form in **children** have not been established.

Preparation and administration
• Follow hazardous drug guidelines for handling, preparation, and administration. (See "Managing hazardous drugs," page 11.)
Cytarabine
• Give dexamethasone eyedrops before high-dose cytarabine, and continue for at least 24 hours after administration to prevent conjunctivitis.
• High-dose cytarabine is highly emetogenic; use aggressive antiemetic therapy.
• Reconstitute each 100 mg with 5 ml bacteriostatic water for injection for I.V. infusion with benzyl alcohol 0.945% weight/volume added as preservative. Resulting solution contains 20 mg/ml.
• For intrathecal administration, reconstitute with preservative-free normal saline solution for injection; use immediately. Do not use bac-

teriostatic water for injection with benzyl alcohol.

- For infusion, may further dilute with normal saline solution or D_5W and give over 30 minutes to 24 hours, depending on dose and amount of solution.
- Patients can tolerate higher total doses when given conventional form by rapid I.V. injection rather than slow infusion.
- Do not give high doses as continuous I.V. infusion.
- Store at 68° to 77° F (20° to 25° C).

Cytarabine liposome
- Administer dexamethasone 4 mg twice daily P.O. or I.V. for 5 days, starting on day of liposome injection.
- Administer by intrathecal route only. Further dilution is not recommended.
- Allow drug to warm to room temperature before withdrawing from vial.
- Withdraw from vial immediately before administration and use within 4 hours. Avoid aggressive agitation. Do not mix with other drugs or save unused portions.
- Do not use in-line filters. Administer directly into CSF through intraventricular reservoir or by direct injection into lumbar sac. Inject slowly over 1 to 5 minutes. After administration by lumbar puncture, instruct patient to lie flat for 1 hour. Observe patient and watch for immediate toxic reactions.
- Refrigerate at 36° to 46° F (2° to 8° C). Do not freeze.

Adverse reactions

CNS: neuritis, dizziness, headache, personality changes, ataxia, mechanical dysphagia, coma, chemical arachnoiditis
CV: thrombophlebitis, chest pain, cardiopathy
EENT: conjunctivitis, sore throat
GI: nausea, vomiting, diarrhea, anorexia, stomatitis, abdominal pain, hematemesis, GI hemorrhage
GU: urinary retention, hyperuricemia, renal failure
Hematologic: bleeding, thrombocytopenia, leukopenia, bone marrow depression, anemia

Hepatic: hepatotoxicity
Musculoskeletal: bone pain
Respiratory: pneumonia, dyspnea, pulmonary edema (with high doses)
Skin: rash, fever, freckling, cellulitis
Other: anaphylaxis, cytarabine syndrome (malaise 6 to12 hours after administration, including fever, myalgia, bone pain, chest pain, rash, and conjunctivitis)

Interactions
Cytarabine
Drug-drug. *Blood dyscrasia–causing drugs:* increased leukopenia and thrombocytopenia
Bone marrow depressants: additive bone marrow depression
Cyclophosphamide: increased risk of cardiomyopathy
Other immunosuppressants (such as azathioprine, chlorambucil, corticosteroids, cyclophosphamide, cyclosporine, glucocorticoids, mercaptopurine, muromonab CD-3, and tacrolimus): increased risk of infection
Methotrexate: synergistic cytotoxic effect
Drug-diagnostic tests. *ALP, AST, bilirubin:* increased
Drug-herb. *Alpha-lipoic acid, coenzyme Q10:* decreased chemotherapy efficacy
Glutamine: possible enhanced tumor growth
Thuja: possible decreased seizure threshold

Toxicity and overdose
- Signs and symptoms of overdose include nausea, vomiting, bone marrow depression, CNS toxicity, and megoblastosis.
- No antidote for overdose exists. Treatment is supportive and may include transfusions.

Special considerations
- Monitor patient closely. Frequent platelet and WBC counts and bone marrow examinations are mandatory.
- Periodically check liver and kidney function test results.
- Perform neurologic evaluations and cerebellar assessment in patients receiving high doses.

Only common or life-threatening adverse reactions are listed.

- Carefully interpret CSF results after liposome administration; liposome particles resemble WBCs in size and appearance.

Patient education
- Instruct patient to seek immediate medical attention for mouth ulcers, tiredness, unusual bleeding or bruising, frequent infections, or seizures.
- Inform patient receiving liposomal form that drug may cause headache, nausea, vomiting, and fever. Emphasize importance of taking concurrent dexamethasone at start of each treatment cycle. Instruct patient to seek medical attention for signs and symptoms of neurotoxicity, including personality changes and staggering gait.
- Tell patient who is pregnant or has childbearing potential that drug may harm fetus. Discuss whether pregnancy continuation is advisable. Inform her that fetal risk decreases when therapy starts during second or third trimester. Caution women receiving liposomal form to avoid pregnancy.
- Provide guidance to help breastfeeding patient decide whether to discontinue breastfeeding or stop drug.

dacarbazine (DTIC)
DTIC-Dome

Classification: Antineoplastic, alkylating agent, triazene, imidazole carboxamide
Pregnancy risk category C

Pharmacology
Dacarbazine alkylates and inhibits DNA and RNA synthesis. It also inhibits enzymes that allow amino acid synthesis in proteins and is responsible for cross-linking DNA strands. It appears to form methylcarbonium ions that attack nucleophilic groups in DNA. Exact mechanism of action is unknown. Activity is cell cycle phase-nonspecific.

Pharmacokinetics
Drug is activated by microsomal liver enzymes and further metabolized rapidly in liver to inactive forms. Elimination half-life is 3 to 5 hours. It is excreted mainly in urine.

How supplied
Powder for injection: 100 mg, 200 mg, 500 mg

Indications and dosages

FDA-APPROVED
➡ Metastatic malignant melanoma
Adults: 2 to 4.5 mg/kg I.V. daily for 10 days, repeated at 4-week intervals; or 250 mg/m^2 I.V. daily for 5 days, repeated every 3 weeks. Or, in CVD regimen (cisplatin, vinblastine, and dacarbazine), 800 mg/m^2 I.V. on day 1, repeated every 21 days.
➡ Hodgkin's lymphoma
Adults: 150 mg/m^2 I.V. for 5 days in combination with other effective drugs, repeated every 4 weeks. Or 375 mg/m^2 I.V. on day 1 in combination with other effective drugs every 15 days (ABVD regimen).

OFF-LABEL USES (SELECTED)
➡ Soft-tissue sarcoma
Adults: MAID regimen (mesna 2,500 mg/m^2 daily, doxorubicin 20 mg/m^2 daily, ifosfamide 2,500 mg/m^2 daily, and dacarbazine 300 mg/m^2 daily), all by continuous I.V. infusion for 3 days, plus an additional dose of mesna 2,500 mg/m^2 on fourth day
➡ Islet-cell carcinoma and carcinoid tumors
Adults: Doxorubicin 60 mg/m^2 on day 1 and dacarbazine 250 mg/m^2 on days 1 to 5, alternating every 4 weeks with streptozocin 500 mg/m^2 and fluorouracil 400 mg/m^2 daily for 5 days, all by continuous I.V. infusion
➡ Malignant pheochromocytoma
Adults: ACVD regimen (Adriamycin, cyclophosphamide, vincristine, and dacarbazine), with doxorubicin 40 mg/m^2 given on day 1, cyclophosphamide 750 mg/m^2 on day 1, vincristine 1.4 mg/m^2 on day 1, and dacarbazine 250 mg/m^2 on days 1 to 5 every 3 to 4 weeks;

or traditional regimen (CVD without adriamycin), all by continuous I.V. infusion

DOSAGE MODIFICATIONS

• Hematopoietic toxicity may warrant temporary suspension or cessation of therapy.
• Reduce dosage in patients with impaired renal and hepatic function.

⊠ WARNINGS

• Hematopoietic depression is most common
toxic event. Hepatic necrosis has been reported.
• Carefully weigh potential benefits against
risk of toxicity.

Contraindications and precautions

Contraindicated in hypersensitivity to drug or
its components.
   Use cautiously in concurrent radiation
therapy, pregnancy or breastfeeding, and in
elderly patients, especially those with renal
impairment. Safety and efficacy in *children*
have not been established.

Preparation and administration

≫ Follow hazardous drug guidelines for
handling, preparation, and administration.
(See "Managing hazardous drugs," page 11.)
• Give prophylactic antiemetics. Prophylactic
antibiotics may be indicated for febrile neutropenic patient, depending on culture and
sensitivity test results.
• Reconstitute with sterile water for injection
to yield 10 mg/ml.
• Reconstituted solution may be diluted further with 50 to 250 ml D_5W or normal saline
solution, and given as I.V. infusion.
• Infuse total dose over 30 to 60 minutes.
• Subcutaneous extravasation during I.V. administration may cause tissue damage and severe pain. Apply hot packs to relieve local
pain, burning sensation, and irritation at injection site.

• After reconstitution, unused solution may
be stored at 39° F (4° C) for up to 72 hours or
at normal room temperature and lighting for
up to 8 hours. If further diluted, resulting solution may be stored at 39° F for up to 24
hours or at normal room conditions for up to
8 hours.

Adverse reactions

CNS: facial paresthesia, malaise
GI: nausea, vomiting, anorexia
Hematologic: thrombocytopenia, leukopenia,
anemia
Hepatic: hepatotoxicity (rare)
Skin: alopecia, dermatitis, pain at injection
site, extravasation, severe photosensitivity re-
actions
Other: anaphylaxis, flushing, fever

Interactions

Drug-drug. *Blood dyscrasia–causing drugs:* increased leukopenia and thrombocytopenia
Bone marrow depressants: additive bone marrow depression
CYPIA2 and 2E1 inhibitors: increased dacarbazine levels and effects
CYPIA2 and 2E1 inducers: decreased dacarbazine levels and effects
Hepatic enzyme inducers: enhanced dacarbazine metabolism
Drug-diagnostic tests. *ALP, ALT, AST, bilirubin:* increased, indicating possible hepatotoxicity
BUN: increased (transient)
Drug-herb. *Alpha-lipoic acid, coenzyme Q10:*
decreased chemotherapy efficacy
Glutamine: possible enhanced tumor growth

Toxicity and overdose

• Signs and symptoms of overdose include
bone marrow depression and diarrhea.
• No specific antidote exists. Provide supportive treatment and monitor blood counts.
Whole blood products may be administered.

Only common or life-threatening adverse reactions are listed.

Special considerations
• Possibility of bone marrow depression necessitates careful WBC, RBC, and platelet monitoring.

Patient education
• Tell patient to seek immediate medical attention for fever, chills, sore throat, or other infection symptoms; yellowing of eyes or skin; dark urine; light-colored stools; or unusual bleeding or bruising.
• Caution patient not to use tanning bed or sunlamp on treatment day or few days afterward. Urge him to use sunscreen or sunblock if he will be exposed to strong sunlight.
• Advise patient who is pregnant or may become pregnant that drug may harm fetus.
• Provide guidance to help breastfeeding patient decide whether to discontinue breastfeeding or stop drug.

dactinomycin (ACT, actinomycin D)
Cosmegen

Classification: Antineoplastic, antitumor antibiotic
Pregnancy risk category C

Pharmacology
Dactinomycin is derived from *Streptomyces parvulus* and inhibits DNA, RNA, and protein synthesis. It decreases replication by binding to DNA, which causes strand splitting. Activity is cell cycle phase-nonspecific.

Pharmacokinetics
Drug is metabolized in liver and distributed widely throughout body (except cerebrospinal fluid), with highest levels found in bone marrow. It peaks in 2 to 5 minutes; elimination half-life is 30 to 40 hours. It is excreted in bile and urine.

How supplied
Powder for injection, lyophilized: 500-mcg vial

Indications and dosages

FDA-APPROVED

➡ Wilms' tumor, childhood rhabdomyosarcoma, Ewing's sarcoma (combination therapy)
Children: 15 mcg/kg I.V. daily for 5 days given in various combinations and schedules with other chemotherapeutic agents (not to exceed 0.5 mg/day)
➡ Metastatic nonseminomatous testicular cancer
Adults: 1,000 mcg/m² I.V. on day 1 as part of combination regimen with cyclophosphamide, bleomycin, vinblastine, and cisplatin
➡ Gestational trophoblastic neoplasia (monotherapy or combination therapy)
Adults: 12 mcg/kg I.V. daily for 5 days as single agent. Or 500 mcg I.V. on days 1 and 2 as part of combination regimen with etoposide, methotrexate, folinic acid, vincristine, cyclophosphamide, and cisplatin.
➡ Locally recurrent or locoregional solid cancers
Adults: 50 mcg (0.05 mg)/kg I.V. for lower extremity or pelvis; 35 mcg (0.035 mg)/kg I.V. for upper extremity
➡ Osteosarcoma
Adults: 0.6 mg/m² I.V. for 2 days on weeks 2, 13, 26, 39, and 42 after surgery. Used in combination with high-dose methotrexate (12 g/m²).

DOSAGE MODIFICATIONS

• Dosage may vary depending on patient's tolerance, neoplasm size and location, and use of other therapies.
• Dosage is calculated in micrograms. Dose intensity per 2-week cycle (for adults or children) should not exceed 15 mcg/kg daily or 400 to 600 mcg/m² I.V. daily for 5 days. Alternative dosing of 2.5 mg/m² may be given in divided doses over 1 week.

- Base dosage for obese or edematous patients on body surface area in effort to more closely relate it to lean body mass.
- For patients taking blood dyscrasia–causing drugs, base dosage adjustment, if necessary, on hematologic parameters.
- Reduce dosage by one-third to one-half in patients with hyperbilirubinemia.

⊠ WARNINGS

- Drug is highly toxic. Both powder and solution must be handled and administered with care. Dust or vapor inhalation and contact with skin, mucous membranes, or eyes must be avoided. Avoid exposure during pregnancy. Because of drug's toxic properties (corrosivity, carcinogenicity, mutagenicity, and teratogenicity), special handling procedures should be reviewed before handling and followed diligently.
- Extravasation during I.V. administration causes severe damage to soft tissues, possibly leading to contracture of arms.

Contraindications and precautions

Contraindicated in chickenpox and herpes zoster infection.

Use cautiously in concurrent radiation therapy, pregnancy or breastfeeding, *elderly patients* (in whom bone marrow depression may be more frequent), and *children*. Greater frequency of toxic effects in infants suggests drug should be given only to infants older than age 12 months.

Preparation and administration

- Follow hazardous drug guidelines for handling, preparation, and administration. (See "Managing hazardous drugs," page 11.)
- Antiemetics usually are given before therapy begins.
- Do not give I.M. or subcutaneously.
- Dilute each 0.5-mg vial with preservative-free sterile water for injection to yield 0.5 mg/ml. May further dilute with 50 ml D$_5$W or normal saline solution.

- Give single I.V. dose by injection over 2 to 3 minutes. Give single I.V. dose by infusion over 20 to 30 minutes
- In suspected extravasation, apply ice to site for 15 minutes intermittently four times a day for 3 days. Close observation and plastic surgery consultation are recommended. Blistering, ulceration, or persistent pain may require wide excision surgery, followed by split-thickness skin grafting.
- Store at 77° F (25° C); excursions are permitted to 59° to 86° F (15° to 30° C). Protect from light and humidity.

Adverse reactions

CNS: malaise, fatigue, lethargy, fever
EENT: cheilitis, dysphagia, esophagitis
GI: nausea, vomiting, diarrhea, anorexia, stomatitis, abdominal pain
Hematologic: thrombocytopenia, leukopenia, anemia, aplastic anemia
Hepatic: hepatotoxicity
Skin: rash, reversible alopecia, folliculitis, acne, desquamation, extravasation, "radiation recall"
Other: pain at injection site

Interactions

Drug-drug. *Blood dyscrasia–causing drugs:* increased leukopenia and thrombocytopenia
Doxorubicin: increased cardiotoxicity
Other bone marrow depressants: additive effects, including GI toxicity, bone marrow depression, and skin erythema and tanning
Drug-diagnostic tests. *Bioassays for determining antibacterial drug concentrations:* interference
Liver enzymes: increased (rare)
Serum and urine uric acid: increased
Drug-herb. *Alpha-lipoic acid, coenzyme Q10:* decreased chemotherapy efficacy
Glutamine: possible enhanced tumor growth

Toxicity and overdose

- Signs and symptoms of overdose include nausea, vomiting, bone marrow depression, stomatitis, and mouth ulcers.

Only common or life-threatening adverse reactions are listed.

• Treatment is supportive. Whole blood products may be given.

Special considerations

• Frequently evaluate renal, hepatic, and bone marrow function.
• Do not give drug to patients with chickenpox or herpes zoster because of risk of severe generalized disease, which may result in death.
• Incidence of second primary tumors (including leukemia) may increase after therapy.
• Carefully observe patient for adverse reactions, which may involve any tissue but most commonly affect hematopoietic system, causing bone marrow depression. Anaphylactoid reaction may also occur.
• Observe patient daily for toxic effects when using combination chemotherapy because full course of therapy occasionally is not tolerated. If stomatitis, diarrhea, or severe hematopoietic depression occurs, discontinue chemotherapeutic agents until patient recovers.
• Dactinomycin and radiation used concomitantly may cause increased incidence of GI toxicity and bone marrow depression.
• Administer extremely cautiously within 2 months of radiation therapy for right-sided Wilms' tumor because hepatomegaly and elevated AST levels have occurred.

Patient education

• Tell patient to seek immediate medical attention for fever, chills, sore throat, or other infection symptoms; yellowing of eyes or skin; dark urine; or light-colored stools.
• Inform patient that prescriber may need to change dosage several times for best effect.
• Instruct patient to avoid persons with chickenpox or herpes zoster because of risk of severe generalized disease (possibly leading to death).
• Caution women with childbearing potential to avoid pregnancy.
• Provide guidance to help breastfeeding patient decide whether to discontinue breastfeeding or stop drug.

darbepoetin alfa
Aranesp

Classification: Hematopoietic, hormone modifier, colony-stimulating factor, recombinant human erythropoietin, antianemic
Pregnancy risk category C

Pharmacology

Darbepoetin alfa stimulates erythropoiesis in bone marrow by same mechanism as endogenous erythropoietin (primary growth factor for erythroid development). Ultimately, this effect enhances RBC production, leading to increased hematocrit and hemoglobin about 2 to 6 weeks after therapy starts.

Pharmacokinetics

Absorption is slow and dose-limiting. Drug peaks in about 90 hours. Terminal half-life is 21 hours with I.V. dose and 49 hours with subcutaneous dose.

How supplied

Prefilled syringe (albumin or polysorbated solution): 25 mcg/0.42 ml, 40 mcg/0.4 ml, 60 mcg/0.3 ml, 100 mcg/0.5 ml, 150 mcg/ 0.3 ml, 200 mcg/0.4 ml, 300 mcg/0.6 ml, 500 mcg/1 ml
Solution for injection (albumin): 25 mcg, 40 mcg, 60 mcg, 100 mcg, 200 mcg, and 300 mcg/1-ml single-dose vials; 150 mcg/0.75 ml
Solution for injection (polysorbate): 25 mcg, 40 mcg, 60 mcg, 100 mcg, and 200 mcg/1-ml single-dose vials

Indications and dosages

FDA-APPROVED

➡ Anemia in patients with nonmyeloid malignancies when anemia results from concomitant chemotherapy
Adults: 2.25 mcg/kg subcutaneously given as weekly injection

➼ Anemia associated with chemotherapy
Adults: 200 mcg subcutaneously every 2
weeks; if response is inadequate, may increase
to 300 mcg every 2 weeks. Or 3 mcg/kg every
2 weeks; if response inadequate, increase to 5
mcg/kg every 2 weeks. Or 4.5 mcg/kg every
week as loading dose until desired hemoglobin level achieved, then maintenance dosage
of 4.5 mcg/kg every 3 weeks.

DOSAGE MODIFICATIONS

• Adjust dosage to achieve and maintain target hemoglobin no higher than 12 g/dl. If hemoglobin increases by less than 1 g/dl after 6
weeks, increase dosage up to 4.5 mcg/kg. If
hemoglobin increases by more than 1 g/dl in
2-week period or exceeds 12 g/dl, reduce
dosage by about 25%. If hemoglobin exceeds
13 g/dl, temporarily withhold drug until hemoglobin falls to 12 g/dl. Then reinitiate at
dosage about 25% below previous.
• For patients who respond to drug with rapid increase in hemoglobin (for example, more
than 1 g/dl in any 2-week period), reduce
dosage.
• Closely monitor and control blood pressure.
Urge patients to comply with antihypertensive
therapy and dietary restrictions. If pharmacologic or dietary measures fail to control blood
pressure, reduce dosage or withhold drug.
• Do not increase dosage more frequently
than once a month.

Contraindications and precautions
Contraindicated in hypersensitivity to drug or
its components and in uncontrolled hypertension.
    Use cautiously in seizure disorder, por-
phyria, hypertension, and pregnancy or
breastfeeding. Safety and efficacy in *children*
have not been established.

Preparation and administration
• Blood pressure should be controlled adequately before therapy begins.

• Evaluate iron status before and during treatment because most patients will require supplemental iron therapy if serum ferritin level
is below 100 mcg/L or serum transferrin saturation is below 20%.
• Do not shake or dilute drug.
• After administration using prefilled syringe,
activate UltraSafe needle guard by placing
hands behind needle, grasping guard with one
hand, and sliding guard forward until needle
is completely covered and guard clicks into
place.
• Store at 36° to 46° F (2 to 8° C). Do not
freeze. Protect from light.

Adverse reactions
CNS: seizures, headache, fatigue, dizziness,
transient ischemic attack, cerebrovascular accident
CV: hypertension, hypotension, cardiac arrest,
angina pectoris, thrombosis, heart failure,
acute myocardial infarction, arrhythmias,
chest pain, edema
GI: nausea, vomiting, diarrhea, abdominal
pain, constipation
Musculoskeletal: bone pain, myalgia, limb
pain, back pain
Respiratory: upper respiratory tract infection,
dyspnea, cough, bronchitis
Skin: sweating, local injection site pain
Other: infection, fever, fluid overload, vascular access hemorrhage, allergic reaction, anaphylaxis, death

Interactions
Drug-diagnostic tests. *Serum ferritin, transferrin saturation:* decreased

Toxicity and overdose
• Cardiovascular and neurologic adverse
events have been associated with excessive or
rapid rises in hemoglobin.
• No known antidote exists. Treatment is supportive. If polycythemia occurs, drug should
be temporarily withheld. If indicated, phlebotomy may be performed.

Only common or life-threatening adverse reactions are listed.

Special considerations

- Darbepoetin alfa and other erythropoietic therapies may increase risk of cardiovascular events, including death. Higher risk of cardiovascular events may be associated with higher hemoglobin or higher rates of hemoglobin increase.
- Thrombotic events have occurred in patients treated with erythropoietic agents.
- Closely monitor renal function and fluid and electrolyte balance.
- Drug increases RBCs and decreases plasma volume, which could reduce dialysis efficacy; patients who are marginally dialyzed may require dialysis adjustments.

Patient education

- Inform patient of possible side effects; tell him to report these promptly.
- Stress importance of complying with drug therapy, dietary and dialysis prescriptions, and blood pressure and hemoglobin monitoring.
- Instruct patient to seek immediate medical attention for pain, tightness in chest, or irregular heartbeat.
- When patient can self-administer drug at home safely and effectively, provide instructions on proper use and administration (including careful review of "Information for Patients" insert). Caution patient or caregiver not to shake drug or reuse needles, syringes, or drug product. Provide instruction on proper needle and syringe disposal, including how to obtain puncture-resistant container for disposal.
- Tell patient not to use drug with abnormal color.
- Inform pregnant patient that drug should be used during pregnancy only if potential benefit justifies potential risk to fetus.

daunorubicin citrate liposome
DaunoXome

Classification: Antineoplastic, anthracycline
Pregnancy risk category D

Pharmacology

Daunorubicin citrate liposome protects entrapped daunorubicin from chemical and enzymatic degradation, minimizing protein binding and decreasing uptake by normal tissues. Specific action is unknown; however, direct DNA binding and inhibition of DNA repair (topoisomerase II inhibition) appear to block DNA and RNA synthesis and fragmentation.

Pharmacokinetics

Parent drug distributes slowly from peripheral tissues to liver for metabolism. Drug is not widely distributed; it clears rapidly from plasma into peripheral tissues. Half-life is about 4 hours. It is excreted in feces and to lesser extent in urine.

How supplied

Solution: 2 mg/ml in single-use vials. DaunoXome provides daunorubicin citrate equivalent to 50 mg of daunorubicin base.

Indications and dosages

FDA-**approved**

➥ Advanced HIV-associated Kaposi's sarcoma
Adults: 40 mg/m^2 I.V. over 60 minutes, with doses repeated every 2 weeks; total dose not to exceed 400 mg/m^2

Off-**label** (**selected**)

➥ Acute leukemias
Adults: 60 to 150 mg/m^2 I.V. daily for 3 days (monotherapy); for combination therapy, see specific regimen (range is 60 to 135 mg/m^2 I.V. daily for 3 days).

➠ Multiple myeloma
Adults: See specific regimen; for combination therapy, range is 80 to 100 mg/m² I.V. daily for 1 day.
➠ Metastatic colon cancer, adjunct in lymphoma
Adults: See specific regimen.

DOSAGE MODIFICATIONS

• Determine blood counts before each dose. Withhold drug if absolute granulocyte count is less than 750 cells/mm³.
• For patients with serum bilirubin level of 1.2 to 3 mg/dl, reduce usual dosage by 25%; if serum bilirubin or creatinine level exceeds 3 mg/dl, reduce usual dosage by 50%.
• For patients receiving blood dyscrasia–causing drugs, base dosage adjustment, if necessary, on hematologic parameters.
• Dosage reduction may be required when two or more bone marrow depressants (including radiation) are used concurrently or consecutively with this drug.

WARNINGS

• Cardiac function should be monitored regularly in patients receiving daunorubicin because of potential risk of cardiotoxicity and heart failure. Cardiac monitoring is advised, especially in patients who have received previous anthracyclines or have preexisting cardiac disease.
• Severe bone marrow depression may occur.
• Dosage should be reduced in hepatic impairment.
• Triad of back pain, flushing, and chest tightness has occurred. Triad generally arises during first 5 minutes of infusion, subsides with interruption of infusion, and does not recur if infusion resumes at slower rate.

Contraindications and precautions

Contraindicated in serious hypersensitivity reaction to drug or its components.

Use cautiously in renal or hepatic impairment, with concurrent radiation to mediastinal area, and in pregnancy. Safety and efficacy in **elderly patients** and **children** have not been established.

Preparation and administration

⟫ Follow hazardous drug guidelines for handling, preparation, and administration. (See "Managing hazardous drugs," page 11.)
• Dilute single dose with equal amount of D₅W to yield 1 mg/ml.
• Withdraw calculated dose from vial and transfer to infusion bag containing equal volume of D₅W.
• Do not mix with other drugs.
• Do not use in-line filters for infusion. Infuse over 60 minutes.
• Drug is translucent red liposomal dispersion. Do not use if opaque.
• Diluted solution is stable for 24 hours at room temperature and 48 hours when refrigerated.
• Store in refrigerator at 36° to 46° F (2° to 8° C). Do not freeze. Protect from light.

Adverse reactions

CNS: fatigue, headache, depression, insomnia, dizziness, malaise, neuropathy
CV: chest pain, edema
GI: cramps, diarrhea, constipation, stomatitis
Musculoskeletal: arthralgia, back pain
Skin: sweating, pruritus

Interactions

Drug-drug. *Blood dyscrasia–causing drugs:* increased leukopenia and thrombocytopenia
Cyclophosphamide: increased cardiotoxicity
Other bone marrow depressants: additive bone marrow depression
Other hepatotoxic drugs: increased risk of toxicity
Previous use of daunorubicin, doxorubicin, or other anthracycline antineoplastics: increased risk of cardiotoxicity
Drug-diagnostic tests. *Cardiac function tests:* decreased left ventricular ejection fraction

---

Only common or life-threatening adverse reactions are listed.

Hematocrit, hemoglobin, platelets, WBCs: decreased

Drug-herb. *Alpha-lipoic acid, coenzyme Q10:* decreased chemotherapy efficacy
Glutamine: possible enhanced tumor growth

Toxicity and overdose
• Signs and symptoms of acute overdose include increased severity of adverse reactions, bone marrow depression (especially granulocytopenia), fatigue, and nausea and vomiting.
• Treatment is supportive.

Special considerations
• Careful hematologic monitoring is required for bone marrow depression; patient must be observed carefully for evidence of intercurrent or opportunistic infections.
• Carefully evaluate cardiac function, particularly in patients with preexisting cardiac disease and in those who received previous anthracycline therapy.

Patient education
• Inform patient that heart function will be monitored regularly and that drug may cause severe decrease in blood cell counts.
• Urge patient to immediately report back pain, flushed skin, or tightness in chest during infusion.
• Tell patient to seek immediate medical attention for difficulty breathing; unusual bleeding or bruising; chest pain; ankle or foot swelling; or fever, chills, sore throat, or other infection symptoms.
• Inform pregnant patient that drug may harm fetus.
• Caution women with childbearing potential to avoid becoming pregnant during therapy.

daunorubicin hydrochloride
Cerubidine

Classification: Antineoplastic, anthracycline
Pregnancy risk category D

D

Pharmacology
Daunorubicin hydrochloride appears to bind directly to DNA, which inhibits DNA repair (topoisomerase II inhibition) and blocks DNA and RNA synthesis and fragmentation. Exact mechanism of action is unclear.

Pharmacokinetics
Drug is metabolized in liver to active and inactive metabolites, and is widely distributed. Initial half-life is 45 minutes; terminal half-life, 18.5 hours. Parent drug is eliminated in 18 hours; active metabolite (daunorubicinol), in about 25 hours. Roughly 40% is excreted in bile and 15% to 25% in urine.

How supplied
Liquid for infusion: 5 mg/ml
Powder for injection: 20 mg

Indications and dosages

FDA-APPROVED

➥ Acute nonlymphocytic leukemia
Adults: 45 mg/m² I.V. daily on days 1, 2, and 3 of first course and days 1 and 2 of subsequent courses, and cytosine arabinoside 100 mg/m² I.V. infusion daily for 7 days for first course and for 5 days for subsequent courses, if required
➥ Acute lymphocytic leukemia
Adults: 45 mg/m² I.V. daily on days 1, 2, and 3 and vincristine 2 mg I.V. on days 1, 8, and 15, and prednisone 40 mg/m² P.O. daily on days 1 to 22, then tapered between days 22 and 29; L-asparaginase 500 international units/kg daily for 10 days on days 22 to 32
Children older than age 2: 25 mg/m² I.V. on day 1 every week, vincristine 1.5 mg/m² I.V.

on day 1 every week, prednisone 40 mg/m^2 P.O. daily. (Multiple dosing strategies exist; see specific regimens.)

OFF-LABEL USES (SELECTED)

➡ Chronic myelogenous leukemia in blastic phase
Adults: Treated as above, depending on myeloid vs lymphoid lineage

DOSAGE MODIFICATIONS

• Reduce dosage in patients with hepatic or renal impairment. Three-quarters of normal dosage is recommended for patients with serum bilirubin level of 1.2 to 3 mg/100 ml, and half of normal dosage for patients with serum bilirubin or creatinine level above 3 mg/100 ml.
• For patients age 60 and older, reduce dosage to 30 mg/m^2 daily and use same regimen as for patients younger than age 60.
• For children younger than age 2 or less than 0.5 m^2 body surface area (BSA), base dosage on weight (1 mg/kg), not BSA.
• Dosage reduction may be required when two or more bone marrow depressants (including radiation) are used concurrently or consecutively with this drug.

☒ WARNINGS

• Drug must be given into rapidly flowing I.V. infusion. It must never be administered I.M. or subcutaneously. Extravasation causes severe local tissue necrosis.
• Total cumulative dosage above 550 mg/m^2 in adults, 300 mg/m^2 in children older than age 2, or 10 mg/kg in children younger than age 2 may cause myocardial toxicity. This effect may occur during therapy or several months afterward. Most severe form manifests as potentially fatal heart failure.
• Therapeutic doses cause severe bone marrow depression.
• Drug should be administered only by physician experienced in leukemia chemotherapy

and in facilities with laboratory and supportive resources adequate to monitor drug tolerance and protect and maintain patient compromised by drug toxicity. Physician and facility must be capable of responding rapidly and completely to severe hemorrhagic conditions or overwhelming infection.
• Dosage should be reduced in patients with hepatic or renal impairment.

Contraindications and precautions

Contraindicated in hypersensitivity to drug or its components.

Use cautiously in renal or hepatic impairment, bone marrow depression, concurrent or consecutive radiation therapy, current or recent chickenpox, herpes zoster, gout, urate renal calculi, heart disease, heart failure, arrythmias, infection, tumor cell infiltration of bone marrow, inadequate bone marrow reserves, pregnancy or breastfeeding, and *elderly patients* and *children.* Infants and children appear to be more susceptible to anthracycline-induced cardiotoxicity than adults, in whom cardiotoxicity is more clearly dose-related.

Preparation and administration

≫ Follow hazardous drug guidelines for handling, preparation, and administration. (See "Managing hazardous drugs," page 11.)
• Do not mix with other drugs or heparin.
• Do not give I.M. or subcutaneously.
• Dilute each 20 mg with 4 ml sterile water for injection to yield 5 mg/ml. Agitate gently to dissolve completely. Further dilute each dose with 10 to 15 ml normal saline solution.
• Inject into tubing or sidearm of rapidly flowing I.V. infusion of D$_5$W or normal saline solution.
• For infusion, dilute further with 100 ml normal saline solution.
• Give single dose by I.V. injection over 3 to 5 minutes or by I.V. infusion over 30 to 45 minutes.
• Be extremely careful to avoid extravasation

at I.V. site, which can cause severe local tissue necrosis.

• Store at 59° to 77° F (15° to 25° C).

Adverse reactions

CV: peripheral edema, acute cardiotoxicity (transient ECG findings), chronic cardiotoxicity (heart failure, arrhythmia, pericarditis, myocarditis)

GI: nausea, vomiting, anorexia, mucositis

GU: discolored urine, erectile dysfunction, sterility, amenorrhea, gynecomastia, hyperuricemia

Hematologic: thrombocytopenia, leukopenia, anemia

Hepatic: hepatotoxicity

Skin: rash, dermatitis, reversible alopecia, extravasation, cellulitis, thrombophlebitis at injection site

Other: anaphylaxis, fever, chills

Interactions

Drug-drug. *Blood dyscrasia–causing drugs:* increased leukopenia and thrombocytopenia

Cyclophosphamide: increased cardiotoxicity

Other bone marrow depressants: additive bone marrow depression

Other hepatotoxic drugs: increased risk of toxicity

Previous use of daunorubicin, doxorubicin, or other anthracycline antineoplastics: increased risk of cardiotoxicity

Drug-diagnostic tests. *Cardiac function tests:* decreased left ventricular ejection fraction

Hematocrit, hemoglobin, platelets, WBCs: decreased

Drug-herb. *Alpha-lipoic acid, coenzyme Q10:* decreased chemotherapy efficacy

Glutamine: possible enhanced tumor growth

Toxicity and overdose

• Signs and symptoms of acute overdose include increased severity of adverse reactions, bone marrow depression (especially granulocytopenia), fatigue, nausea, and vomiting.

• Treatment is supportive.

Special considerations

• To eradicate leukemic cells and induce complete remission, profound bone marrow suppression is usually required. Both peripheral blood and bone marrow must be evaluated to form appropriate treatment.

• Attaining normal-appearing bone marrow may require up to three induction courses.

• Therapy requires close patient observation and frequent CBC determinations. Evaluate cardiac, renal, and hepatic function before each treatment course.

• Drug may induce hyperuricemia secondary to rapid lysis of leukemic cells. As a precaution, allopurinol administration usually begins before antileukemic therapy starts. Monitor blood uric acid level and initiate appropriate therapy if hyperuricemia develops.

• Take appropriate measures to control systemic infection before beginning therapy.

• Bone marrow depression occurs in all patients given therapeutic doses. Do not start drug in patients with preexisting drug-induced bone marrow depression unless benefit warrants risk.

• Carefully observe patients (particularly infants and children) for cardiotoxicity. Monitor ECG before each course.

• In adults, incidence of drug-induced heart failure increases at cumulative dosages exceeding 550 mg/m². (Cumulative dosage may differ, depending on renal function and other conditions).

• Significant hepatic or renal impairment can enhance toxicity at recommended dosages. Before administration, evaluate hepatic and renal function using conventional clinical laboratory tests.

Patient education

• Tell patient drug may turn urine red.

• Inform patient that drug may cause severe heart problems and extremely low blood counts.

• Urge patient to immediately report difficulty breathing or swallowing; wheezing; lightheadedness or fainting; sudden swelling of

face, lips, tongue, legs, or arms; rash, pain, or inflammation at injection site; unusual bleeding or bruising; or fever, chills, sore throat, or other infection symptoms.
• Caution pregnant patient that drug may harm fetus.
• Advise women with childbearing potential to avoid becoming pregnant during therapy.

denileukin diftitox
Ontak

Classification: Biological response modifier
Pregnancy risk category C

Pharmacology
Denileukin diftitox, a recombinant DNA–derived cytotoxic protein, directs cytocidal action of diphtheria toxin to cancer cells expressing interleukin-2 (IL-2) receptor on activated T and B lymphocytes and macrophages. It interacts with high-affinity IL-2 receptors on cell surface and inhibits cellular protein synthesis, causing cytolysis within hours.

Pharmacokinetics
Drug is metabolized in liver by proteolytic degradation. Distribution half-life is 2 to 5 minutes; plasma half-life, about 80 minutes. Onset, peak, and duration vary.

How supplied
Solution for I.V. injection (frozen): 150 mcg/ml (300 mcg in 2 ml) single-use vial

Indications and dosages

FDA-approved

➡ Persistent or recurrent cutaneous T-cell lymphoma in which cancer cells express CD25 component of IL-2 receptor
Adults: 9 or 18 mcg/kg I.V. daily for 5 consecutive days, repeated every 21 days

Off-label uses (selected)

➡ Chronic lymphocytic lymphoma with CD25 expression, non-Hodgkin's lymphoma
Adults: 18 mcg/kg I.V. daily for 5 days, repeated every 21 days
➡ Steroid-refractory graft-versus-host disease (GVHD)
Adults: 4.5 mcg/kg I.V. daily on days 1 through 5; then weekly on days 8, 15, 22, and 29 or until GVHD resolves

Dosage modifications

• Delay administration until serum albumin level reaches at least 3 g/dl.

WARNINGS

• Patients receiving drug should be managed by physicians experienced in antineoplastic therapy and care of cancer patients, and in facility equipped for close monitoring and cardiopulmonary resuscitation as necessary.

Contraindications and precautions
Contraindicated in hypersensitivity to drug or its components (diphtheria toxin, IL-2, or excipients).
Use cautiously in infection, hypoalbuminemia, pregnancy or breastfeeding, and *elderly patients.* Safety and efficacy in *children* have not been established.

Preparation and administration
• Follow hazardous drug guidelines for handling, preparation, and administration. (See "Managing hazardous drugs," page 11.)
• Before giving drug, cancer cells should be tested for CD25 expression.
• Obtain CBC, blood chemistry panel (including hepatic and renal function), and serum albumin levels before and weekly during therapy.
• To minimize infusion-related events, premedicate with acetaminophen, nonsteroidal anti-inflammatory drugs, and antihistamines.

- Do not give by I.V. bolus or mix with other drugs.
- Do not administer through in-line filter.
- Thaw at room temperature. Gently swirl vial to mix. Use solution only if it is clear, colorless, and without visible particulates.
- Prepare diluted drug in plastic syringe or soft plastic I.V. bag. Diluted concentration should yield at least 15 mcg/ml solution. For each 1 ml of drug from vial, add no more than 9 ml sterile saline solution without preservative to I.V. bag. Infuse over at least 15 minutes.
- Give prepared solution within 6 hours; discard unused portion.
- During infusion, observe closely for hypersensitivity reaction. Keep appropriate drugs and resuscitative equipment at hand.
- If infusion reaction occurs, discontinue drug or reduce infusion rate, depending on reaction severity. No clinical experience exists with infusion times beyond 80 minutes.
- Store frozen at 14° F (–10° C) or below. Do not refreeze after thawing.

Adverse reactions

CNS: asthenia, headache, dizziness, paresthesia, nervousness, confusion, insomnia
CV: vascular leak syndrome, thrombotic events, chest pain, hypotension, hypertension, vasodilation, tachycardia, arrhythmias
EENT: rhinitis, pharyngitis, visual impairment
GI: diarrhea, nausea, vomiting, constipation, anorexia, dyspepsia, dysphagia, pancreatitis
GU: acute renal insufficiency, microscopic hematuria, albuminuria, pyuria
Hematologic: thrombocytopenia, leukopenia, anemia
Musculoskeletal: myalgia, joint pain
Metabolic: hypoalbuminemia, hyperthyroidism, hypothyroidism, hypocalcemia, hypokalemia, dehydration
Respiratory: dyspnea, increased cough, lung disorder
Skin: pruritus, rash (generalized maculopapular, petechial, vesicular bullous, urticarial, or eczematous; possible acute or delayed onset)

Other: infection (possibly severe), pain, chills, fever, sweating, edema, weight loss, injection site reactions, flulike symptom complex (possible acute or delayed onset), hypersensitivity reactions including anaphylaxis

Interactions

Drug-diagnostic tests. *Serum calcium, potassium:* decreased
Serum and urine creatinine, serum transaminases: increased
Drug-herb. *Coenzyme Q10:* possible decreased chemotherapy efficacy

Toxicity and overdose

- No clinical experience with accidental overdose exists. With dosage of 31 mcg/kg daily, reported dose-limiting toxicities include moderate to severe nausea, vomiting, fever, chills, and persistent asthenia. Higher daily dosages have not been evaluated.
- No known antidote exists. If overdose occurs, closely monitor hepatic and renal function and overall fluid balance.

Special considerations

- Evaluate patient for vascular leak syndrome, marked by at least two of following: edema, hypotension, and hypoalbuminemia. Monitor weight, edema, blood pressure, and serum albumin levels carefully. Preexisting low albumin levels and history of cardiovascular disease seem to predispose patients to syndrome.
- Monitor patients carefully for infection; cutaneous T-cell lymphoma predisposes patients to cutaneous infection.
- Loss of visual acuity, usually with or without pigment mottling, has occurred.

Patient education

- Instruct patient to increase fluid intake.
- Advise patient to avoid crowds and exposure to illness because drug increases susceptibility to infection.
- Urge patient to immediately report chest pain, difficulty breathing, chills, burning at infusion site, rash, signs and symptoms of

thrombosis, throat tightness, redness, swelling, and pain.
• Advise breastfeeding patient to stop breastfeeding during therapy.

dexamethasone
Adrenocot, Cortastat, Cortastat LA, Cortastat 10, Dalalone, Dalalone D.P., Dalalone L.A., Decadron, Decadron 5-12 Pak, Decaject, De-Sone LA, Dexacen-4, Dexamethasone Intensol, Dexasone, Dexasone LA, Dexpak Taperpak, Hexadrol, Hexadrol Phosphate, Solurex, Solurex LA

dexamethasone acetate

dexamethasone sodium phosphate
AK-Dex, Decadron Phosphate

Classification: Glucocorticoid, anti-inflammatory
Pregnancy risk category C

Pharmacology
Dexamethasone has unclear antineoplastic action. It is used mainly for potent anti-inflammatory effects and ability to modify immune responses to diverse stimuli, to stimulate bone marrow, and to promote protein, fat, and carbohydrate metabolism.

Pharmacokinetics
All forms are metabolized in kidney, with some biliary component. Action is fairly rapid, with a short duration; however, suspension form is long-acting. Elimination half-life is 3 to 4 hours. Drug is excreted primarily by kidneys, with some biliary component.

How supplied
Concentrate (oral): 1 mg/ml (contains 30% alcohol)

Elixir: 0.5 mg/5 ml
Solution for I.V., I.M., intra-articular, intralesional, or soft-tissue injection (sodium phosphate): 4 mg/ml, 10 mg/ml
Solution for I.V. injection only (sodium phosphate): 24 mg/ml
Suspension for I.M., intra-articular, intralesional, or soft-tissue injection (acetate): 8 mg/ml
Tablets (dexamethasone): 0.25 mg, 0.5 mg, 0.75 mg, 1 mg, 1.5 mg (also available in taper pack), 2 mg, 4 mg, 6 mg

Indications and dosages

FDA-APPROVED

➟ Palliative management of leukemia and lymphoma
Adults: Dosage varies and must be individualized.
➟ Palliative management of acute leukemia
Children age 12 and older: Dosage varies with drug regimen, response, comorbidities, and other factors.
➟ Palliative management of cerebral edema associated with primary or metastatic brain tumor
Adults: 10 mg I.V. (phosphate) followed by 4 mg every 6 hours I.M. until cerebral edema symptoms subside

OFF-LABEL USES (SELECTED)

➟ Prostatic carcinoma (second-line treatment)
Adults: 0.5 to 1.5 mg P.O. daily for suppression of adrenal androgen production
➟ Multiple myeloma (before bone marrow transplantation)
Adults: When used as part of VAD (vincristine, doxorubicin [Adriamycin], dexamethasone) regimen, 40 mg P.O. daily on days 1 through 4, 9 through 12, and 17 through 20, repeated every 28 to 35 days. Or when used with thalidomide, 20 mg P.O. daily on days 1 through 4, 9 through 12, and 17 through 20, repeated every 28 days. Or when used with bortezomib, 20 mg P.O. daily on days 1, 2, 4, 5, 8, 9, 11, and 12, given every 21 days.

➥ Multiple myeloma (after bone marrow transplantation)
Adults: Dosage ranges from 40 mg daily for 5 days every 28 days to 20 mg/m² P.O. daily on days 1 through 4, 9 through 12, and 17 through 20; repeated every 28 days.

➥ Primary brain tumor (treatment adjunct)
Adults: Dosage ranges from 2 mg P.O. every 24 hours to 10 mg P.O. every 6 hours.

➥ Fever secondary to cancer
Adults: 2 to 10 mg P.O twice daily

➥ Antiemetic in cancer chemotherapy (prophylaxis for acute nausea and vomiting)
Adults: 10 to 20 mg P.O. or I.V. 30 to 60 minutes before first chemotherapy dose. With twice-daily chemotherapy, divide daily dose in two, and administer one dose before each chemotherapy dose.
Children ages 1 to 12: 10 to 14 mg/m² P.O. (dexamethasone) or I.V. (sodium phosphate) 30 to 60 minutes before first chemotherapy dose. With twice-daily chemotherapy, divide daily dose into two, and give one dose before each chemotherapy dose.

➥ Antiemetic in cancer chemotherapy (treatment of nausea and vomiting)
Adults: 10 to 20 mg P.O or I.V. every 4 to 6 hours
Children ages 1 to 12: Initially, 10 mg/m² P.O. or I.V. (maximum dose, 20 mg); then 5 mg/m² P.O or I.V. every 6 hours

➥ Antiemetic in cancer chemotherapy (prophylaxis for delayed nausea and vomiting)
Adults: 8 mg P.O. twice daily for 3 days in combination with continuously administered dopamine antagonist
Children ages 1 to 12: 4 to 6 mg P.O. twice daily for 3 days in combination with continuously administered dopamine antagonist

➥ Antiemetic in radiation therapy for cancer (prophylaxis for acute nausea and vomiting)
Adults: 2 mg P.O. three times daily
Children ages 1 to 12: 2 to 4 mg/m² P.O. twice daily

➥ Premedication before docetaxel administration (to prevent fluid retention and reduce severity of hypersensitivity reactions)

Adults: 8 to 10 mg P.O. twice daily for 3 to 5 days, starting 1 day before docetaxel

D

• Dosage may need to be increased during stress in patients receiving long-term dexamethasone therapy.
• Dosage may need to be adjusted in patients receiving concomitant phenytoin, phenobarbital, ephedrine, or rifampin.
• For palliative management of cerebral edema linked to primary or metastatic brain tumor, response usually occurs within 12 to 24 hours; dosage may be reduced after 2 to 4 days and gradually discontinued over 5 to 7 days.
• For primary brain tumor, dosage of 10 mg P.O. every 6 hours is commonly used but provides no antineoplastic activity. Use lowest dosage that controls symptoms.

Contraindications and precautions

Contraindicated in hypersensitivity to drug or its components (including sulfites in sodium phosphate form) and in systemic fungal infections.

Use cautiously in prolonged therapy, hypothyroidism, cirrhosis, ocular herpes simplex, psychic derangements, emotional instability or psychotic tendency, other corticosteroid use, nonspecific ulcerative colitis, abscess or other pyogenic infection, diverticulitis, fresh intestinal anastomoses, active or latent peptic ulcer disease, renal insufficiency, hypertension, osteoporosis, myasthenia gravis, fat embolism, signs of peritoneal irritation, pregnancy or breastfeeding, and *children younger than age 12.*

Preparation and administration

• In patients receiving large oral doses, drug may be given with meals and antacids between meals to prevent peptic ulcer.
• Maintain or adjust initial dosages until patient response is satisfactory. If such a response does not occur after reasonable period,

---

discontinue tablets or elixir and switch patient to other therapy.

• Acetate suspension is a sterile white suspension (pH 5 to 7.5) that settles on standing but is easily resuspended by mild shaking. Give I.M. when oral therapy is not feasible. Do not inject I.V. because this may cause atrophy at injection site. To reduce risk or severity of atrophy, do not inject subcutaneously, avoid injection into deltoid muscle, and avoid repeated I.M. injections into same site, if possible.

• Drug is not recommended as initial therapy in acute, life-threatening situations.

• Sodium phosphate form may be given undiluted or added to D_5W or normal saline solution and administered as infusion. Give 24-mg/ml product I.V. only. Drug is sensitive to heat; do not autoclave vial. Protect from freezing and light. Store container in carton until contents have been used.

• Store tablets at controlled temperature of 59° to 86° F (15° to 30° C).

Adverse reactions

CNS: depression, headache, mood changes, seizures, vertigo, increased intracranial pressure with papilledema (pseudotumor cerebri)
CV: heart failure, hypertension, tachycardia, thromboembolism, thrombophlebitis
EENT: cataracts, decreased visual acuity, glaucoma exacerbation, increased intraocular pressure, increased risk of corneal infection, optic nerve damage, poor corneal wound healing
GI: abdominal distention, diarrhea, nausea, peptic ulcer disease (possibly leading to perforation and hemorrhage), pancreatitis, ulcerative esophagitis
GU: hypercalciuria
Metabolic: cushingoid state, decreased glucose tolerance, growth suppression in children, hypothalamic-pituitary-adrenal suppression, hyperglycemia, hypokalemic alkalosis, sodium retention
Musculoskeletal: aseptic necrosis of femoral and humeral heads, osteoporosis, muscle weakness, steroid myopathy, muscle mass loss, vertebral compression fractures, patho-

logic long-bone fracture, tendon rupture
Skin: acne, bruising, ecchymosis, petechiae, poor wound healing, striae, thin fragile skin, allergic dermatitis, angioneurotic edema
Other: weight gain, appetite increase, anaphylactoid or hypersensitivity reactions

Interactions

Drug-drug. *Aspirin:* increased hypoprothrombinemia risk
Coumarin anticoagulants: altered anticoagulant response
Ephedrine, phenobarbital, phenytoin, rifampin: possible increase in metabolic clearance of dexamethasone
Potassium-depleting diuretics: increased risk of hypokalemia
Drug-diagnostic tests. *Dexamethasone suppression test (DST):* false negative (with concomitant indomethacin, phenytoin, phenobarbital, ephedrine, or rifampin therapy)
Nitroblue-tetrazolium test: false negative
Serum calcium, serum sodium: increased
Skin test reactions: suppressed
Thyroxine: decreased
Drug-food. *Grapefruit juice:* increased dexamethasone level
Drug-herb. *Echinacea:* possible decrease in dexamethasone action
Ephedra (ma huang): possible increase in dexamethasone clearance
Licorice: possible decrease in dexamethasone clearance
Rhubarb: possible increased corticosteroid-induced potassium loss (with overuse)

Toxicity and overdose

• Reports of acute toxicity and death after overdose are rare. With long-term use, hypothalamic-pituitary-adrenal suppression, muscle weakness, or osteoporosis may signify toxicity.

• No specific antidote exists. Provide supportive and symptomatic treatment.

Only common or life-threatening adverse reactions are listed.

Special considerations

• Check prothrombin time frequently in patients receiving drug comcomitantly with coumarin anticoagulants.

• Interpret DST results cautiously for patients receiving concomitant indomethacin, phenytoin, phenobarbital, rifampin, or ephedrine.

• Observe patient closely for hypokalemia when giving drug concomitantly with potassium-depleting diuretics.

• Sodium phosphate injection contains sodium bisulfite, which may cause allergic-type reactions (including anaphylaxis and life-threatening asthmatic episodes in certain susceptible patients).

• Rule out latent or active amebiasis before starting therapy if patient has spent time in tropics or has unexplained diarrhea. Drug may exacerbate diarrhea.

• To minimize drug-induced adrenocortical insufficiency from too-rapid drug withdrawal, reduce dosage gradually.

• Inactivated viral or bacterial vaccines may not cause expected serum antibody response in patients receiving immunosuppressive dexamethasone doses.

• Watch for signs of hypoadrenalism in infants born to women who received substantial doses during pregnancy.

• Carefully monitor growth and development of infants and children on prolonged therapy.

Patient education

• Instruct patient on long-term therapy to wear or carry medical alert information. Caution him not to stop taking drug abruptly.

• Advise patient to restrict sodium intake, as necessary.

• Recommend potassium and calcium supplements, as necessary.

• Instruct patient to report vision changes. Advise patient on chronic therapy to have eye examination at least twice yearly.

• Caution patient on immunosuppressive doses to avoid exposure to chickenpox or measles; if exposure occurs, tell him to seek medical attention without delay.

• If patient is pregnant, discuss drug's anticipated benefits in light of possible hazards to mother, embryo, or fetus.

• Advise breastfeeding patient to stop breastfeeding during therapy.

D

dexrazoxane hydrochloride
Zinecard

Classification: Chelator, cytoprotective agent
Pregnancy risk category C

Pharmacology

Dexrazoxane is a cyclic ethylenediamene tetra-acetic acid–derivative that readily penetrates cell membranes. Exact action is unknown. However, drug is thought to undergo intracellular conversion to ring-opened chelating agent that interferes with iron-mediated free radical generation (which is partly responsible for anthracycline-induced cardiomyopathy).

Pharmacokinetics

Drug is metabolized mainly in liver. Distribution is wide and rapid, with highest concentrations in liver and kidney. Terminal half-life is 3 to 4 hours. Parent drug and metabolite are excreted by kidney.

How supplied

Powder for injection: 250-mg and 500-mg single-use vials

Indications and dosages

FDA-APPROVED

⊖ To reduce incidence and severity of cardiomyopathy associated with doxorubicin in women with metastatic breast cancer who have received cumulative doxorubicin doses of 300 mg/m² and will continue to receive doxorubicin to maintain tumor control
Adults: 10:1 ratio of dexrazoxane:doxorubicin (for example, 500 mg/m² dexrazoxane to 50

mg/m^2 doxorubicin) by slow I.V. push or rapid I.V. infusion, followed by doxorubicin within 30 minutes of starting dexrazoxane

OFF-LABEL USES (SELECTED)

⮞ Anthracycline extravasation during chemotherapy
Adults: 1,000 mg/m^2 I.V. every 24 hours for two doses, with first dose given within 5 hours of extravasation; then 500 mg/m^2 I.V. on day 3 in extremity opposite to extravasation site
➡ Prophylaxis for anthracycline-induced cardiotoxicity
Adults: For doxorubicin-related cardiotoxicity, 10:1 ratio of dexrazoxane:doxorubicin by slow I.V. push or rapid I.V. infusion, followed by anthracycline within 30 minutes of starting dexrazoxane. For epirubicin-related cardiotoxicity, 10:1 ratio of dexrazoxane:epirubicin by slow I.V. push or rapid I.V. infusion, followed by anthracycline within 30 minutes of starting dexrazoxane.
Children: For doxorubicin-related cardiotoxicity, 10:1 ratio of dexrazoxane:doxorubicin by slow I.V. push or rapid I.V. infusion, followed by anthracycline within 30 minutes of starting dexrazoxane. For epirubicin-related cardiotoxicity, 10:1 ratio of dexrazoxane:epirubicin by slow I.V. push or rapid I.V. infusion, followed by anthracycline within 30 minutes of starting dexrazoxane.

DOSAGE MODIFICATIONS

• Because reduced doxorubicin dosage is recommended in hyperbilirubinemia, dexrazoxane dosage should be reduced proportionately (maintaining 10:1 ratio) in patients with hepatic impairment.

Contraindications and precautions

Contraindicated with chemotherapy regimens that do not contain an anthracycline.

Use cautiously in combination with other cytotoxic drugs, in pregnancy or breastfeeding, and in **elderly patients**. Long-term safety

and efficacy in **children** have not been established.

Preparation and administration

• Do not mix with other drugs.
• Reconstitute with 0.167 molar (M/6) sodium lactate injection to yield concentration of 10 mg/ml sodium lactate. Further dilute reconstituted solution in I.V. infusion bags with either normal saline injection or D$_5$W to concentration range of 1.3 to 5 mg/ml.
• Give reconstituted solution by slow I.V. push or rapid I.V. infusion.
• After completing dose by I.V. push or infusion, and before total elapsed time of 30 minutes (from beginning of dexrazoxane administration), give doxorubicin I.V. injection. Do not give doxorubicin before I.V. dexrazoxane injection.
• Dexrazoxane is not recommended for use at time of doxorubicin initiation.
• Store at 77° F (25° C); excursions are permitted to 59° to 86° F (15° to 30° C). Reconstituted solutions remain stable for 6 hours at controlled room temperature or refrigerated at 36° to 46° F (2° to 8° C). Discard unused solution.

Adverse reactions

CNS: fatigue, malaise, neurotoxicity
CV: phlebitis
GI: nausea, vomiting, diarrhea, anorexia, stomatitis, dysphagia
Skin: alopecia, streaking or erythema with injection
Other: fever, infection, pain with injection

Interactions

Drug-drug. FAC (fluorouracil, doxorubicin [Adriamycin], and cyclophosphamide) regimen: interference with FAC antitumor efficacy
Other cytotoxic drugs: increased myelosuppressive effects
Drug-diagnostic tests. CBC: bone marrow depression

Only common or life-threatening adverse reactions are listed.

Toxicity and overdose

- No known cases of overdose have occurred. Expected primary toxic effect is bone marrow depression.
- No known antidote exists. Manage suspected overdose with supportive care until bone marrow depression and related conditions resolve.

Special considerations

- Observe for bone marrow depression.
- Monitor cardiac function because of possible anthracycline-induced cardiotoxicity.

Patient education

- Inform patient that alopecia usually reverses 2 to 3 months after last dose. Tell him that new hair growth may differ in color or texture.
- Instruct patient to report fever, signs and symptoms of local infection, or sore throat.
- Urge patient to practice fastidious oral hygiene.
- Inform pregnant patient that use during pregnancy is indicated only if potential benefit justifies potential fetal risk.
- Advise breastfeeding patient to stop breastfeeding during therapy.

dextroamphetamine sulfate
Dexedrine, Dexedrine Spansule, Dextrostat

Classification: Amphetamine, anorexigenic, CNS stimulant
Controlled substance schedule II
Pregnancy risk category C

Pharmacology

Dextroamphetamine releases nerve terminal stores of norepinephrine, stimulating CNS and respiratory centers. Anorexigenic effects occur in hypothalamus. Peripheral actions include blood pressure elevation and weak bronchodilatory and respiratory stimulation.

Pharmacokinetics

Immediate-release form is absorbed from GI tract within 3 hours; sustained-release form, within 8 to 10 hours. Sustained-release form delivers smaller dose immediately, with remainder of dose delivered over 24 hours. Urine alkalization may prolong duration.

How supplied

Capsules (sustained-release): 5 mg, 10 mg, 15 mg
Tablets: 5 mg, 10 mg

Indications and dosages

OFF-LABEL USES (SELECTED)

⇥ Stimulant for fatigue
Adults: 5 to 15 mg (sustained-release) P.O., using lowest dosage that achieves desired results

WARNINGS

- Drug has high potential for abuse.
- Long-term use may lead to drug dependence and should be avoided.
- Possibility of patients obtaining drug for nontherapeutic use or distributing it to others requires particular attention. Drug should be prescribed and dispensed sparingly.

Contraindications and precautions

Contraindicated in hypersensitivity or idiosyncratic reaction to sympathomimetic amines, advanced arteriosclerosis, symptomatic cardiovascular disease, moderate to severe hypertension, hyperthyroidism, glaucoma, agitated states, history of drug abuse, and within 14 days of MAO inhibitors.

Use cautiously in tartrazine sensitivity, mild hypertension, motor and phonic tics, Tourette's syndrome, pregnancy or breastfeeding, and *children*.

⊖ Orphan drug   ≫ Potentially carcinogenic

Preparation and administration
- Prescribe or dispense smallest amount feasible at one time to minimize overdose risk.
- Store at 59° to 86° F (15° to 30° C) in tightly closed, light-resistant container.

Adverse reactions
CNS: aggressiveness, dizziness, dysphoria, headache, hyperactivity, insomnia, irritability, restlessness, stimulation, talkativeness, tremor
CV: cardiomyopathy, decreased heart rate, arrhythmias, hypertension, palpitations, tachycardia
GI: anorexia, constipation, diarrhea, dry mouth, metallic taste
GU: libido changes, erectile dysfunction
Skin: urticaria
Other: addiction, dependence, chills, weight loss

Interactions
Drug-drug. *Adrenergic blockers:* inhibited adrenergic blocker action
Antihistamines: reduced sedative effect of antihistamine
Antihypertensives: enhanced hypotensive effect
Chlorpromazine, haloperidol: blocked dopamine and norepinephrine reuptake, which inhibits dextroamphetamine's central stimulant effect
Ethosuximide: delayed intestinal absorption of ethosuximide
GI acidifiers (such as ascorbic acid, glutamic acid, guanethidine, and reserpine): decreased dextroamphetamine absorption and efficacy
GI alkalizers: increased dextroamphetamine absorption and efficacy
Linezolid: increased dextroamphetamine effects
Lithium carbonate: inhibited stimulatory effect of dextroamphetamine
MAO inhibitors: slowed dextroamphetamine metabolism with increased risk of hypertensive crisis, neurologic toxic effects, and malignant hyperpyrexia
Meperidine: potentiated analgesic effect of meperidine

Methenamine, urinary acidifiers (such as ammonium chloride and sodium acid phosphate): increased urinary excretion and decreased efficacy of dextroamphetamine
Norepinephrine: enhanced adrenergic effects
Phenobarbital, phenytoin: delayed intestinal absorption of these drugs
Propoxyphene: increased CNS stimulation, possibly causing fatal seizures in propoxyphene overdose
Tricyclic antidepressants: enhanced tricyclic or sympathomimetic activity, marked and sustained increase in dextroamphetamine brain concentration, potentiated cardiovascular effects
Urinary alkalizers (such as acetazolamide and some thiazides): decreased urinary excretion and increased efficacy of dextroamphetamine
Veratrum alkaloids: inhibited hypotensive effects of these drugs
Drug-diagnostic tests. *Plasma corticosteroids:* elevated levels
Urinary steroid tests: possible interference
Drug-food. *Acidic foods and beverages:* possible decrease in drug absorption
Caffeine: increased CNS stimulant effects
Drug-herb. *Ephedra (ma huang), guarana:* possible drug potentiation
Yohimbe: increased risk of hypertensive crisis

Toxicity and overdose
- Signs and symptoms of acute overdose include restlessness, tremor, hyperreflexia, rhabdomyolysis, rapid respirations, hyperpyrexia, confusion, assaultiveness, hallucinations, and panic states. Psychosis is most severe manifestation of chronic intoxication. Fatigue and depression usually follow central stimulation. Cardiovascular effects include arrhythmias, hypertension, hypotension, and circulatory collapse. Other symptoms include nausea, vomiting, diarrhea, and abdominal cramps. Seizures and coma usually precede fatal poisoning.
- Management of acute toxicity is largely symptomatic and includes gastric lavage, activated charcoal and cathartics, and sedation.

Only common or life-threatening adverse reactions are listed.

- Urine acidification increases drug excretion but may magnify risk of acute renal failure. For acute severe hypertension, I.V. phentolamine has been suggested; however, blood pressure usually decreases gradually when sufficient sedation has been achieved. Chlorpromazine antagonizes drug's central stimulant effects. Hemodialysis or peritoneal dialysis is ineffective.

Special considerations

- Concomitant phenobarbital may cause synergistic anticonvulsant action.
- Watch for signs and symptoms of drug abuse.
- Monitor patient's caloric intake to ensure adequate nutritional status.
- Monitor patients with tartrazine sensitivity (especially those with aspirin hypersensitivity); they may experience allergic-type reactions (including bronchial asthma).
- Infants born to women dependent on drug have increased risk of premature delivery and low birth weight. They may exhibit such withdrawal symptoms as dysphoria, agitation, and lassitude.

Patient education

- Advise patient to take drug early in day to avoid insomnia.
- Instruct patient to swallow sustained-release capsules whole without chewing or crushing.
- Caution patient not to stop using drug abruptly after prolonged high-dosage use; doing so may cause extreme fatigue, mental depression, and sleep EEG changes.
- Inform patient that drug may mask signs and symptoms of extreme fatigue.
- Caution patient to avoid driving and other hazardous activities until drug's effects are known.
- Inform patient who is pregnant or becomes pregnant during therapy that drug is advised only if potential benefit justifies potential fetal risk.
- Caution breastfeeding patient to stop breastfeeding during therapy.

diphenhydramine hydrochloride
Banaril, Benadryl, Diphedryl, Dytan, Hyrexin, Q-Dryl, Trux-Adryl, Valu-Dryl

D

Classification: H_1 antihistamine, antiemetic, antivertigo agent
Pregnancy risk category B

Pharmacology
Diphenhydramine, a first-generation ethanolamine antihistamine, binds nonselectively to central and peripheral H_1 receptors, causing CNS stimulation or depression. Binding to central muscarinic receptors causes antiemetic effects.

Pharmacokinetics
Drug is absorbed quickly, with maximum activity in about 1 hour. It is widely distributed throughout body, including CNS. Duration is 4 to 8 hours. Metabolites appear as degradation products of metabolic transformation in liver and are excreted almost completely within 24 hours.

How supplied
Capsules: 25 mg, 50 mg
Liquid (oral): 25 mg/5 ml
Solution for injection: 10 mg/ml, 50 mg/ml
Tablets: 25 mg, 50 mg
Tablets (chewable): 25 mg

Indications and dosages

Off-label uses (selected)

➥ Premedication for cytotoxic agents
Adults: 25 to 50 mg P.O. 1 hour before administration of monoclonal antibody (such as rituximab or alemtuzumab) and paclitaxel
➥ Nausea or vomiting
Adults: Individualize dosage according to patient needs and response. Usual dosage is 25 to 50 mg P.O. three or four times daily; or 10

to 50 mg I.V. or deep I.M.; maximum daily dosage is 400 mg.

Children weighing more than 9.1 kg (20 lb): Individualize dosage according to patient needs and response. Usual dosage is 12.5 to 25 mg P.O. three or four times daily; or 5 mg/kg or 150 mg/m² per 24 hours, not to exceed 300 mg daily; or 5 mg/kg or 150 mg/m² per 24 hours I.V. or deep I.M in four divided doses, with maximum daily dosage of 300 mg.

Contraindications and precautions

Contraindicated in hypersensitivity to diphenhydramine or other antihistamines of similar chemical structure, when used as local anesthetic (parenteral form), during breastfeeding, and in newborn and premature infants.

Use cautiously in lower respiratory tract disease, increased intraocular pressure, angle-closure glaucoma, stenosing peptic ulcer disease, pyloroduodenal obstruction, symptomatic prostatic hypertrophy, bladder-neck obstruction, hyperthyroidism, hypertension, cardiovascular disease, within 14 days of MAO inhibitors, pregnancy, and *elderly patients* and *children.*

Preparation and administration

• Use injectable form only when oral forms are impractical.

• Check for incompatibility before giving I.V. Administer at a rate of 25 mg (or fraction thereof) over 1 minute. Extend injection time in nonemergency situations and children.

• Inject I.M. deep into large muscle mass.

• Do not administer subcutaneously.

• Drug may be given undiluted.

• Drug is commonly combined with phenothiazine or butyrophenone to enhance antiemetic properties and reduce risk of extrapyramidal symptoms.

• Store capsules and injection at controlled room temperature of 59° to 86° F (15° to 30° C) protected from moisture, freezing, and light.

Adverse reactions

CNS: anxiety, confusion, dizziness, drowsiness, euphoria, fatigue, neuritis, paresthesia, poor coordination

CV: palpitation, tachycardia, hypotension

EENT: blurred vision, dilated pupils, tinnitus, nasal stuffiness, dry nose and throat

GI: anorexia, constipation, diarrhea, dry mouth, nausea, vomiting, epigastric distress

GU: dysuria, urinary frequency, urinary retention, erectile dysfunction

Hematologic: bone marrow depression, hemolytic anemia

Respiratory: chest tightness, increased thick secretions, wheezing

Skin: photosensitivity, rash, urticaria

Other: diaphoresis, chills

Interactions

Drug-drug. *Anticholinergics:* enhanced anticholinergic and CNS effects

CNS depressants: additive effects

MAO inhibitors: prolonged and intensified anticholinergic effects

Drug-diagnostic tests. *Serum and urine tricyclic antidepressants, urine methadone:* false positive

Skin allergy tests: false negative

Drug-herb. *Ginkgo:* possible seizure risk

Ginseng (Siberian), L-tryptophan, melatonin, sassafras, stinging nettle, valerian, yerba mansa: increased sedation

Toxicity and overdose

• Overdose signs and symptoms may vary from CNS depression to stimulation. Stimulation is particularly likely in children. Drug may cause hallucinations, seizures, or death (especially in infants and children). Atropine-like signs and symptoms, dry mouth, fixed and dilated pupils, flushing, and GI symptoms also may occur.

• Do not give stimulants to treat overdose. Vasopressors may be used to treat hypotension. If vomiting does not occur spontaneously after oral diphenhydramine administration, induce vomiting (preferably by having patient drink a glass of water or milk and then stimulating the gag reflex). Take precautions against aspiration, especially in infants and children. If vomiting is unsuccessful, gastric lavage is indicated within 3 hours of ingestion (or later if large amounts of milk or cream were given previously). Isotonic or half-isotonic saline solution is preferred lavage solution. Saline cathartics (such as milk of magnesia) draw water into bowel and therefore can aid in rapid dilution of bowel contents.

Special considerations

- Monitor patient for excess drowsiness.
- Drug is more likely to cause dizziness, sedation, and hypotension in elderly patients.
- Drug may diminish mental alertness in children or cause excitation in young children.

Patient education

- Inform patient that drug may cause drowsiness.
- Advise patient not to use drug with alcohol; additive effect may occur.
- Caution patient not to drive or perform other hazardous activities requiring mental alertness.
- Advise women with childbearing potential to avoid getting pregnant during therapy.
- Instruct breastfeeding patient to stop breastfeeding while taking drug.

diphenoxylate hydrochloride and atropine sulfate
Logen, Lomanate, Lomotil, Lonox

Classification: Antidiarrheal
Controlled substance schedule V
Pregnancy risk category C

Pharmacology

Diphenoxylate is a constipating meperidine congener with no analgesic activity. It inhibits GI motility and prolongs GI transit time. Substherapeutic amount of atropine is added to reduce abuse potential.

Pharmacokinetics

Drug is metabolized rapidly and extensively in liver. Onset is 1 hour; peak, 2 hours; and duration, 3 to 4 hours. Elimination half-life of diphenoxylic acid (drug's major metabolite) is about 12 to 14 hours. Drug is excreted in bile and urine.

How supplied

Liquid: 2.5 mg diphenoxylate and 0.025 mg atropine/5 ml
Tablets: 2.5 mg diphenoxylate and 0.025 mg atropine

Indications and dosages

FDA-APPROVED

➥ Adjunctive therapy in management of diarrhea
Adults: Initially, two tablets P.O. four times daily (20 mg daily) or 10 ml of liquid P.O. four times daily, reduced to meet individual requirements
Children age 2 and older: Initially, 0.3 to 0.4 mg/kg liquid P.O. in four divided doses

Contraindications and precautions

Contraindicated in hypersensitivity to drug or atropine, obstructive jaundice, and diarrhea associated with pseudomembranous enterocolitis or enterotoxin-producing bacteria.

Use cautiously in advanced hepatorenal disease and abnormal hepatic function (hepatic coma may result); toxigenic *Escherichia coli*, *Salmonella*, *Shigella*, and pseudomembranous enterocolitis associated with broad-spectrum antibiotics; acute ulcerative colitis; concomitant use of MAO inhibitors (may precipitate hypertensive crisis), alcohol, barbiturates, or tranquilizers; and pregnancy or breastfeeding. Drug is not recommended for *children younger than age 2*; it should be used with special caution in young children because of possible delayed toxicity and greater variability of response. Also consider child's nutritional status and degree of dehydration.

Preparation and administration

- Control often can be maintained with as little as 5 mg (two tablets or 10 ml of liquid) daily.
- Use oral solution, not tablets, in children younger than age 13.
- Use plastic dropper only when measuring drug.
- Store at controlled temperature of 59° to 86° F (15° to 30° C) in well-closed, light-resistant, child-resistant container.

Adverse reactions

CNS: euphoria, depression, malaise, lethargy, confusion, sedation, drowsiness, dizziness, restlessness, headache, numb extremities
CV: tachycardia
EENT: blurred vision
GI: nausea, vomiting, toxic megacolon, paralytic ileus, pancreatitis, dry mouth, abdominal discomfort, anorexia
GU: urinary retention
Skin: urticaria, pruritus, dry skin and mucous membranes
Other: swelling of gums, hyperthermia, flushing, anaphylaxis, angioneurotic edema

Interactions

Drug-drug. *Barbiturates, tranquilizers:* increased actions of these drugs
MAO inhibitors: possible hypertensive crisis

Toxicity and overdose

- Initial signs and symptoms of overdose may include dry skin and mucous membranes, mydriasis, restlessness, flushing, hyperthermia, and tachycardia, followed by lethargy or coma, hypotonic reflexes, nystagmus, pinpoint pupils, and respiratory depression. Respiratory depression may occur as late as 30 hours after ingestion, and may recur despite initial response to narcotic antagonists.
- Treat all overdoses as serious, and monitor patient closely for at least 48 hours, preferably

under continuous hospital care. Induce vomiting and gastric lavage. Activated charcoal may significantly decrease diphenoxylate bioavailability. In noncomatose patients, slurry of 100 g activated charcoal can be given immediately after induction of vomiting or gastric lavage. Use pure narcotic antagonist (such as naloxone) to treat respiratory depression. After initial improvement, repeated naloxone doses may be used to counteract recurrent respiratory depression.

Special considerations

- Acute diarrhea usually improves clinically within 48 hours. If no improvement occurs after reaching maximum daily dose of 20 mg within 10 days, further administration is unlikely to control symptoms.
- Carefully observe patients with acute ulcerative colitis. Discontinue drug promptly if abdominal distention or other untoward symptoms develop. Toxic megacolon has been reported with agents that inhibit intestinal motility or prolong intestinal transit time.
- Do not exceed recommended dosage. At high doses, drug exhibits codeine-like effects. Dosage producing antidiarrheal action is widely separated from dosage that causes CNS effects.
- Drug use should be accompanied by appropriate fluid and electrolyte therapy, when indicated. If patient has severe dehydration or electrolyte imbalance, withhold drug until appropriate corrective therapy has been initiated. Drug-induced inhibition of peristalsis may cause fluid retention in intestine, which may further aggravate dehydration and electrolyte imbalances.

Patient education

- Caution patient not to exceed recommended dosage.
- Instruct patient to keep drug in child-resistant container out of reach of children.
- Inform patient, parent, or guardian that overdose may cause severe respiratory depres-

---

Only common or life-threatening adverse reactions are listed.

sion and coma, possibly leading to permanent brain damage or death.

- Advise patient to use caution when driving or performing other activities requiring mental alertness because drug may cause drowsiness or dizziness.
- Instruct patient with acute ulcerative colitis to notify prescriber promptly and discontinue drug if abdominal distention or other untoward symptoms develop.
- Inform patient to avoid using alcohol, barbiturates, and tranquilizers while taking this drug.

docetaxel
Taxotere

Classification: Antineoplastic, antimitotic agent
Pregnancy risk category D

Pharmacology
Docetaxel binds to free tubulin and promotes assembly of tubulin into stable microtubules while inhibiting their disassembly. This effect leads to production of dysfunctional microtubule bundles and stabilization of microtubules, which blocks cell cycle at mitosis phase. Drug is twice as potent as paclitaxel on per-mg basis.

Pharmacokinetics
Drug is metabolized primarily in liver and distributed widely throughout body. It is highly protein-bound. Onset is rapid, and duration is 7 days. Half-life is about 11 hours, Elimination is triphasic; drug is excreted primarily in feces.

How supplied
Viscous solution for injection (40 mg/ml): 20 mg and 80 mg in single-dose vials containing 40 mg docetaxel (anhydrous) and 1,040 mg polysorbate 80

Indications and dosages

FDA-APPROVED

➥ Monotherapy of locally advanced or metastatic breast cancer after chemotherapy failure
Adults: 60 to 100 mg/m^2 I.V. over 1 hour every 3 weeks; or 35 mg/m^2 I.V. infusion over 1 hour every week for 6 weeks, followed by 2-week rest period
➥ Treatment adjunct in node-positive breast carcinoma
Adults: 75 mg/m^2 I.V. 1 hour after doxorubicin 50 mg/m^2 I.V. and cyclophosphamide 500 mg/m^2 I.V. every 3 weeks for 6 courses
➥ First-line therapy in combination with cisplatin for unresectable locally advanced or metastatic non-small-cell lung cancer without previous chemotherapy
Adults: 75 mg/m^2 I.V. over 1 hour every 3 weeks
➥ Monotherapy for locally advanced or metastatic non-small-cell lung cancer after platinum-based chemotherapy failure
Adults: 75 mg/m^2 I.V. over 1 hour every 3 weeks
➥ Unresectable locally advanced or metastatic non-small-cell lung cancer in chemotherapy-naive patients, in combination with cisplatin, in patients with good performance status (ECOG 0-2)
Adults: 75 mg/m^2 I.V. over 1 hour, immediately followed by cisplatin 75 mg/m^2 I.V. over 30 to 60 minutes every 3 weeks
➥ Hormone-refractory metastatic prostate cancer, in combination with prednisone
Adults: 75 mg/m^2 I.V. over 1 hour once every 3 weeks for five to ten cycles, with prednisone 5 mg P.O. twice daily given continuously

OFF-LABEL USES (SELECTED)

➥ Small-cell lung cancer after failure of first-line chemotherapy; ovarian cancer after failure of platinum-based therapy
Adults: 100 mg/m^2 I.V. over 1 hour every 3 weeks

➡ Advanced or metastatic esophageal, gastric, or gastroesophageal junction carcinomas, including adenocarcinomas and squamous cell carcinomas

Adults: As monotherapy, 75 to 100 mg/m^2 I.V. infusion over 1 hour every 21 days; in combination with other agents, such as cisplatin, fluorouracil, or gemcitabine, and with concurrent radiation therapy, 60 to 85 mg/m^2 I.V. over 1 hour every 21 to 28 days

➡ Advanced, recurrent, or metastatic head and neck carcinoma, alone or in combination

Adults: 60 to 100 mg/m^2 I.V. over 1 hour every 3 to 4 weeks for two to six cycles

➡ Bladder (urothelial) carcinoma

Adults: 75 to 100 mg/m^2 I.V. over 1 hour every 21 days for up to six cycles

➡ Ovarian carcinoma after failure of platinum-based therapy

Adults: 100 mg/m^2 I.V. over 1 hour every 21 days

DOSAGE MODIFICATIONS

• Adjust dosage from 100 mg/m^2 to 75 mg/m^2 in breast cancer patients who experience febrile neutropenia, neutrophil count below 500/mm^3 for more than 1 week, or severe or cumulative cutaneous reactions. If these reactions persist, decrease dosage from 75 mg/m^2 to 55 mg/m^2 or discontinue drug. If patient experiences Grade 4 neutropenia (neutrophil count below 500/mm^3) lasting 7 days or more, febrile neutropenia, or Grade 4 infection during cycle, reduce dosage by 25% for subsequent cycles.

• Dosage adjustments in patients with neurosensory symptoms (paresthesia, dysesthesia, pain) typically are not necessary; these symptoms tend to reverse after drug withdrawal. Such symptoms correlate with cumulative doses. Drug should be discontinued entirely in patients who develop Grade 3 or above peripheral neuropathy.

• Withhold drug until toxicity resolves in patients with non-small-cell lung cancer receiving drug as monotherapy, patients receiving

initial dosage of 75 mg/m^2 who experience febrile neutropenia, those with neutrophil count below 500/mm^3 for more than 1 week, those with severe or cumulative cutaneous reactions, or those experiencing other Grade 3 or 4 nonhematologic toxic effects. Once symptoms resolve, drug may be resumed at dosage of 55 mg/m^2.

• For patients with non-small-cell lung cancer receiving combination therapy with cisplatin, if platelet-count nadir during previous course was below 25,000/mm^3 or if febrile neutropenia or serious nonhematologic toxic effects occur, reduce dosage to 65 mg/m^2. In patients requiring further dosage reduction, 50 mg/m^2 is recommended.

• For patients who experience Grade 3 or 4 stomatitis, decrease dosage to 60 mg/m^2.

☒ WARNINGS

• Higher incidence of treatment-related deaths have occurred in patients with abnormal hepatic function, those receiving higher doses, and those with non-small-cell lung cancer who received previous treatment with platinum-based chemotherapy and received docetaxel as monotherapy at dosage of 100 mg/m^2.

• Do not give drug if patient has bilirubin level above ULN or AST or ALT level more than 1.5 × ULN concomitant with ALP level above 2.5 × ULN. Patients with bilirubin elevations or transaminase abnormalities concurrent with ALP are at increased risk for Grade 4 neutropenia, febrile neutropenia, infections, severe thrombocytopenia, severe stomatitis, severe skin toxicity, and toxic death. Patients with isolated transaminase elevations above 1.5 × ULN also have higher rate of febrile neutropenia Grade 4, but no increased incidence of toxic death. Bilirubin, AST or ALT, and ALP values should be obtained before each docetaxel cycle and reviewed by treating physician.

Only common or life-threatening adverse reactions are listed.

• Drug should not be given to patients with neutrophil counts below 1,500/mm³. Frequent blood cell counts should be obtained for all patients.

Contraindications and precautions

Contraindicated in history of severe hypersensitivity reaction to docetaxel or other drugs formulated with polysorbate 80, neutrophil count below 1,500/mm³, bilirubin level above ULN, or AST or ALT above 1.5 × ULN concomitant with ALP above 2.5 × ULN.

Use cautiously in women with childbearing potential, pregnancy or breastfeeding, and *elderly patients*. Safety and efficacy in *children younger than age 16* have not been established.

Preparation and administration

• Follow hazardous drug guidelines for preparation, handling, and administration. (See "Managing hazardous drugs," page 11.)
• To reduce severity of fluid retention and hypersensitivity reactions, premedicate all patients with oral corticosteroids, such as dexamethasone 16 mg daily (for instance, 8 mg twice daily for 3 days, starting 1 day before docetaxel therapy begins).
• If patient has preexisting pleural or cardiac effusions, monitor closely from start of therapy for possible exacerbation.
• Do not let concentrate come into contact with plasticized PVC equipment or devices used to prepare solutions for infusion. Store final dilution for infusion in glass or polypropylene bottles or polypropylene or polyolefin plastic bags, and administer through polyethylene-lined administration sets.
• Reconstitute initially with diluent provided, to yield solution of 10 mg/ml. Rotate gently to mix; do not shake. Further dilute in at least 250 ml normal saline solution or D₅W. Infuse over 1 hour.
• If patient experiences hypersensitivity reaction within several minutes of starting drug,

discontinue therapy immediately and treat aggressively if more severe reactions occur.
• Infusion solution remains stable for 4 hours when stored at 36° to 77° F (2° to 25° C). Use fully prepared infusion solution (in either normal saline solution or D₅W) within 4 hours (including 1-hour I.V. infusion).
• Keep in original package until ready to use, and protect from bright light. Freezing does not adversely affect product.

Adverse reactions

CNS: severe paresthesia, dysesthesia, pain, severe asthenia
CV: severe fluid retention, peripheral edema
GI: nausea, vomiting, diarrhea, stomatitis, anorexia, GI hemorrhage (secondary to thrombocytopenia)
Hematologic: neutropenia, febrile neutropenia, leukopenia, thrombocytopenia, anemia
Musculoskeletal: myalgia, arthralgia
Respiratory: pleural effusion
Skin: nail disorders, alopecia, skin disorders, severe skin toxicity
Other: infection, fever, weight gain, hypersensitivity reactions ranging from minor to severe, death

Interactions

Drug-drug. *Cisplatin:* increased incidence and severity of peripheral neuropathy
CYP450 3A4 inhibitors: increased docetaxel blood level
Drugs that induce, inhibit, or are metabolized by CYP450 3A4 (such as erythromycin, ketoconazole, nifedipine, and troleandomycin): altered docetaxel metabolism
Drug-diagnostic tests. *ALP, ALT, AST, bilirubin, BUN, serum creatinine:* increased
Neutrophils, platelets, WBCs: reduced
Drug-food. *Grapefruit juice:* possible altered levels of drugs cleared by CYP450 3A4 enzymes
Drug-herb. *Coenzyme Q10:* possible decreased chemotherapy efficacy
Echinacea: possible increased docetaxel level

Toxicity and overdose

• Anticipated overdose complications include bone marrow depression, peripheral neurotoxicity, and mucositis.

• No known antidote exists. Treatment is supportive. Keep patient in specialized unit where vital functions can be monitored closely. Give therapeutic granulocyte-colony stimulating factor to prevent neutropenia, and use other appropriate symptomatic measures.

Special considerations

• Perform frequent peripheral blood cell counts on all patients. Patient should not receive subsequent cycles until neutrophil count rises above 1,500/mm³ and platelet count rises above 100,000/mm³.

• Severe fluid retention may occur despite 3-day dexamethasone premedication regimen. If peripheral edema occurs, treat with standard measures.

• Closely monitor patients with preexisting effusions for possible exacerbation, starting from first dose.

• Continuously monitor patient for hypersensitivity reactions.

• Patients who respond to therapy may not show improved performance status, and may even show worsening, during therapy.

Patient education

• Inform patient that alopecia reverses within 2 to 3 months after last dose, but that new hair growth may differ in color or texture.

• Stress importance of maintaining fastidious oral hygiene.

• Caution women with childbearing potential to avoid becoming pregnant during therapy because drug can harm fetus.

• Advise breastfeeding patient to stop breastfeeding before therapy begins.

dolasetron mesylate
Anzemet

Classification: Antiemetic
Pregnancy risk category B

Pharmacology

Dolasetron mesylate and its active metabolite, hydrodolasetron (MDL 74,156), are highly specific and selective serotonin 5-hydroxytryptamine (5-HT₃) receptor antagonists with no activity at other known serotonin receptors and with low affinity for dopamine receptors. Drug blocks action of serotonin 5-HT₃ receptors on nerve terminals of vagus peripherally and centrally in chemoreceptor trigger zone of the area postrema, preventing stimulation of vomiting reflex.

Pharmacokinetics

Drug is rapidly metabolized to active metabolite. After I.V. dose, it peaks in less than 1 hour; after oral dose, in 1.5 hours, with 60% to 80% bioavailability. Half-life of I.V. dose is about 10 minutes for parent drug and 8 hours for active metabolite. Drug is excreted unchanged mostly in urine, with some in feces.

How supplied

Injection: 20 mg/ml in 5-ml vial (single-use) or 25-ml vial (multidose)
Tablets: 50 mg, 100 mg

Indications and dosages

FDA-APPROVED

➡ Prevention of nausea and vomiting associated with initial and repeated courses of emetogenic cancer chemotherapy
Adults: 1.8 mg/kg I.V. as single dose approximately 30 minutes before chemotherapy; or fixed dose of 100 mg I.V. over 30 seconds; or 100 mg P.O. as single dose 1 hour before chemotherapy

Only common or life-threatening adverse reactions are listed.

Children ages 2 to 16: 1.8 mg/kg I.V. as single dose approximately 30 minutes before chemotherapy, to maximum of 100 mg; or 1.8 mg/kg injection solution P.O., to maximum 100-mg dose given within 1 hour before chemotherapy

OFF-LABEL USES (SELECTED)

➥ Radiation-induced nausea and vomiting
Adults: 100 mg P.O. daily on radiation therapy days
Children ages 2 to 16: 1.8 mg/kg P.O. or I.V. on radiation therapy days

Contraindications and precautions

Contraindicated in hypersensitivity to drug.

Use cautiously in previous treatment with other selective 5-HT$_3$ receptor antagonists, preexisting or possibility of prolonged cardiac conduction intervals, congenital QT syndrome, use of concomitant antiarrhythmics or other drugs that prolong QT interval, cumulative high-dose anthracycline therapy, and pregnancy or breastfeeding. Safety and efficacy in *children younger than age 2* have not been established.

Preparation and administration

• Mix injection form in apple or apple-grape juice for children's oral doses.
• Single I.V. injection (up to 100 mg) may be infused over 30 seconds, or diluted in 50 ml of compatible I.V. solution (normal saline injection, D$_5$W injection, 5% dextrose and half-normal saline injection, 5% dextrose and lactated Ringer's injection, lactated Ringer's injection, or 10% mannitol injection) and infused over 15 minutes.
• Do not mix injection form with other drugs.
• Flush infusion line before and after administering.
• After dilution, injection form is stable under normal lighting conditions at room temperature for 24 hours or refrigerated for 48 hours.
• Store at controlled room temperature of 68° to 77° F (20° to 25° C) protected from light.

Adverse reactions

CNS: headache, fatigue, light-headedness, dizziness
CV: hypertension, hypotension, ECG changes
GI: diarrhea, abdominal pain, constipation
Hepatic: abnormal hepatic function
Other: fever, pain, chills, shivering, increased appetite

D

Interactions

Drug-drug. *Atenolol:* decreased hydrodolasetron clearance
Cimetidine: increased hydrodolasetron blood level
Drugs that prolong QTc interval: possible increase in QTc prolongation
Drug-diagnostic tests. *Transaminases:* elevated
Drug-food. *Grapefruit juice:* possible altered levels of drugs cleared by CYP450 3A4 enzymes
Drug-herb. *St. John's wort:* possible altered levels of drugs cleared by CYP450 3A4 enzymes

Toxicity and overdose

• Signs and symptoms of acute toxicity include tremors, depression, and seizures. Other symptoms may include prolonged PR, QRS, and QTc intervals and second-degree or complete atrioventricular conduction block. Individual doses as large as 5 mg/kg I.V. or 400 mg P.O. have been given safely.
• No known specific antidote exists. Patients with suspected overdose should be monitored by telemetry and managed with supportive therapy. Treatment may include infusion of plasma expander, dopamine, and atropine.

Special considerations

• Monitor cardiac status, especially in patients receiving other drugs that may prolong QTc interval (including patients with hypokalemia or hypomagnesemia and those taking diuretics that may cause electrolyte abnormalities).
• Monitor liver function tests.

Patient education

• Instruct patient to take oral dose 1 hour before chemotherapy.
• Tell patient to report irregular heartbeats or other heart problems.

doxorubicin hydrochloride
Adriamycin, Adriamycin PFS, Adriamycin RDF

Classification: Antineoplastic, anthracycline antibiotic
Pregnancy risk category D

Pharmacology

Doxorubicin has nucleotide base intercalation and cell-membrane lipid-binding activities, which may explain its cytotoxic effects on cancer cells and toxic effects on various organs. Intercalation inhibits nucleotide replication and action of DNA and RNA polymerases. Drug also may cause free-radical damage to DNA.

Pharmacokinetics

Drug is metabolized in liver to active and inactive forms. It is widely distributed to all body tissues; 75% is protein-bound. Onset is rapid, peak occurs within 2 hours, and duration is 24 to 36 days. Initial distribution half-life is approximately 5 minutes; terminal half-life, 20 to 48 hours. Drug is excreted primarily in bile, with small amount in urine.

How supplied

Injection (Adriamycin PFS): 10-, 20-, 50-, 75-, and 150-mg single-dose vials; 200-mg single-dose Cytosafe vial; 150- and 200-mg multi-dose vials
Powder for injection, lyophilized (Adriamycin RDF): 10-, 20-, and 50-mg single-dose vials; 150-mg multidose vial

Indications and dosages

➡ To produce regression in disseminated neoplastic conditions, such as acute lymphoblastic leukemia, acute myeloblastic leukemia, Wilms' tumor, neuroblastoma, soft-tissue and bone sarcomas, breast carcinoma, ovarian carcinoma, transitional cell bladder carcinoma, thyroid carcinoma, gastric carcinoma, Hodgkin's disease, malignant lymphoma, and bronchogenic carcinoma in which small-cell histologic type is more responsive than other cell types
Adults: As single agent, 60 to 75 mg/m^2 by slow I.V. infusion at 21-day intervals; in combination, 40 to 60 mg/m^2 by slow I.V. infusion every 21 to 28 days
➡ Ewing's sarcoma
Adults: In combination with vincristine and cyclophosphamide, alternating with ifosfamide, mesna, and etoposide, 40 to 60 mg/m^2 I.V. by slow I.V. infusion every 21 to 28 days

➡ Carcinoid tumors
Adults: Dosages vary. Drug is often mixed with other antineoplastics for use in hepatic embolization, but rarely given as systemic chemotherapy.
➡ Bladder carcinoma (prophylaxis)
Adults: In combination with other chemotherapeutic agents, 30 to 50 mg/m^2 I.V. per cycle; or 50 to 80 mg by bladder instillation, retained 1 to 2 hours, weekly for 4 weeks, then monthly
➡ Primary hepatocellular carcinoma
Adults: In combination with cisplatin, 30 mg/m^2 I.V. on days 2 and 3 every 21 days for four cycles; or mixed with iodized oil and given as chemoembolization
➡ Cervical, endometrial, head, neck, pancreatic, prostatic, or testicular carcinoma; germcell tumors; multiple myeloma
Adults: As single agent, 60 to 75 mg/m^2 by slow I.V. infusion at 21-day intervals; in combination with other chemotherapy agents, 40

to 60 mg/m² by slow I.V. infusion every 21 to 28 days
➦ Retinoblastoma
Children: In combination with other chemotherapeutics agents as first-line treatment, 30 to 60 mg/m² I.V. every 21 to 42 days

DOSAGE MODIFICATIONS

• Use lower range of recommended dosages as single I.V. injection at 21-day intervals for patients with inadequate bone marrow reserves due to old age, previous therapy, or neoplastic marrow infiltration.
• Reduce dosage in patients with hepatic impairment.
• Hyperbilirubinemia necessitates dosage reduction. For serum bilirubin level of 1.2 to 3 mg/dl, reduce dosage by 50%; for level of 3.1 to 5 mg/dl, reduce by 75%.

⊠ WARNINGS

• Drug is for I.V. use only.
• Severe local tissue necrosis results if extravasation occurs during administration. Drug must not be given I.M. or subcutaneously.
• Myocardial toxicity, including potentially fatal heart failure, may occur during therapy or even years later. Probability of developing impaired myocardial function is roughly 1% to 2% at total cumulative dose of 300 mg/m², 3% to 5% at dose of 400 mg/m², 5% to 8% at dose of 450 mg/m², and 6% to 20% at dose of 500 mg/m². Risk of developing heart failure rises rapidly with increasing total cumulative doses exceeding 450 mg/m². Toxicity may occur at lower cumulative doses in patients on concurrent cyclophosphamide therapy and in those with preexisting heart disease or previous mediastinal irradiation. Children are at increased risk for delayed cardiotoxicity.
• Secondary acute myelogenous leukemia (AML) has been reported. Refractory secondary leukemia is more common when drug is given in combination with DNA-damaging antineoplastic agents, when patient has been heavily pretreated with cytotoxic drugs, or

when doxorubicin doses have been escalated. Children also are at risk for developing secondary AML.
• Dosage should be reduced in patients with impaired hepatic function.
• Severe bone marrow depression may occur.

Contraindications and precautions

Contraindicated in marked bone marrow depression induced by radiotherapy or previous treatment with other antitumor agents and in previous treatment with complete cumulative doses of doxorubicin, daunorubicin, idarubicin, other anthracyclines, and anthracenes.

Use cautiously in rapidly growing tumors, previous treatment with doxorubicin or other topoisomerase II inhibitors, impaired hepatic function, history of cardiovascular disease, pregnancy or breastfeeding, and in ***children***.

Preparation and administration

⟫ Follow hazardous drug guidelines for preparation, handling, and administration. (See "Managing hazardous drugs," page 11.)
• Consider pretreatment with allopurinol because of hyperuricemia risk.
• To prevent inadvertent overdose, do not interchange formulations or confuse with liposomal form.
• Drug is a vesicant and may cause tissue damage if extravasation occurs. Don't give I.M. or subcutaneously.
• Reconstitute 10-, 20-, 50-, and 150-mg vials with 5, 10, 25, and 75 ml (respectively) of normal saline injection, yielding final concentration of 2 mg/ml. Bacteriostatic diluents are not recommended.
• After adding diluent, shake vial and let contents dissolve.
• Attach tubing to butterfly needle inserted in large vein.
• Slowly administer in tubing of free-running I.V. infusion of normal saline injection or D$_5$W.
• Administration rate depends on dosage and vein size. However, dose should be administered over no less than 3 minutes.

• Do not mix drug with heparin or fluoro-uracil; these drugs are incompatible, and precipitate may form. Until specific compatibility data are available, it is not recommended that doxorubicin be mixed with other drugs.

• Local erythematous streaking along vein, as well as facial flushing, may indicate too-rapid administration.

• Stop infusion immediately and restart in another vein if patient complains of burning or stinging sensation (which may indicate perivenous infiltration). Perivenous infiltration also may occur painlessly even if blood returns well on needle aspiration.

• With suspected extravasation, intermittent ice applied to site for 15 minutes four times a day for 3 days may be useful. Benefit of local drug administration has not been clearly established. Because extravasation reactions commonly are progressive, close observation and plastic surgery consultation are recommended. Blistering, ulceration, and persistent pain are indications for wide-excision surgery followed by split-thickness skin grafting.

• Store single-dose and multidose vials in cartons at controlled temperature of 59° to 86° F (15° to 30° C) protected from light.

• Refrigerate single-dose and multidose glass and Cytosafe vials in cartons at 36° to 46° F (2° to 8° C) protected from light. Reconstituted solution is stable for 7 days at room temperature under normal light, and for 15 days under refrigeration (36° to 46° F). Protect from sunlight. Discard unused solution from 10-, 20-, and 50-mg single-dose vials. Also discard unused solutions of multidose vials remaining beyond recommended storage times.

Adverse reactions

CV: cardiotoxicity
EENT: esophagitis (possibly occurring 5 to 10 days after administration)
GI: diarrhea; acute, severe nausea and vomiting; stomatitis (possibly occurring 5 to 10 days after administration); colon ulceration and necrosis (possibly leading to fatal infection or bleeding)

GU: urine discoloration
Hematologic: secondary AML (when given with DNA-damaging antineoplastics), bone marrow depression
Skin: reversible complete alopecia, hyperpigmentation of nail beds and dermal crease (mainly in children); severe cellulitis, vesication, and tissue necrosis with extravasation
Other: facial flushing (with too-rapid injection), erythematous streaking along vein proximal to injection site

Interactions

Drug-drug. *Carbamazepine, phenytoin:* decreased levels of these drugs
Cyclosporine: potential AUC increase (possibly from decreased clearance of parent drug and decreased doxorubicinol metabolism), causing more profound and prolonged hematologic toxicity along with coma and seizures
Paclitaxel: decreased doxorubicin clearance, leading to profound neutropenic and stomatitis episodes
Phenobarbital: increased doxorubicin elimination
Progesterone: increased neutropenia and thrombocytopenia
Streptozocin: inhibited hepatic metabolism of doxorubicin
Traztuzumab: increased risk of cardiotoxicity
Verapamil: initially increased doxorubicin peak concentration in heart, with higher incidence and severity of degenerative cardiac tissue changes
Drug-diagnostic tests. *Blood uric acid:* increased
CBC: bone marrow depression
Drug-food. *Grapefruit and pomegranate juice:* possible inhibition of CYP3A4 metabolism of doxorubicin, causing increased drug levels and increased risk of adverse effects
Drug-herb. *Coenzyme Q10:* possible decreased chemotherapy efficacy
Glucosamine: reduced doxorubicin effect (from decreased expression of intracellular topoisomerase II)

Only common or life-threatening adverse reactions are listed.

Toxicity and overdose

- Acute overdose may present as mucositis, leukopenia and thrombocytopenia, and cardiomyopathy with resultant heart failure.
- Severely myelosuppressed patients require hospitalization, antimicrobials, platelet transfusions, and symptomatic mucositis treatment. Consider use of hematopoietic growth factor (G-CSF, GM-CSF). Treatment of cardiomyopathy consists of vigorous management of heart failure with digitalis preparations, diuretics, beta blockers, spironolactone, and afterload reducers (such as ACE inhibitors).

Special considerations

- Because severe bone marrow depression may occur, frequently monitor CBC with differential.
- Frequently monitor liver function tests and left ventricular ejection fraction, especially as patient approaches lifetime cumulative maximum dose.
- Carefully monitor cardiac function to minimize cardiotoxicity risk. In adult patients, severe cardiotoxicity may occur precipitously without antecedent ECG changes.
- Acute life-threatening arrhythmias have been reported during or within a few hours after administration.
- Drug may induce tumor lysis syndrome in patients with rapidly growing tumors. Appropriate supportive and pharmacologic measures may prevent or relieve this complication.
- Children are at increased risk for delayed cardiotoxicity; periodic follow-up cardiac evaluations are recommended.
- As component of intensive chemotherapy regimens for children, drug may contribute to prepubertal growth failure. It may also contribute to gonadal impairment (which is usually temporary, though infertility may be permanent).

Patient education

- Inform patient that drug discolors urine for 1 to 2 days after administration.
- Counsel caregivers of children receiving drug to take such precautions as wearing latex gloves to prevent contact with patient's urine and other body fluids for at least 5 days after each treatment.
- Caution women with childbearing potential to avoid pregnancy.
- Advise breastfeeding patient to stop breastfeeding during therapy.

doxorubicin hydrochloride, liposomal (liposomal encapsulated doxorubicin [LED])
Doxil

Classification: Antineoplastic, anthracycline
Pregnancy risk category D

Pharmacology

Liposomal doxorubicin is encapsulated in long-circulating stealth liposomes that prevent detection of liposomes by mononuclear phagocyte system and increase blood circulation time. Exact action is unclear, but liposomes are thought to persist in circulation, penetrating often-compromised tumor vasculature and ultimately inhibiting mitotic activity and nucleic acid synthesis.

Pharmacokinetics

Drug is metabolized in liver and distributed primarily to vascular fluid in intravascular space. Significant levels of doxorubicinol (principal metabolite) do not occur, probably because of slow distribution of free doxorubicin to liver. Half-life is approximately 55 hours. Drug is excreted primarily in bile.

How supplied

Sterile, translucent, red liposomal dispersion for I.V. injection: 2 mg/ml (equal to 20 mg doxorubicin hydrochloride) in 10-ml single-use vial;

2 mg/ml (equal to 50 mg doxorubicin hydrochloride) in 25-ml single-use vial

Indications and dosages

FDA-APPROVED

⊖ Metastatic ovarian carcinoma in patients with disease refractory to platinum-based chemotherapy (disease that has progressed during treatment or within 6 months of completing treatment)
Adults: 50 mg/m² (doxorubicin hydrochloride equivalent) by slow I.V. infusion at initial rate of 1 mg/minute; repeat once every 4 weeks for at least four courses as long as patient fails to progress, shows no evidence of cardiotoxicity, and continues to tolerate treatment.
➡ AIDS-related Kaposi's sarcoma in patients with disease that progressed on previous combination chemotherapy or who do not tolerate such therapy
Adults: 20 mg/m² (doxorubicin hydrochloride equivalent) by slow I.V. infusion at initial rate of 1 mg/minute; repeat once every 3 weeks, for as long as patient responds satisfactorily and tolerates treatment.

OFF-LABEL USES (SELECTED)

➡ Alone or as adjunct for advanced nonovarian gynecologic cancer, solid tumors, metastatic head and neck cancer, hormone-refractory prostate cancer, glioblastoma, and metastatic brain tumor
Adults: 40 to 80 mg/m² I.V. every 3 to 4 weeks
➡ Locally advanced and metastatic breast carcinoma
Adults: As monotherapy, various regimens are used, including 45 to 60 mg/m² I.V. every 3 to 4 weeks for maximum of six cycles; or 35 to 70 mg/m² I.V. every 3 to 6 weeks; or 50 mg/m² I.V. as 1-hour infusion every 4 weeks.
⊖ Multiple myeloma
Adults: One regimen consists of liposomal doxorubicin 40 mg/m² I.V. infusion over 2 to 3 hours with vincristine 2 mg I.V. on day 1 of

each cycle. Then, dexamethasone 40 mg P.O. on days 1 through 4 of each cycle. A second regimen adds thalidomide 50 mg P.O. daily initially, increased by 50 mg P.O. daily every week to maximum tolerated dose, not to exceed 400 mg daily. Regimen repeats every 4 weeks for minimum of six cycles and for two cycles after best response.

DOSAGE MODIFICATIONS

• Because drug exhibits nonlinear pharmacokinetics at 50 mg/m², dosage adjustments may cause nonproportionally greater change in plasma level and drug exposure.
• If Grade 2 or higher adverse events occur, decrease dosage or delay therapy; do not increase dosage later.
• In hepatic impairment, reduce normal dosage by 50% if serum bilirubin level is 1.2 to 3 mg/dl or by 25% if bilirubin level exceeds 3 mg/dl.
Modifications according to toxicity level
• *Grade 1 palmar-plantar erythrodysesthesia (hand-foot syndrome [HFS]):* Continue dosing. If patient previously had Grade 3 or 4 toxicity, delay dosing up to 2 weeks and decrease dosage by 25%.
• *Grade 2 HFS:* Delay dosing up to 2 weeks or until resolved to Grade 0 to 1. If no resolution occurs after 2 weeks, discontinue drug. If resolved to Grade 0 to 1 within 2 weeks and there are no Grade 3 to 4 HFS toxicities, continue treatment at previous dosage and return to original dosing interval. If patient previously experienced Grade 3 to 4 toxicity, continue treatment with 25% dosage reduction and return to original dosing interval.
• *Grade 3 HFS:* Delay dosing up to 2 weeks or until resolved to Grade 0 to 1. Decrease dosage by 25% and return to original dosing interval. If no resolution occurs after 2 weeks, discontinue drug.
• *Grade 4 HFS:* Delay dosing up to 2 weeks or until resolved to Grade 0 to 1. Decrease dosage by 25% and return to original dosing interval. If no resolution occurs after 2 weeks, discontinue drug.

• *Grade 1 hematologic toxicity* (absolute neutrophil count [ANC] 1,500 to 1,900/mm^3; platelets, 75,000 to 150,000/mm^3): No dosage reduction is necessary.

• *Grade 2 hematologic toxicity* (ANC 1,000 to less than 1,500/mm^3; platelets, 50,000 to less than 75,000/mm^3): Wait until ANC is 1,500/mm^3 or above and platelet count is 75,000/mm^3 or above; then redose with no dosage reduction.

• *Grade 3 hematologic toxicity* (ANC 500 to 999/mm^3; platelets, 25,000 to less than 50,000/mm^3): Wait until ANC is 1,500/mm^3 or above and platelet count is 75,000/mm^3 or above; then redose with no dosage reduction.

• *Grade 4 hematologic toxicity* (ANC below 500/mm^3; platelets below 25,000/mm^3): Wait until ANC is 1,500/mm^3 or above and platelet count is 75,000/mm^3 or above; then redose at 25% dosage reduction or continue full dose with cytokine support.

• *Grade 1 stomatitis:* Redose unless patient experienced previous Grade 3 or 4 toxicity. If so, delay dosing up to 2 weeks and decrease dosage by 25%. Return to original dosing interval.

• *Grade 2 stomatitis:* Delay dosing up to 2 weeks or until resolved to Grade 0 to 1. If no resolution occurs after 2 weeks, discontinue drug. If resolved to Grade 0 to 1 within 2 weeks and there is no Grade 3 to 4 stomatitis, continue treatment at previous dosage and return to original dosing interval. If patient previously experienced Grade 3 to 4 toxicity, continue treatment with 25% dosage reduction and return to original dosing interval.

• *Grade 3 stomatitis:* Delay dosing up to 2 weeks or until resolved to Grade 0 to 1. Decrease dosage by 25% and return to original dosing interval. If no resolution occurs after 2 weeks, discontinue drug.

• *Grade 4 stomatitis:* Delay dosing up to 2 weeks or until resolved to Grade 0 to 1. Decrease dosage by 25% and return to original dosing interval. If no resolution occurs after 2 weeks, discontinue drug.

 WARNINGS

• Irreversible myocardial toxicity leading to heart failure may occur as total dosage approaches 550 mg/m^2. Previous use of other anthracyclines or anthracenediones increases risk of cardiotoxicity and reduces total dose that can be given without cardiotoxicity. Cardiotoxicity also may occur at lower cumulative doses in patients who have had previous mediastinal irradiation or are receiving cyclophosphamide concurrently.

• Drug should be given to patients with history of cardiovascular disease only when benefit outweighs risk.

• Acute infusion-related reactions have occurred in up to 10% of patients. These reactions usually resolve within several hours to 1 day after infusion is slowed or terminated. Serious and sometimes life-threatening or fatal allergic infusion reactions have been reported. Drugs to treat such reactions, as well as emergency equipment, should be available for immediate use.

• Drug should be given at initial rate of 1 mg/minute to minimize risk of infusion reactions.

• Severe bone marrow depression may occur.

• Dosage should be reduced in patients with impaired hepatic function.

• Accidental substitution of drug for doxorubicin hydrochloride has caused severe side effects. Doxorubicin liposomal should not be substituted for conventional doxorubicin on per-mg basis.

Contraindications and precautions

Contraindicated in hypersensitivity to drug or its components and in breastfeeding.

Use cautiously in previous treatment with other anthracyclines, previous radiation therapy, cardiovascular disease, hepatic impairment, pregnancy, and **elderly patients** and **children**.

Preparation and administration

>> Follow hazardous drug guidelines for preparation, handling, and administration. (See "Managing hazardous drugs," page 11.)

• Consider pretreatment with allopurinol because of hyperuricemia risk.

• Drug causes lower incidence of emesis than doxorubicin hydrochloride, but patients still require pretreatment with or concomitant use of antiemetics.

• Liposomal encapsulation can substantially affect drug's functional properties. Also, different liposomal products may vary in chemical composition and physical form. Do not substitute.

• Drug is not a clear solution but a translucent, red liposomal dispersion.

• Do not give drug I.M. or subcutaneously or as bolus injection or undiluted solution. Do not mix with other drugs or use bacteriostatic agents (such as benzyl alcohol). Do not use in-line filters.

• Dilute appropriate dose (to maximum of 90 mg) in 250 ml D_5W. Do not use other diluents. Strictly observe aseptic technique (drug contains no preservative or bacteriostatic agent). Refrigerate diluted drug at 36° to 46° F (2° to 8° C) and administer within 24 hours.

• Rapid infusion may increase risk of infusion-related reactions (most of which occur during first infusion). Administer at initial rate of 1 mg/minute to help minimize risk of infusion reactions. If no infusion reaction occurs, increase rate to complete infusion over 1 hour.

• Always administer into free-flowing I.V. line with good blood return.

• Drug is irritant (but not vesicant). Take precautions to avoid extravasation. With I.V. use, extravasation may occur with or without accompanying stinging or burning sensation, even if blood returns well on needle aspiration. If signs or symptoms of extravasation occur, stop infusion immediately and restart in another vein. Applying ice over extravasation site for 30 minutes may help relieve local reaction.

• Refrigerate at 36° to 46° F (2° to 8° C). Prolonged freezing may adversely affect drug, but freezing for less than 1 month does not.

Adverse reactions

CNS: asthenia, paresthesia, headache, malaise, somnolence, dizziness, depression, insomnia, anxiety, emotional lability

CV: cardiotoxicity, chest pain, peripheral edema, hypotension, tachycardia

EENT: conjunctivitis, retinitis, rhinitis, pharyngitis

GI: nausea, vomiting, diarrhea, constipation, anorexia, abdominal pain, enlarged abdomen, stomatitis, dyspepsia, oral candidiasis, mouth ulceration, glossitis, esophagitis, dysphagia, taste perversion

GU: albuminuria

Hematologic: bone marrow depression, hemolysis, increased prothrombin time

Hepatic: hyperbilirubinemia

Metabolic: dehydration, hypocalcemia, hyperglycemia

Musculoskeletal: back pain, myalgia

Respiratory: dyspnea, increased cough, pneumonia

Skin: alopecia; rash; dry skin; pruritus; skin discoloration; skin disorder; vesiculobullous rash; maculopapular rash; exfoliative dermatitis; herpes zoster; herpes simplex; erythematous streaking along vein proximal to injection site; severe cellulitis, vesication, and tissue necrosis with extravasation

Other: HFS, mucous membrane disorder, pain, fever, allergic reaction, chills, infection, diaphoresis, weight loss, allergic reaction, infusion-related reactions (including flushing, dyspnea, facial swelling, headache, chills, chest pain, back pain, tightness in chest and throat, fever, tachycardia, pruritus, rash, cyanosis, syncope, bronchospasm, asthma, apnea, and hypotension)

Interactions

Drug-drug. *Carbamazepine, phenytoin:* decreased levels of these drugs

---

Only common or life-threatening adverse reactions are listed.

Cyclosporine: potential AUC increase for doxorubicin and doxorubicinol, resulting in more profound and prolonged hematologic toxicity, coma, and seizures

Paclitaxel: decreased doxorubicin clearance, leading to profound neutropenic and stomatitis episodes

Phenobarbital: increased doxorubicin elimination

Progesterone: increased doxorubicin-induced neutropenia and thrombocytopenia

Streptozocin: inhibited hepatic metabolism of doxorubicin

Trastuzumab: increased cardiotoxicity risk

Verapamil: possible increase in initial peak doxorubicin concentration in heart, with higher incidence and severity of degenerative cardiac tissue changes

Drug-diagnostic tests. *AST, blood glucose, calcium, serum bilirubin, uric acid, urine albumin:* increased

CBC: bone marrow depression

WBCs: decreased

Drug-food. *Grapefruit and pomegranate juice:* possible inhibition of CYP3A4 metabolism of doxorubicin, causing increased drug levels and increased risk of adverse effects

Drug-herb. *Coenzyme Q10:* possible decreased chemotherapy efficacy

Glucosamine: possible reduced doxorubicin effects

Toxicity and overdose

• Acute overdose causes increased mucositis, leukopenia, and thrombocytopenia.

• Treat severely myelosuppressed patient with hospitalization, antibiotics, platelet and granulocyte transfusions, and symptomatic treatment of mucositis.

Special considerations

• Monitor patient carefully. Most adverse events can be managed by reducing dosage or delaying dosing.

• Monitor liver function tests frequently.

• Carefully monitor cardiac function to minimize cardiotoxicity risk. In adults, severe car-

diotoxicity may occur precipitously, without antecedent ECG changes.

• Although bone marrow depression may be moderate and reversible, monitor CBC with differential frequently.

• Observe for signs and symptoms of HFS (swelling, pain, erythema and, for some patients, skin desquamation on hands and feet), which may become severe, requiring drug withdrawal.

Patient education

• Inform patient and caregiver of expected adverse reactions.

• Tell patient to report signs and symptoms of HFS (including tingling or burning, redness, flaking, bothersome swelling, small blisters, or small sores on palms or soles), stomatitis symptoms (including painful redness, swelling, or sores in mouth), infection symptoms (such as temperature of 100.5° F [38° C] or higher), nausea or vomiting, tiredness, weakness, rash, or mild hair loss.

• Advise women with childbearing potential to avoid pregnancy and breastfeeding.

dronabinol
Marinol

Classification: Antiemetic, antivertigo agent, appetite stimulant
Controlled substance schedule IV
Pregnancy risk category B

Pharmacology

Dronabinol, an orally active cannabinoid, has complex effects on CNS, including central sympathomimetic activity. Cannabinoid receptors in neural tissues may play a role in mediating drug effects. Drug has reversible effects on appetite, mood, cognition, memory, and perception. These effects appear to be dose-related, increasing in frequency with higher dosages, and vary greatly among patients.

Pharmacokinetics
Drug is almost completely absorbed. Because of high first-pass effect, only 10% to 20% reaches systemic circulation. Drug is highly protein-bound and exhibits high lipid solubility. With oral dose, onset is approximately 0.5 to 1 hour and peak is 2 to 4 hours. Duration of psychoactive effects is 4 to 6 hours; appetite stimulant effect may last 24 hours or longer.

How supplied
Capsules (soft gelatin): 2.5 mg, 5 mg, 10 mg

Indications and dosages

FDA-APPROVED
➤ Nausea and vomiting associated with chemotherapy in patients unresponsive to conventional antiemetic therapy
Adults: Initially, 5 mg/m² P.O. 1 to 3 hours before chemotherapy, then every 2 to 4 hours for total of four to six doses daily; increase dosage by 2.5-mg/m² increments to maximum of 15 mg/m²/dose.
Children: 5 mg/m² starting 1 to 3 hours before chemotherapy, then 5 mg/m²/dose every 2 to 4 hours after chemotherapy for total of four to six doses daily; escalate dosage by 2.5-mg/m² increments to maximum of 15 mg/m²/dose.

OFF-LABEL USES (SELECTED)
➤ Appetite stimulant for cancer-related cachexia
Adults: Initially, 2.5 mg P.O. twice daily before lunch and supper, increased to maximum of 20 mg daily in divided doses

DOSAGE MODIFICATIONS
• For use as appetite stimulant and for patients unable to tolerate 5 mg daily, reduce dosage to 2.5 mg daily as single dose in evening or at bedtime. If indicated and no significant adverse effects have occurred, gradually increase dosage to maximum of 20 mg daily given in divided doses.

Contraindications and precautions
Contraindicated in hypersensitivity to cannabinoid or sesame oil.
Use cautiously in history of substance abuse (including alcohol abuse and dependence); cardiac disorders; concomitant use of sedatives, hypnotics, or other psychoactive drugs; mania; depression; schizophrenia; pregnancy or breastfeeding; and *children*.

Preparation and administration
• When using as appetite stimulant, give before lunch and dinner.
• To minimize CNS side effects, entire daily dose may be given at bedtime.
• Use caution when escalating dosage because of increased frequency of dose-related adverse reactions at higher dosages.
• Store in well-closed container in cool environment between 46° and 59° F (8° and 15° C); protect from freezing.

Adverse reactions
CNS: anxiety, dizziness, euphoria, poor concentration, mood changes, paranoia, suicidal ideation
CV: palpitations, tachycardia
GI: abdominal pain, nausea and vomiting
Other: asthenia, facial flushing

Interactions
Drug-drug. *Amitriptyline, amoxapine, desipramine, other tricyclic antidepressants:* additive tachycardia, hypertension, drowsiness
Amphetamines, sympathomimetics: additive hypertension, tachycardia, possible cardiotoxicity
Antihistamines, atropine, scopolamine, other anticholinergics: additive or superadditive tachycardia, drowsiness
Antihistamines, barbiturates, benzodiazepines, buspirone, lithium, muscle relaxants, opioids, other CNS depressants: additive drowsiness and CNS depression
Disulfiram: possible hypomanic reaction
Theophylline: increased theophylline metabolism

Drug-herb. *Aloe, rhubarb*: possible reduced drug absorption
Eucalyptus: possible increased drug level

Toxicity and overdose

• Signs and symptoms of mild intoxication include drowsiness, euphoria, heightened sensory awareness, altered time perception, reddened conjunctiva, dry mouth, and tachycardia. Moderate intoxication causes memory impairment, depersonalization, mood alteration, urinary retention, and reduced bowel motility. Severe intoxication causes decreased motor coordination, lethargy, slurred speech, and orthostatic hypotension. Apprehensive patients may experience panic reactions; patients with preexisting seizure disorders may experience seizures.

• Manage potentially serious oral ingestion (if recent) with gut decontamination. In unconscious patient with secure airway, instill activated charcoal (30 to 100 g in adults or 1 to 2 g/kg in infants) through nasogastric tube. Saline cathartic or sorbitol may be added to first activated charcoal dose. Place patient experiencing depressive, hallucinatory, or psychotic reaction in quiet area and offer reassurance. Benzodiazepines (5 to 10 mg diazepam P.O.) may be used to treat extreme agitation.

Special considerations

• Evaluate and monitor vital signs for hypotension and tachycardia.
• Monitor patient for adverse CNS reactions, especially confusion.
• Use with caution and careful psychiatric monitoring in patients with mania, depression, or schizophrenia; drug may exacerbate these conditions.
• Monitor fluid intake and output to prevent dehydration.

Patient education

• Inform patient about potential for additive CNS depression if drug is used with alcohol or other CNS depressants (such as benzodiazepines and barbiturates).

• Caution patient not to drive or engage in other hazardous activities until drug's effects are known.
• Advise patient of possible mood changes and other behavioral effects, to avoid panic in case such events occur. Tell him or caregiver that he should remain under supervision of responsible adult during initial drug use and after dosage adjustments.
• Instruct breastfeeding patient not to use drug while breastfeeding.

droperidol
Inapsine

Classification: Antiemetic
Pregnancy risk category C

Pharmacology

Droperidol, a butyrophenone antipsychotic, antagonizes dopamine action at subcortical CNS levels, causing marked tranquilization and sedation. It produces antiemetic effect by binding centrally to dopamine receptors (primarily dopamine$_2$ receptors) in chemoreceptor trigger zone and blocking dopamine's effect. Drug also causes peripheral vasodilation and reduces pressor effect of epinephrine.

Pharmacokinetics

Drug is metabolized in liver. With single I.M. and I.V. doses, onset occurs in 3 to 10 minutes, though drug may not peak for up to 30 minutes. Duration of tranquilizing and sedative effects is 2 to 4 hours, but alertness may remain altered up to 12 hours. Drug is excreted in urine (75%) and feces (22%).

How supplied

Solution for injection: 2.5 mg/ml in 1- and 2-ml vials

Indications and dosages

FDA-APPROVED

➥ Adjunct to control nausea and vomiting associated with emetogenic chemotherapy
Adults: Recommended initial maximum dosage is 2.5 mg I.M or slow I.V. infusion. Additional 1.25-mg doses may be given to achieve desired clinical effect.

➥ To prevent chemotherapy-induced nausea and vomiting
Adults: 2.5 to 5 mg I.V. 30 to 60 minutes before chemotherapy; same or one-half I.V. dose may be given I.M. after chemotherapy as needed but no more than once every hour.
Children ages 2 to 12: 0.05 to 0.06 mg/kg I.V. or I.M. every 3 to 4 hours as needed; maximum dosage is 0.1 mg/kg.

DOSAGE MODIFICATIONS

• Dosage may be individualized. Factors to consider include patient's age, weight, physical status, underlying pathologic condition, and use of other drugs.
• Initiate drug at low dosage and adjust upward with caution in patients older than age 65 and those who abuse alcohol, and when given concomitantly with such agents as benzodiazepines, volatile anesthetics, and I.V. opioids.

⊠ WARNINGS

• Drug is for I.M. or I.V. use only.
• QT prolongation and torsades de pointes have been reported in patients receiving drug at doses at or below recommended dosages (including some with no known risk factors for QT prolongation). Some cases have been fatal. All patients should undergo 12-lead ECG before administration to detect prolonged QTc interval. Do not administer if QT interval is prolonged.
• Because of potential for serious proarrhythmic effects and death, drug should be reserved for patients who fail to show acceptable response to other antiemetics (from insufficient drug efficacy or intolerable adverse effects of those drugs).
• Drug should be given with extreme caution in patients at risk for prolonged QT syndrome, such as in heart failure, bradycardia, diuretic use, cardiac hypertrophy, hypokalemia, hypomagnesemia, administration of other drugs known to increase QTc interval (such as MAO inhibitors), or electrolyte imbalance (particularly hypokalemia and hypomagnesemia). Other risk factors may include age over 65, alcohol abuse, and use of such agents as benzodiazepines, volatile anesthetics, and I.V. opioids.

Contraindications and precautions

Contraindicated in hypersensitivity to drug and known or suspected QTc prolongation (including congenital long-QT syndrome). Use cautiously in cardiovascular, renal, and hepatic disease; Parkinson's disease; electrolyte imbalance; pheochromocytoma; pregnancy or breastfeeding; and *elderly patients* and *children.* Safety and efficacy have not been established for *children younger than age 2.*

Preparation and administration

• For patients at risk for potentially serious arrhythmias, begin ECG monitoring before drug therapy starts and continue for 2 to 3 hours after therapy ends. Use caution in giving additional doses following initial dosage because of risk of arrhythmias.
• Droperidol is not recommended other than in treating perioperative nausea and vomiting in patients for whom other treatments are ineffective or inappropriate.
• Store at 59° to 77° F (15° to 25° C) protected from light.

Adverse reactions

CNS: drowsiness
CV: prolonged QTc interval, cardiac arrest, torsade de pointes, ventricular tachycardia, hypertension, hypotension

---

Only common or life-threatening adverse reactions are listed.

Respiratory: apnea, bronchospasm, respiratory arrest, respiratory depression

Interactions
Drug-drug. *Antiarrhythmics (Class I or II), antidepressants, antihistamines, antimalarials, calcium channel blockers, neuroleptics:* prolonged QTc interval
Barbiturates, general anesthetics, opioids, tranquilizers: additive or potentiated droperidol effects
Centrally acting anticholinergics, metoclopramide: increased risk of extrapyramidal symptoms
Drug-diagnostic tests. *ECG:* abnormal
Drug-herb. *Ephedra (ma huang):* increased risk of QTc prolongation
L-tryptophan, melatonin, sassafras: increased sedation

Toxicity and overdose
• Signs and symptoms of overdose include exaggerated sedation.
• No treatment should be needed. Otherwise, treat symptomatically.

Special considerations
• Monitor vital signs frequently for orthostatic hypotension and tachycardia.
• Keep I.V. fluids at hand to treat hypotension.
• Monitor ECG for prolonged QTc interval.
• Evaluate respiratory status frequently if drug is used with opioids or depressants.
• Patients older than age 65 may be at greater risk for cardiac adverse effects.

Patient education
• Advise patient to avoid alcohol use during therapy.
• Instruct patient to avoid abrupt position changes to prevent orthostatic hypotension.
• Caution patient to avoid driving and other activities requiring mental alertness until drug's effects are known.

epirubicin hydrochloride
Ellence

Classification: Anthracycline antibiotic
Pregnancy risk category D

E

Pharmacology
Epirubicin is a cytotoxic agent derived from doxorubicin. Anthracyclines can interfere with biochemical and biological functions within eukaryotic cells. However, precise mechanism of drug's cytotoxic and antiproliferative properties are unclear. Drug has a more favorable therapeutic index than doxorubicin, with less hematologic toxicity and cardiotoxicity at equimolar doses. Activity is cell cycle phase-nonspecific.

Pharmacokinetics
Drug is extensively and rapidly metabolized primarily by liver; epirubicinol is principal active metabolite. With I.V. dose, drug is rapidly and widely distributed, and binds strongly to plasma proteins. Half-life is approximately 30 to 35 hours. Parent drug and metabolites are glucuronidated and excreted in bile to a much larger extent than in kidney.

How supplied
Solution for injection: 50 mg/25 ml, 200 mg/dl in single-use vials

Indications and dosages

FDA-APPROVED

⊖ Adjuvant therapy in patients with evidence of axillary-node tumor involvement after resection of primary breast cancer
Adults: Initially, 100 to 120 mg/m² by I.V infusion; repeated in 3- to 4-week cycles

OFF-LABEL USES (SELECTED)

➡ Esophageal carcinoma, esophagogastric junction carcinoma, and adenocarcinoma in combination with other agents

---

Adults: In combination with cisplatin and 5-fluorouracil, 50 mg/m^2 I.V. every 3 weeks
➡ Locally unresectable and metastatic gastric carcinoma
Adults: As single agent or in combination, 50 mg/m^2 I.V. every 21 days; or 30 mg/m^2 I.V. on days 1 and 5 every 28 days
➡ Non-small-cell lung carcinoma
Adults: 120 mg/m^2 I.V. every 3 weeks; or 35 to 60 mg/m^2 I.V. daily for 3 days every 3 weeks
➡ Limited and extensive small-cell lung carcinoma
Adults: 20 to 25 mg/m^2 I.V. weekly; or 50 to 150 mg/m^2 I.V. every 3 to 4 weeks
➡ Stage III and IV (FIGO) ovarian carcinoma
Adults: As single agent, 90 mg/m^2 by I.V. push every 3 weeks for maximum of 12 courses; in combination, 65 to 75 mg/m^2 I.V. every 28 days
➡ Hodgkin's lymphoma
Adults: In combination, 60 to 90 mg/m^2 I.V. every 21 days
➡ Non-Hodgkin's lymphoma
Adults: As single agent or in combination, 75 to 90 mg/m^2 I.V. every 21 days
➡ Soft-tissue sarcoma
Adults: In combination with other agents or instead of doxorubicin, 60 mg/m^2 I.V. for 2 to 3 days every 3 weeks for five cycles; or 75 to 90 mg/m^2 I.V. on day 1 every 3 weeks
➡ Bladder cancer
Adults: 50 mg in 50 ml normal saline solution by intravesicular instillation for 1 to 2 hours weekly for 8 weeks; then monthly
➡ Prostate cancer
Adults: 25 mg/m^2 I.V. weekly; or in combination with estramustine, 100 mg/m^2 I.V. every 21 days
➡ Primary hepatocellular carcinoma
Adults: In combination with other agents, 50 mg/m2 I.V. on day 1 every 21 days

DOSAGE MODIFICATIONS

• For patients who have had primary breast cancer resection, total dose may be given on day 1 of each treatment cycle, or divided equally and given on days 1 and 8 of each cycle.
• After first cycle, dosage adjustments should be based on hematologic and nonhematologic toxicities. Patients with treatment-cycle nadir platelet counts below 50,000/mm^3, absolute neutrophil count (ANC) below 250/mm^3, neutropenic fever, or Grade 3 or 4 nonhematologic toxicity should receive day-1 dosage in subsequent cycles reduced to 75% of day-1 dosage given in current cycle. In subsequent courses, day-1 chemotherapy should be delayed until platelet count is at least 100,000/mm^3, ANC is at least 1,500/mm^3, and nonhematologic toxicities recover to below Grade 1.
• For patient receiving divided dose on days 1 and 8, day-8 dosage should be 75% of day-1 dosage if platelet count is 75,000 to 100,000/mm^3 and ANC is 1,000 to 1,499/mm^3. If day-8 platelet count is below 75,000/mm^3, ANC is below 1,000/mm^3, or Grade 3 or 4 nonhematologic toxicity has occurred, day-8 dose should be omitted.
• Consider lower starting dosages for heavily pretreated patients, preexisting bone marrow depression, or existing neoplastic bone marrow infiltration.
• Reduce dosage in hepatic impairment. No definitive recommendations for use in patients with hepatic impairment are available. In patients with elevated serum AST or total bilirubin level, dosage reductions have been recommended as follows: For serum bilirubin level of 1.2 to 3 mg/dl or AST level 2 to 4 × ULN, give 50% of recommended starting dose; for serum bilirubin level above 3 mg/dl or AST more than 4 × ULN, give 25% of recommended starting dose.
• Consider lower dosages in patients with severe renal impairment (serum creatinine level above 5 mg/dl).

⊠ WARNINGS

• Drug is a vesicant and can cause severe local tissue necrosis with extravasation. It should be administered into a free-flowing I.V. with good blood return.

- Drug must not be given I.M. or subcutaneously.
- Myocardial toxicity (including potentially fatal heart failure) may occur during therapy or years afterward. Probability of clinically evident heart failure is approximately 0.9% at cumulative dose of 550 mg/m^2, 1.6% at 700 mg/m^2, and 3.3% at 900 mg/m^2. In adjuvant treatment for breast cancer, maximum cumulative dose used in clinical trials was 720 mg/m^2. Risk of heart failure increases rapidly with increasing total cumulative doses above 900 mg/m^2; this cumulative dose should be exceeded only with extreme caution. Active or dormant cardiovascular disease, previous or concomitant radiotherapy to mediastinal or pericardial area, previous therapy with other anthracyclines or anthracenediones, or concomitant use of other cardiotoxic drugs may increase cardiotoxicity risk. Cardiotoxicity may occur at lower cumulative doses whether or not cardiac risk factors are present.
- Secondary acute myelogenous leukemia (AML) has been reported in patients with breast cancer treated with epirubicin and other anthracyclines. Refractory secondary leukemia is more common when such drugs are given in combination with DNA-damaging antineoplastic agents, when patients have been heavily pretreated with cytotoxic drugs, or when anthracycline doses have been escalated.
- Dosage should be reduced in patients with impaired hepatic function.
- Severe bone marrow depression may occur.

Contraindications and precautions

Contraindicated in hypersensitivity to drug or other anthracyclines or anthracenediones, baseline neutrophil count below 1,500/mm^3, severe myocardial insufficiency, recent myocardial infarction, and previous treatment with anthracyclines up to maximum cumulative dose.

Use cautiously in risk factors for cardiomyopathy (active or dormant cardiovascular disease, previous therapy with other anthracyclines or anthracenediones, or concomitant use of other drugs that can suppress cardiac contractility), serum creatinine level below 5 mg/dl, thrombophlebitis and thromboembolic phenomena, hepatic impairment, before or after radiation therapy, pregnancy or breastfeeding, and *elderly patients* (especially women older than age 70). Safety and efficacy in *children* have not been established.

Preparation and administration

- Follow hazardous drug guidelines for handling, preparation, and administration. (See "Managing hazardous drugs," page 11.)
- Before initial treatment and during each cycle, perform careful baseline assessment of blood counts; serum total bilirubin, AST, and creatinine; and cardiac function (measured by baseline cardiac evaluation with ECG and MUGA scan or echocardiogram), as well as evaluation of left ventricular ejection fraction (LVEF), especially in patients with risk factors for increased cardiotoxicity. Repeated MUGA or echocardiographic evaluation of LVEF should be performed, particularly with higher cumulative doses.
- Before starting treatment, patients should recover from acute toxicities (such as stomatitis, neutropenia, thrombocytopenia, and generalized infections).
- Consider giving antiemetic before therapy begins, particularly when administering drug in conjunction with other emetogenic drugs.
- If drug is administered with paclitaxel, give paclitaxel after epirubicin. Paclitaxel may significantly increase epirubicin bioavailability and slow recovery from neutropenia if given first.
- Do not exceed cumulative dose of 900 mg/m^2 because of cardiomyopathy risk.
- Patients who receive 120 mg/m^2 regimen as component of combination chemotherapy may also require prophylactic antibiotic thera-

py with trimethoprim-sulfamethoxazole or fluoroquinolone.
• Drug is intended for I.V. infusion only (except off-label intravesicular use). Do not administer I.V. push because of risk of extravasation, which may occur even if blood return is adequate.
• Avoid prolonged contact with alkaline solutions, which cause hydrolysis. Do not mix with other drugs (particularly heparin and 5-fluorouracil) because of chemical incompatibility that may lead to precipitation.
• Drug can be used in combination with other antitumor agents but should not be mixed with other drugs in same syringe.
• Administer slowly into free-running I.V. infusion of normal saline solution or 5% glucose solution. Infusion should take 3 to 20 minutes, depending on dosage and solution volume. This technique helps minimize risk of thrombosis and perivenous extravasation, which could lead to local pain, severe cellulitis, vesication, and tissue necrosis.
• Facial flushing and local erythematous streaking along vein may indicate excessively rapid administration and may precede local phlebitis or thrombophlebitis.
• Burning or stinging sensation may indicate perivenous infiltration. Immediately stop infusion and restart in another vein. Perivenous infiltration may occur without pain.
• Use drug within 24 hours after rubber stopper is first penetrated; discard unused solution.
• Store refrigerated between 36° and 46° F (2° and 8° C) protected from light.

Adverse reactions

CNS: lethargy
CV: myocardial toxicity (cardiomyopathy, heart failure), thrombophlebitis and thromboembolic phenomena including pulmonary embolism (in some cases fatal)
EENT: conjunctivitis, keratitis
GI: nausea, vomiting, diarrhea, anorexia, mucositis

GU: amenorrhea, hot flashes, red urine, chromosomal sperm damage
Hematologic: leukopenia, neutropenia, anemia, thrombocytopenia, severe bone marrow depression
Metabolic: hyperuricemia (from tumor lysis syndrome)
Skin: alopecia, rash, itching, skin changes, local toxicity (injection site pain, severe cellulitis, vesication, tissue necrosis), inflammatory recall reaction at site of previous irradiation
Other: fever, infection, secondary AML

Interactions

Drug-drug. *Cimetidine:* 50% increase in mean AUC (100 mg/m^2) and 30% decrease in plasma clearance of epirubicin
Other cardioactive compounds that could cause heart failure (such as calcium channel blockers): possible cardiac dysfunction
Other cytotoxic drugs: additive toxicity, especially hematologic and GI effects
Paclitaxel: significantly increased bioavailability and slowed recovery from epirubicin-induced neutropenia (when given before epirubicin)
Traztuzumab: increased risk of cardiomyopathy
Verapamil: increased epirubicin AUC
Drug-diagnostic tests. *Neutrophils, platelets, WBCs:* decreased
Serum uric acid: increased
Transaminases: grade 1 or 2 changes (more common when drug is given with other antineoplastics)
Drug-herb. *Coenzyme Q10:* possible decreased chemotherapy efficacy

Toxicity and overdose

• Overdose may cause adverse events similar to known epirubicin toxicities, and may progress to multisystem failure and death.
• If overdose occurs, provide supportive treatment (including antibiotics, blood and platelet transfusions, colony-stimulating factors, and intensive care as needed) until recovery. Delayed heart failure may occur months after ad-

---

Only common or life-threatening adverse reactions are listed.

ministration. Observe patient carefully over time for indications of heart failure, and provide appropriate supportive therapy.

Special considerations

• Monitor CBC and platelet count before and during each cycle. In most cases, WBC nadir occurs 10 to 14 days after administration. Neutropenia is usually transient, with WBC and neutrophil counts generally returning to normal by day 21.
• Evaluate serum total bilirubin and AST levels before and during therapy. Patients with elevated bilirubin or AST may experience slower drug clearance with increased toxicity. Patients with severe hepatic impairment have not been evaluated and should not receive drug.
• Evaluate serum creatinine level before and during therapy.
• Monitor serum uric acid, potassium, calcium phosphate, and creatinine levels immediately after initial therapy. Hydration, urine alkalization, and prophylaxis with allopurinol to prevent hyperuricemia may minimize potential complications of tumor lysis syndrome.
• Carefully monitor patient for clinical complications of bone marrow depression. Supportive care may be necessary to treat severe neutropenia and severe infectious complications.
• Monitor patient for thrombophlebitis and thromboembolic phenomena, including pulmonary embolism.
• Monitor patient for potential cardiotoxicity, especially with greater cumulative drug exposure. Watch for signs and symptoms of early cardiotoxicity.
• Monitor patient for delayed cardiotoxicity. Life-threatening heart failure is most severe form of drug-induced cardiomyopathy and depends on cumulative dose. If it occurs, delayed cardiotoxicity usually develops late in course of therapy or within 3 months afterward. However, later events (including several months to years after termination) have been reported.

• Drug may cause inflammatory recall reaction at radiation sites.
• During epirubicin therapy, substitute cimetidine with alternative H_2-antagonist, such as ranitidine or famotidine.

Patient education

• Inform patient about expected adverse effects, including GI symptoms (nausea, vomiting, diarrhea, and stomatitis) and potential neutropenic complications.
• Instruct patient to report signs and symptoms of dehydration, fever, infection, or heart failure or injection site pain.
• Tell patient he will almost certainly experience alopecia.
• Inform patient that urine may appear red for 1 to 2 days but that this is harmless.
• Tell patient drug may cause irreversible myocardial damage and leukemia.
• Because drug may cause chromosomal damage in sperm, advise males to use effective contraception.
• Inform female patients that drug may cause irreversible amenorrhea or premature menopause.
• Caution women with childbearing potential to avoid pregnancy.
• Advise breastfeeding patient to stop breastfeeding before therapy begins.

epoetin alfa
Epogen, Procrit

Classification: Hematopoietic agent, hormone/hormone modifier
Pregnancy risk category C

Pharmacology

Epoetin alfa, a glycoprotein manufactured by recombinant DNA technology, induces RBC production by stimulating division and differentiation of committed erythroid progenitor cells. It causes release of reticulocytes from bone marrow into bloodstream, where they mature to erythrocytes. In anemic patients undergoing chemotherapy, drug increases hematocrit and reduces transfusion requirements after first month of therapy (months 2 and 3).

Pharmacokinetics

Drug is well absorbed. Half-life is 4 to 13 hours.

How supplied

Solution for injection: 2,000, 3,000, 4,000, and 10,000 units/ml in single-dose, preservative-free vials; 10,000 and 20,000 units/ml in multidose preserved vials

Indications and dosages

FDA-APPROVED

➡ Anemia in patients with nonmyeloid cancers, when anemia results from effects of concomitantly administered chemotherapy; to decrease need for transfusions in patients receiving concomitant chemotherapy for at least 2 months
Adults: 150 units/kg subcutaneously three times weekly, with dosage adjusted to response after 8 weeks; or 40,000 units subcutaneously weekly, with dosage adjusted to response after 4 weeks

OFF-LABEL USES (SELECTED)

➡ Chronic anemia associated with neoplastic disease and cancer
Adults: Initially, 40,000 units subcutaneously each week, with dosage adjusted to response after 4 weeks
➥ Anemia associated with myelodysplastic syndromes (MDS) in selected patients
Adults: Initially, 40,000 to 80,000 units subcutaneously each week, with dosage adjusted to response after 4 weeks

DOSAGE MODIFICATIONS

• Patients with MDS commonly need higher-than-usual dosages to achieve response.

• If initial dosage induces rapid hematocrit response (such as increase of more than 4 percentage points in any 2-week period), reduce dosage.
• If response is unsatisfactory, increase dosage up to 300 units/kg three times weekly or 60,000 units weekly. If this dosage also causes unsatisfactory response, patient is unlikely to respond to higher dosages.
• If hematocrit exceeds 40%, withhold drug until level falls to 36%. Reduce dosage by 25% when treatment resumes, and adjust dosage to maintain desired hematocrit.
• If hematocrit increase exceeds 4 points in 2-week period, decrease dosage because of possible seizures and exacerbation of hypertension. See table below.

Hgb or Hct (obtained every 4 weeks of therapy)	Has patient required transfusion in last 4 weeks?	Dosage adjustment after 4 weeks of therapy	Dosage adjustment after 12 weeks of therapy
Hgb below 11 g/dl or Hct above 33 g/dl	N/A	Increase to 60,000 units/ week.	If Hgb increases less than 1 g/dl, discontinue drug.
Hgb 11 to 11.9 g/dl or Hct 33 to 35.9 g/dl	No	Maintain current dosage.	Maintain current dosage.
	Yes	Increase to 60,000 units/ week.	If Hgb increases less than 1 g/dl, discontinue drug.
Hgb above 11.9 g/dl or Hct above 35.9 g/dl	N/A	Withhold dose until Hgb is below 12 g/dl or Hct is below 36 g/dl; then restart at 40,000 units given at 2-week intervals.	Withhold dose until Hgb is below 12 g/dL or Hct is below 36 g/dl; then restart at 40,000 units given at 2-week intervals.

Key: Hgb = hemoglobin; Hct = hematocrit

Only common or life-threatening adverse reactions are listed.

Contraindications and precautions

Contraindicated in hypersensitivity to mammalian cell-derived products or albumin (human) and in uncontrolled hypertension.

Use cautiously in history of seizure disorder or underlying hematologic disease (such as sickle cell anemia, MDS, or hypercoagulable disorders); porphyria; chronic renal failure; hypertension; cardiovascular disease; thrombotic events; iron deficiency; underlying infectious, inflammatory, or malignant processes; occult blood loss; vitamin deficiencies; hemolysis; aluminum intoxication; osteitis fibrosa cystica; myeloid cancers; and pregnancy or breastfeeding. Multidose preserved formulations contain benzyl alcohol, linked to increased incidence of potentially fatal neurologic and other complications in premature infants. Safety and efficacy have not been established in *children*.

Preparation and administration

• Do not shake vial; doing so may denature glycoprotein, rendering drug inactive.
• Administer dose slowly to decrease stinging at injection site.
• Store at 36° to 46° F (2° to 8° C).

Adverse reactions

CNS: headache, seizures
CV: hypertension, tachycardia
GI: diarrhea, nausea, vomiting
Metabolic: hyperkalemia
Musculoskeletal: arthralgia, myalgia
Respiratory: dyspnea
Other: injection site stinging

Interactions

Drug-diagnostic tests. *Serum BUN, creatinine, phosphorus, potassium, uric acid:* increased
Drug-herb. *Ginkgo:* possible seizure risk

Toxicity and overdose

• Doses of up to 1,500 units/kg three times weekly for 3 to 4 weeks have been given without direct toxic effects. Therapy can cause polycythemia if hematocrit is not monitored carefully and dosage adjusted appropriately. Anticipated toxic effects include polycythemia, exacerbation of hypertension, and seizures.
• If polycythemia is a concern, phlebotomy may be indicated to decrease hematocrit.

Special considerations

• Measure hematocrit once weekly until stabilized; then measure periodically.
• Monitor patient for iron deficiency; underlying infectious, inflammatory, or malignant processes; occult blood loss; underlying hematologic disease (such as thalassemia, refractory anemia, or other myelodysplastic disorders); vitamin deficiencies (of folic acid or vitamin B_{12}); hemolysis; aluminum intoxication; and osteitis fibrosa cystica (especially if patient fails to respond or maintain response to recommended dosages).
• Monitor blood pressure carefully, particularly in patients with underlying history of hypertension, chronic renal failure, or cardiovascular disease.
• In patients with chronic renal failure who are on hemodialysis and have clinically evident ischemic heart disease or heart failure, manage hematocrit carefully (not to exceed 36%).
• Drug is not indicated for anemia in cancer patients because of such factors as iron or folate deficiencies, hemolysis, or GI bleeding (which should be managed appropriately).
• Both Epogen and Procrit contain albumin.
• Reimbursement may be lower than normal or withheld if patient receives dose with hemoglobin of 12 g/dl or higher or hematocrit of 36% or higher, if treatment starts with hemoglobin of 12 g/dl or higher or hematocrit of 36% or higher, or if hemoglobin is 11 to 11.9 g/dl in absence of fatigue, cold intolerance, or cardiac symptoms.

Patient education

• If home use is prescribed, instruct patient or caregiver in proper administration and importance of proper disposal. Caution against reusing needles and syringes.

• Stress importance of complying with anti-hypertensive therapy and dietary restrictions during therapy.

• As hematocrit increases and patient's sense of well-being and quality of life improve, reinforce importance of dietary compliance.

• Inform patients who do not want to take blood products for religious or other purposes that product contains albumin, a component of human blood.

erlotinib

Tarceva

Classification: Antineoplastic, miscellaneous
Pregnancy risk category D

Pharmacology

Erlotinib is a human epidermal growth factor receptor type 1/epidermal growth factor receptor (HER1/EGFR) that inhibits intracellular phosphorylation of tyrosine kinase associated with EGFR. EGFR is expressed on cell surface of normal and cancer cells.

Pharmacokinetics

Drug is about 60% absorbed after administration on empty stomach; food increases bioavailability to almost 100%. It is metabolized in liver and peaks 4 hours after dosing. Half-life is about 36 hours. Drug is cleared predominantly by CYP3A4 metabolism and excreted in bile.

How supplied

Tablets: 25 mg, 100 mg, 150 mg

Indications and dosages

FDA-APPROVED

➥ Locally advanced or metastatic non-small-cell lung cancer after failure of at least one chemotherapy regimen
Adults: 150 mg P.O. at least 1 hour before or 2 hours after food ingestion, continued until disease progression or unacceptable toxicity occurs. There is no evidence that treatment beyond progression is beneficial.

⊝ First-line treatment for locally advanced, unresectable, or metastatic pancreatic cancer (with gemcitabine)
Adults: 100 mg P.O. daily at least 1 hour before or 2 hours after food ingestion, continued until disease progression or unacceptable toxicity occurs

OFF-LABEL USES (SELECTED)

➥ Colorectal and renal cell cancer
Adults: Various dosing regimens
⊝ Malignant glioma
Adults: 100 to 150 mg P.O. daily at least 1 hour before or 2 hours after food ingestion. Early clinical use suggests benefit when used with other antineoplastics.

DOSAGE MODIFICATIONS

• When dosage reduction is necessary, reduce in 50-mg decrements.

• If patient develops acute onset of new or progressive pulmonary symptoms (such as dyspnea, cough, or fever), withhold drug pending evaluation.

• If interstitial lung disease develops, discontinue drug and provide appropriate treatment as necessary.

• Patients with severe diarrhea who do not respond to loperamide, those who become dehydrated, and those with severe skin reactions may require dosage reduction or temporary drug withdrawal.

• In patients concomitantly receiving strong CYP3A4 inhibitors, dosage reduction should be considered if serious adverse reactions occur.

• Pretreatment with CYP3A4 inducers decreases drug's AUC by about two-thirds. Alternative treatments without CYP3A4-inducing activity should be considered; if such treatment is unavailable, erlotinib dosage greater than 150 mg should be considered. If dosage

is adjusted upward, it must be reduced on withdrawal of rifampin or other inducers.
• Consider reducing dosage or interrupting therapy if severe adverse reactions occur.

Contraindications and precautions

No known contraindications exist.

Use cautiously in concomitant warfarin therapy, hepatic dysfunction, suspected interstitial lung disease (such as pneumonitis, interstitial pneumonia, obliterative bronchiolitis, pulmonary fibrosis, adult respiratory distress syndrome, or lung infiltration), and pregnancy or breastfeeding. Safety and efficacy in *children* have not been established.

Preparation and administration

• Administer drug at least 1 hour before or 2 hours after food ingestion.
• No clinical benefit has been shown with concurrent administration of erlotinib with platinum-based chemotherapy; use is not recommended for first-line patients with locally advanced or metastatic non-small-cell lung cancer.
• Store at 77° F (25° C); excursions are permitted to 59° to 86° F (15° to 30° C).

Adverse reactions

CNS: fatigue
EENT: conjunctivitis, keratoconjunctivitis sicca
GI: diarrhea, anorexia, nausea, vomiting, stomatitis, abdominal pain
Respiratory: dyspnea, cough, interstitial lung disease (possibly fatal)
Skin: rash, pruritus, dry skin
Other: infection

Interactions

Drug-drug. *CYP3A4 inducers (including carbamazepine, phenobarbital, phenytoin, rifabutin, rifampin, rifapentin):* decreased erlotinib AUC
CYP3A4 inhibitors (including atanazavir, clarithromycin, indinavir, itraconazole, ketoconazole, nefazodone, nelfinavir, ritonavir, saquinavir, trole-

andomycin, voriconazole): increased erlotinib AUC
Warfarin and other coumarin anticoagulants: elevated INR, possibly increased bleeding risk
Drug-diagnostic tests. *Serum ALT, AST, bilirubin:* increased
Drug-food. *Any food:* increased erlotinib bioavailability
Drug-herb. *Coenzyme Q10:* possible decreased chemotherapy efficacy
St. John's wort: possible decreased erlotinib AUC

Toxicity and overdose

• Severe adverse reactions (such as diarrhea, rash, and liver transaminase elevations) may occur with therapy above recommended dosage of 150 mg daily.
• In suspected overdose, withhold drug and provide symptomatic treatment.

Special considerations

• Periodically monitor liver function tests (ALP, bilirubin, and transaminases).
• Monitor INR and prothrombin time regularly in patients receiving warfarin, other coumarin anticoagulants, or nonsteroidal antiinflammatory drugs.

Patient education

• Urge patient to seek prompt medical advice for severe or persistent diarrhea, nausea, anorexia, vomiting, eye irritation, or onset or worsening of unexplained shortness of breath or cough.
• Caution women with childbearing potential to avoid becoming pregnant while taking drug.
• Advise breastfeeding patient to stop breastfeeding during therapy.

E

estramustine phosphate sodium
Emcyt

Classification: Antineoplastic, alkylating agent
Pregnancy risk category D

Pharmacology
Estramustine phosphate sodium (a combination of estrogen and nitrogen mustard compound) reduces testosterone levels, increases levels of estrogen and testosterone-estradiol binding globulin, and may exert cytostatic effects.

Pharmacokinetics
Drug is well absorbed (approximately 75%); some foods affect absorption. It is highly localized in prostatic tissue and rapidly dephosphorylated during absorption into peripheral circulation. It is metabolized in liver; terminal half-life is about 20 hours. Excretion route is not clear, but biliary excretion dominates.

How supplied
Capsules: 140 mg

Indications and dosages

FDA-APPROVED

➡ Palliation of metastatic or progressive prostatic cancer
Adults: 14 mg/kg P.O. in three or four divided doses with water at least 1 hour before or 2 hours after meals; continued for 30 to 90 days before deciding whether to continue therapy

OFF-LABEL USES (SELECTED)

➡ Hormone-refractory prostatic cancer
Adults: Various dosing regimens, including combination with vinblastine, docetaxel, or etoposide

Contraindications and precautions
Contraindicated in hypersensitivity to estradiol or nitrogen mustard, active thrombophlebitis, and thromboembolic disorders (except when tumor mass is cause of thromboembolic phenomenon and benefits may outweigh risks).

Use cautiously in fluid retention; hepatic impairment; cerebrovascular or coronary artery disease; hypertension; metabolic bone diseases associated with hypercalcemia; renal insufficiency; diabetes mellitus; and history of thrombophlebitis, thrombosis, or thromboembolic disorders.

Preparation and administration
• Follow hazardous drug guidelines for handling, preparation, and administration. (See "Managing hazardous drugs," page 11.)
• Give drug with water at least 1 hour before or 2 hours after meals.
• Treat patients for 30 to 90 days before determining possible benefits of continued therapy. Therapy should continue as long as favorable response lasts. Some patients have been maintained for more than 3 years at doses ranging from 10 to 16 mg/kg daily.
• Store in refrigerator at 36° to 46° F (2° to 8° C).

Adverse reactions
CNS: hypertension
CV: peripheral edema
GI: diarrhea, flatulence, nausea, minor GI upset
GU: breast tenderness or enlargement
Respiratory: dyspnea

Interactions
Drug-drug. *Hepatotoxic drugs:* increased hepatotoxicity
Drug-diagnostic tests. *AST, lactate dehydrogenase:* abnormal results
Glucose tolerance: decreased
Drug-food. *Calcium-rich foods, milk, milk products:* impaired drug absorption

---

Only common or life-threatening adverse reactions are listed.

Drug-herb. *Coenzyme Q10:* possible decreased chemotherapy efficacy

Toxicity and overdose
- Although overdose has not been reported, anticipated signs and symptoms are manifestations of known adverse reactions.
- If overdose occurs, use gastric lavage and treat symptomatically. Monitor hematologic and hepatic parameters for at least 6 weeks afterward.

Special considerations
- Monitor patients with history of thrombophlebitis, thrombosis, or thromboembolic disorders or with cerebrovascular or coronary artery disease.
- Monitor diabetic patients carefully; drug may decrease glucose tolerance.
- Drug may exacerbate preexisting or incipient peripheral edema or heart failure. These and other conditions that might be influenced by fluid retention (such as epilepsy, migraine, or renal dysfunction) require careful observation.
- Monitor liver function tests at appropriate intervals during therapy, and repeat 2 months after drug withdrawal.
- Monitor blood pressure; drug may cause hypertension.

Patient education
- Instruct patient to take drug with water.
- Tell patient not to consume milk, milk products, calcium-rich foods, or such preparations as calcium-containing antacids simultaneously with drug.
- Advise patients with childbearing potential to use effective contraception because of drug's possible mutagenic effects.

estrogens, conjugated
Premarin, Premarin Intravenous

Classification: Hormone/hormone modifier, antineoplastic
Pregnancy risk category X

Pharmacology
Conjugated estrogens diffuse through cell membranes, distribute throughout cell, and bind to and activate nuclear estrogen receptor (DNA-binding protein in females' estrogen-responsive tissues, including reproductive tract, breast, pituitary, hypothalamus, liver, and bone). Activated estrogen receptor binds to specific DNA sequences or hormone-response elements, enhancing transcription of adjacent genes and in turn leading to adequate functioning of female reproductive system.

Pharmacokinetics
Drug is well-absorbed from GI tract, metabolized to active compounds in liver, widely distributed, and protein-bound. Peak occurs 8 hours after oral dose and persists for 3 to 4 hours until estrogen levels slowly return to baseline. I.V. dose produces rapid response. Drug is excreted primarily in urine.

How supplied
Powder for injection: 25 mg/5-ml vial
Tablets: 0.3 mg, 0.625 mg, 0.9 mg, 1.25 mg, 2.5 mg

Indications and dosages

FDA-APPROVED

➡ Palliation of inoperable breast cancer in appropriately selected postmenopausal women and men with metastatic disease
Adults: 10 mg P.O. three times daily for 3 months or longer

➡ Palliation of advanced androgen-dependent prostatic cancer
Adults: 1.25 to 2.5 mg P.O. three times daily

OFF-LABEL USES (SELECTED)

➡ Salvage treatment of hemorrhagic cystitis caused by cyclophosphamide or ifosfamide
Adults: 2.5 mg P.O. twice daily until hemorrhaging stops

DOSAGE MODIFICATIONS

• Patients with end-stage renal failure should receive 25% to 50% of usual dosage.

☒ WARNINGS

• Drug increases risk of endometrial carcinoma. Risk seems to depend on treatment duration and dosage. When drug is used in treating menopausal symptoms, lowest dosage that controls symptoms should be used, and drug should be discontinued as soon as possible. When prolonged treatment is medically indicated, patient should be reassessed at least twice yearly to determine need for continued therapy. Although evidence must be considered preliminary, one study suggests that cyclic administration of low doses may carry less risk than continuous administration. Thus, it appears prudent to use such a regimen.
• Close clinical surveillance of women receiving estrogens is important. In all cases of undiagnosed persistent or recurring abnormal vaginal bleeding, adequate diagnostic measures should be taken to rule out cancer. No evidence suggests that "natural" estrogens are more or less hazardous than "synthetic" estrogens at equiestrogenic doses.
• Drug should not be used during pregnancy. If used during pregnancy, or if patient becomes pregnant while taking it, she should be told of potential risks to fetus and counseled on risks of continuing pregnancy.

Contraindications and precautions

Contraindicated in hypersensitivity to estrogens or their ingredients, undiagnosed abnormal genital bleeding, known or suspected breast cancer (except in appropriately selected patients being treated for metastatic disease), known or suspected estrogen-dependent neoplasia, active thrombophlebitis or thromboembolic disorders, and known or suspected pregnancy.

Use cautiously in women with strong family history of breast cancer or who have breast nodules, fibrocystic disease, or abnormal mammograms; women with gallbladder disease; cerebrovascular or coronary artery disease; diabetes mellitus; hypercalcemia; hepatic impairment; conditions that might be influenced by fluid retention; familial lipoprotein metabolism defects; history of mental depression or jaundice during pregnancy; and breastfeeding. Safety and efficacy in *children* have not been established.

Preparation and administration

• Follow hazardous drug guidelines for handling, preparation, and administration. (See "Managing hazardous drugs," page 11.)
• Obtain complete medical and family history before starting therapy. During pretreatment and periodic physical examinations, pay special attention to blood pressure, breasts, abdomen, and pelvic organs and obtain a Papanicolaou smear. Generally, estrogens should not be prescribed longer than 1 year without another physical examination being performed.
• Do not administer drug I.V. for injection with other agents.
• I.V. drug is compatible with normal saline solution, dextrose, and invert sugar solutions. It is also incompatible with protein hydrolysate, ascorbic acid, and acidic solutions.
• Diluent (5-ml ampule) for injection contains 2% benzyl alcohol in sterile water.
• Give parenteral form by slow I.V. infusion.
• Store tablets at 77° F (25° C).

Only common or life-threatening adverse reactions are listed.

- Before reconstitution, store injection in package refrigerated at 36° to 46° F (2° to 8° C).

Adverse reactions

CNS: depression, migraine, emotional lability, cerebrovascular accident
CV: hypertension, edema, arterial thromboembolism, venous thrombosis, myocardial infarction
EENT: contact lens intolerance, retinal thrombosis
GI: nausea, vomiting, gallbladder disease, bloating, mesenteric thrombosis, pancreatitis
GU: breakthrough bleeding, spotting, amenorrhea, change in cervical secretions, breast enlargement, breast tenderness, endometrial cancer
Hepatic: benign hepatic tumors
Metabolic: hyperglycemia, hypertriglyceridemia, hypercalcemia, fluid retention
Respiratory: pulmonary embolism
Skin: melasma

Interactions

Drug-drug. *Amprenavir:* decreased serum amprenavir level
Azole antifungals: increased estrogen levels
Benzodiazepines: increased or decreased benzodiazepine level
Corticosteroids: increased corticosteroid effect
Cyclosporine: increased risk of cyclosporine toxicity
CYP450 inducers (such as rifampin and barbiturates): decreased estrogen levels
Paclitaxel: possible increase in paclitaxel exposure (from decreased paclitaxel metabolism)
Phenytoin: loss of seizure control, decreased estrogen levels
Tricyclic antidepressants: attenuation of antidepressant efficacy and tricyclic toxicity
Warfarin: theoretically increased risk of thromboembolism
Drug-diagnostic tests. *Antithrombin, lactate dehydrogenase, serum cholesterol:* decreased
Factors VII, VIII, IX, and X; prothrombin; triglycerides and phospholipid concentrations; thyroid-binding globulin (TBG); total thyroid hormone: increased (with large estrogen dosages)
Free triiodothyronine resin uptake: decreased, reflecting increased TBG (with large estrogen dosages)
Glucose tolerance: impaired (with large estrogen dosages)
High-density lipoproteins, norepinephrine-induced platelet aggregability, serum calcium, serum glucose: increased
Metapyrone test: reduced response (with large estrogen dosages)
Pregnanediol excretion, serum folate: decreased (with large estrogen dosages)
Drug-herb. *Ginseng:* additive estrogenic effects
St. John's wort: decreased estrogen level

Toxicity and overdose

- Based on many reports of children accidentally ingesting large doses of estrogen-containing oral contraceptives, acute serious ill effects do not occur. Overdose may cause nausea and withdrawal bleeding in females.
- Treatment, if indicated, is supportive.

Special considerations

- If hypercalcemia occurs, withdraw drug and take appropriate measures to reduce serum calcium level.
- Oral contraceptives may be associated with hepatic adenoma. Although benign and rare, such adenomas may rupture and cause death from intra-abdominal hemorrhage. Such lesions have not been linked to other estrogen or progestin preparations, but should be considered in estrogen users with abdominal pain and tenderness, abdominal mass, or hypovolemic shock.
- In patients with familial lipoprotein metabolism defects, drug may trigger massive plasma triglyceride elevations, leading to pancreatitis and other complications.
- Large doses used to treat prostate or breast cancer are more likely to cause thrombolytic adverse reactions. Also, men receiving estrogens for prostate cancer are at increased risk for thrombosis.

- If feasible, discontinue drug at least 4 weeks before surgery associated with increased risk for thromboembolism or during prolonged immobilization period.
- Carefully monitor patients with diabetes mellitus or history of depression.
- If jaundice develops, discontinue drug while cause of jaundice is investigated.
- Inform pathologist of estrogen therapy when submitting relevant specimens.

Patient education

- Instruct patient to report signs and symptoms of serious side effects, such as thromboembolic events.
- If patient is pregnant or becomes pregnant while taking drug, discuss potential risks to fetus and advisability of continuing pregnancy.
- Provide guidance to help breastfeeding patient decide whether to discontinue breastfeeding or stop drug.

etoposide (VP-16)
Toposar, VePesid

etoposide phosphate
Etopophos

Classification: Antineoplastic, epipodophyllotoxin

Pregnancy risk category D

Pharmacology

Etoposide, a semisynthetic podophyllotoxin derivative, delays cell transit through S phase, which is followed by arrest in late S or early G2 phase. At high concentrations (10 mcg/ml or more), it causes lysis of cells entering mitosis. At low concentrations (0.3 to 10 mcg/ml), it inhibits cells from entering prophase. Phosphate form is a water-soluble etoposide ester that decreases risk of precipitation after dilution and during I.V. administration; it rapidly converts to etoposide after I.V. infusion and has same mechanism of action as etoposide.

Pharmacokinetics

Oral dose is about 50% absorbed by GI tract, necessitating oral dosages twice as high as parenteral dosages. (However, oral doses above 200 mg exhibit markedly less absorption, suggesting saturable absorption process.) Drug is metabolized in liver and extensively protein-bound. Elimination half-life is about 10 hours. It is excreted unchanged in urine (roughly 30% of dose) and as metabolites in bile (10% to 15% of parent drug).

How supplied
etoposide
Capsules: 50 mg
Solution for injection: 20 mg/ml
etoposide phosphate
Solution for injection (water-soluble): 100 mg/ml

Indications and dosages

FDA-APPROVED

➡ Refractory testicular tumors in patients who have received appropriate surgical, chemotherapeutic, and radiotherapeutic therapy
Adults: In combination with other approved chemotherapeutic agents, 50 to 100 mg/m² I.V. (etoposide for injection or equivalent doses of phosphate form) daily on days 1 through 5; or 100 mg/m² I.V. daily on days 1, 3, and 5; repeated at 3- to 4-week intervals after adequate recovery from any toxicity
➡ Small-cell lung cancer as first-line treatment
Adults: In combination with other approved chemotherapeutic agents, dosage range is 35 mg/m² I.V. (etoposide for injection or equivalent doses of phosphate form) daily for 4 days to 50 mg/m² daily for 5 days, or etoposide capsules P.O. at twice the I.V. dosage and rounded to nearest 50 mg.

Only common or life-threatening adverse reactions are listed.

E

OFF-LABEL USES (SELECTED)

➥ Carcinoma of unknown primary site
Adults: In combination with platinum agent, 100 mg/m² I.V. on days 1 to 3, repeated every 21 days

➥ First-line treatment of carcinoma of unknown primary site
Adults: In combination with paclitaxel and carboplatin, 50 mg P.O. alternating with 100 mg P.O. on days 1 to 10, repeated every 21 days

➥ Ewing's sarcoma
Adults: 100 mg/m² I.V. over 5 days in combination with vincristine, doxorubicin, and cyclophosphamide alternating with ifosfamide with mesna
Children: Various dosages, alternating with an anthracycline and cyclophosphamide regimen

➥ Hodgkin's lymphoma, high-dose chemotherapy with stem-cell rescue
Adults: In combination, 150 mg/m² I.V. every 12 hours from day −7 to day −4, with stem cells administered on day 0

➥ High-dose conditioning regimens for allogeneic bone marrow transplantation
Children: 60 mg/kg I.V. as single dose

➥ Bone marrow transplantation conditioning regimen for patients with rhabdomyosarcoma or neuroblastoma
Children: 160 mg/m² by continuous I.V. infusion for 4 days

➥ Non-small-cell lung carcinoma
Adults: As single agent or in combination with platinum agent, 100 mg/m² I.V. on days 1 to 3, repeated every 21 days

➥ Brain tumors
Children: 150 mg/m² I.V. daily on days 2 and 3 of treatment course

➥ Advanced neuroblastoma
Children: In combination, 100 mg/m² I.V. on day 1, alternating with another multiagent cycle using etoposide 200 mg/m² I.V. on day 3

➥ Osteosarcoma and soft-tissue sarcoma, in combination with ifosfamide and platinum
Adults: 80 to 100 mg/m² I.V on days 1 to 3, repeated every 21 to 28 days

➥ Acute myelocytic leukemia
Children: For remission induction, 150 mg/m² I.V. daily for 2 to 3 days for two to three cycles; for intensification or consolidation, 250 mg/m² I.V. for 3 days on courses two to five. (Several different courses, including ones using other chemotherapeutic agents, are given.)

DOSAGE MODIFICATIONS

• Dosage should be modified if patient is receiving other drugs with myelosuppressive effects or has had previous radiation therapy or chemotherapy (which may have compromised bone marrow reserves). If platelet count is below 50,000/mm³ or absolute neutrophil count is below 500/mm³, withhold drug until counts have sufficiently recovered.
• In renal impairment, initial dosage modification is based on creatinine clearance. For clearance below 50 ml/minute, give 100% of recommended dosage; for clearance of 15 to 50 ml/minute, give 75% of recommended dosage. Base subsequent dosages on patient tolerance and clinical effect. Data are not available for patients with creatinine clearance below 15 ml/minute; consider further dosage reduction.
• In hepatic impairment, reduce dosage to 50% of recommended dose in patients with bilirubin level 1 to 2 × ULN; reduce dosage to 25% of recommended dose in patients with bilirubin level 2 to 4 × ULN; and stop drug in patients with bilirubin level above 4 × ULN.

⊠ WARNINGS

• Drug should be given under supervision of qualified physician experienced in use of chemotherapeutic agents.
• Severe bone marrow depression with resulting infection or bleeding may occur.

Contraindications and precautions

Contraindicated in hypersensitivity to drug or its components.

Use cautiously in low serum albumin level, renal impairment, and pregnancy or breast-feeding. Safety and efficacy in *children* have not been established. Injection contains poly-sorbate 80, associated with life-threatening syndrome involving hepatic and renal failure, pulmonary deterioration, thrombocytopenia, and ascites in premature infants receiving in-jectable vitamin E product containing polysor-bate 80.

Preparation and administration

• Follow hazardous drug guidelines for han-dling, preparation, and administration. (See "Managing hazardous drugs," page 11.)
• Plastic devices made of acrylic or ABS (com-posed of acrylonitrile, butadiene, and styrene) may crack and leak when used with undiluted etoposide injection.
• If solution contacts skin or mucosa, imme-diately and thoroughly wash skin with soap and water, and flush mucosa with water.
• Dilute etoposide for injection before use with D_5W or normal saline injection, for final concentration of 0.2 to 0.4 mg/ml. Precipita-tion may occur in solutions prepared at con-centrations above 0.4 mg/ml.
• Administer solution over 30 to 60 minutes; hypotension may follow rapid I.V. administra-tion. Use longer duration if volume to be in-fused is a concern. Do not give by rapid I.V. injection.
• Unopened vials are stable for 24 months at temperature of 77° F (25° C). Vials diluted as recommended to concentration of 0.2 and 0.4 mg/ml are stable for 96 and 24 hours, re-spectively, in glass or plastic containers kept at room temperature under normal room fluo-rescent lights.
• Before use, reconstitute contents of each etoposide phosphate vial with 5 ml or 10 ml sterile water for injection, D_5W, normal saline injection, sterile bacteriostactic water for in-jection with benzyl alcohol, or bacteriostatic sodium chloride for injection with benzyl al-cohol, to concentration equivalent to 20 mg/ml or 10 mg/ml etoposide (22.7 mg/ml or 11.4 mg/ml etoposide phosphate), respective-ly. After reconstitution, give solution without further dilution. Alternatively, it can be dilut-ed further to concentrations as low as 0.1 mg/ml etoposide with D_5W or normal saline in-jection.
• Administer etoposide phosphate solutions over as little as 5 minutes or up to 210 min-utes.
• If anaphylactoid-like reaction occurs, imme-diately stop infusion and administer pressors, corticosteroids, antihistamines, and volume expanders as appropriate.
• When refrigerated at 36° to 46° F in original package, unopened vials of etoposide phos-phate for injection are stable until date indi-cated on package.
• When reconstituted or diluted as directed, store etoposide phosphate solution in glass or plastic container at controlled room tempera-ture of 68° to 77° F (20° to 25° C) or refriger-ated at 36° to 46° F (2° to 8° C) for 24 hours, protected from light. Use refrigerated solu-tions immediately on return to room tempera-ture.
• Refrigerate capsules at 36° to 46° F (2° to 8° C); they remain stable for 24 months.

Adverse reactions

CNS: malaise, dizziness (phosphate form only)
CV: transient hypotension (with rapid I.V. administration)
GI: mucositis, constipation, abdominal pain, diarrhea, taste alteration (phosphate form only); nausea, vomiting, anorexia
Hematologic: anemia, bone marrow depres-sion, neutropenia, leukopenia, thrombocyto-penia, acute leukemia
Skin: reversible alopecia
Other: chills, fever, extravasation, phlebitis (phosphate form only); asthenia; anaphylac-tic-like reactions (chills, fever, tachycardia, bronchospasm, dyspnea, or hypotension)

Only common or life-threatening adverse reactions are listed.

Interactions

Drug-drug. *Aprepitant:* increased etoposide concentrations
Cyclosporine (high-dose): increased etoposide exposure with decreased total body clearance compared to etoposide alone (phosphate form only)
Levamisole and similarly acting drugs: inhibited phosphatase activity (phosphate form only)
Drug-diagnostic tests. *CBC:* decreased
Drug-food. *Grapefruit juice:* decreased oral etoposide absorption
Drug-herb. *Coenzyme Q10, glucosamine, St. John's wort:* reduced etoposide effects

Toxicity and overdose

• Neurotoxicity is most common sign of overdose.
• No proven antidote exists.

Special considerations

• Monitor CBC with differential frequently, and observe for bone marrow depression during and after therapy.
• Monitor patients with low serum albumin because of increased risk of drug toxicities.
• Consider drug a potential carcinogen. Acute leukemia with or without preleukemic phase has been reported rarely in patients treated with etoposide alone or in association with other neoplastic agents. Risk of developing preleukemic or leukemic syndrome is unclear.

Patient education

• Inform patient who uses drug during pregnancy or becomes pregnant while receiving it that it may harm fetus. Advise women with childbearing potential to avoid becoming pregnant.
• Provide guidance to help breastfeeding patient decide whether to discontinue breastfeeding or stop drug.

exemestane
Aromasin

Classification: Antineoplastic, aromatase inhibitor, hormone/hormone modifier
Pregnancy risk category D

Pharmacology

Exemestane, structurally related to the natural substrate androstenedione, acts as false substrate for aromatase enzyme. It is processed to an intermediate that binds irreversibly to active site of enzyme, causing its inactivation ("suicide inhibition"). Drug significantly lowers circulating estrogen concentrations in postmenopausal women but has no detectable effect on adrenal biosynthesis of corticosteroids or aldosterone.

Pharmacokinetics

Drug is rapidly absorbed from GI tract, with faster absorption in women with breast cancer than in healthy women; high-fat meal increases absorption. It is metabolized in liver by CYP450 3A4 and aldoketoreductase and is extensively distributed in tissues. It is highly plasma protein-bound. Peak occurs in 3 to 7 days; mean terminal half-life is approximately 24 hours. Drug is eliminated equally in urine and feces.

How supplied

Tablets: 25 mg

Indications and dosages

FDA-APPROVED

⊖ Advanced breast cancer in postmenopausal women whose disease progresses after tamoxifen therapy
Adults: 25 mg P.O. once daily after a meal, continued until tumor progression appears

DOSAGE MODIFICATIONS

• For patients receiving drug with potent

CYP3A4 inducer (such as rifampin or phenytoin), give 50 mg P.O. once daily after a meal.

Contraindications and precautions

Contraindicated in hypersensitivity to drug or its components.

Use cautiously in moderate to severe hepatic insufficiency, renal insufficiency (creatinine clearance below 35 ml/minute/1.73 m²), premenopausal women, concurrent use with estrogen-containing agents, and pregnancy or breastfeeding. Safety and efficacy in *children* have not been established.

Preparation and administration

• Follow hazardous drug guidelines for handling, preparation, and administration. (See "Managing hazardous drugs," page 11.)
• Administer drug after meal. (Fatty meal may increase drug absorption.)
• Store at 77° F (25° C); excursions are permitted to 59° to 86° F (15° to 30° C).

Adverse reactions

CNS: fatigue, depression, insomnia, anxiety, dizziness, headache
CV: edema (including peripheral edema, leg edema), hypertension
GI: nausea, increased appetite, anorexia, vomiting, abdominal pain, constipation, diarrhea
Respiratory: dyspnea, coughing
Other: hot flashes, increased sweating, weight gain, pain, flulike symptoms

Interactions

Drug-drug. *CYP3A4 inducers (such as carbamazepine, phenobarbital, phenytoin, and rifampin):* possible decrease in exemestane effect
CYP3A4 inhibitors (such as azole antifungals and statin antihyperlipidemics): possible increase in exemestane effect
Drug-food. *Fatty foods:* increased drug absorption
Drug-herb. *CYP3A4 inducers (such as St. John's wort):* possible significant decrease in drug exposure
Dehydroepiandrosterone: possible interference

with antiestrogen effects of exemestane
Glutamine: possible enhanced tumor growth

Toxicity and overdose

• Most common signs and symptoms of overdose are those associated with adverse reactions.
• No specific antidote exists; treatment is symptomatic. Provide general supportive care, including frequent monitoring of vital signs and close observation.

Special considerations

• Monitor renal and hepatic function.
• Drug is indicated only for postmenopausal women. Use caution if breastfeeding patient is inadvertently exposed to drug.

Patient education

• Instruct patient to take drug after meal.
• If patient becomes pregnant during therapy, advise her that drug may harm fetus and cause pregnancy loss.
• Instruct breastfeeding patient not to breastfeed during therapy.

fentanyl citrate
fentanyl transdermal system
Duragesic

fentanyl transmucosal
Actiq

Classification: Opioid analgesic
Controlled substance schedule II
Pregnancy risk category C

Pharmacology

Fentanyl, a pure opioid agonist, acts primarily by binding to opioid mu-receptors in brain, spinal cord, and smooth muscle. These actions alter pain perception and produce analgesia and sedation.

Only common or life-threatening adverse reactions are listed.

Pharmacokinetics

Drug is metabolized in liver. Transdermal form releases drug from reservoir at nearly constant amount per unit of time. Serum concentrations reach steady state between 12 and 24 hours; drug peaks between 24 and 72 hours. With transmucosal dose (lozenge), onset is 5 to 15 minutes, peak is 20 to 30 minutes, and duration is several hours. Drug is excreted in urine.

How supplied

Transdermal systems: 25-mcg/hour, 50-mcg/hour, 75-mcg/hour, and 100-mcg/hour patches
Transmucosal lozenges (oral): 200 mcg, 400 mcg, 600 mcg, 800 mcg, 1,200 mcg, and 1,600 mcg in protective foil pouches

Indications and dosages

FDA-APPROVED

➡ Breakthrough cancer pain in opioid-tolerant patients
Adults: One 200-mcg transmucosal lozenge unit dissolved in mouth over 15 minutes, repeated in 15 minutes if necessary; maximum daily dosage is 4 units.
➡ Moderate to severe chronic pain in patients who require continuous opioid analgesia
Adults and children older than age 2: Dosage must be individualized based on patient's status, and evaluated at regular intervals after transdermal application. Initially, for opioid-tolerant patients, 25-mcg/hour system transdermally, with system changed every 72 hours. Some patients may require dosing every 48 hours. Children must be receiving at least 60 mg oral morphine equivalent daily when converting to intradermal system.

DOSAGE MODIFICATIONS

• Dosage may be increased after 3 days, if needed. Thereafter, 6 days should elapse between dosage increases.
• Reduce transdermal dosage in elderly and

debilitated patients. In elderly patients, do not start Duragesic at doses above 25 mcg/hour unless patient is already receiving more than 135 mg oral morphine daily or equivalent dose of another opioid.
• Oral-form dosage is usually increased when patients need more than one dosage unit per breakthrough cancer pain episode for several consecutive episodes.
• For patients using transdermal form, dosage of additional opioids or other CNS depressants (including benzodiazepines) should be decreased by at least 50%.
• Dosage of transdermal form should be adjusted in patients who develop fever. Serum fentanyl level may increase by about one-third in patients with body temperature of 104° F (40° C).
• Recommended initial transdermal dosage based on daily oral morphine dosage is conservative; 50% of patients are likely to require dosage increase after initial application. Multiple systems may be used for delivery rates exceeding 100 mcg/hour.
• After transdermal dosage increase, patient may take up to 6 days to reach equilibrium on new dosage. Therefore, patient should wear higher dosage through two applications before further dosage increase is made on basis of average daily use of supplemental analgesic.

⊠ WARNINGS

• Fentanyl transmucosal (Actiq) and fentanyl transdermal (Duragesic) should be used only in opioid-tolerant patients. Patients considered opioid-tolerant are those receiving at least 60 mg morphine daily, 25 mcg/hour transdermal fentanyl, 30 mg oxycodone P.O. daily, 8 mg hydromorphone P.O. daily, or equianalgesic dose of another opioid for 1 week or longer.
• Actiq should be given only to cancer patients. Use should be restricted to oncologists and pain specialists experienced in use of Schedule II opioids to treat cancer pain. Patients and caregivers must be instructed that

Actiq can be fatal to children and that they must keep all units out of children's reach and discard open units properly.

• Duragesic is contraindicated in acute or postoperative pain, mild or intermittent pain responsive to p.r.n. or nonopioid therapy, and initial doses above 25 mcg/hour. Give only to patients who require total daily dose at least equivalent to 25 mcg/hour.

Contraindications and precautions

Contraindicated in hypersensitivity to drug or opioid intolerance. Oral form is contraindicated in opioid intolerance and breastfeeding. Duragesic is contraindicated in doses exceeding 25 mcg/hour at initiation of opioid therapy and hypersensitivity to transdermal adhesives.

Use cautiously in respiratory compromise or susceptibility to respiratory depression, hepatic or renal impairment, bradycardia, drug or alcohol abuse, and pregnancy. Transdermal form may be given to *children age 2 and older* who are opioid-tolerant. Dosage and safety of oral form in opioid-tolerant *children younger than age 16* who have breakthrough cancer pain have not been established.

Preparation and administration

• Patient should dissolve lozenge over 15 minutes.
• Use of Duragesic in opioid-intolerant patients may lead to fatal respiratory depression.
• Clip (rather than shave) hair before applying Duragesic. If site needs to be cleaned, use clear water only and let skin dry completely before applying system. Apply system immediately after removing from sealed package, firmly pressing it in place with palm for 30 seconds. Make sure contact is complete, especially around edges. Apply system only to nonirritated, nonirradiated skin on flat surface (such as chest, back, flank, or upper arm). Rotate site if patient needs analgesia beyond 72 hours.

• Store oral form at 77° F (25° C); excursions are permitted between 59° and 86° F (15° and 30° C) until ready to use. Do not store Actiq or Duragesic above 77° F; protect from freezing and moisture.

Adverse reactions

CNS: headache, confusion, dizziness, drowsiness
GI: nausea, vomiting, diarrhea, constipation, decreased appetite
Respiratory: dyspnea, respiratory depression
Skin: itching, diaphoresis

Interactions

Drug-drug. *Azole antifungals (such as ketoconazole and itraconazole), CYP3A4 inhibitors (such as macrolide antibiotics, including erythromycin), protease inhibitors (such as ritonavir):* decreased fentanyl clearance, prolonged opioid effects
Benzodiazepines, CNS depressants: increased respiratory depression, hypotension
CYP3A4 inducers (such as carbamazepine, phenytoin, rifampin): increased fentanyl clearance
Drug-herb. *St. John's wort:* increased sedation, increased analgesia

Toxicity and overdose

• Signs and symptoms of toxicity include respiratory and CNS depression, bradycardia, shock, apnea, hypotension, seizures, and cardiac arrest.
• If patient experiences muscle rigidity that impedes respirations, provide ventilatory assistance, administer opioid antagonist, and as final alternative, give neuromuscular blocker. Administer fluids if severe or persistent hypotension occurs in hypovolemic patient. Perform gastric lavage or administer activated charcoal after patient's airway is secure.

Special considerations

• Opioid withdrawal symptoms, such as nausea, vomiting, diarrhea, anxiety, and shivering, may occur after conversion or dosage adjustment.

Only common or life-threatening adverse reactions are listed.

- Evaluate for muscle rigidity in patients on high doses; neuromuscular blockers may be needed.
- If patient is at high risk for bradycardia, consider premedicating with anticholinergic (such as atropine) to minimize bradycardia risk.

Patient education

- Caution patient not to drive or perform hazardous activities unless he can tolerate adverse reactions.
- Advise patient to keep oral transmucosal units and transdermal systems out of children's reach. Drug may be fatal to children if ingested.
- Allow patient and caregiver to watch patient safety video (available from manufacturer) on proper product use, storage, handling, and disposal directions.
- Instruct patient to dispose of transdermal unit and partially consumed transmucosal unit according to package insert.
- Inform patient of possible side effects. Tell him to contact health care professional if effects persist.
- Caution patient to avoid alcohol use.

filgrastim
Neupogen

Classification: Hematopoietic agent, antineutropenic agent, colony-stimulating factor
Pregnancy risk category C

Pharmacology

Filgrastim, a human granulocyte colony-stimulating factor produced by recombinant DNA technology, binds to granulocyte surface, stimulating activity, proliferation, and differentiation of these progenitor cells. This enhances neutrophil chemotaxis and phagocytosis, which increases cytotoxicity and ultimately reduces fever and infection risk in neutropenic

patients. After single subcutaneous dose, absolute neutrophil count (ANC) decreases 50% to 75% for 30 minutes before rising to maximum 8 to 10 hours later. After drug withdrawal, ANC normalizes in 24 to 48 hours.

Pharmacokinetics

Drug is metabolized in liver and kidney. Onset occurs in 5 to 60 minutes with subcutaneous or I.V. dose. Drug peaks 2 to 6 hours after subcutaneous dose and 24 hours after I.V. dose. Elimination half-life is 7 hours or less.

How supplied

Solution for injection: 300 mcg/ml and 480 mcg/1.6 ml (300 mcg/ml) in single-dose vials; 300 mcg/0.5 ml and 480 mcg/0.8 ml in pre-filled syringes

Indications and dosages

FDA-APPROVED

➥ To decrease incidence of infection in patients with nonmyeloid cancers who are receiving myelosuppressive chemotherapy; to reduce time to neutrophil recovery and fever duration after chemotherapy treatment of adults with acute myeloid leukemia
Adults: Initially, 5 mcg/kg subcutaneously or by I.V. infusion daily over 15 to 30 minutes, with first dose no sooner than 24 hours after chemotherapy ends; continue therapy every day for up to 2 weeks until ANC reaches 10,000/mm^3
⊖ Neutropenia and neutropenia-related sequelae in patients with nonmyeloid cancers who are undergoing myeloablative chemotherapy followed by bone marrow transplantation
Adults: Initially, 10 mcg/kg by I.V. infusion daily over 4 or 24 hours or as continuous 24-hour subcutaneous infusion, given no sooner than 24 hours after chemotherapy and bone marrow infusion
➥ Mobilization of hematopoietic progenitor cells into peripheral blood for collection by leukapheresis

Adults: 10 mcg/kg subcutaneously daily as bolus or continuous infusion for at least 4 days before first leukapheresis procedure; continued until last leukapheresis
➥ To reduce incidence and duration of neutropenia sequelae in symptomatic patients with congenital, cyclic, or idiopathic neutropenia
Adults: Initially, for patients with congenital neutropenia, 6 mcg/kg subcutaneously twice daily; for patients with cyclic or idiopathic neutropenia, 5 mcg/kg subcutaneously daily

Off-label uses (selected)

➥ AIDS-associated neutropenia
Adults: Various dosages, including 5 to 10 mcg/kg subcutaneously daily for 2 to 4 weeks
➥ Myelodysplastic syndrome
Adults: Various dosages, including 0.3 to 10 mcg/kg subcutaneously daily; individualized to patient response

Dosage modifications

• For myelosuppressive chemotherapy, dosage may be increased in increments of 5 mcg/kg for each cycle, according to duration and severity of ANC nadir. Discontinue drug if ANC exceeds 10,000/mm³ after expected chemotherapy-induced neutrophil nadir.
• During neutrophil recovery after bone marrow transplantation, adjust daily dosage to neutrophil response. When ANC exceeds 1,000/mm³ for 3 consecutive days, reduce dosage to 5 mcg/kg daily. Then, if ANC remains above 1,000/mm³ for 3 more days, discontinue drug. If ANC drops below 1,000/mm³, resume drug at 5 mcg/kg daily. If ANC decreases below 1,000/mm³ at any time during administration of 5 mcg/kg daily, increase dosage to 10 mcg/kg daily.
• Monitor neutrophil counts for 4 days after administration; consider dosage adjustment for patients with WBC count above 100,000/mm³.
• Patients with severe, chronic neutropenia require long-term daily administration to maintain clinical benefit. ANC should not be used as sole indicator of efficacy; adjust dosage based on both clinical course and ANC. Patients may experience clinical benefit with ANC below 1,500/mm³. Reduce dosage if ANC persistently exceeds 10,000/mm³.

Contraindications and precautions

Contraindicated in hypersensitivity to drug, its components, or *Escherichia coli*–derived proteins.

Use cautiously in simultaneous administration of cytotoxic chemotherapy, concurrent radiation, chemotherapy associated with delayed bone marrow depression (such as nitrosoureas or mitomycin C), or myelosuppressive doses of antimetabolites (such as 5-fluorouracil); in patients receiving drugs that may potentiate neutrophil release (such as lithium), and in pregnancy or breastfeeding. Serious long-term risks have not been identified in *children ages 4 months to 17 years* with severe, chronic neutropenia. Safety and efficacy in neonates and neutropenia of infancy have not been established.

Preparation and administration

• If necessary, drug may be diluted in D₅W. Do not dilute with saline solution; product may precipitate.
• If drug is diluted to concentrations between 5 and 15 mcg/ml, protect from adsorption to plastic materials by adding albumin (human) to final concentration of 2 mg/ml. Do not dilute to final concentration below 5 mcg/ml.
• When diluted in D₅W or D₅W plus albumin (human), drug is compatible with glass bottles, PVC and polyolefin I.V. bags, and polypropylene syringes.
• Patients who experience local site reactions from subcutaneous administration may benefit from local ice application for 10 to 15 minutes before injection.
• Bring drug to room temperature for maximum of 24 hours before administering. Do not shake vial.

Only common or life-threatening adverse reactions are listed.

- Discard vial after 24 hours when left at room temperature. Refrigerate at 36° to 46° F (2° to 8° C).

Adverse reactions

GI: nausea, vomiting, diarrhea
Hematologic: chronic neutropenia (with long-term use), splenomegaly
Musculoskeletal: mild to severe bone pain (more frequent with high I.V. doses)
Skin: alopecia
Other: fever, fatigue

Interactions

Drug-drug. None known, but not fully evaluated
Drug-diagnostic tests. *ALP, lactate dehydrogenase, leukocyte ALP score, uric acid:* possible increases
ANC (in patients with congenital or idiopathic neutropenia): cyclic fluctuations
Platelets: decreased (usually temporary)

Toxicity and overdose

- Maximum tolerated dosage has not been determined. Excessive leukocytosis is most common toxic effect.
- If overdose occurs, discontinue drug and provide supportive therapy.

Special considerations

- In patients receiving chemotherapy, monitor CBC before chemotherapy and twice weekly during chemotherapy to check for excessive leukocytosis.
- Monitor hematocrit, CBC, and platelet count at least three times weekly after bone marrow transplantation.
- In patients with severe, chronic neutropenia, obtain CBC with differential and platelet count twice weekly during first 4 weeks of therapy and for 2 weeks after any dosage adjustment. After patient becomes clinically stable, monitor monthly.
- Rare cases of splenic rupture (some fatal) have been reported. Closely evaluate patients with abdominal or shoulder pain.

Patient education

- If patient does not wish to receive blood products for religious or other reasons, inform him that product contains albumin, a component of human blood (if albumin is added during dilution).
- If home use is prescribed, provide thorough instructions on proper administration; stress importance of proper disposal of materials. Caution patient against reusing needles and syringes.
- Tell patient drug may cause GI symptoms and bone pain. Urge him to contact health care professional if symptoms persist.
- Inform patient that he will undergo regular testing during therapy.

floxuridine
FUDR

Classification: Antineoplastic, antimetabolite
Pregnancy risk category D

Pharmacology

Floxuridine quickly converts to 5-fluorouracil. It deactivates thymidylate synthetase, an enzyme that interferes with DNA synthesis and inhibits RNA formation. This effect causes cells to rupture and die.

Pharmacokinetics

Drug is metabolized in liver. Onset is rapid; elimination half-life is 30 minutes. It is excreted by kidney.

How supplied

Powder for injection: 500-mg vial

Indications and dosages

> FDA-APPROVED

➥ Metastatic primary malignant neoplasm of GI tract; adenocarcinoma and secondary malignant neoplasm of liver in patients considered incurable by surgery or other means

Adults: 0.1 to 0.6 mg/kg daily by continuous arterial infusion; or 0.4 to 0.6 mg/kg daily usually by hepatic artery infusion

OFF-LABEL USES (SELECTED)

➥ Palliative management of colorectal adenocarcinoma with hepatic metastasis
Adults: Various dosing schedules
➥ Ovarian carcinoma not responsive to other antimetabolites
Adults: Various dosing schedules
➥ Metastatic renal carcinoma
Adults: 0.75 mg/kg daily as constant I.V. infusion for 14 days followed by 14-day infusion of heparinized saline in 28-day cycle. In circadian 14-day protocol, 68% of daily dose is given during late daily activity phase (between 3 P.M. and 9 P.M.). Total daily dose by continuous I.V. infusion is divided into four segments (15%, 68%, 15%, and 2%) lasting 6 hours each, with first dose starting at 9:00 A.M.
➥ Solid tumors
Adults: 500 mcg/kg to 1 mg/kg I.V. daily for 6 to 15 days or until toxicity occurs. Alternatively, 30 mg/kg I.V. injection daily for 5 days, followed by 15 mg/kg I.V. injection every other day up to 11 days or until toxicity occurs.

DOSAGE MODIFICATIONS

• Discontinue therapy promptly if any of these toxicity signs appears: myocardial ischemia, stomatitis or esophagopharyngitis, leukopenia (WBC count below 3,500/mm^3) or rapidly falling WBC count, intractable vomiting, diarrhea, frequent bowel movements, watery stools, GI ulceration and bleeding, thrombocytopenia (platelet count below 100,000/mm^3), or hemorrhage from any site.
• Discontinue therapy promptly if patient receiving hepatic arterial infusion develops obstructive jaundice.

⊠ WARNINGS

• Drug is approved for intra-arterial infusion only.
• Because severe toxic reactions may occur, all patients should be hospitalized for first course.
• Drug should be given only by or under supervision of qualified physician experienced with this drug and intra-arterial therapy.

Contraindications and precautions

Contraindicated in poor nutritional status, bone marrow depression, potentially serious infections, and pregnancy or breastfeeding.
Use cautiously in poor-risk patients with hepatic or renal impairment, history of high-dose pelvic irradiation, or previous use of alkylating agents. Safety and efficacy in *children* have not been established.

Preparation and administration

• Follow hazardous drug guidelines for handling, preparation, and administration. (See "Managing hazardous drugs," page 11.)
• For disease extending beyond area capable of infusion by single artery, consider systemic therapy with other chemotherapeutic agents.
• Reconstitute by adding 5 ml sterile water for injection to yield solution containing approximately 100 mg/ml of drug.
• Dilute intra-arterial calculated daily doses with D$_5$W or normal saline injection to volume appropriate for infusion apparatus.
• Use infusion pump suitable for overcoming pressure in large arteries and ensuring uniform infusion rate.
• Store sterile powder at 59° to 86° F (15° to 30° C). Refrigerate reconstituted vials at 36° to 46° F (2° to 8° C) for no more than 2 weeks.

Adverse reactions

CNS: lethargy, malaise, weakness
CV: myocardial ischemia
EENT: pharyngitis
GI: nausea, vomiting, diarrhea, enteritis, stomatitis, duodenal ulcer, duodenitis, gastritis, bleeding, gastroenteritis, glossitis, anorexia, cramps, abdominal pain, intrahepatic or extrahepatic biliary sclerosis, acalculous cholecystitis

Hematologic: anemia, leukopenia, thrombocytopenia
Skin: localized erythema, alopecia, dermatitis, nonspecific skin toxicity, rash
Other: fever, procedural complications of regional arterial infusion (arterial aneurysm, ischemia, or thrombosis; embolism; fibromyositis; thrombophlebitis; hepatic necrosis; abscesses; infection or bleeding at catheter site; blocked, displaced, or leaking catheter)

Interactions

Drug-drug. *Bone marrow suppressants:* increased bone marrow depression
Drug-diagnostic tests. *Liver function tests:* elevated
Platelets, RBCs, WBCs: decreased
Prothrombin time, sedimentation rate, total protein: abnormal

Toxicity and overdose

• Toxicity signs include myocardial ischemia, stomatitis, esophagopharyngitis, leukopenia, intractable vomiting, diarrhea, GI ulceration, GI bleeding, thrombocytopenia (platelets below 100,000/mm³), and hemorrhage from any site. Therapies that increase stress, interfere with nutrition, or depress bone marrow function increase risk of drug toxicity.
• No specific antidote exists. Discontinue drug promptly and provide supportive therapy. Monitor patient's hematologic status for at least 4 weeks.

Special considerations

• Carefully monitor patient's hematologic status, including WBC and platelet counts and renal and hepatic function.
• Drug may cause severe hematologic toxicity, GI hemorrhage, and even death despite careful patient selection and dosage adjustment.

Patient education

• Instruct patient to report persistent side effects, such as nausea, vomiting, diarrhea, enteritis, and stomatitis.

• Urge women with childbearing potential to use effective contraception.
• Caution breastfeeding patient to avoid breastfeeding during therapy.

fludarabine phosphate
Fludara

F

Classification: Antineoplastic, antimetabolite
Pregnancy risk category D

Pharmacology

Fludarabine is rapidly dephosphorylated to 2-fluoro-ara-A and then phosphorylated to active triphosphate 2-fluoro-ara-ATP. This metabolite inhibits DNA synthesis by inhibiting DNA polymerase alpha, ribonucleotide reductase, and DNA primase. Complete mechanism of action is unclear.

Pharmacokinetics

Drug is widely distributed and peaks in 1 hour. Elimination half-life is 9 to 10 hours. Drug is eliminated mainly by kidney.

How supplied

Powder for injection, lyophilized: 25 mg and 50 mg in single-dose vials

Indications and dosages

FDA-APPROVED

⊖ Refractory B-cell chronic lymphocytic leukemia (CLL) after treatment with at least one standard alkylating-agent regimen
Adults: 25 mg/m² I.V. over 30 minutes daily for 5 consecutive days, with each 5-day cycle starting every 28 days

OFF-LABEL USES (SELECTED)

➥ Relapsed non-Hodgkin's lymphoma
Adults: 25 mg/m² I.V. over 30 minutes daily for 5 consecutive days, with each 5-day course starting every 3 to 4 weeks

➡ Acute lymphocytic leukemia in children and adults ages 1 to 21

Children and adults ages 1 to 21: 10.5 mg/m² I.V. loading bolus, followed by 30.5 mg/m² continuous I.V. infusion daily for 5 days

➡ Solid tumors in children and adults ages 1 to 21

Children and adults ages 1 to 21: 7 mg/m² loading bolus, followed by 20 mg/m² continuous I.V. infusion daily for 5 days

DOSAGE MODIFICATIONS

• Dosage should be decreased or delayed if hematologic or nonhematologic toxicity occurs.

• Dosage may need to be decreased in renal insufficiency or bone marrow impairment.

• In adults with moderate renal impairment (creatinine clearance of 30 to 70 ml/minute/1.73 m²), dosage should be decreased by 20%. Drug should not be administered to patients with severe renal impairment (creatinine clearance below 30 ml/minute/1.73 m²).

• Optimal treatment duration for refractory CLL and non-Hodgkin's lymphoma have not been determined. It is recommended that three additional cycles be given after maximal response; drug should then be discontinued.

☒ WARNINGS

• Drug may severely suppress bone marrow function.

• Life-threatening autoimmune hemolytic anemia may occur after one or more cycles. Monitor patient closely for hemolysis.

• Drug given in combination with pentostatin is not recommended because of high incidence of fatal pulmonary toxicity.

Contraindications and precautions

Contraindicated in hypersensitivity to drug and in pregnancy or breastfeeding.

Use cautiously in risk for tumor lysis syndrome, renal impairment, and *elderly pa-*

tients. Safety and efficacy in *children* have not been established.

Preparation and administration

• Follow hazardous drug guidelines for handling, preparation, and administration. (See "Managing hazardous drugs," page 11.)

• If solution contacts skin or mucous membranes, wash thoroughly with soap and water; if it contacts eyes, rinse eyes thoroughly with plain water.

• Reconstitute by adding 2 ml of sterile water for injection. Use within 8 hours.

• Avoid exposure by inhalation.

• Store drug refrigerated at 36° to 46° F (2° to 8° C).

Adverse reactions

GI: nausea, vomiting, diarrhea
Hematologic: neutropenia, thrombocytopenia, anemia
Respiratory: pneumonia
Other: fever, chills, infection, fatigue

Interactions

Drug-drug. *Antigout drugs:* decreased effects of these drugs
Bone marrow suppressants: increased risk of bone marrow depression
Pentostatin: severe pulmonary toxicity
Drug-diagnostic tests. *ALP, AST, serum uric acid:* possible increases
Drug-herb. *Alpha-lipoic acid, coenzyme Q10:* possible decreased chemotherapy efficacy

Toxicity and overdose

• Signs and symptoms of CNS toxicity include lethargy, coma, blindness, and bone marrow depression. When used at high doses (roughly four times greater than recommended) in acute leukemia, drug may cause severe neurologic effects, including blindness, coma, and death.

• No known specific antidote exists. If overdose occurs, discontinue drug and provide supportive therapy.

Only common or life-threatening adverse reactions are listed.

Special considerations
- Monitor CBC and platelet counts regularly during treatment to determine degree of hematopoietic suppression. Duration of clinically significant cytopenia ranges from approximately 2 months to 1 year.
- Drug may lead to tumor lysis syndrome, marked by flank pain, hematuria, hyperuricemia, hyperphosphatemia, hypocalcemia, metabolic acidosis, hyperkalemia, hematuria, urate crystalluria, and renal failure.
- Monitor for excessive toxicity in patients with renal insufficiency or bone marrow impairment.

Patient education
- Instruct patient about signs and symptoms of bone marrow depression (such as unusual bleeding or bruising) and infection.
- Advise patient to avoid crowds and exposure to infection.
- Inform patient that some side effects begin 60 days after therapy ends.
- Caution women with childbearing potential to avoid pregnancy.
- Advise breastfeeding patient not to breastfeed during therapy.

fluorouracil (5-fluorouracil, 5-FU)
Adrucil, Carac, Efudex, Fluoroplex

Classification: Antineoplastic, antimetabolite
Pregnancy risk category D

Pharmacology
Fluorouracil blocks conversion of deoxyuridylic acid to thymidylic acid, thus impeding DNA synthesis (and to a lesser extent, RNA synthesis). Because DNA and RNA are crucial for cell division and growth, thymine deficiency causes unbalanced growth and death of cell. Effects are most marked on rapidly growing cells and those that take up drug at a more rapid rate.

Pharmacokinetics
About 7% to 20% of drug is excreted in urine in 6 hours, with more than 90% excreted during first hour. Remainder is metabolized in liver and excreted by kidneys. Elimination half-life is 20 minutes.

How supplied
Solution for injection: 50 mg/ml
Topical cream and solution: 5%

Indications and dosages

FDA-APPROVED

➥ Palliative management of colon, rectum, breast, stomach, or pancreas carcinoma
Adults: Various dosing regimens
➥ Superficial basal cell carcinoma when conventional methods are impractical
Adults: 5% cream or solution topically twice daily in amount sufficient to cover lesions, continued for at least 3 to 6 weeks

DOSAGE MODIFICATIONS

- Obliteration of superficial basal cell lesions may require 10 to 12 weeks of therapy.
- If patient is obese or has had spurious weight gain from edema, ascites, or other fluid retention, base dosage on estimated lean body mass (dry weight), not body weight.

⊠ WARNINGS

- Patients should be hospitalized for first course of therapy due to potential for severe toxic reactions.

Contraindications and precautions
Contraindicated in hypersensitivity to drug or its components, poor nutritional status, bone marrow depression, and serious infection.

Use cautiously in poor-risk patients with history of high-dose pelvic radiation therapy or previous use of alkylating agents, widespread bone marrow involvement by metastatic tumors, hepatic or renal impairment, and in pregnancy or breastfeeding. Safety and efficacy in *children* have not been established.

Preparation and administration

• Follow hazardous drug guidelines for handling, preparation, and administration. (See "Managing hazardous drugs," page 11.)

• Obtain WBC count before each parenteral dose.

• Dosages given by I.V. injection do not require dilution. Administer drug by direct I.V. through Y-tube or three-way stopcock of free-flowing infusion over 1 to 2 minutes.

• Drug may be diluted in normal saline solution or D_5W for continuous infusion, usually given over 24 hours.

• If precipitate forms from exposure to low temperatures, resolubilize by heating to 171° F (77° C) and shaking vigorously. Allow to cool to body temperature before using.

• Store solution at room temperature protected from light.

• Apply topical form with care near eyes, nose, and mouth. Wash hands immediately after administering.

• Topical application causes erythema, usually followed by vesiculation, erosion, ulceration, necrosis, and epithelialization.

• Use porous gauze dressing for topical form to avoid inflammatory reactions in adjacent normal skin.

• Store topical form at room temperature of 59° to 86° F (15° to 30° C). Protect from light and keep in carton until ready to use.

Adverse reactions

GI: stomatitis, esophagopharyngitis, diarrhea, anorexia, nausea, vomiting
Hematologic: leukopenia (usually within 9 to 14 days after I.V. administration, but may occur as late as day 25), thrombocytopenia (occasionally occurs 7 to 17 days after I.V. administration)
Skin: alopecia, photosensitivity, pruritic dermatitis (usually pruritic maculopapular rash on extremities but sometimes on trunk); local

reactions including pain, pruritus (topical form)

Interactions

Drug-drug. *Bone marrow suppressants:* increased bone marrow depression
Leucovorin calcium: possible increase in fluorouracil toxicity
Metronidazole: increased fluorouracil concentrations
Phenytoin: increased phenytoin level
Tamoxifen: increased risk of thromboembolism
Warfarin: increased bleeding
Drug-diagnostic tests. *Albumin, platelets, WBCs:* decreased
Eosinophils: increased
5-HIAA: increased excretion
Liver function tests: elevated
Prothrombin time, sedimentation rate, total protein: abnormal results
Drug-herb. *Alfalfa:* increased photosensitivity (with excessive alfalfa doses)

Toxicity and overdose

• Overdose is unlikely. Anticipated effects include nausea, vomiting, diarrhea, GI ulceration and bleeding, and bone marrow depression (including thrombocytopenia, leukopenia, and agranulocytosis).

• No specific antidote exists. If overdose occurs, monitor patient's hematologic status for at least 4 weeks, and treat as needed.

Special considerations

• Carefully monitor patient, including CBC with differential and platelet count.

• Monitor renal and hepatic function.

• Dipyrimidine dehydrogenase deficiency has been associated with rare, severe toxicity, which may involve stomatitis, diarrhea, neutropenia, and neurotoxicity. Lack of this enzyme results in prolonged 5-fluorouracil clearance.

• Therapeutic response is unlikely without some evidence of toxicity.

• Monitor patient closely; drug can cause severe hematologic toxicity, GI hemorrhage, and

Only common or life-threatening adverse reactions are listed.

even death despite meticulous patient selection and careful dosage adjustment.
• Drug has been associated with palmar-plantar erythrodysesthesia (hand-foot syndrome). Drug withdrawal brings gradual resolution over 5 to 7 days. Pyridoxine may ease symptoms, but its safety and efficacy have not been established
• Drug may cause angina and coronary vasospasms. Treat with nitrates and morphine to relieve pain. For prevention, use calcium-channel blocker therapy.

Patient education

• Instruct patient to avoid prolonged exposure to ultraviolet rays; drug may increase risk of skin reactions.
• Inform patient of toxic reactions, particularly mucosal erythema, ulcers on inner margin of lips, and difficulty swallowing.
• Advise patient to perform fastidious oral hygiene.
• Tell patient that drug may cause alopecia but that this usually reverses.
• Inform patient that treated skin may be unsightly during therapy and possibly for several weeks afterward.
• Lesions may not heal completely until 1 to 2 months after therapy.
• Teach patients about signs and symptoms of bone marrow depression (such as unusual bleeding or bruising) and infection.
• Instruct patient to avoid crowds and exposure to infection.
• Caution women with childbearing potential to use contraception and to avoid becoming pregnant during therapy.
• Advise breastfeeding patient not to breastfeed during therapy.

flutamide
Eulexin

Classification: Antineoplastic, antiandrogen, hormone/hormone modifier
Pregnancy risk category D

F

Pharmacology
Flutamide, a nonsteroidal antiandrogen, blocks testosterone activity by inhibiting androgen uptake or binding in target tissues. Prostate carcinoma responds to treatment that counteracts effects, or removes source, of testosterone. Plasma testosterone and estradiol elevations have occurred after administration.

Pharmacokinetics
Drug has good oral availability and is metabolized in liver. It peaks 1 to 2 hours after dose. Onset varies. Duration is about 72 hours, and elimination half-life is 8 to 10 hours. Drug is excreted primarily in urine.

How supplied
Capsules: 125 mg

Indications and dosages

FDA-APPROVED

➡ Locally confined stage B2-C and stage D2 metastatic carcinoma of prostate
Adults: In combination with luteinizing hormone-releasing hormone (LHRH) agonists, two capsules (250 mg) P.O. every 8 hours, for total daily dose of 750 mg

WARNINGS

• Drug has caused death from hepatic failure, usually within first 3 months of therapy. Evidence of hepatic injury includes elevated serum transaminase levels, jaundice, and hepatic encephalopathy. Hepatic injury may reverse on withdrawal. Obtain liver function tests at first sign of hepatic dysfunction.

• Drug is not recommended for patients whose ALT exceeds 2 × ULN.
• If jaundice occurs or ALT increases above 2 × ULN, drug should be withdrawn immediately and patient's liver function tests should be followed closely.

Contraindications and precautions

Contraindicated in hypersensitivity to drug or its components and severe hepatic impairment.
Use cautiously in women. Drug has not been studied in *children*.

Preparation and administration

• Follow hazardous drug guidelines for handling, preparation, and administration. (See "Managing hazardous drugs," page 11.)
• In stage B2-C prostate carcinoma, flutamide and LHRH agonist should start 8 weeks before radiation therapy and continue during therapy.
• Measure serum transaminase levels before treatment, monthly for first 4 months of therapy, and then periodically.
• Leuprolide acetate is most commonly used LHRH in combination therapy.
• Capsule may be opened and contents mixed with soft food, such as applesauce or pudding.
• Store between 36° and 86° F (2° and 30° C).

Adverse reactions

GI: diarrhea, constipation, nausea
GU: nocturia, loss of libido, erectile dysfunction
Hematologic: anemia, hemolytic anemia
Hepatic: hepatic encephalopathy
Skin: rash, photosensitivity
Other: asthenia, hot flashes, generalized pain

Interactions

Drug-drug. *Warfarin:* prolonged prothrombin time (PT)
Drug-diagnostic tests. *ALT, AST, bilirubin, creatinine, glucose, serum estradiol, testosterone:* possible increases

Hemoglobin, platelets, WBCs: decreased
Drug-herb. *Eucalyptus, skullcap, valerian:* possible increased risk of hepatotoxicity

Toxicity and overdose

• Dosages up to 1,500 mg daily for up to 36 weeks have been used with no serious adverse effects. Overdose signs and symptoms include hypoactivity, piloerection, bradypnea, ataxia, lacrimation, anorexia, tranquilization, emesis, and methemoglobinemia.
• Dialysis does not clear drug. If patient does not vomit spontaneously, induce vomiting (if patient is alert). Provide general supportive measures, including frequent monitoring of vital signs and close patient observation.

Special considerations

• Reduced sperm counts occurred during 6-week study of flutamide monotherapy in normal humans.
• Carefully monitor PT in patients also receiving warfarin. Downward adjustments of warfarin dosage may be necessary.
• Closely monitor liver function test results.
• In patients susceptible to aniline toxicity (such as those with G6PD, hemoglobin M disease, or smokers), consider monitoring methomoglobin levels.
• Drug is highly protein-bound and is not cleared by hemodialysis.
• For patient with objective disease progression and elevated prostate-specific antigen (PSA) level, consider initiating treatment-free period of antiandrogen while continuing LHRH.
• Breast cancer has been reported in men treated with drug.
• Antiandrogen withdrawal response may occur in patients initially managed with combination of flutamide and LHRH agonist analogues or orchiectomy. Discontinue flutamide if patient has evidence of clinical or PSA progression when receiving this combination, while maintaining castrate testosterone levels with either LHRH agonist analogues or orchiectomy.

Patient education

- Inform patient that drug may color urine amber or yellow-green.
- Because of photosensitivity risk, caution patient to wear clothing to guard against ultraviolet light exposure until tolerance is known. Caution patient to avoid prolonged sun exposure and tanning beds.
- Urge patient to immediately report nausea, vomiting, abdominal pain, or yellowing of skin or eyes.

fulvestrant
Faslodex

Classification: Antineoplastic, antiestrogen, hormone/hormone modifier
Pregnancy risk category D

Pharmacology

Fulvestrant, an estrogen receptor (ER) antagonist, binds to estrogen receptors on tumors and other target cells. Drug down-regulates ER protein in human breast cancer cells and inhibits growth. It also decreases Ki67 labeling index, a cell proliferation marker.

Pharmacokinetics

Drug is metabolized in liver. It is 99% protein-bound. It peaks in about 7 days and maintains peak for at least 1 month; half-life is 40 days. It is excreted primarily in feces, with small amount excreted in urine.

How supplied

Solution for injection: 250 mg/5 ml (50 mg/ml) and 125 mg/2.5 ml (50 mg/ml) in prefilled syringes

Indications and dosages

FDA-approved

➡ Hormone receptor–positive metastatic breast cancer in postmenopausal women with disease progression after antiestrogen therapy
Adults: 250 mg I.M. monthly as single 5-ml injection or two concurrent 2.5-ml injections

Contraindications and precautions

Contraindicated in hypersensitivity to drug or its components, bleeding diatheses, thrombocytopenia, anticoagulant use, and pregnancy.

Use cautiously in moderate to severe hepatic impairment and in breastfeeding. Safety and efficacy in *children* have not been established.

Preparation and administration

- Follow hazardous drug guidelines for handling, preparation, and administration. (See "Managing hazardous drugs," page 11.)
- Exclude pregnancy before starting therapy.
- Administer I.M. injection slowly into large muscle (gluteal).
- Do not give subcutaneously, I.V., or intra-arterially.
- Refrigerate at 36° to 46° F (2° to 8° C).
- To protect from light, store in original carton until ready to use.

Adverse reactions

CNS: headache
CV: vasodilation
EENT: pharyngitis
GI: nausea, vomiting, constipation, abdominal pain
Musculoskeletal: back pain
Other: asthenia, hot flashes

Interactions

Drug-drug: *Anticoagulants:* increased bleeding risk

Toxicity and overdose

- No known signs and symptoms of toxicity exist.
- If overdose occurs, provide supportive treatment.

Special considerations

- Obtain estrogen receptor assay before starting therapy.

F

- Monitor blood chemistries and plasma lipids.
- Monitor liver function studies.

Patient education

- Inform patient that drug may cause hot flashes, asthenia, or vaginal bleeding. Tell her to report these symptoms if they persist.
- Caution patients with childbearing potential to avoid pregnancy during therapy. Urge them to use effective contraception. Advise them to contact physician immediately if pregnancy occurs.
- Advise breastfeeding patient not to breastfeed during therapy.

gefitinib
Iressa

Classification: Antineoplastic, signal transduction inhibitor
Pregnancy risk category D

Pharmacology

Gefitinib may inhibit activity of many tyrosine kinases associated with transmembrane cell surface receptors, including those associated with epidermal growth factor receptor (EGFR)-TK. This effect ultimately blocks cell growth and reproduction. EGFR is expressed on cell surface of many normal cells and cancer cells, including those in colon, lung, head, and neck.

Pharmacokinetics

Drug is metabolized in liver. It peaks in 3 to 7 hours and achieves steady-state plasma concentrations in 10 days. Elimination half-life is 48 hours. It is excreted primarily in feces.

How supplied

Tablets: 250 mg

Indications and dosages

FDA-APPROVED

➡ Locally advanced or metastatic non-small-cell lung cancer after failure of platinum-based and docetaxel chemotherapies
Adults: 250 mg P.O. daily

DOSAGE MODIFICATIONS

- Drug is administered on continuous schedule over 28 days. It is given for 14 days on and 14 days off in patients with poorly tolerated diarrhea and adverse skin reactions.
- If patient experiences acute onset or worsening of pulmonary symptoms (such as dyspnea, cough, and fever), stop drug and initiate appropriate treatment. Discontinue drug if interstitial lung disease is confirmed.
- For patients receiving potent CYP3A4 inducers (such as rifampin or phenytoin), consider increasing dosage to 500 mg daily in absence of severe adverse reactions.

WARNINGS

- Drug should be used only in cancer patients who have already taken it and whose physicians believe it is benefiting them. New patients should not receive it; large study found that it did not extend life. Currently, new patients can obtain drug only through special allocation by manufacturer.

Contraindications and precautions

Contraindicated in hypersensitivity to drug or its components.

Use cautiously in hepatic impairment, cardiac disease, severe renal impairment, and pregnancy or breastfeeding. Safety and efficacy in *children* have not been established.

Preparation and administration

- Do not crush or break film-coated tablet. Tablets can be dispersed only in half-glass of noncarbonated drinking water. Drop tablet into water without crushing it, and stir until it

Only common or life-threatening adverse reactions are listed.

disperses. Have patient drink immediately, then rinse glass with water and drink again.
• Drug may be given by nasogastric tube if patient cannot swallow.
• Store at temperature of 68° to 77° F (20° to 25° C).

Adverse reactions
EENT: conjunctivitis
GI: diarrhea, nausea, vomiting, anorexia
Skin: rash, acne, dry skin

Interactions
Drug-drug. *CYP3A4 inducers (such as rifampin, phenytoin):* increased gefitinib metabolism and decreased plasma concentration
CYP3A4 inhibitors (such as ketoconazole, itraconazole): decreased gefitinib metabolism and increased plasma concentration
Histamine$_2$-receptor antagonists (such as ranitidine, cimetidine): decreased gefitinib plasma concentration
Warfarin: increased INR, bleeding events
Drug-diagnostic tests. *ALP, ALT, AST, serum bilirubin:* possible increases

Toxicity and overdose
• Anticipated overdose effects include increased frequency and severity of some adverse reactions—mainly diarrhea and rash.
• Provide symptomatic treatment. In particular, manage severe diarrhea appropriately.

Special considerations
• Monitor INR or prothrombin time regularly in patients receiving warfarin.
• Observe closely for interstitial lung disease; incidence is 1%, with one-third of cases fatal.

Patient education
• Inform patient that drug may cause nausea, anorexia, vomiting, or persistent diarrhea. Tell him to report these symptoms promptly if they persist.
• Advise patient to report eye irritation.
• Instruct patient to consume adequate fluids, especially if diarrhea occurs.

• Tell patient to promptly report new or worsening pulmonary symptoms, such as dyspnea, cough, and fever.
• Advise women with childbearing potential to use effective contraception.
• Caution breastfeeding patient not to breastfeed during therapy.

gemcitabine hydrochloride
Gemzar

Classification: Antineoplastic, antimetabolite, pyrimidine nucleoside analogue
Pregnancy risk category D

Pharmacology
Gemcitabine kills malignant cells undergoing DNA synthesis (S-phase) and blocks cells' progression through G1/S-phase boundary. Cytotoxic effect results from combined actions of diphosphate and triphosphate nucleosides, causing inhibition of DNA synthesis.

Pharmacokinetics
Drug is metabolized throughout body and distributed rapidly. Half-life is less than 2 hours. Maximum serum concentration occurs within 30 minutes. Drug is excreted mainly in urine.

How supplied
Powder for injection: 200 mg (10-ml vial), 1 g (50-ml vial)

Indications and dosages

FDA-APPROVED

➡ Locally advanced (nonresectable Stage II or III) or metastatic (Stage IV) adenocarcinoma of pancreas in patients previously treated with fluorouracil
Adults: 1,000 mg/m^2 I.V. over 30 minutes once weekly for up to 7 weeks, followed by 1 week without treatment; subsequent cycles of weekly infusions for 3 consecutive weeks out of every 4 weeks

➤ Inoperable locally advanced (Stage IIIA or IIIB) or metastatic (Stage IV) non-small-cell lung cancer

Adults: In combination with cisplatin, 1,000 mg/m^2 I.V. over 30 minutes on days 1, 8, and 15 of 28-day cycle, with cisplatin 100 mg/m^2 I.V. given on day 1 after gemcitabine infusion; or 1,250 mg/m^2 I.V. over 30 minutes on days 1 and 8 of 21-day cycle, with cisplatin 100 mg/m^2 I.V. given on day 1 after gemcitabine infusion

➤ Breast cancer

Adults: In combination with paclitaxel, 1,250 mg/m^2 I.V. over 30 minutes on days 1 and 8 of each 21-day cycle, with paclitaxel 175 mg/m^2 given before gemcitabine on day 1 of each cycle

OFF-LABEL USES (SELECTED)

➤ Locally advanced, unresectable, or metastatic gallbladder carcinomas or biliary tract carcinomas (such as cholangiocarcinoma, biliary tree carcinoma, or bile duct carcinoma)

Adults: Several dosages and regimens are showing activity for this indication.

➤ Metastatic bladder (urothelial) carcinoma

Adults: 1,000 to 1,200 mg/m^2 I.V. over 30 minutes once weekly for 3 weeks, followed by 1 week without treatment; repeat up to six cycles

➤ Advanced or relapsed epithelial ovarian carcinoma

Adults: 800 to 1,250 mg/m^2 I.V. over 30 minutes once weekly for 2 or 3 weeks, followed by 1 to 2 weeks without treatment

➤ Hodgkin's and non-Hodgkin's lymphomas

Adults: 1,000 to 1,250 mg/m^2 I.V. over 30 minutes on days 1, 8, and 15 of 28-day cycle, for up to nine cycles

➤ Relapsed, refractory, progressive, metastatic, or nonseminomatous gonadal cancer (including testicular and ovarian cancer) and extragonadal germ cell tumor

Adults: Several dosages and regimens are showing activity for this indication.

DOSAGE MODIFICATIONS

• Dosage may be increased by 25% in patients who complete entire cycle of therapy, provided that absolute granulocyte count (AGC) and platelet nadirs exceed 1,500 × 10^6/L and 100,000 × 10^6/L, respectively, and nonhematologic toxicity has not exceeded WHO Grade 1.

• Dosage may be increased further by 20% in patients who tolerate subsequent course at increased dosage, provided that AGC and platelet nadirs exceed 1,500 × 10^6/L and 100,000 × 10^6/L, respectively, and nonhematologic toxicity has not exceeded WHO Grade 1.

• *Pancreatic cancer treatment:* If bone marrow depression occurs, therapy should be modified or suspended based on degree of hematologic toxicity, according to guidelines in table below.

Absolute granulocyte count (× 10^6/L)		Platelet count (× 10^6/L)	% of full dose
1,000 or more	and	100,000 or more	100
500 to 999	or	50,000 to 99,000	75
Below 500	or	Below 50,000	Withhold

• *Non-small-cell lung cancer treatment:* Patients may require dosage adjustments for hematologic toxicity for both gemcitabine and cisplatin. Gemcitabine dosage adjustment is based on granulocyte and platelet counts obtained on day of therapy, based on guidelines in table above. For Grade 3 or 4 nonhematologic toxicity (except alopecia, nausea, or vomiting), combination therapy with gemcitabine and cisplatin should be withheld or dosage decreased by 50%.

• *Breast cancer treatment:* Dosage adjustments for hematologic toxicity are based on granulocyte and platelet counts obtained on day 8 of therapy. If bone marrow depression occurs, dosage should be modified according to the following table. For Grade 3 or 4 nonhematologic toxicity (except alopecia, nausea, or vomiting), drug should be withheld or dosage decreased by 50%. For paclitaxel dosage adjustments, see manufacturer's prescribing information.

Absolute granulocyte count ($\times 10^6$/L)		Platelet count ($\times 10^6$/L)	% of full dose
1,200 or more	and	Above 75,000	100
1,000 to 1,199	or	50,000 to 75,000	75
700 to 999	and	50,000 or more	50
Below 700	or	Above 50,000	Withhold

Contraindications and precautions

Contraindicated in hypersensitivity to drug.

Use cautiously in concurrent radiation therapy, significant renal or hepatic impairment, and pregnancy or breastfeeding. Thrombocytopenia (Grade 3 or 4) is more common in **elderly patients**. Safety and efficacy in **children** have not been established.

Preparation and administration

• Follow hazardous drug guidelines for handling, preparation, and administration. (See "Managing hazardous drugs," page 11.)
• Monitor CBC with differential and platelet count before each dose.
• When giving drug with cisplatin, follow manufacturer's guidelines regarding hydration.
• If solution contacts skin or mucosa, immediately wash skin thoroughly with soap and water, or rinse mucosa with copious amounts of water.
• Reconstitute by adding 5 ml normal saline solution injection to 200-mg vial or 25 ml normal saline solution injection to 1-g vial. Do not reconstitute at concentrations above 40 mg/ml.
• Give drug as prepared or dilute further with normal saline solution injection to concentration as low as 0.1 mg/ml. Infuse over 30 minutes. Toxicity risk increases with infusion times beyond 60 minutes and dosing more frequent than weekly.

• Do not refrigerate reconstituted solution; crystallization may occur.
• Reconstituted solution is stable for 24 hours at 68° to 77° F (20° to 25° C). Discard unused portion.
• Store powder at room temperature at 68° to 77° F.

Adverse reactions

GI: nausea, vomiting, constipation, diarrhea
Respiratory: mild to moderate dyspnea
Skin: mild to moderate pruritic rash
Other: generalized pain, peripheral edema

Interactions

Drug-drug. *Other antineoplastics:* increased risk of bone marrow depression
Drug-diagnostic tests. *Serum ALP, ALT, AST, bilirubin, BUN, and creatinine:* possible increases
Drug-herb. *Alpha-lipoic acid, coenzyme Q10:* possible decreased chemotherapy efficacy

Toxicity and overdose

• Bone marrow depression, paresthesia, and severe rash are primary signs and symptoms of toxicity.
• No known antidote exists. In suspected overdose, monitor appropriate blood counts and provide supportive therapy.

Special considerations

• Monitor CBC with differential and platelet count throughout therapy.
• Evaluate renal and hepatic function before each dose and periodically afterward.
• Monitor patient for bone marrow depression (marked by leukopenia, thrombocytopenia, and anemia).
• Monitor serum creatinine, potassium, calcium, and magnesium levels in patients receiving combination therapy with cisplatin.

Patient education

• Inform patient that drug may cause nausea, vomiting, constipation, dyspnea, and other

side effects. Tell him to report symptoms promptly if they persist.
- Counsel patient to avoid crowds and exposure to infection.
- Advise women with childbearing potential to use effective contraception.
- If patient becomes pregnant while receiving drug, discuss potential risk to fetus and risk of pregnancy loss.
- Provide guidance to help breastfeeding patient decide whether to discontinue breastfeeding or stop drug, based on drug's importance to patient and potential risk to infant.

gemtuzumab ozogamicin
Mylotarg

Classification: Antineoplastic, monoclonal antibody
Pregnancy risk category D

Pharmacology
Gemtuzumab ozogamicin contains recombinant humanized monoclonal antibody and calicheamicin, a cytotoxic antitumor antibiotic. This antibody binds to CD33 antigen on surface of leukemic cells (including myeloid stem cells, erythrocytes, thrombocytes, monocytes, macrophages, and neutrophils), which occur in more than 80% of patients with acute myeloid leukemia. Binding results in formation of complex that releases antibiotic into lysomes of myeloid cells, causing DNA double-strand breaks and, ultimately, cell death.

Pharmacokinetics
Drug is metabolized in liver. Half-life is 45 hours for first dose and 60 hours for second.

How supplied
Powder for injection: 5 mg

Indications and dosages

FDA-APPROVED
CD33-positive acute myeloid leukemia in patients ages 60 and older who are not considered candidates for other cytotoxic chemotherapy
Adults: 9 mg/m^2 I.V. infusion over 2 hours; repeated 14 days later

DOSAGE MODIFICATIONS
- Second dose may be given before patient recovers fully from hematologic toxicities.

WARNINGS
- Drug is for I.V. use only. Use only as a single agent. No controlled trials demonstrate safety and efficacy for combination therapy.
- Drug may cause severe bone marrow depression when used at recommended doses.
- Monitor patient carefully for signs and symptoms of hepatotoxicity.
- Drug can cause severe hypersensitivity reactions (including anaphylaxis) and other infusion-related reactions (including severe pulmonary events). These reactions may be fatal.

Contraindications and precautions
Contraindicated in hypersensitivity to drug or its components.
Use cautiously in hepatic impairment, pregnancy, and breastfeeding. Safety and efficacy in *children* have not been established.

Preparation and administration
- Follow hazardous drug guidelines for handling, preparation, and administration. (See "Managing drug guidelines," page 11.)
- Because patients with high peripheral blast counts may be at greater risk for pulmonary events and tumor lysis syndrome, consider leukoreduction with hydroxyurea or leukapheresis to reduce peripheral WBC count below 30,000/mm^3 before starting therapy.

- Reassess liver function studies before second dose.
- Do not administer as I.V. push or bolus.
- Allow drug to reach room temperature before reconstituting.
- Reconstitute vial contents with 5 ml sterile water for injection, yielding 1 mg/ml. Dilute by injecting into 100-ml I.V. bag of normal saline solution injection. Place bag into UV protective bag. Use solution immediately.
- Infuse reconstituted solution over 2 hours through separate peripheral or central I.V. line with low protein-binding, 1.2-micron terminal filter.
- Interrupt infusion if patient experiences dyspnea or clinically significant hypotension.
- In most cases, infusion-related symptoms occur during or within 24 hours of infusion. To reduce incidence of such reactions, give diphenhydramine 50 mg P.O. and acetaminophen 650 to 1,000 mg P.O. 1 hour before therapy. Thereafter, give acetaminophen 650 to 1,000 mg P.O every 4 hours as needed, for two doses. Steroids also may be given before infusion.
- Monitor vital signs during infusion and for 4 hours afterward.
- Protect drug from direct or indirect sunlight and unshielded fluorescent light during preparation and administration.
- Reconstituted drug in vial may be refrigerated at 36° to 46° F (2° to 8° C) and protected from light for up to 8 hours.

Adverse reactions

CNS: headache
CV: hypotension, hypertension
EENT: epistaxis
GI: diarrhea, abdominal pain, stomatitis, nausea, vomiting
Hematologic: severe bone marrow depression (neutropenia, anemia, thrombocytopenia) in 98% of patients
Hepatic: hepatotoxicity (including severe veno-occlusive disease [VOD])
Respiratory: dyspnea
Skin: rash

Other: asthenia, sepsis, postinfusion syndrome (fever, chills, nausea, and vomiting that resolve within 2 to 4 hours with supportive therapy)

Interactions

Drug-diagnostic tests. *Hematocrit, hemoglobin, platelets, serum magnesium and potassium, WBCs:* decreased
Serum ALT, AST, bilirubin: increased
Drug-herb. *Alpha-lipoic acid, coenzyme Q10:* possible decreased chemotherapy efficacy

Toxicity and overdose

- No cases of overdose have been reported.
- If overdose occurs, provide supportive measures and carefully monitor blood pressure and blood counts. Drug is not dialyzable.

Special considerations

- Closely monitor electrolytes, CBC and platelet counts, and liver function test results.
- Monitor patients carefully for signs and symptoms of hepatotoxicity—particularly those of VOD. Deaths from hepatic failure and VOD have been reported.
- Patients who receive drug before or after hematopoietic stem cell transplantation, those with underlying hepatic disease or abnormal liver function, and those receiving drug in combination chemotherapy may be at increased risk for severe VOD.
- Drug has not been studied in patients with renal failure. It is not dialyzable.

Patient education

- Inform patient about signs and symptoms of bone marrow depression (such as unusual bleeding or bruising) and infection.
- Instruct patient to avoid crowds and exposure to infection.
- Advise women with childbearing potential to use contraception because drug may harm fetus.
- Caution breastfeeding patient not to breastfeed during therapy.

goserelin acetate
Zoladex

Classification: Antineoplastic, gonadotropin-releasing hormone analogue, luteinizing hormone (LH)–releasing analogue
Pregnancy risk category X; D (advanced breast cancer)

Pharmacology

Goserelin, a synthetic analogue of luteinizing hormone-releasing hormone (LHRH), stimulates release of LH and follicle-stimulating hormone from anterior pituitary, causing sustained pituitary-gonadal suppression. In men, drug decreases serum testosterone levels to ranges that normally occur in surgically castrated men roughly 21 days after therapy begins. In women, drug decreases estradiol to postmenopausal levels. Drug also binds to LHRH receptors in breast cancer tissue.

Pharmacokinetics

Drug is released slowly over 28 days after administration; metabolism is insignificant. Drug peaks in 12 to 15 days. Elimination half-life is 4.2 hours, prolonged to 12 hours in impaired renal function. It is excreted in urine.

How supplied

Implant (subcutaneous): 3.6 mg and 10.8 mg in preloaded syringes

Indications and dosages

FDA-APPROVED

➡ Palliative treatment of advanced prostate carcinoma
Adults: 3.6 mg subcutaneously into upper abdominal wall every 28 days; or 10.8 mg subcutaneously into upper abdominal wall every 12 weeks
➡ Treatment of locally confined Stage T2b to T4 (Stage B2-C) prostate carcinoma (in combination with flutamide and radiotherapy)

Adults: Starting 8 weeks before and continuing during radiotherapy, goserelin 3.6 mg subcutaneously with flutamide; followed in 28 days by goserelin 10.8 mg subcutaneously. Alternatively, four injections of 3.6 mg subcutaneously can be administered at 28-day intervals as two depots preceding and two during radiotherapy.
➡ Palliative treatment of advanced breast cancer
Adults: 3.6 mg subcutaneously into upper abdominal wall every 28 days

DOSAGE MODIFICATIONS

• For palliative treatment of advanced breast cancer, dosage may be increased to 7.2 mg every 4 weeks if serum estradiol level does not fall to postmenopausal level after 8 weeks of therapy.
• In obese patients, AUC decreases by 1% to 2.5% with 1-kg weight increase.

Contraindications and precautions

Contraindicated in hypersensitivity to drug, its components, or LHRH agonist analogues; women of childbearing age (except for 3.6 mg-dose in advanced breast cancer); and breastfeeding.
Safety and efficacy in *children* have not been established.

Preparation and administration

• Follow hazardous drug guidelines for handling, preparation, and administration. (See "Managing hazardous drugs," page 11.)
• Local anesthetic may be used to reduce injection discomfort.
• Goserelin syringe cannot be used for aspiration. If needle penetrates vessel, blood will appear in syringe chamber. In this case, withdraw needle and inject elsewhere with new syringe.
• Follow manufacturer's instructions for syringe use and special injection technique.
• Store at room temperature, not to exceed 77° F (25° C).

Only common or life-threatening adverse reactions are listed.

Adverse reactions

CNS: headache, depression, spinal cord compression
GI: nausea, diarrhea
GU: sexual dysfunction, decreased erection, lower urinary tract symptoms, ureteral obstruction
Skin: diaphoresis
Other: hot flashes, vasodilation, anaphylaxis

Interactions

Drug-diagnostic tests. *Calcium, estrogen:* misleading results
Serum acid phosphatase, testosterone: possible increases
Drug-herb. *Alpha-lipoic acid, coenzyme Q10:* possible decreased chemotherapy efficacy

Toxicity and overdose

• Drug's pharmacologic properties and administration mode make overdose unlikely. Anticipated signs and symptoms of overdose are endocrine-related, such as hot flashes.
• In suspected overdose, provide supportive treatment.

Special considerations

• Although rare, hypersensitivity reactions (including anaphylactic reactions) have been reported.
• Drug is alternative when orchiectomy or estrogen therapy is not indicated or unacceptable to patient.
• Watch for transient worsening of symptoms, signs and symptoms of increased testosterone level in men or increased estrogen level in women, and signs and symptoms of worsening prostate or breast cancer (which may develop during first few weeks of therapy).
• Monitor testosterone level closely in obese patients who have not responded clinically to 10.8-mg dose.
• Drug may reduce bone mineral density, which may be partly irreversible. Weigh benefits and risks of therapy for patients with history of previous treatment causing bone density loss and those with major risk factors for this condition.
• Ureteral obstruction and spinal cord compression may occur in patients with prostate cancer. Hypercalcemia may occur in patients with metastatic prostate or breast cancer. Watch for weakness, paresthesia, and urinary tract obstruction.

Patient education

• Advise premenopausal women to use effective nonhormonal contraception during therapy and for 12 weeks afterward. Missing one or more successive doses may lead to breakthrough menstrual bleeding or ovulation, increasing potential for conception.
• Instruct patient to notify health care professional if regular menstruation persists.
• Inform patients that drug may cause hot flashes, headaches, depression, and other side effects. Tell them to report symptoms promptly if they persist.
• Advise patient on reducing risk factors for bone density loss, such as chronic alcohol abuse, tobacco abuse, or long-term use of drugs that can reduce bone density (including anticonvulsants and corticosteroids).
• Teach patient at risk for ureteral obstruction or spinal cord compression about symptoms of these conditions. Tell him to report these promptly.

granisetron hydrochloride
Kytril

Classification: Antiemetic, selective 5-HT$_3$ receptor antagonist
Pregnancy risk category B

Pharmacology

Granisetron blocks serotonin stimulation at receptor sites on abdominal vagal afferent nerve and in chemoreceptor trigger zone. This blockade has an antiemetic effect.

Pharmacokinetics

Drug is metabolized in liver, and is 65% plasma protein–bound. Onset is rapid (usually within 1 to 3 minutes), duration is 24 hours, and half-life is 3 to 14 hours. Drug is excreted in urine and feces.

How supplied

Solution (oral): 1 mg/5 ml
Solution for injection: 1 mg/ml
Tablets: 1 mg

Indications and dosages

FDA-APPROVED

➡ Prevention of nausea and vomiting associated with emetogenic cancer therapy
Adults: For oral dosing only on chemotherapy days—With 2-mg once-daily regimen, give two 1-mg tablets or 10 ml of oral solution (2 tsp, equivalent to 2 mg granisetron) up to 1 hour before chemotherapy. With 1-mg twice-daily regimen, give first 1-mg tablet or 1 tsp (5 ml) of oral solution up to 1 hour before chemotherapy, and give second tablet or second tsp (5 ml) of oral solution 12 hours after first.
Adults and children older than age 2: 10 mcg/kg I.V. within 30 minutes before start of chemotherapy and only on chemotherapy days
➡ Nausea and vomiting associated with radiation, including total body irradiation and fractionated abdominal radiation
Adults: 2 mg P.O. daily within 1 hour of radiation

Contraindications and precautions

Contraindicated in hypersensitivity to drug or its components.

Use cautiously in pregnancy or breastfeeding. Safety and efficacy have not been established for I.V. use in *children younger than age 2* or for P.O. use in *children younger than age 18.*

Preparation and administration

• Injection solution may be given I.V. undiluted over 30 seconds or diluted with normal saline solution or D_5W and infused over 5 minutes.
• Prepare I.V. infusion just before administering. Injection form is stable for at least 24 hours when diluted in normal saline solution or D_5W and stored at room temperature under normal lighting.
• Do not mix injection form with other drugs.
• Store oral solution, single-dose vials, and multidose vials at 77° F (25° C); excursions are permitted to 59° to 86° F (15° to 30° C). After multidose vial is penetrated, use contents within 30 days. Do not freeze. Protect from light.
• Store tablets at 59° to 86° F protected from light.
• Keep oral solution bottle closed tightly, stored upright, and protected from light.

Adverse reactions

CNS: headache, somnolence
GI: constipation, nausea, vomiting
Hematologic: leukopenia, thrombocytopenia
Other: asthenia

Interactions

Drug-drug. *CYP450 inducers (including carbamazepine, phenobarbital, phenytoin, rifabutin, rifampin, and rifapentin) and CYP450 inhibitors (including atanazavir, clarithromycin, indinavir, itraconazole, ketoconazole, nefazodone, nelfinavir, ritonavir, saquinavir, troleandomycin, and voriconazole):* altered granisetron clearance and half-life
Drug-diagnostic tests. *ALT, AST:* possible increases
Hematocrit, hemoglobin, platelets, WBCs: possible decreases
Drug-herb. *Horehound:* possible increased granisetron effects

Toxicity and overdose

• Overdose may cause no symptoms or slight headache only.

Only common or life-threatening adverse reactions are listed.

• No specific antidote exists. Treat symptomatically.

Special considerations
• Monitor liver function and CBC with differential.
• When given to patients after abdominal surgery or to patients with chemotherapy-induced nausea and vomiting, drug may mask progressive ileus or gastric distention.

Patient education
• Inform patient that transient taste disorder may occur.
• Advise patient that orthostatic hypotension, drowsiness, dizziness, headache, GI upset, or stomach pain may occur, and to contact prescriber if these symptoms persist.

histrelin acetate implant
Vantas

Classification: Antineoplastic, gonadotropin-releasing hormone (GnRH) analogue, hormone/hormone modifier
Pregnancy risk category X

Pharmacology
Histrelin acetate is a synthetic, nonapeptide agonist of naturally occurring GnRH or luteinizing hormone-releasing hormone (LHRH). It stimulates release of LH and follicle-stimulating hormone from anterior pituitary, causing sustained pituitary gonadotropin suppression. In men, this effect reduces serum testosterone levels to those normally seen in surgically castrated men.

Pharmacokinetics
Drug peaks in 12 hours and is released continuously throughout 52-week dosing period. Half-life is 12 hours.

How supplied
Implant: 50-mg drug core inside nonbiodegradable hydrogel reservoir

Indications and dosages

FDA-approved

➡ Palliative treatment of advanced prostate cancer
Adults: One implant subcutaneously in inner aspect of upper arm every 12 months to provide continuous drug release for 12 months

Contraindications and precautions
Contraindicated in hypersensitivity to drug components, GnRH, or GnRH-agonist analogues; women who are or who may become pregnant during therapy; breastfeeding women; and *children*.
   Use cautiously in hepatic insufficiency.

Preparation and administration
• Adhere to insertion and removal procedures supplied with implant.
• Insert implant subcutaneously into inner aspect of upper arm.
• Implant is not radiopaque. If it is difficult to locate by palpation, use ultrasound or CT scan.
• Keep implant in opaque plastic bag and carton, and refrigerate at 36° to 46° F (2° to 8° C) until day of procedure.

Adverse reactions
CNS: headache, insomnia
GI: constipation
GU: erectile dysfunction, testicular atrophy
Skin: redness, swelling, itching at injection site; mild local reactions (such as pain, soreness, and tenderness) after insertion
Other: hot flashes, fatigue

Interactions
None significant

⊖ Orphan drug ⠀⠀⠀⠀⠀⠀⠀⠀⠀⠀⠀⠀⠀⠀⠀⠀⠀⠀⠀⠀ ≫ Potentially carcinogenic

Toxicity and overdose

• Administration mode makes overdose unlikely. Anticipated symptoms include endocrine-related adverse reactions, such as hot flashes.
• In suspected overdose, manage symptoms supportively.

Special considerations

• Monitor serum testosterone and prostate-specific antigen (PSA) levels periodically.
• Closely observe patients with metastatic vertebral lesions or urinary tract obstruction during first few weeks of therapy. Ureteral or bladder-outlet obstruction and spinal cord compression may occur and contribute to paralysis, with or without fatal complications.
• Drug causes transient testosterone increase during first week of therapy. Patient may experience new onset or worsening of symptoms, such as bone pain, neuropathy, or hematuria.

Patient education

• Caution patient not to get arm wet. Tell him to avoid heavy lifting or strenuous arm exertion for 7 days after implant insertion.
• Inform patient he may experience pain, bruising, and redness at insertion site for 2 weeks after insertion.
• Tell patient implant has been known to expel from insertion site. Instruct him to contact prescriber if this occurs.
• Give patient product information leaflet.
• Inform patient that he will undergo regular blood tests (PSA and testosterone levels) to determine response to treatment.

hydrocodone bitartrate and ibuprofen
Vicoprofen

Classification: Opioid analgesic, nonsteroidal anti-inflammatory (NSAID)
Controlled substance schedule III
Pregnancy risk category C

Pharmacology

Hydrocodone bitartrate is a semisynthetic opioid analgesic whose precise mechanism of action is unknown. Experts believe it may combine with CNS opiate receptors to cause drowsiness, mood changes, mental clouding, and altered perception and response to pain. Ibuprofen is a peripherally acting NSAID analgesic with no known effects on opiate receptors; it also has antipyretic action. Mechanism of action is not completely understood but may relate to inhibition of cyclo-oxygenase activity and prostaglandin synthesis.

Pharmacokinetics

Hydrocodone peaks in 1.7 hours, is not extensively protein-bound, and has a half-life of 4.5 hours. Ibuprofen peaks in 1.8 hours, is 99% protein-bound, and has a half-life of 2.2 hours. Both drugs are excreted in urine.

How supplied

Tablets: 7.5 mg hydrocodone/200 mg ibuprofen

Indications and dosages

FDA-APPROVED

➡ Short-term management of acute pain
Adults: 1 tablet P.O. every 4 to 6 hours, as needed, not to exceed 5 tablets in 24 hours

OFF-LABEL USES (SELECTED)

➡ Chronic cancer pain
Adults: 1 to 2 tablets P.O. every 6 to 8 hours, as needed, for up to 4 weeks

---

Only common or life-threatening adverse reactions are listed.

- Reduce dosage in elderly patients.
- If given with another CNS depressant, reduce dosage of one or both drugs.

Contraindications

Contraindicated in hypersensitivity to hydrocodone or ibuprofen and in history of asthma, urticaria, or allergic-type reactions to aspirin or other NSAID.

Use cautiously in hepatic or renal impairment, hypothyroidism, Addison's disease, prostatic hypertrophy, urethral stricture, history of GI ulceration or bleeding, conditions that increase risk of GI bleeding, hypertension, heart failure, postoperative patients with pulmonary disease, smoking, alcoholism, poor general health, oral corticosteroid or anticoagulant therapy, NSAID therapy, within 14 days of MAO inhibitors, and pregnancy or breastfeeding. Use special care with *elderly patients;* spontaneous reports of fatal GI events have occurred. Safety and efficacy in *children younger than age 16* have not been established.

Preparation and administration

- Before starting therapy, rehydrate patient who is considerably dehydrated.
- Do not administer with aspirin.
- Store in light-resistant container at 77° F (25° C); excursions are permitted to 59° to 86° F (15° to 30° C).

Adverse reactions

CNS: drowsiness, dizziness, headache, somnolence
CV: hypotension
GI: nausea, vomiting, constipation, dyspepsia, abdominal pain ·
Skin: diaphoresis, facial flushing

Interactions

Drug-drug. *ACE inhibitors:* reduced antihypertensive effect
Anticholinergics: paralytic ileus

Antidepressants: increased effect of either drug
CNS depressants (such as antihistamines or anti-anxiety drugs): respiratory depression
Furosemide: reduced diuretic effect (from ibuprofen)
Lithium: reduced clearance and increased plasma concentration of lithium
MAO inhibitors: severe or even fatal reactions
Methotrexate: possible increase in methotrexate toxicity (from ibuprofen)
Warfarin: increased risk of GI bleeding
Drug-diagnostic tests. *Hemoglobin:* decreased
Liver enzymes: increased
Drug-herb. *Chamomile, kava, valerian:* possible increased hydrocodone effect
St. John's wort: increased sedation, increased analgesia

H

Toxicity and overdose

- Overdose signs and symptoms include respiratory depression, irregular breathing, and coma.
- Provide supportive treatment, such as by reversing significant respiratory depression with I.V. naloxone. Consider gastric lavage (unless consciousness is impaired), alkali administration, diuresis induction, and oral activated charcoal (to reduce ibuprofen absorption and reabsorption). Dialysis is unlikely to remove ibuprofen effectively .

Special considerations

- Monitor kidney and liver function in patients with renal or hepatic impairment. Discontinue drug if abnormal liver function test results persist or worsen, patient develops clinical signs and symptoms of hepatic disease, or systemic manifestations (such as eosinophilia or rash) occur.
- Psychic dependence, physical dependence, and tolerance may develop. Physical dependence is clinically significant only after several weeks of continued use, although mild degree of physical dependence may develop after a few days.
- Serious GI toxicity (such as inflammation, bleeding, ulceration, and perforation of stom-

ach, small intestine, or large intestine) can occur at any time with NSAIDs, with or without warning and even with short-term therapy.

Patient education

- Inform patient that drug may be taken with food.
- Caution patient that drug is habit-forming.
- Instruct patient to avoid alcohol while using drug.
- Counsel patient about signs and symptoms of serious GI toxicity and what steps to take if these occur.
- Advise patient to change position slowly to avoid sudden blood pressure decrease.
- Inform patient drug may impair ability to drive and perform other hazardous activities.
- Caution women to avoid pregnancy and breastfeeding during therapy.

hydromorphone hydrochloride

Dilaudid, Dilaudid-5, Dilaudid-HP, Hydrostat IR

Classification: Opioid analgesic
Controlled substance schedule II
Pregnancy risk category C

Pharmacology

Hydromorphone binds to CNS opiate receptors and alters pain response, providing analgesia and sedation. It is eight times more potent than morphine. It acts on medullary cough center to depress cough reflex and on brainstem respiratory centers to depress respirations. It also affects organs with smooth muscles (including stomach), decreasing GI motility. Drug may stimulate histamine release, contributing to orthostatic hypotension.

Pharmacokinetics

Drug is metabolized in liver. With I.V. dose, onset is 15 minutes; with oral dose, 30 min-

utes. Peak is 30 to 120 minutes; duration, 2 to 5 hours; and half-life, 1 to 3 hours. A small amount is excreted in urine.

How supplied

Powder for injection (high-potency solution): 250 mg
Rectal suppository: 3 mg
Solution (oral): 5 ml/5 mg
Solution for injection: 1 mg/ml, 2 mg/ml, 3 mg/ml, 4 mg/ml, 10 mg/ml
Tablets: 1 mg, 2 mg, 3 mg, 4 mg, 8 mg

Indications and dosages

FDA-APPROVED

➥ Relief of moderate to severe pain
Adults: 2 to 10 mg P.O. every 3 to 6 hours, as needed; or 3 mg P.R. every 6 to 8 hours for acute pain and 3 to 6 mg P.R. every 3 to 4 hours for chronic pain, as needed; or 2.5 to 10 mg oral solution P.O. every 3 to 6 hours, as needed; or 2 to 4 mg I.V., subcutaneously, or I.M. every 4 to 6 hours, as needed
➥ Relief of moderate to severe pain in opioid-tolerant patients who require larger-than-usual opioid doses for adequate pain relief (high-potency solution)
Adults weighing more than 50 kg (110 lb): 0.2 to 0.6 mg I.V. every 2 to 3 hours
➥ Chronic cancer pain
Adults: 3 to 4 mg I.M., subcutaneously, or I.V. every 3 to 4 hours, as needed

DOSAGE MODIFICATIONS

- Initial dosage should be reduced in elderly patients; debilitated patients; those with severe hepatic, pulmonary, or renal impairment; myxedema or hypothyroidism; adrenocortical insufficiency; CNS depression; coma; toxic psychoses; prostatic hypertrophy; urethral stricture; gallbladder disease; acute alcoholism; delirium tremens; or kyphoscoliosis.
- When combining drug with other CNS depressants, dosage of one or both drugs should be reduced.

Only common or life-threatening adverse reactions are listed.

• Dosage should be increased gradually if analgesia is inadequate, tolerance develops, or pain severity increases. Reduced duration of effect is usually first sign of tolerance.

⊠ WARNINGS

• High-potency injection is highly concentrated solution intended for use only in opioid-tolerant patients. Do not confuse it with standard parenteral formulations of injections. Overdose and death could result.

Contraindications and precautions

Contraindicated in hypersensitivity to drug, respiratory depression and status asthmaticus, as obstetric analgesia, and in patients who have previously received large amounts of parenteral opioids.

Use cautiously in chronic obstructive pulmonary disease, cor pulmonale, substantially decreased respiratory reserve, hypoxia, hypercapnia, preexisting respiratory depression, circulatory shock, alcoholism, risk of addiction, within 14 days of MAO inhibitors, and pregnancy or breastfeeding. *Elderly patients* are at greater risk for oversedation. Safety and efficacy in *children* have not been established.

Preparation and administration

• Use high-potency form only in opioid-tolerant patients. Do not confuse it with standard hydromorphone or other opioids; overdose and death could result.
• Use equivalency chart when switching patient from another opioid to hydromorphone.
• Experience with I.V. use of high-potency form is limited. If I.V. use is necessary, give injection slowly, over at least 2 to 3 minutes.
• In case of accidental skin exposure to oral liquid, remove contaminated clothing and rinse affected area with water.
• Slight yellowish discoloration may develop in ampules without potency loss.
• Injection form is chemically stable for at

least 24 hours when stored at 77° F (25° C) and protected from light.
• Store oral liquid and tablets at 59° to 77° F (15° to 25° C). Store parenteral forms at 59° to 86° F (15° to 30° C). Protect both forms from light.
• Refrigerate suppositories between 36° and 46° F (2° and 8° C) and protect from light.

Adverse reactions

CNS: sedation, anxiety, dizziness, lethargy
CV: hypotension, bradycardia
EENT: cataracts, glaucoma (with long-term use)
GI: nausea, vomiting, abdominal pain, constipation
GU: urinary retention
Respiratory: respiratory depression, apnea, decreased cough reflex
Skin: diaphoresis, pruritus
Other: physical dependence

Interactions

Drug-drug. *CNS depressants (such as sedatives or hypnotics), general anesthetics, phenothiazines, tranquilizers:* increased respiratory depression, hypotension, sedation
MAO inhibitors: severe and possibly fatal reactions
Neuromuscular blockers: increased respiratory depression
Drug-diagnostic tests. *Amylase, lipase:* increased
Drug-herb. *St. John's wort:* increased sedation, increased analgesia

Toxicity and overdose

• Serious overdose causes respiratory depression, somnolence progressing to stupor or coma, skeletal muscle flaccidity, cold and clammy skin, constricted pupils, and in some cases bradycardia and hypotension. Especially after I.V. injection, apnea, circulatory collapse, cardiac arrest, and death may occur.
• To treat overdose, establish airway, begin assisted or controlled ventilation, and administer naloxone (usually 0.4 to 2.0 mg I.V.) to re-

verse respiratory depression (dose can be repeated in 3 minutes). Do not give naloxone unless patient has clinically significant respiratory or circulatory depression. Give naloxone cautiously to persons with known or suspected physical dependence on hydromorphone; in such cases, abrupt or complete reversal of opioid effects may trigger acute abstinence syndrome.

Special considerations
• High-potency dosing may cause severe hypotension in patients with impaired ability to maintain blood pressure because of such factors as depleted blood volume, certain drugs, or general anesthesia. Drug may cause orthostatic hypotension in ambulatory patients.
• Observe for signs and symptoms of dependence. Patients receiving high-potency form may develop psychic or physical dependence and tolerance after repeated administration. Drug should be prescribed and administered with same degree of caution as that used for morphine.
• Abrupt discontinuation is likely to cause withdrawal syndrome, resulting in anorexia, nausea, fever, headache, sudden severe joint pain, rebound inflammation, fatigue, weakness, lethargy, dizziness, and orthostatic hypotension.

Patient education
• Advise patient not to drink alcohol while using drug.
• Caution patient not to drive or perform other hazardous activities while using drug.
• Instruct patient and family to flush leftover oral liquid and tablets down toilet.
• Caution women to avoid pregnancy and breastfeeding while using drug.

hydroxyurea
Droxia, Hydrea, Mylocel

Classification: Antineoplastic, antimetabolite
Pregnancy risk category D

Pharmacology
Hydroxyurea immediately inhibits DNA synthesis by acting as ribonucleotide reductase inhibitor. It does not interfere with RNA or protein synthesis.

Pharmacokinetics
Drug is well absorbed and is metabolized in liver. It peaks in 2 hours; duration is 24 hours, and half-life is 2 to 5 hours. It is excreted in urine.

How supplied
Capsules: 200 mg, 250 mg, 300 mg, 400 mg, 500 mg
Tablets: 1,000 mg

Indications and dosages

FDA-APPROVED

➡ Melanoma and recurrent, metastatic, or inoperable ovarian carcinoma
Adults: 80 mg/kg P.O. every 3 days or 20 to 30 mg/kg P.O. every day
➡ Local control of primary squamous cell (epidermoid) carcinomas of head and neck, excluding lips
Adults: In combination with radiation therapy, 80 mg/kg P.O. as single dose every 3 days beginning 7 days before start of radiation; then continuing during and after radiation therapy
➡ Resistant, chronic myelocytic leukemia
Adults: 20 to 30 mg/kg P.O. daily

DOSAGE MODIFICATIONS

• Initial dosage may be based on patient's actual or ideal weight, whichever is lower.
• Elderly patients require lower dosages.

Only common or life-threatening adverse reactions are listed.

• Dosage should be adjusted as necessary in patients receiving drug with other myelosuppressants.

• In patients with renal impairment, dosage should be decreased up to 50% for creatinine clearance of 10 to 50 ml/minute, and up to 75% for creatinine clearance below 10 ml/minute.

• If WBC count falls below 2,500/mm^3 or platelet count drops below 100,000/mm^3, interrupt therapy until values rise significantly toward normal. If blood counts are between acceptable and toxic range, do not increase dosage.

• Acceptable ranges include neutrophil count of 2,500 cells/mm^3 or more, platelet count of 95,000/mm^3 or more, reticulocyte count of 95,000/mm^3 or more, and hemoglobin above 5.3 g/dl.

• Toxic ranges include neutrophil count below 2,000 cells/mm^3, platelet count below 80,000/mm^3, hemoglobin below 4.5 g/dl, and reticulocyte count below 80,000/mm^3 if hemoglobin is below 9 g/dl.

• If blood counts are within toxic range, discontinue drug until hematologic recovery occurs. Drug may be resumed after reducing dosage by 2.5 mg/kg daily from dosage linked to hematologic toxicity. Then dosage may be adjusted up or down every 12 weeks in increments of 2.5 mg/kg daily until patient is at stable dosage that does not cause hematologic toxicity for 24 weeks.

• If patient develops hematologic toxicity twice on specific dosage, do not use same dosage again.

WARNINGS

• Drug is genotoxic and a presumed transspecies carcinogen, implying it poses carcinogenic risk to humans. In patients receiving long-term therapy for myeloproliferative disorders, secondary leukemia may occur.

Contraindications and precautions

Contraindicated in hypersensitivity to drug or its components, marked bone marrow depression (WBC count below 2,500/mm^3), thrombocytopenia, platelet count below 100,000/mm^3), severe anemia, and HIV infection.

Use cautiously in pregnancy or breastfeeding and in *elderly patients*. Safety and efficacy in *children* have not been established.

Preparation and administration

≫ Follow hazardous drug guidelines for handling, preparation, and administration. (See "Managing hazardous drugs," page 11.)

• Capsules may be opened and mixed in water.

• Administer prophylactic folic acid as indicated; drug causes macrocytosis, which may mask folic acid deficiency.

• Keep patient hydrated (10 to 12 glasses of water daily).

• Keep container tightly closed and store at 77° F (25° C); excursions are permitted to 59° to 86° F (15° to 30° C).

Adverse reactions

GI: nausea, vomiting, anorexia, constipation, diarrhea
GU: renal toxicity
Hematologic: leukopenia, thrombocytopenia, anemia, megaloblastic erythropoiesis
Other: fever, chills, malaise

Interactions

Drug-drug. *Bone marrow depressants:* increased risk of bone marrow depression
Drug-diagnostic tests. *BUN, creatinine, liver enzymes, uric acid:* increased
Hemoglobin, platelets, RBCs, WBCs: decreased
Drug-herb. *Alpha-lipoic acid, coenzyme Q10:* possible decreased chemotherapy efficacy

Toxicity and overdose

• Overdose signs and symptoms include violet erythema, edema of palms and soles followed by scaling of hands and feet, severe

generalized skin hyperpigmentation, and stomatitis.
• In overdose or toxicity, discontinue therapy and treat symptomatically.

Special considerations

• Closely monitor blood counts and kidney and liver function tests before and during therapy; obtain hemoglobin and total WBC and platelet counts as least once weekly and obtain bone marrow examination as indicated.
• Manage severe anemia with whole blood replacement without stopping hydroxyurea therapy.
• Neutropenia is usually first and most common indicator of hematologic suppression. Thrombocytopenia and anemia occur less often and are rare without preceding leukopenia.

Patient education

• Inform patient about signs and symptoms of bone marrow depression (such as unusual bleeding or bruising) and infection.
• Instruct patient to avoid crowds and exposure to infection.
• Tell patient capsules may be opened and mixed with water.
• Caution patient and caregiver not to expose others to drug. If powder from capsule spills, instruct them to wipe it up immediately with damp, disposable towel and discard towel in closed container (such as plastic bag).
• Advise women with childbearing potential to avoid pregnancy. If patient becomes pregnant while receiving drug, discuss potential fetal hazards and risk of pregnancy loss.
• Caution breastfeeding patient not to breastfeed during therapy.

ibritumomab tiuxetan
In-111 Zevalin, Y-90 Zevalin

Classification: Antineoplastic, monoclonal antibody
Pregnancy risk category D

Pharmacology

Ibritumomab binds to CD20 antigen on malignant B lymphocytes and induces apoptosis. Tiuxetin binds the radionuclides In (indium)-111 or Y (yttrium)-90 and is covalently linked to amino groups of lysines and argines in antibody. Beta emission from Y-9 causes cell damage by stimulating free radical formation in target and neighboring cells.

Pharmacokinetics

Physical half-life is 64 hours; biological half-life (determined by radioactivity detection) is 30 hours. Drug is excreted to slight degree by kidney.

How supplied

Solution for injection: Two kits, each containing one 3-ml glass vial containing 2 ml (3.2 mg) ibritumomab at 1.6 mg/ml in low-metal normal saline solution, one 3-ml glass vial containing 2 ml low-metal 50 mM sodium acetate, one 10-ml glass vial containing 10 ml formulation buffer (PPBS containing 7.5% human serum albumin and 1 mM DTPA), and one empty 10-ml glass vial.

Indications and dosages

FDA-APPROVED

➡ Relapsed or refractory low-grade, follicular, or transformed B-cell non-Hodgkin's lymphoma, including patients with rituximab-refractory follicular non-Hodgkin's lymphoma
Adults: Therapy requires two steps. *Step 1:* Single I.V. infusion of rituximab 250 mg/m², followed by In-111 Zevalin 5.0 mCi (1.6 mg

total antibody dose) I.V. *Step 2:* After 7 to 9 days, second I.V. infusion of rituximab 250 mg/m² given before Y-90 Zevalin 0.4 mCi/kg I.V.

DOSAGE MODIFICATIONS

• Y-90 Zevalin dosage should be reduced to 0.3 mCi/kg (11.1 MBq/kg) in patients with baseline platelet count of 100,000 to 149,000/mm³.

☒ WARNINGS

• Deaths have occurred from infusion reactions within 24 hours of rituximab infusion, with roughly 80% following first infusion. Associated signs and symptoms include hypoxia, pulmonary infiltrate, adult respiratory distress syndrome, myocardial infarction, ventricular fibrillation, and cardiogenic shock. If infusion reaction occurs, discontinue rituximab, In-111 Zevalin, and Y-90 Zevalin, and provide supportive treatment.
• Y-90 Zevalin administration causes severe, prolonged cytopenia in most patients. Do not administer regimen to patients with 25% or greater lymphoma bone marrow involvement or impaired bone marrow function, as seen in previous myeloablative therapy, platelet count below 100,000/mm³, neutrophil count below 1,500/mm³, and hypocellular bone marrow (marked by 15% or less cellularity or marked reduction in bone marrow precursors).
• Do not exceed maximum Y-90 Zevalin dose, which is 32.0 mCi (1184 MBq).
• Do not give Y-90 Zevalin to patients with altered biodistribution, as determined by imaging with In-111 Zevalin.

Contraindications and precautions
Contraindicated in hypersensitivity to drug or its components and anaphylactic reactions to murine proteins.

Use cautiously in pregnancy, breastfeeding, and *elderly patients*. Safety and efficacy in *children* have not been established.

Preparation and administration
• Follow hazardous drug guidelines for handling, preparation, and administration. (See "Managing hazardous drugs," page 11.)
• In-111 Zevalin and Y-90 Zevalin are not available in Zevalin kits. Isotopes must be ordered from separate manufacturers at same time that ibritumomab tiuxetan kits are ordered.
• Do not mix any regimen component with other drugs.
• Administer ibritumomab tiuxetan in a two-step process.
– *Step 1:* Administer rituximab 250 mg/m² I.V. at 50 mg/hour. If hypersensitivity or infusion-related event does not occur, increase infusion rate in 50-mg/hour increments every 30 minutes to maximum of 400 mg/hour. If hypersensitivity or infusion-related event occurs, temporarily slow or stop infusion. Infusion can continue at 50% of previous rate when symptoms improve. Within 4 hours after completing rituximab infusion, give In-111 Zevalin 5.0 mCi I.V. over 10 minutes. Evaluate biodistribution by obtaining whole-body scan at 2 to 24 hours and again 48 to 72 hours after In-111 Zevalin injection. Third image at 90 to 120 hours may be necessary. If biodistribution is unacceptable, do not proceed. If biodistribution is acceptable, 7 to 10 days later proceed with Step 2.
– *Step 2:* Administer rituximab 250 mg/m² I.V. at 50 mg/hour if infusion-related event occurred with first rituximab administration. Increase dosage in 100-mg/hour increments at 30-minute intervals to maximum of 400 mg/hour, as tolerated. Within 4 hours of completing rituximab infusion, administer Y-90 Zevalin I.V. over 10 minutes at a dosage of 0.4 mCi/kg (14.8 MBq/kg) actual body weight for patients with platelet count above 150,000/mm³, and 0.3 mCi/kg (11.1 MBq/kg) actual body weight for patients with platelet count of 100,000 to 149,000/mm³.
• Observe for signs and symptoms of severe infusion reaction, such as hypotension, angio-

edema, hypoxia, and bronchospasm, which may require administration interruption.
• Take precautions to avoid extravasation, and observe closely for signs of extravasation during infusion. If extravasation occurs, stop infusion immediately and restart in another vein.
• Drug is given as one-time only regimen.
• Store at 36° to 46° F (2° to 8° C). Do not freeze.

Adverse reactions
CNS: dizziness
EENT: rhinitis
GI: nausea, vomiting, diarrhea, abdominal pain
Hematologic: thrombocytopenia, neutropenia, anemia, hemorrhage
Respiratory: apnea, bronchospasm, cough
Skin: rash, pruritus, urticaria
Other: asthenia chills, infection, fever

Interactions
Drug-drug. *Anticoagulants, drugs that impede platelet function:* increased risk of prolonged, severe thrombocytopenia
Bone marrow depressants: increased risk of bone marrow depression
Drug-diagnostic tests. *Hematocrit, hemoglobin, platelets, WBCs:* severely decreased

Toxicity and overdose
• In clinical trials, Y-90 Zevalin doses as high as 0.52 mCi/kg (19.2 MBq/kg) caused severe hematologic toxicities.
• Some patients require autologous stem cell support to manage hematologic toxicity.

Special considerations
• Monitor for thrombocytopenia and neutropenia. Median time to nadir is 7 to 9 weeks; median cytopenia duration is 22 to 35 days.
• Monitor CBC and platelet count weekly after regimen ends, and continue until levels recover. Continue monitoring for cytopenias for up to 3 months after therapy ends.

• Whole-body scans should be whole-body planar view anterior and posterior gamma images. If third image is needed, use large field-of-view gamma camera with medium energy collimator.
• Although solid-organ toxicity has not been directly attributed to radiation from adjacent tumors, consider this potential carefully before treating patients with very high tumor uptake next to critical organs or structures.
• Regimen results in significant radiation dose to testes. Radiation dose to ovaries has not been established.
• Drug contains human albumin, posing remote risk of viral disease transmission (including theoretical risk of contracting Creutzfeldt-Jakob disease).

Patient education
• Inform patient that drug is administered in two visits 7 to 9 days apart.
• Advise patient of signs and symptoms of bone marrow depression (such as unusual bleeding or bruising) and infection.
• Tell patient to avoid crowds and exposure to infection.
• Inform patient that side effects can occur up to 3 months after therapy ends.
• Advise patient to use effective contraception during treatment and for up to 12 months afterward.
• Caution women with childbearing potential not to become pregnant during therapy because drug may harm fetus and cause pregnancy loss.
• Advise breastfeeding patient not to breastfeed during therapy.

idarubicin hydrochloride
Idamycin PFS

Classification: Antineoplastic, anthracycline antitumor antibiotic
Pregnancy risk category D

Pharmacology
Idarubicin inhibits nucleic acid synthesis and interacts with enzyme topoisomerase II. These effects disrupt RNA and DNA, resulting in cell death. Because of its high lipophilicity, drug has greater rate of cellular uptake than other anthracyclines.

Pharmacokinetics
Drug is widely distributed in blood and bone marrow. Onset is immediate, and drug peaks within a few minutes. Estimated half-life is 4 to 22 hours. Drug is eliminated mainly by biliary tract and to much lesser degree by kidney.

How supplied
Powder for infusion: 5-, 10-, and 20-mg vials

Indications and dosages

FDA-approved

➡ Acute myeloid leukemia in adults
Adults: Initially, 12 mg/m^2 daily by slow I.V. injection over 10 to 15 minutes for 3 days in combination with cytarabine. Cytarabine may be given as 100 mg/m^2 continuous I.V. infusion daily for 7 days, or as 25 mg/m^2 I.V. bolus followed by cytarabine 200 mg/m^2 by continuous I.V. infusion daily for 5 days. Repeat once, depending on initial response.

Off-label uses (selected)

➡ Acute lymphocytic leukemia
Adults: Variable dosing
➡ Advanced breast cancer
Adults: Variable dosing, including 8 mg/m^2 I.V. daily for 5 days, repeated every 3 weeks;

or 12 mg/m^2 I.V. daily for 3 days, repeated every 3 weeks

Dosage modifications

• For patients with hepatic impairment and bilirubin level of 2.6 to 5 mg/dl, dosage should be reduced by 50%. If bilirubin level is below 5 mg/dl, drug should not be given.
• Drug should not be given if bilirubin level exceeds 5 mg/dl.
• For patients with renal impairment and serum creatinine level below 2.5 mg/dl, dosage decrease should be considered.
• Drug should not be given if bilirubin level exceeds 5 mg/dl.
• If second course of therapy is indicated, course should be delayed in patients who experienced severe mucositis after first course, until recovery occurs; then dosage should be reduced by 25%.

WARNINGS

• Drug should be given I.V. slowly—never I.M. or subcutaneously. Severe local tissue necrosis can result from extravasation.
• Drug can cause myocardial toxicity, leading to heart failure. This is more common in patients who have received previous anthracyclines or who had preexisting cardiac disease.
• Severe bone marrow depression can occur when drug is used at effective, therapeutic doses.
• Dosage should be reduced in patients with impaired hepatic or renal function.

Contraindications and precautions
No known contraindications exist.
   Use cautiously in bone marrow depression, renal or hepatic impairment, preexisting cardiac disease, previous therapy with anthracyclines at high cumulative doses, previous therapy with other potentially cardiotoxic drugs, pregnancy or breastfeeding, and in *elderly patients*. Safety and efficacy in *children* have not been established.

Preparation and administration

- Follow hazardous drug guidelines for handling, preparation, and administration. (See "Managing hazardous drugs," page 11.)
- Monitor serum bilirubin and creatinine levels closely before and during therapy.
- Maximum lifetime dose is 150 mg/m^2.
- Reconstitute 20-mg powder vials with 20 ml sterile water for injection to yield final concentration of 1 mg/ml.
- Administer I.V. slowly over 10 to 15 minutes into tubing of free-running I.V. infusion of normal saline solution injection or D$_5$W injection.
- Do not mix with other drugs. Precipitation occurs with heparin.
- If extravasation occurs, place ice packs over area for 30 minutes immediately and then for 30 minutes four times daily for 3 days. Elevate affected extremity. For ulceration or severe persistent pain at extravasation site, consider early wide excision of involved area.
- Reconstituted solutions are physically and chemically stable for 72 hours when refrigerated at 36° to 46° F (2° to 8° C) or at controlled room temperature of 59° to 86° F (15° to 30°C). Discard unused solution.
- Store in carton under refrigeration (36° to 46° F) protected from light.

Adverse reactions

CNS: headache
CV: arrhythmias, heart failure, cardiomyopathy
GI: nausea, vomiting, abdominal cramping, diarrhea, mucositis
Hematologic: leukopenia, anemia, thrombocytopenia
Skin: alopecia (usually partial), rash

Interactions

Drug-drug. *Alkaline solutions, heparin:* I.V. incompatibility
Antigout drugs: decreased antigout efficacy
Bone marrow depressants: increased risk of bone marrow depression
Trastuzumab: increased cardiotoxicity risk

Drug-diagnostic tests. *ALP, ALT, AST, bilirubin, uric acid:* increased
ECG: changes including arrhythmias, bundle-branch block, and depressed T waves
Drug-herb. *Alpha-lipoic acid, coenzyme Q10:* possible decreased chemotherapy efficacy

Toxicity and overdose

- Overdose effects are severe and prolonged and include bone marrow depression, increased GI toxicity, and possible arrhythmia.
- Provide supportive care, including platelet transfusion, antibiotics, and symptomatic treatment of mucositis. Conventional peritoneal or hemodialysis is unlikely to be effective. No known antidote exists.

Special considerations

- Drug may induce hyperuricemia. Take appropriate steps to prevent hyperuricemia and control systemic infections before starting therapy.
- Monitor patient closely for severe bone marrow depression, which occurs in all patients receiving drug—typically within 10 to 15 days of initial dose. Obtain frequent CBC and platelets counts.
- Monitor patient for cardiotoxicity (including arrhythmia, heart failure, and cardiomyopathy), and treat appropriately. Cardiotoxicity is usually associated with left ventricular ejection fraction decreased from pretreatment baseline values. Myocardial toxicity risk may be higher with concomitant or previous radiation to mediastinal-pericardial area or in patients with anemia, bone marrow depression, infection, leukemic pericarditis, or myocarditis.

Patient education

- Instruct patient about signs and symptoms of bone marrow depression (such as unusual bleeding or bruising) and infection.
- Advise patient to avoid crowds and exposure to infection.
- Inform patient that complete alopecia is likely to occur but is reversible. New hair

Only common or life-threatening adverse reactions are listed.

growth typically resumes 2 to 3 months after last dose and may differ in color or texture.

• Instruct patient to practice fastidious oral hygiene.

• Inform patient that drug may turn urine pink or red.

• Caution women with childbearing potential to avoid pregnancy. If patient becomes pregnant while receiving drug, discuss potential hazards to fetus and risk of pregnancy loss.

• Advise breastfeeding patient not to breast-feed during therapy.

ifosfamide
Ifex, Ifex/Mesnex

Classification: Antineoplastic, alkylating agent
Pregnancy risk category D

Pharmacology

Ifosfamide, a synthetic cyclophosphamide analogue, is chemically related to nitrogen mustards. It is activated by hepatic enzymes, causing production of alkylated metabolites that interact with DNA to form crosslinks, thus breaking DNA chain and preventing cell synthesis. Urinary metabolites are not cytotoxic.

Pharmacokinetics

Drug is metabolized in liver. Onset occurs at end of infusion. Drug peaks in 1 to 6 hours. Elimination half-life is 7 to 15 hours. Drug is excreted in urine.

How supplied

Powder for injection: 1 g, 3 g

Indications and dosages

FDA-approved

➥ Second-line chemotherapy for germ-cell testicular cancer
Adults: 1.2 g/m^2 I.V. infusion daily for 5 con-

secutive days; repeated every 3 weeks or after recovery from hematologic toxicity (platelet count at or above 100,000/mm^3 and WBC count at or above 4,000/mm^3); typically in combination with vinblastine and cisplatin and administered with mesna or other prophylactic agent for hemorrhagic cystitis

Off-label uses (selected)

➥ Ewing's and soft-tissue sarcoma
Adults: As part of MAID protocol (mesna, Adriamycin, ifosfamide, and dacarbazine), 2,500 mg/m^2 I.V. infusion daily over 24 hours for 3 days (with mesna at same dosage); on day 4, give mesna only.

➥ Hodgkin's and non-Hodgkin's lymphoma
Adults: As part of MIME protocol (mesna or mitoguazon, ifosfamide, methotrexate, and etoposide), 1 g/m^2 I.V. infusion daily on days 1 through 5, with cycle repeated every 3 weeks for up to 1 year

➥ Non-small-cell lung cancer
Adults: In combination with carboplatin, 1,500 mg/m^2 I.V. infusion on days 1, 3, and 5, with cycle repeated every 28 days until progression or for maximum of six courses

➥ Head and neck carcinoma; breast, cervical, endometrial, or ovarian epithelial and germ-cell carcinoma; neuroblastoma; osteosarcoma; acute lymphocytic lymphoma; bladder carcinoma; relapsed or refractory thymoma and thymic carcinoma
Adults: Various dosing schedules

Dosage modifications

• Dosage may need to be adjusted if drug is used in combination with other myelosuppressants.

• Drug has been given to patients with compromised hepatic and renal function, although optimal dosing schedules have not been determined.

⊠ WARNINGS

• If patient experiences urotoxic adverse effects (particularly hemorrhagic cystitis) or

CNS toxicities (such as confusion and coma), therapy may need to be discontinued.
- Severe bone marrow depression may occur.
- Patients previously treated with cisplatin are at increased risk for nephrotoxicity.

Contraindications and precautions

Contraindicated in hypersensitivity to drug or its components, bone marrow depression, and pregnancy or breastfeeding.

Use cautiously in renal impairment, leukopenia, granulocytopenia, extensive bone marrow metastases, or previous therapy with radiation or other cytotoxic agents. Safety and efficacy in *children* have not been established.

Preparation and administration

- Follow hazardous drug guidelines for handling, preparation, and administration. (See "Managing hazardous drugs," page 11.)
- For 5-day regimen, obtain urinalysis before each dose and regularly throughout therapy. If results show microscopic hematuria with more than 10 RBCs/high-power field, withhold therapy until hematuria resolves.
- Obtain hemoglobin level and WBC and platelet counts before each dose and at appropriate intervals. Unless clinically essential, do not give drug to patients with WBC count below 2,000/mm^3 or platelet count below 50,000/mm^3.
- To prevent bladder toxicity, hydrate patient with at least 2 L of oral or I.V. fluid daily.
- Administer uroprotectant such as mesna to prevent hemorrhagic cystitis. Typically, mesna is given at same time as ifosfamide. Initial mesna dosage is 20% of ifosfamide dosage. Then, give two additional mesna doses at 40% of initial ifosfamide dosage 2 hours and 6 hours after initial ifosfamide dose.
- Reconstitute by adding 20 ml sterile water for injection or bacteriostatic water for injection to 1-g vial (or 60 ml to 3-g vial) to yield final concentration of 50 mg/ml.
- Solution may be diluted further to achieve concentration of 0.6 to 20 mg/ml in D$_5$W in-

jection, normal saline solution injection, Lactated ringer's injection, or sterile water for injection.
- Administer as slow I.V. infusion over at least 30 minutes.
- Refrigerate reconstituted solution or admixture and use within 24 hours.
- Admixtures are stable for at least 1 week at 86° F (30° C) or 6 weeks at 41° F (5° C).

Adverse reactions

CNS: somnolence, confusion, coma, seizures, hallucinations, psychosis
GI: nausea, vomiting
GU: hemorrhagic cystitis, hematuria, nephrotoxicity, urinary frequency
Hematologic: bone marrow depression, leukopenia, thrombocytopenia
Metabolic: metabolic acidosis
Skin: alopecia

Interactions

Drug-drug. *Aprepitant:* possible increase in ifosfamide plasma concentration
Other bone marrow suppressants: increased bone marrow depression
Phenytoin, phenobarbital: increased ifosfamide effects
Warfarin: increased bleeding risk
Drug-diagnostic tests. *ALT, AST, bilirubin, BUN, creatinine, lactate dehydrogenase, uric acid:* increased
Hematocrit, hemoglobin, platelets, WBCs: decreased
Drug-herb. *Alpha-lipoic acid, coenzyme Q10:* possible decreased chemotherapy efficacy

Toxicity and overdose

- Toxicity signs and symptoms include bone marrow depression, nausea, vomiting, and hemorrhagic cystitis.
- No known antidote exists. In suspected overdose, provide supportive measures.

Special considerations

- Drug may cause somnolence, confusion, hallucinations and, in some cases, coma. Dis-

---

Only common or life-threatening adverse reactions are listed.

continue therapy if these occur.
- Hematuria incidence and severity can be significantly reduced through vigorous hydration, fractionated dosing schedule, and use of protector (such as mesna).
- Drug may interfere with normal wound healing.
- In patients on warfarin, monitor prothrombin time and INR closely for 3 to 4 days during initiation and withdrawal of therapy.

Patient education
- Advise patient that nausea, vomiting, and other side effects may occur and to report these symptoms promptly if they persist.
- Teach patient about signs and symptoms of bone marrow depression (such as unusual bleeding or bruising) and infection.
- Advise patient to drink at least 2 L of fluid daily during therapy and for 3 days thereafter.
- Tell patient who is not receiving mesna to stay alert for signs and symptoms of hemorrhagic cystitis.
- Instruct patient to avoid crowds and exposure to infection.
- Urge both men and women to use effective contraception while taking drug.
- If patient becomes pregnant while receiving drug, discuss potential hazards to fetus and risk of pregnancy loss.
- Caution breastfeeding patient not to breastfeed during therapy.

imatinib mesylate
Gleevec

Classification: Antineoplastic, signal transduction inhibitor
Pregnancy risk category D

Pharmacology
Imatinib mesylate inhibits Bcr-Abl tyrosine kinase, an abnormal tyrosine kinase created by Philadelphia chromosome abnormality in chronic myeloid leukemia (CML). Drug inhibits proliferation, induces apoptosis, and inhibits tumor growth in Bcr-Abl–positive cell lines and fresh leukemic cells in Philadelphia chromosome–positive (Ph+) CML.

Pharmacokinetics
Drug is metabolized in liver and peaks in 3 hours. Elimination half-life is 18 hours. It is excreted primarily in feces.

How supplied
Capsules: 100 mg
Tablets: 100 mg, 400 mg

Indications and dosages

FDA-APPROVED

➲ Initial treatment of Ph+ CML in chronic phase
Adults: 400 to 600 mg P.O. daily
➥ Ph+ CML in blast crisis, accelerated phase, or chronic phase after failure of interferon alfa therapy
Adults: For chronic phase, 400 mg P.O. daily; for blast crisis or accelerated phase, 600 mg P.O. daily
➥ Kit (CD117)-positive, unresectable or metastatic malignant GI stromal tumor (GIST)
Adults: 400 to 600 mg P.O. daily
➥ Recurrent Ph+ CML in chronic phase after stem cell transplant, or patients resistant to interferon alfa therapy
Children older than age 3: 260 mg/m^2 P.O. daily (tablets only)

OFF-LABEL USES (SELECTED)

➥ Acute lymphocytic leukemia, glioma, refractory prostate cancer, small-cell lung cancer, soft-tissue sarcoma
Adults: Various dosing schedules

DOSAGE MODIFICATIONS

- Dosage increase from 400 to 600 mg may be considered in patients with chronic-phase CML, or from 600 to 800 mg (400 mg twice daily) in adults in accelerated phase or blast crisis. The following conditions apply to this decision: no severe adverse reactions or severe non-leukemia-related neutropenia or thrombocytopenia, no disease progression, failure to achieve satisfactory hematologic response after at least 3 months of treatment, failure to achieve cytogenetic response after 6 to 12 months, or loss of previously achieved hematologic or cytogenetic response.

• For children with chronic-phase CML, increased daily dosages may be considered (under circumstances similar to those for adults in chronic phase) from 260 to 340 mg/m^2 daily, as clinically indicated.

• Increase dosage by at least 50% in patients receiving drug with potent CYP3A4 inducer (such as rifampin or phenytoin).

• For adults, if elevation in bilirubin level is above 3 × institutional upper limit of normal (IULN) or liver transaminase levels are above 5 × IULN, withhold drug until bilirubin level drops below 1.5 × IULN and transaminase levels drop below 2.5 × IULN; thereafter, continue at reduced daily dosage. For children, daily dosages of tablets can be reduced from 260 to 200 mg/m^2 daily or from 340 to 260 mg/m^2 daily if bilirubin level is above 3 × IULN or liver transaminase levels exceed 5 × IULN.

• Reduce dosage or interrupt therapy in patients with severe neutropenia and thrombocytopenia, according to the following recommendations:

– *Chronic-phase CML (starting dosage of 400 mg) or GIST (starting dosage of either 400 or 600 mg):* Absolute neutrophil count (ANC) below 1.0 × 10^9/L and/or platelet count below 50 × 10^9/L

1. Stop drug until ANC is at or above 1.5 × 10^9/L and platelets are at or above 75 × 10^9/L.

2. Resume drug at original starting dosage of 400 or 600 mg (260 mg/m^2 in children).

3. If ANC recurrence is below 1 × 10^9/L and/or platelets are below 50 × 10^9/L, repeat step 1 and resume drug at reduced dosage (300 mg [200 mg/m^2 in children]

if starting dosage was 400 mg [260 mg/m^2 in children], 400 mg if starting dosage was 600 mg).

– *Accelerated-phase CML and blast crisis (starting dosage of 600 mg):* ANC below 0.5 × 10^9/L and/or platelets above 10 × 10^9/L (after at least 1 month of therapy)

1. Determine if cytopenia is related to leukemia (perform marrow aspirate or biopsy).

2. If cytopenia is unrelated to leukemia, reduce dosage to 400 mg.

3. If cytopenia persists for 2 weeks, reduce dosage further to 300 mg.

4. If cytopenia persists for 4 weeks and is still unrelated to leukemia, stop drug until ANC reaches or exceeds 1 × 10^9/L and platelets reach or exceed 20 × 10^9/L; then resume therapy at 300 mg.

• If patient experiences severe nonhematologic adverse reactions (such as severe hepatotoxicity or fluid retention), withhold drug until event resolves. Then resume as appropriate, depending on initial severity of event.

Contraindications and precautions

Contraindicated in hypersensitivity to drug or its components.

Use cautiously in patients with hepatic or renal impairment and in pregnancy or breastfeeding. Edema risk increases in *elderly patients*. Safety and efficacy in *children younger than age 3* have not been established.

Preparation and administration

• Follow hazardous drug guidelines for handling, preparation, and administration. (See "Managing hazardous drugs," page 11.)

• Monitor liver function (transaminases, bilirubin, and ALP) before therapy begins and then monthly, or as clinically indicated.

• Administer with meal and large glass of water.

• In adults, give daily doses above 600 mg in two divided doses. In children, give daily doses above 400 mg in two divided doses (one in morning and one in evening).

Only common or life-threatening adverse reactions are listed.

• For patient unable to swallow film-coated tablets, mix tablets in glass of water or apple juice and give immediately after tablets have disintegrated completely.
• Store at 77° F (25° C); excursions are permitted to 59° to 86° F (15° to 30° C). Protect from moisture.

Adverse reactions

CNS: headache, fatigue, weakness, cerebral hemorrhage
CV: fluid retention (in periorbital area or lower extremities)
GI: anorexia, nausea, diarrhea, vomiting, abdominal pain, dyspepsia, GI hemorrhage
Hematologic: neutropenia, thrombocytopenia, anemia
Metabolic: hypokalemia
Musculoskeletal: musculoskeletal pain, muscle cramps, arthralgia
Respiratory: cough, dyspnea, pneumonia, pleural effusion, pulmonary edema, pericardial effusion
Skin: rash, petechiae, photosensitivity reaction
Other: night sweats, fever, ascites

Interactions

Drug-drug. *CYP3A4 inducers (such as carbamazepine, dexamethasone, phenytoin, rifampin):* decreased imatinib plasma concentration
CYP3A4 inhibitors (such as clarithromycin, erythromycin, itraconazole, ketoconazole): increased imatinib plasma concentration
CYP3A4-metabolized drugs (such as calcium channel blockers, dihydropyridine, certain HMG-CoA reductase inhibitors, triazolobenzodiazepines): increased plasma concentration of these drugs
CYP3A4 substrates with narrow therapeutic window (such as cyclosporine, pimozide): potentially altered therapeutic effect of these drugs
Drug-diagnostic tests. *Bilirubin, transaminases:* possible increases
Platelets, potassium, WBCs: possible decreases

Drug-herb. *Alpha-lipoic acid, coenzyme Q10:* possible decreased chemotherapy efficacy
St. John's wort: decreased imatinib plasma concentration

Toxicity and overdose

• Experience with dosages above 800 mg is limited. Anticipated toxicity symptoms are drug-related adverse reactions, such as nausea, vomiting, diarrhea, fluid retention, and muscle cramps.
• If overdose occurs, provide supportive treatment.

Special considerations

• Obtain CBC weekly for first month, biweekly for second month, and periodically thereafter as clinically indicated.
• Cytopenia occurs more often in patients with accelerated-phase CML or blast crisis than in those with chronic-phase CML.
• Do not give warfarin; it is metabolized by CYP2C9 and CYP3A4. Patients requiring anticoagulation should receive low-molecular-weight or standard heparin.
• Closely monitor patient receiving drug concomitantly with potent CYP3A4 inducers.
• Weigh patient regularly and monitor for signs and symptoms of fluid retention, which may be severe. Higher doses increase edema risk.
• Monitor patient for GI bleeding.
• Drug may cause liver and kidney toxicities and increased rate of opportunistic infections.
• Patients taking total daily dosage of 1,200 mg may have increased iron levels and require treatment to lower iron exposure.

Patient education

• Instruct patient to take drug with food and large glass of water.
• Advise patient to check weight daily and to report swelling or rapid weight gain promptly.
• Inform patient about signs and symptoms of bone marrow depression (such as unusual bleeding or bruising) and infection.

- Instruct patient to avoid prolonged exposure to sunlight and to use sunscreen and wear protective clothing when outdoors because drug may cause photosensitivity.
- Instruct patient to avoid crowds and exposure to infection.
- Caution women with childbearing potential to use effective contraception. If patient becomes pregnant while receiving drug, discuss potential hazards to fetus and risk of pregnancy loss.
- Advise breastfeeding patient not to breastfeed during therapy.

interferon alfa-2a, recombinant (IFLrA, rIFN-A)
Roferon-A

Classification: Antineoplastic, antiviral, immunomodulator, biological response modifier (recombinant DNA origin)
Pregnancy risk category C

Pharmacology
Recombinant interferon alfa-2a exerts direct antiproliferative action against tumor cells by inhibiting virus replication and modulating host immune response. Mechanism for antitumor and antiviral activity is poorly understood.

Pharmacokinetics
Drug is metabolized in liver and kidney. Levels peak in 3 to 12 hours. Drug is excreted through glomeruli and undergoes rapid proteolytic degradation during tubular reabsorption, causing negligible reappearance of intact drug in systemic circulation.

How supplied
Solution (single-use prefilled syringes): 3 million, 6 million, and 9 million international units

Indications and dosages

FDA-APPROVED

➡ Hairy cell leukemia
Adults: For induction, 3 million international units subcutaneously daily for 16 to 24 weeks. For maintenance, 3 million international units I.M. or subcutaneously three times weekly. Dosages above 3 million international units are not recommended.
➡ Chronic myelogenous leukemia (CML, Philadelphia-chromosome positive)
Adults: Initially, 9 million international units subcutaneously daily. Short-term tolerance may improve by gradually increasing dosage over first week from 3 million international units daily for 3 days to 6 million international units daily for 3 days, to target dosage of 9 million international units daily for duration of therapy.
Children: 2.5 to 5 million international units/m^2 subcutaneously daily

OFF-LABEL USES (SELECTED)

➡ Renal-cell carcinoma
Adults: Usually 9 million international units with 12 million international units interleukin-2 subcutaneously on days 1 to 4 during weeks 1 to 4. Repeat cycle every 6 weeks.
➡ Carcinoid tumors
Adults: One dosage schedule is 3 to 6 million international units subcutaneously three times weekly.
➡ Cutaneous T-cell lymphoma
Adults: Initial dosage usually is escalated to 18 million international units subcutaneously daily for a total of 12 weeks. *Recommended escalation schedule*—On days 1 to 3, 3 million international units daily; on days 4 to 6, 9 million international units daily; on days 7 to 10, 18 million international units daily. For maintenance, give drug subcutaneously three times weekly at maximum dosage acceptable to patient, but not exceeding 18 million international units.
➡ Non-Hodgkin's lymphoma (low and intermediate grades)

Only common or life-threatening adverse reactions are listed.

Adults: For typical monotherapy induction regimen, give up to 6 million international units subcutaneously daily. For typical combination regimen, give up to 6 million international units subcutaneously three times weekly. For maintenance, 3 million international units subcutaneously three times weekly may be appropriate.

DOSAGE MODIFICATIONS

• If severe reactions occur in patients with Kaposi's sarcoma or hairy cell leukemia, dosage should be reduced by 50% or drug stopped temporarily until reactions abate.

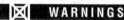 **WARNINGS**

• Depression and suicidal behavior have occurred in some patients. Monitor patient's neuropsychiatric status closely.

Contraindications and precautions

Contraindicated in hypersensitivity to drug or its components and in benzyl alcohol allergy.

Use cautiously in myelosuppression; concurrent use of potentially myelosuppressive drugs; immunosuppression; neurotoxic, hematotoxic, or cardiotoxic effects of previous or concurrent drugs; severe preexisting cardiac disease; severe renal or hepatic disease; diabetes mellitus; seizure disorders; compromised CNS function; mental depression; cardiac disease or history of cardiac disease; GI bleeding; pregnancy; and breastfeeding. Drug should not be given to patients with preexisting thyroid abnormalities whose thyroid function cannot be maintained in normal range by drugs; patients with visceral AIDS-related Kaposi's sarcoma associated with rapidly progressive or life-threatening disease; autoimmune hepatitis or a history of autoimmune disease; or immunosuppressed transplant recipients. When reconstituted with diluent provided, powder for injection contains benzyl alcohol and is not indicated for infants. Except in

CML treatment, safety and efficacy in *children younger than age 18* have not been established.

Preparation and administration

• Follow hazardous drug guidelines for handling, preparation, and administration. (See "Managing hazardous drugs," page 11.)
• Ensure that patient is well hydrated (especially during initial treatment) to reduce risk of hypotension associated with fluid depletion.
• Drug is indicated for subcutaneous use only. (Many forms of this drug have been discontinued.)
• Avoid using different brands in single-treatment regimen; dosage and adverse reactions vary.
• Swirl vial gently to dissolve drug.
• Store prefilled syringes at 36° to 46° F (2° to 8° C). Do not freeze or shake.

Adverse reactions

CNS: depression, dizziness, decreased mental status, confusion, paresthesia, seizures, headache, fatigue, suicidal ideation
CV: hypotension
GI: taste changes, anorexia, nausea, vomiting
GU: erectile dysfunction
Hematologic: neutropenia, thrombocytopenia, leukopenia, anemia
Hepatic: hepatotoxicity
Musculoskeletal: myalgia
Skin: rash, dry skin, pruritus, alopecia
Other: flulike syndrome, chills, fever, weight loss, edema

Interactions

Drug-drug. *Cardiotoxic, hematotoxic, and neurotoxic drugs:* increased effects of these drugs
Centrally acting drugs: possible additive adverse effects
Drugs metabolized by CYP450: possible change in oxidative metabolism of these drugs
Interleukin-2: increased risk of renal failure
Myelosuppressants: additive myelosuppression
Theophylline: reduced theophylline clearance

Drug-diagnostic tests. *ALP, ALT, AST, bilirubin, BUN, calcium, creatinine, fasting glucose, INR, lactate dehydrogenase, neutralizing antibodies, phosphate, uric acid, hemoglobin, platelets, prothrombin time, partial thromboplastin time, WBCs:* altered

Toxicity and overdose
• No overdose cases have been reported. However, repeated large doses may be associated with profound lethargy, fatigue, prostration, and coma.
• If severe reactions occur, reduce dosage or stop drug and begin appropriate corrective measures. Reinstitute drug cautiously, considering patient's further need. Be alert for toxicity recurrence.

Special considerations
• Monitor standard hematologic tests (including CBC with differential, hemoglobin, and platelets), blood chemistries, hairy cells, and bone marrow hairy cells at baseline and periodically during therapy.
• In patients with Kaposi's sarcoma, obtain indicator lesion measurements and total lesion count at baseline and then monthly.
• Monitor patient closely for depression; consider stopping drug if it occurs. Although dosage reduction or drug withdrawal may resolve depressive symptoms, depression may persist (suicides have occurred after withdrawal).
• Monitor periodic liver function tests.
• Monitor ECG before and during therapy in patients with advanced cancer or preexisting cardiac disease.
• Interferon-alphas have been associated with serious or fatal GI hemorrhage.

Patient education
• Instruct patient to drink plenty of fluids, especially during initial stages of therapy.
• Advise patient to seek medical attention at once if depression or suicidal thoughts occur.
• Caution patient to avoid activities requiring mental alertness until drug effects are known.
• Urge patient to report unusual bruising or

bleeding, chest pain, respiratory difficulty, swelling of extremities, unusual weight gain, or other unusual symptoms.
• If patient will be using drug at home, provide appropriate instructions, including review of Patient Information Sheet, proper administration, importance of not changing brands without medical consultation, importance of never reusing syringes and needles, use of puncture-resistant container for discarding used syringes and needles, and proper container disposal.
• Caution women with childbearing potential not to take drug unless they use effective contraception.
• Provide guidance to breastfeeding patient to help her decide whether to discontinue breastfeeding or stop drug.

interferon alfa-2b, recombinant (IFN-alfa 2)
Intron A

Classification: Antineoplastic, antiviral, immunomodulator, biological response modifier (recombinant DNA origin)
Pregnancy risk category C

Pharmacology
Recombinant interferon alfa-2b exerts cellular activity by binding to specific cell-surface membrane receptors. This action suppresses cell proliferation, enhances macrophagic phagocytic activity, augments specific cytotoxicity of lymphocytes for target cells, and inhibits virus replication in virus-infected cells.

Pharmacokinetics
With I.V. use, drug levels peak in 15 to 60 minutes, with undetectable concentrations 4 hours after administration; elimination half-life is roughly 2 hours. With I.M. and subcutaneous use, elimination half-life is about 2 to 3 hours.

Only common or life-threatening adverse reactions are listed.

How supplied

Powder for injection (with diluent): 10 million, 18 million, and 50 million international units/vial
Solution for injection (multidose pens): 18 million, 30 million, and 60 million international units
Solution for injection (vials): 3 million international units/0.5 ml, 5 million international units/0.5 ml, and 10 million international units/1 ml

Indications and dosages

⊜ Hairy cell leukemia
Adults: 2 million international units/m^2 I.M. or subcutaneously three times weekly for up to 6 months. Responding patients may benefit from continued treatment.

⊜ Adjuvant to surgical treatment for malignant melanoma in patients who are free of disease but at increased risk of systemic recurrence within 56 days of treatment
Adults: 20 million international units/m^2 by I.V. infusion over 20 minutes for 5 consecutive days per week for 4 weeks, followed by maintenance dosage of 10 million international units/m^2 subcutaneously three times weekly for 48 weeks

⊜ Clinically aggressive follicular non-Hodgkin's lymphoma
Adults: 5 million international units subcutaneously three times weekly for up to 18 months with anthracycline-containing chemotherapy regimen

⊜ AIDS-related Kaposi's sarcoma
Adults: 30 million international units/m^2 subcutaneously or I.M three times weekly until severe intolerance or maximum response has occurred after 16 weeks of therapy. (For this indication, only 50-million international units strength should be used.)

➥ Renal-cell carcinoma
Adults: One dosage regimen included 5 million international units/m^2 subcutaneously on day 1 of therapy. For typical induction therapy before day 1, 1.25 million international units/m^2 3 days before, 2.5 million international units/m^2 2 days before, and 3.75 million international units/m^2 on day before treatment; then 5 million international units/ m^2 subcutaneously each Monday, Wednesday, and Friday until tumor progresses.

➥ Chronic myelogenous leukemia
Adults: One dosage schedule is 4 to 5 million international units/m^2 subcutaneously daily. When WBC count is controlled, dosage may be given three times weekly. Adjust dosage according to tolerance. Maintain this regimen unless disease progresses rapidly or severe intolerance occurs.

➥ Follicular non-Hodgkin's lymphoma
Adults: One dosage schedule is 5 million international units subcutaneously three times weekly (every other day).

• *For patients with hairy cell leukemia:* If severe adverse reactions develop, interrupt therapy until reactions abate; then restart therapy at 50% of initial dosage. Discontinue drug permanently if severe adverse reactions continue or recur after dosage adjustment, if disease progresses, or if patient fails to respond after 6 months.

• *For patients with malignant melanoma:* Discontinue drug temporarily if granulocyte count falls below 500/mm^3 or if ALT or AST level rises above 5 to 10 × ULN. When adverse reactions abate, restart at 50% of previous dosage. Withdraw permanently if toxicity persists after temporary withdrawal, severe adverse effects recur after dosage decrease, granulocyte count drops below 250/mm^3, or ALT or AST level rises to 10 × ULN.

• *For patients with follicular lymphoma:* Modify regimen for evidence of serious toxicity. Delay chemotherapy regimen if neutrophil count is below 1,500/mm^3 or platelet count is below 75,000/mm^3. Interrupt therapy temporarily if neutrophil count is below 1,000/mm^3 or

---

⊜ Orphan drug   ≫ Potentially carcinogenic

platelet count is below 50,000/mm³; reduce dosage by 50% to 2.5 million international units three times weekly if neutrophil count is above 1,000/mm³ but below 1,500/mm³. Stop therapy permanently if AST level exceeds 5 × ULN or serum creatinine level exceeds 2 mg/dl.
• *For patients with AIDS-related Kaposi's sarcoma:* Maintain selected dosage regimen unless disease progresses rapidly or severe intolerance occurs. For severe adverse reactions, decrease dosage by 50% or stop drug temporarily until adverse reactions abate. Discontinue drug permanently if adverse effects persist, or if they recur after dosage decrease.

⊠ WARNINGS

• Drug can cause or aggravate fatal or life-threatening neuropsychiatric, autoimmune, ischemic, and infectious disorders. Patients should be monitored closely through periodic clinical and laboratory evaluations. Therapy should be withdrawn if patient experiences persistently severe or worsening signs or symptoms of these conditions (which often resolve after discontinuation).

Contraindications and precautions

Contraindicated in hypersensitivity to drug or its components and in combination with ribavirin in pregnant women, males with pregnant female partners, and patients with autoimmune hepatitis.

Use cautiously and select carefully among various drug forms and strengths in debilitating medical conditions; platelet count below 50,000/mm³ (I.M. injection); history of cardiovascular disease; preexisting psychiatric conditions (especially depression); preexisting psoriasis and sarcoidosis; abnormal hepatic function; diabetes mellitus; pulmonary infiltrates or impaired pulmonary function; bone marrow depression; autoimmune disease; coagulation disorders; ophthalmologic conditions; elevated triglyceride levels; concurrent

narcotic or sedative-hypnotic use; breastfeeding; and *elderly patients.* Patients with preexisting thyroid abnormalities whose thyroid function cannot be maintained in normal range by drugs, patients with visceral AIDS-related Kaposi's sarcoma associated with rapidly progressive or life-threatening disease; autoimmune hepatitis or a history of autoimmune disease; and immunosuppressed transplant recipients should not receive this drug. Combination therapy involving recombinant interferon alfa-2b and ribavirin is not recommended in patients with severe renal impairment and should be used cautiously in patients with moderate renal impairment. When reconstituted with diluent provided, powder for injection contains benzyl alcohol and is not indicated for infants. Safety and efficacy in *children younger than age 18* have not been established.

Preparation and administration

• Follow hazardous drug guidelines for handling, preparation, and administration. (See "Managing hazardous drugs," page 11.)
• Ensure that patient is well hydrated (especially during initial treatment) to reduce risk of hypotension.
• Some forms must not be given for certain indications. Before prescribing and administering, confirm that form and strength are appropriate for patient's indication.
• Do not use different brands in single treatment regimen. Dosage, administration routes, and adverse reactions vary among brands.
• Drug is indicated as adjunctive therapy within 56 days of surgery for patients with malignant melanoma who are disease-free but at high risk for systemic recurrence. It is not intended for induction-phase treatment of malignant melanoma.
• Use multidose pens for subcutaneous injection only.
• Do not use solution for injection for I.V. administration.
• Do not use 50-million international unit strength powder for injection to treat hairy

cell leukemia or follicular lymphoma.
• Do not use multidose pens or multidose vials of solution for injection to treat AIDS-related Kaposi's sarcoma.
• Do not give by I.M. injection to patients with platelet counts below 50,000/mm³; administer subcutaneously instead.
• Immediately before use, reconstitute powder for injection with diluent provided (bacteriostatic water for injection), which contains 0.9% benzyl alcohol as preservative.
• Antipyretics may be used to prevent or relieve fever and headache.
• Store powder for injection (before and after reconstitution), pens, and solution between 36° and 46° F (2° and 8° C).

Adverse reactions

CNS: dizziness, confusion, paresthesia, depression, difficulty thinking or concentrating, insomnia, fatigue, hypoesthesia, asthenia, amnesia, somnolence, malaise, rigors, suicidal ideation
CV: chest pain, bradycardia, arrhythmia, heart failure
EENT: nasal congestion, sinusitis
GI: anorexia, nausea, diarrhea, vomiting, dyspepsia, dry mouth
Hematologic: leukopenia, thrombocytopenia
Hepatic: hepatotoxicity
Musculoskeletal: arthralgia, back pain
Respiratory: dyspnea, coughing, pulmonary embolism
Skin: rash, dryness, pruritus, alopecia, increased diaphoresis, photosensitivity
Other: fever, flulike symptoms

Interactions

Drug-drug. *Myelosuppressants (such as zidovudine):* increased myelosuppression
Theophylline: decreased theophylline clearance
Drug-diagnostic tests. *ALP, ALT, AST, bilirubin, BUN, calcium, creatinine, fasting blood glucose, hemoglobin, INR, platelets, prothrombin time, partial thromboplastin time, thyroid-stimulating hormone (TSH), triglycerides, WBC count with differential:* altered

Toxicity and overdose
No information available

Special considerations
• Monitor standard hematologic tests (including CBC with differential and platelets), blood chemistries, electrolytes, liver function tests, and TSH at baseline and periodically during therapy.
• Perform baseline eye examination; thereafter, perform periodic examination in patients with preexisting eye conditions.
• Obtain chest X-ray if respiratory symptoms occur. If evidence of pulmonary infiltrates or pulmonary impairment appears, consider discontinuing therapy; monitor patient closely.
• Monitor ECG in patients with cardiovascular conditions or advanced cancer.
• Monitor patient closely for depression; consider stopping drug if depression occurs. Dosage reduction or drug withdrawal may resolve depressive symptoms; however, depression may persist and suicides have occurred after withdrawal.
• Hepatotoxicity (including death) has occurred in patients receiving injection form. Closely monitor patient who develops hepatic function abnormalities during treatment; if appropriate, discontinue drug.
• Rarely, drug may cause diabetes mellitus and hyperglycemia. Measure blood glucose levels in symptomatic patients; follow up as appropriate. Diabetic patients may require adjustment of antidiabetic regimen.
• If triglyceride level rises, provide clinically appropriate management. Severe hypertriglyceridemia (triglyceride level above 1,000 mg/dl) may result in pancreatitis. Consider discontinuing drug in patients with triglyceride level persistently above 1,000 mg/dl who develop pancreatitis symptoms, such as abdominal pain, nausea, or vomiting.
• With higher dosages, obtundation and coma may occur (usually in elderly patients). Although these effects usually reverse rapidly when therapy ends, full resolution may take up to 3 weeks in severe episodes.

Patient education

• Advise patient to drink plenty of fluids, especially during initial stages of therapy.

• Urge patient to seek immediate medical attention for depression or suicidal thoughts, easy bruising or bleeding, yellowing of eyes or skin, or other new symptoms.

• Advise patient to report changes in visual acuity or visual field or other eye problems.

• If patient will be using drug at home, provide instructions on appropriate use, including review of Patient Information Sheet, proper administration, importance of not changing brands without medical consultation, importance of not reusing syringes and needles, use of puncture-resistant container for discarding used syringes and needles, and proper container disposal.

• Caution patient receiving high doses not to drive or perform other tasks requiring mental alertness.

• Instruct patient to avoid prolonged exposure to sunlight.

• Caution female patients and female partners of males taking ribavirin in combination with interferon alfa-2b to avoid pregnancy.

• Provide guidance to breastfeeding patient to help her decide whether to discontinue breast-feeding or stop drug.

interferon alfa-n3 (human leukocyte-derived)
Alferon N

Classification: Antineoplastic, immunomodulator, biological response modifier
Pregnancy risk category C

Pharmacology

Interferon alfa-n3, a highly purified mixture of up to 14 natural human alpha-interferon subtypes, is a naturally occurring protein made from pooled units of human leukocytes induced by incomplete infection with avian virus. Drug has antiviral, immunoregulatory, and antiproliferative properties. Exact mechanism of antineoplastic activity is unknown, but may relate to any of the three actions mentioned above. Antiviral and antiproliferative actions presumably relate to changes in synthesis of RNA, DNA, and cellular proteins (including oncogenes).

Pharmacokinetics

Plasma concentrations are below detectable levels; however, systemic effects have been reported, indicating some systemic absorption. Drug is filtered through glomeruli and undergoes rapid proteolytic degradation during tubular reabsorption.

How supplied

Solution for injection: 5 million international units/ml

Indications and dosages

OFF-LABEL USES (SELECTED)

➡ Hairy cell leukemia, AIDS-related Kaposi's sarcoma, bladder carcinoma, renal carcinoma, chronic myelocytic leukemia, non-Hodgkin's lymphoma, malignant melanoma, multiple myeloma, mycosis fungoides, carcinoid tumors, epithelial ovarian carcinoma
Adults: Various dosage schedules have been used for off-label indications. Because these regimens are still largely investigational, prescriber should consult medical literature in choosing specific dosage. In clinical trials, cancer patients received 3 million, 9 million, or 15 million international units I.M. daily for 10 days.

Contraindications and precautions

Contraindicated in hypersensitivity to human interferon alfa or product components and in anaphylactic sensitivity to mouse immunoglobulin (IgG), egg protein, or neomycin.

Use cautiously in debilitating medical conditions (such as cardiovascular disease, including unstable angina and uncontrolled heart failure), severe pulmonary disease (such as chronic obstructive pulmonary disease), diabetes mellitus with ketoacidosis, coagulation disorders, severe myelosuppression, seizure disorders, fertile males and females, pregnancy, breastfeeding, and *elderly patients*. Safety and efficacy in *children younger than age 18* have not been established.

Preparation and administration
• Follow hazardous drug guidelines for handling, preparation, and administration. (See "Managing hazardous drugs," page 11.)
• Ensure that patient is well hydrated (especially during initial treatment) to reduce risk of hypotension.
• If patient has acute, serious hypersensitivity reaction (such as urticaria, angioedema, bronchoconstriction, or anaphylaxis), stop drug at once and begin appropriate medical therapy.
• Store at 36° to 46° F (2° to 8° C). Do not freeze or shake.

Adverse reactions
CNS: headache, fatigue, dizziness, malaise, sleepiness
CV: chest pain, hypotension
EENT: blurred vision
GI: nausea, vomiting, heartburn, diarrhea, constipation, anorexia, stomatitis, dry mouth
Hematologic: neutropenia, thrombocytopenia
Musculoskeletal: myalgia, arthralgia, back pain
Skin: pruritus
Other: fever, chills, flulike symptoms, pain at injection site, anaphylaxis

Interactions
Drug-drug. *Theophylline:* increased theophylline level
Drug-diagnostic tests. *ALP:* altered
WBCs: decreased

Toxicity and overdose
No information available

Special considerations
• Monitor CBC with differential.
• Product is made from human blood and may pose risk of transmitting viruses and other infectious agents.

Patient education
• Instruct patient to drink plenty of fluids, especially during initial stages of therapy.
• Advise patient to immediately report early indications of hypersensitivity reactions, such as hives, generalized itching, tightness of chest, wheezing, and signs or symptoms of low blood pressure (such as dizziness on standing).
• Caution men and women with childbearing potential not to take drug unless they use effective contraception.
• Provide guidance to help breastfeeding patient decide whether to discontinue breastfeeding or stop drug.

irinotecan hydrochloride
Camptosar

Classification: Antineoplastic, topoisomerase I inhibitor
Pregnancy risk category D

Pharmacology
Irinotecan, a camptothecin derivative, relieves torsional strain in DNA by inducing reversible single-strand breaks. Its cytotoxicity may result from double-strand DNA damage produced during DNA synthesis, when replication enzymes interact with ternary complex formed by topoisomerase I, DNA, and either irinotecan or SN-38 (drug's active metabolite).

Pharmacokinetics
Drug is metabolized to SN-38 primarily in liver. SN-38 concentration peaks about 1 hour after end of 90-minute infusion. Drug is 30% to 68% protein-bound and has a terminal

half-life of 6 to 12 hours. SN-38 is 95% protein-bound, with a terminal half-life of 10 to 20 hours. Urinary excretion of drug is 11% to 20%; SN-38, less than 1%; and SN-38 glucuronide, 3%.

How supplied

Solution: 2-ml and 5-ml single-dose amber glass vials. Each ml contains 20 mg irinotecan (based on trihydrate salt), 45 mg sorbitol, and 0.9 mg lactic acid.

Indications and dosages

FDA-APPROVED

➡ First-line therapy with leucovorin and 5-fluorouracil (5-FU) for patients with metastatic carcinoma of colon or rectum
Adults: Administer as I.V. infusion over 90 minutes. For all regimens, give leucovorin immediately after irinotecan, and give 5-FU immediately after leucovorin. Currently recommended irinotecan dosages and modifications for both combination and single-agent therapy are shown in the following tables.

Combination-agent irinotecan regimens and dosage modifications*			
Drug	**Starting dosage**	**Level-1 dose**	**Level-2 dose**
Regimen 1: 6-week cycle with bolus 5-FU and leucovorin (next cycle begins on day 43)			
Irinotecan‡ (125 mg/m² I.V. over 90 minutes)	125 mg/m²	100 mg/m²	75 mg/m²
Leucovorin‡ (20 mg/m² I.V. bolus)	20 mg/m²	20 mg/m²	20 mg/m²
5-FU‡ (500 mg/m² I.V. bolus)	500 mg/m²	400 mg/m²	300 mg/m²

(continued)

Drug	**Starting dosage**	**Level-1 dose**	**Level-2 dose**
Regimen 2: 6-week cycle with infusional 5-FU/ leucovorin (next cycle begins on day 43)			
Irinotecan§ (180 mg/m² I.V. over 90 minutes)	180 mg/m²	150 mg/m²	120 mg/m²
Leucovorin§ (200 mg/m² I.V. over 2 hours)	200 mg/m²	200 mg/m²	200 mg/m²
5-FU‖ bolus (400 mg/m² I.V. bolus)	400 mg/m²	320 mg/m²	240 mg/m²
5-FU‖ infusion† (600 mg/m² I.V. over 22 hours)	600 mg/m²	480 mg/m²	360 mg/m²

* Dosage reductions beyond level-2 dose by decrements of roughly 20% may be needed for patients with continued toxicity. If intolerable toxicity does not develop, continue treatment with additional cycles indefinitely as long as patient continues to experience clinical benefit.

† Infusion follows bolus administration.

‡ Dosing on days 1, 8, 15, and 22

§ Dosing on days 1, 15, and 29

‖ Dosing on days 1, 2, 15, 16, 29, and 30

Single-agent irinotecan regimens and dosage modifications			
Drug	**Starting dosage**	**Level-1 dose**	**Level-2 dose**
*Weekly regimen**			
Irinotecan† (125 mg/m² I.V. over 90 minutes)	125 mg/m²	100 mg/m²	75 mg/m²

(continued)

Drug	Starting dosage	Level-1 dose	Level-2 dose
Once-every-3-weeks regimen‡			
Irinotecan§ (350 mg/m² I.V. over 90 minutes)‖	350 mg/m²	300 mg/m²	250 mg/m²

* Adjust subsequent dosages as high as 150 mg/m² or as low as 50 mg/m² in 25- to 50-mg/m² decrements based on tolerance.

† Dosing on days 1, 8, 15, and 22, followed by 2-week rest.

‡ Adjust subsequent dosages to as low as 200 mg/m² in 50-mg/m² decrements based on tolerance.

§ Once every 3 weeks

‖ Unless intolerable toxicity develops, continue treatment with additional cycles indefinitely as long as patient continues to experience clinical benefit.

➡ Metastatic carcinoma of colon or rectum in patients whose disease has recurred or progressed after initial fluorouracil-based therapy
Adults: Single-dose regimen (see table above) by I.V. infusion once weekly for 4 weeks, followed by 2-week rest period. After adequate recovery, repeat additional doses in similar 6-week cycle; continue indefinitely in patients who achieve response or whose disease remains stable.

OFF-LABEL USES (SELECTED)
➡ Non-small-cell lung cancer
Adults: In one study, 60 mg/m² I.V. was given over 90 minutes on days 1, 8, and 15 with cisplatin 80 mg/m² I.V. over 30 minutes on day 1 of 28-day cycle.
➡ Cervical cancer
Adults: In one study, 350 mg/m² I.V. was given over 30 to 50 minutes every 3 weeks.
➡ Ovarian cancer
Adults: In one study, 250 to 300 mg/m² I.V. was given over 90 minutes every 3 weeks.
➡ Pancreatic cancer
Adults: In one study, 100 mg/m² I.V. was given over 90 minutes, with gemcitabine 1,000 mg/m² I.V. given over 30 minutes on days 1 and 8 of 21-day cycle.

➡ Brain tumors
Adults: In one study, 125 mg/m² I.V. was given over 90 minutes once weekly for 4 weeks, followed by a 2-week rest.
➡ Gastric cancer
Adults: In one study, 180 mg/m² I.V. was given over 90 minutes on day 1, with leucovorin 200 mg/m² I.V. given over 2 hours followed by fluorouracil 400 mg/m² I.V. bolus, then fluorouracil 600 mg/m² by continuous I.V. infusion over 22 hours on days 1 and 2, repeated every 14 days.

DOSAGE MODIFICATIONS

• Patients age 70 and older should receive starting dosage of 300 mg/m² in single-agent, once-every-3-week regimen.
• All dosage modifications should be based on worst preceding toxicity. After first treatment, patients with active diarrhea should have been able to resume pretreatment bowel function without requiring antidiarrheals for at least 24 hours before next chemotherapy administration.
• Monitor patients carefully for toxicity, and evaluate before each treatment. Modify irinotecan and 5-FU dosages as needed according to tolerance. Based on recommended dosage levels, adjust subsequent doses as shown in the following tables.

(Text continues on page 208.)

Recommended dosage modifications for irinotecan/5-FU/leucovorin combination schedules*		
Toxicity NCI CTC Grade† value)	During treatment cycle	At start of subsequent cycles‡
No toxicity	Maintain dose level.	Maintain dose level.
Neutropenia		
1 (1,500 to 1,999/mm³)	Maintain dose level.	Maintain dose level.
2 (1,000 to 1,499/mm³)	Decrease one dose level.	Maintain dose level.

(continued)

⊖ Orphan drug   ≫ Potentially carcinogenic

Recommended dosage modifications for irinotecan/5-FU/leucovorin combination schedules* (continued)

Toxicity NCI CTC Grade[†] (value)	During treatment cycle	At start of subsequent cycles[‡]
Neutropenia (continued)		
3 (500 to 999/mm³)	Omit dose until resolved to Grade 2 or lower; then decrease one dose level.	Decrease one dose level.
4 (below 500/mm³)	Omit dose until resolved to Grade 2 or lower; then decrease two dose levels.	Decrease two dose levels.
Neutropenic fever	Omit dose until resolved; then decrease two dose levels.	
Other hematologic toxicities	Dosage modifications for leukopenia or thrombocytopenia during treatment cycle and at start of subsequent cycles are based on NCI toxicity criteria and are same as recommended for neutropenia above.	
Diarrhea		
1 (2 to 3 stools/day more than pretreatment)	Delay dose until resolved to baseline; then give same dosage.	Maintain dose level.
2 (4 to 6 stools/day more than pretreatment)	Decrease one dose level.	Maintain dose level.
3 (7 to 9 stools/day more than pretreatment)	Omit dose until resolved at or below grade 2; then decrease one dose level.	Decrease one dose level.
4 (10 or more stools/day more than pretreatment)	Omit dose until resolved at or below grade 2; then decrease two dose levels.	Decrease two dose levels.
Other nonhematologic toxicities§		
1	Maintain dose level.	Maintain dose level.

(continued)

Toxicity NCI CTC Grade[†] (value)	During treatment cycle	At start of subsequent cycles[‡]
Other nonhematologic toxicities§ (continued)		
2	Decrease one dose level.	Decrease one dose level.
3	Omit dose until resolved to Grade 2 or lower; then decrease one dose level.	Decrease one dose level.
4	Omit dose until resolved to Grade 2 or lower; then decrease two dose levels.	Decrease two dose levels.

For mucositis or stomatitis, decrease 5-FU only, not irinotecan.

* Patients should have resumed pretreatment bowel function without requiring antidiarrhea medications for at least 24 hours before next chemotherapy administration. New cycle should not begin until granulocyte count recovers to 1,500/mm³ or higher, platelet count recovers to 100,000/mm³ or higher, and treatment-related diarrhea resolves fully. Delay treatment 1 to 2 weeks to allow recovery from toxicities. If patient does not recover after 2-week delay, consider discontinuing therapy.

† National Cancer Institute Common Toxicity Criteria (version 1.0)

‡ Relative to starting dose used in previous cycle

§ Excludes alopecia, anorexia, asthenia

Recommended dosage modifications for single-agent schedules*

Worst toxicity	During treatment cycle	At start of next cycles (after adequate recovery), compared with starting dosage in previous cycle*	
NCI Grade[†] (value)	Weekly	Weekly	Once every 3 weeks
No toxicity	Maintain dose level.	Increase 25 mg/m² up to maximum dosage of 150 mg/m².	Maintain dose level.

(continued)

Only common or life-threatening adverse reactions are listed.

Worst toxicity NCI Grade† (value)	During treatment cycle Weekly	At start of next cycles (after adequate recovery), compared with starting dosage in previous cycle* Weekly	Once every 3 weeks
Neutropenia			
1 (1,500 to 1,999/mm³)	Maintain dose level.	Maintain dose level.	Maintain dose level.
2 (1,000 to 1,499/mm³)	Decrease 25 mg/m².	Maintain dose level.	Maintain dose level.
3 (500 to 999/mm³)	Omit dose until resolved to Grade 2 or lower; then decrease 25 mg/m².	Decrease 25 mg/m².	Decrease 50 mg/m².
4 (below 500/mm³)	Omit dose until resolved to Grade 2 or lower; then decrease 50 mg/m².	Decrease 50 mg/m².	Decrease 50 mg/m².
Neutropenic fever	Omit dose until resolved; decrease 50 mg/m² when resolved.	Decrease 50 mg/m².	Decrease 50 mg/m².
Other hematologic toxicities	Dosage modifications for leukopenia, thrombocytopenia, and anemia during treatment cycle and at start of subsequent cycles are based on NCI toxicity criteria and are same as recommended for neutropenia above.		
Diarrhea			
1 (2 to 3 stools/day more than pretreatment)	Maintain dose level.	Maintain dose level.	Maintain dose level.
2 (4 to 6 stools/day more than pretreatment)	Decrease 25 mg/m².	Maintain dose level.	Maintain dose level.
Diarrhea (continued)			
3 (7 to 9 stools/day more than pretreatment)	Omit dose until resolved to Grade 2 or lower; then decrease 25 mg/m².	Decrease 25 mg/m².	Decrease 50 mg/m².
4 (10 or more stools/day more than pretreatment)	Omit dose until resolved to Grade 2 or lower; then decrease 50 mg/m².	Decrease 50 mg/m².	Decrease 50 mg/m².
Other nonhematologic toxicities‡			
1	Maintain dose level.	Maintain dose level.	Maintain dose level.
2	Decrease 25 mg/m².	Decrease 25 mg/m².	Decrease 50 mg/m².
3	Omit dose until resolved to Grade 2 or lower; then decrease 25 mg/m².	Decrease 25 mg/m².	Decrease 50 mg/m².
4	Omit dose until resolved to Grade 2 or lower; then decrease 50 mg/m².	Decrease 50 mg/m².	Decrease 50 mg/m².

* All dosage modifications should be based on worst preceding toxicity.

† National Cancer Institute Common Toxicity Criteria (version 1.0)

‡ Excludes alopecia, anorexia, asthenia

(continued)

🡒 Orphan drug   🡆 Potentially carcinogenic

WARNINGS

• Drug should be administered only under supervision of physician experienced in using cancer chemotherapeutic agents. Complications can be managed appropriately only when adequate diagnostic and treatment facilities are readily available.

• Drug can cause both early and late forms of diarrhea that appear to be mediated by different mechanisms. Both forms may be severe.

• *Early* diarrhea (occurring during or shortly after irinotecan infusion) may be accompanied by cholinergic symptoms of rhinitis, increased salivation, miosis, lacrimation, diaphoresis, flushing, and intestinal hyperperistalsis (which can cause abdominal cramping). Atropine may prevent or relieve early diarrhea and other cholinergic symptoms.

• *Late* diarrhea (generally occurring more than 24 hours after administration) can be life-threatening because it may be prolonged and cause dehydration, electrolyte imbalance, or sepsis. Late diarrhea should be treated promptly with loperamide. Patients with diarrhea should be monitored carefully and receive fluid and electrolyte replacement if they become dehydrated; they should receive antibiotics if ileus, fever, or severe neutropenia occurs. Drug administration should be interrupted and subsequent dosages reduced if severe diarrhea occurs.

• Severe myelosuppression may occur.

Contraindications and precautions

Contraindicated in hypersensitivity to drug.

Use cautiously in bilirubin level above 2 mg/dl, diarrhea, colitis, neutropenia, volume depletion, patients experiencing cholinergic symptoms, pregnancy, breastfeeding, and *elderly patients.* Safety and efficacy in *children* have not been established.

Preparation and administration

• Follow hazardous drug guidelines for handling, preparation, and administration. (See "Managing hazardous drugs," page 11.)

• Except in well-designed clinical study, do not use drug with Mayo Clinic regimen of 5-FU/leucovorin (administration for 4 to 5 consecutive days every 4 weeks).

• Administering drug to patients with bilirubin level above 2 mg/dl is not recommended (these patients were not included in clinical studies).

• Drug is emetogenic; patient should be premedicated with antiemetics. Most patients receive dexamethasone 10 mg with another type of antiemetic (such as ondansetron, granisetron, or another 5-HT$_3$ blocker). Give antiemetics on treatment day starting at least 30 minutes before irinotecan administration. Consider providing antiemetic regimen (such as prochlorperazine) for subsequent use as needed.

• Consider prophylactic or therapeutic administration of atropine 0.25 to 1 mg I.V. or subcutaneously (unless clinically contraindicated) in patients with cholinergic symptoms, such as rhinitis, increased salivation, miosis, lacrimation, diaphoresis, flushing, abdominal cramping, or diarrhea (occurring during or shortly after irinotecan infusion). These symptoms are more frequent with higher dosages.

• Keep drug vial, backing, and plastic blister in carton until time of use.

• Dilute for infusion with 250 to 500 ml D$_5$W to yield 0.12 to 2.8 mg/ml. Use within 24 hours if kept at controlled room temperature or within 48 hours if refrigerated. If diluted with normal saline solution, use within 6 hours if kept at controlled room temperature; do not refrigerate (precipitate may form).

• Do not add other drugs to infusion solution.

• Administer by I.V. infusion. Take care to avoid extravasation; monitor infusion site for signs of inflammation. If extravasation occurs, flush site with sterile water and apply ice.

• Store undiluted drug at controlled temperature of 59° to 86° F (15° to 30° C). Protect from light and freezing.

Only common or life-threatening adverse reactions are listed.

Adverse reactions

CNS: insomnia, dizziness, asthenia, headache, fever, pain
CV: vasodilation, bradycardia, thromboembolic events
EENT: rhinitis, miosis, lacrimation
GI: severe diarrhea; nausea; vomiting; anorexia; stomatitis; flatulence; dyspepsia; abdominal cramping, pain, or enlargement; hyperperistalsis; colonic ulceration; colitis; salivation
Hematologic: leukopenia, anemia, neutropenia, thrombocytopenia
Hepatic: hepatotoxicity
Metabolic: dehydration
Musculoskeletal: back pain
Respiratory: dyspnea, increased cough
Skin: alopecia, rash, flushing
Other: weight loss, chills, infection, diaphoresis, hypersensitivity reactions including anaphylaxis

Interactions

Drug-drug. *Dexamethasone:* possible lymphocytopenia, hyperglycemia
Diuretics: possible dehydration
Laxatives: increased severity of diarrhea
Other antineoplastics: increased adverse effects
Prochlorperazine: increased risk of akathisia
Drug-diagnostic tests. *ALP, hemoglobin, neutrophils, WBCs:* altered
Drug-herb. *Alpha-lipoic acid, coenzyme Q10:* possible decreased chemotherapy efficacy
Dandelion, St. John's wort: increased clearance of irinotecan or its metabolites
Glutamine: possible enhanced tumor growth

Toxicity and overdose

• No overdose cases have been reported. In clinical trials, adverse reactions with dosages up to 750 mg/m^2 were similar to those reported with recommended dosages.
• No known antidote exists. Provide maximum supportive care to prevent dehydration caused by diarrhea and to treat infectious complications.

Special considerations

• Before each dose, carefully monitor WBC count with differential, hemoglobin, and platelets.
• In clinical trials of irinotecan/5-FU/leucovorin or 5-FU/leucovorin, patients with baseline performance status of 2 had higher rates of hospitalization, neutropenic fever, thromboembolism, first-cycle treatment discontinuation, and early deaths compared to patients with baseline performance status of 0 or 1.
• Carefully monitor patient with diarrhea. Give fluid and electrolyte replacement for dehydration; give antibiotics for ileus, fever, or severe neutropenia. If Grade 2, 3, or 4 late diarrhea occurs, decrease subsequent dosages within current cycle.
• Deaths from sepsis after severe neutropenia have occurred. Manage neutropenic complications promptly with antibiotics. Temporarily omit therapy during treatment cycle if neutropenic fever occurs or absolute neutrophil count (ANC) falls below 1,500/mm^3. After patient recovers to ANC of at least 1,500/mm^3, reduce subsequent dosages based on neutropenia level.
• Monitor hepatic function. Patients with modestly elevated baseline serum total bilirubin levels (1 to 2 mg/dl) are at significantly greater risk for first-cycle Grade 3 or 4 neutropenia. No association between baseline bilirubin elevations and increased risk of late diarrhea has been seen in studies of weekly dosage schedule.
• Closely monitor patients with history of pelvic or abdominal irradiation because of increased risk of myelosuppression.
• Monitor results of UGT1A1 molecular assay test to detect UGT1A1 gene variations that have been associated with increased risk for severe adverse reactions to drug.
• Drug may cause colitis complicated by ulceration, bleeding, ileus, and infection. Provide prompt antibiotic support to patients with ileus.

• Closely monitor elderly patients with co-morbid conditions because of greater risk of late diarrhea.

Patient education

• Inform patient and caregiver of drug's expected toxic effects, particularly GI complications (such as nausea, vomiting, abdominal cramping, diarrhea, and infection). Instruct patient to keep loperamide at hand and to start treatment for late diarrhea (usually occurring more than 24 hours after irinotecan dose) at first episode of poorly formed or loose stools or at earliest onset of unusually frequent bowel movements.

• Instruct patient to report first-time diarrhea during treatment, black or bloody stools, dehydration symptoms (such as dizziness, light-headedness, or fainting), inability to take fluids by mouth due to nausea or vomiting, inability to control diarrhea within 24 hours, or fever or other evidence of infection.

• Instruct patient to avoid using laxatives.

• Counsel women with childbearing potential to avoid pregnancy during therapy. If patient is pregnant or becomes pregnant during therapy, inform her that drug may harm fetus.

• Advise breastfeeding patient to discontinue breastfeeding during therapy.

isotretinoin (13-*cis*-retinoic acid)

Accutane, Amnesteem, Claravis, Sotret

Classification: Retinoid
Pregnancy risk category X

Pharmacology

Isotretinoin has an unknown mechanism of cytotoxic action.

Pharmacokinetics

Drug is highly lipophilic and has enhanced oral absorption when given with high-fat meal. It is metabolized in liver (primarily by CYP450 enzymes 2C8, 2C9, 3A4, and 2B6) and is more than 99.9% bound to plasma proteins (mainly albumin). It peaks at 3 hours. Parent compound and metabolites are excreted in urine and feces.

How supplied

Capsules: 10 mg, 20 mg, 40 mg

Indications and dosages

OFF-LABEL USES (SELECTED)

➡ Squamous-cell cancer of head and neck
Adults: Usually 50 to 100 mg/m^2 P.O. daily
➡ Advanced, refractory lymphoid malignancies (given with interferon alfa)
Adults: Usual starting dosage of 1 mg/kg P.O. daily in two divided doses
➡ Cutaneous T-cell lymphoma
Adults: Usually 1 to 2 mg/kg P.O. daily

DOSAGE MODIFICATIONS

➡ Dosage should be adjusted based on disease response or appearance of adverse effects (some of which may be dose-related).

WARNINGS

• Drug must not be used by pregnant patients even for short periods due to risk of major fetal malformation. Potentially, any fetus exposed during pregnancy can be affected.

• Documented external fetal abnormalities include skull, ear, and eye abnormalities; facial dysmorphia; and cleft palate. Documented internal abnormalities include CNS, cardiovascular, and thymus gland abnormalities and parathyroid hormone deficiency. In some cases, death has occurred. IQ scores less than 85 (with or without obvious CNS abnormalities) also have been reported.

• Drug increases risk of spontaneous abortion and premature birth.

• Drug is contraindicated in women with childbearing potential, unless patient meets all of these conditions: (1) is not pregnant or

---

Only common or life-threatening adverse reactions are listed.

breastfeeding, (2) is capable of complying with mandatory contraceptive measures required for therapy and of understanding behaviors associated with increased pregnancy risk, and (3) can reliably understand and carry out instructions.

• Women with childbearing potential must use two effective contraception methods simultaneously. Effective methods include both primary and secondary contraception forms. *Primary* forms include tubal ligation; partner's vasectomy; intrauterine devices; birth control pills; and injectable, implantable, and insertable hormonal birth control products. *Secondary* forms include diaphragms, latex condoms, and cervical caps (each must be used with spermicide). Caution patient not to take St. John's wort concomitantly with oral contraceptives because it reduces contraceptive efficacy.

• Isotretinoin must be prescribed under iPLEDGE program. Physicians and dispensing pharmacies must be registered with program, and patients must be registered and meet program qualifications.

Contraindications and precautions

Contraindicated in hypersensitivity to drug or its components and in pregnancy.

Use cautiously in psychiatric disorders; hypertriglyceridemia; vision problems; tinnitus or hearing impairment; elevated liver enzyme levels; history of intestinal disorders; genetic predisposition to age-related osteoporosis; history of childhood osteoporosis conditions, osteomalacia, or other bone metabolism disorders; concomitant tetracycline use (should be avoided because of association with pseudotumor cerebri); patients with childbearing potential (unless they meet all iPLEDGE conditions); breastfeeding patients (use not recommended); male partners of females with childbearing potential; *elderly patients;* and *children.* Use in children younger than age 12 has not been studied.

Preparation and administration

• Female patients must have had two negative urine or serum pregnancy tests with a sensitivity of at least 25 mIU/ml before receiving drug.

• Obtain pretreatment liver function tests, as well as blood lipid levels under fasting conditions.

• Administer drug with meal.

• Store at controlled temperature of 59° to 86° F (15° to 30° C). Protect from light.

Adverse reactions

CNS: pseudotumor cerebri, depression, psychosis, suicidal ideation or attempts, suicide, aggressive and violent behavior
CV: palpitations, tachycardia, vascular thrombotic disease, cerebrovascular accident
EENT: conjunctivitis, corneal opacities, decreased night vision, hearing impairment, tinnitus, epistaxis, dry nose, dry mucous membranes
GI: nausea, vomiting, abdominal pain, dry mouth, pancreatitis, inflammatory bowel disease
GU: glomerulonephritis
Hematologic: anemia, thrombocytopenia, neutropenia, agranulocytosis (rare)
Hepatic: hepatitis
Musculoskeletal: rhabdomyolysis, decreased bone mineral density, musculoskeletal symptoms
Skin: cheilosis, rash, dry skin, facial skin desquamation, petechiae, cheilitis, pruritus, skin fragility, brittle nails, photosensitivity
Other: allergic reactions including anaphylaxis

Interactions

Drug-drug. *Corticosteroids (systemic):* possible increased risk of osteoporosis
Hormonal contraceptives: possible decreased contraceptive efficacy
Microdosed progesterone preparations ("minipills" containing no estrogen): possible contraceptive inadequacy
Phenytoin: possible increased risk of osteomalacia

Tetracyclines: increased risk of pseudotumor cerebri
Vitamin A: additive toxic effects
Drug-diagnostic tests. *ALP, ALT, AST, creatine kinase (CK), fasting blood glucose, GGT, lactate dehydrogenase, plasma triglycerides, platelets, sedimentation rate, serum cholesterol, uric acid:* increased
Liver function tests; urinary WBCs, protein, and blood: abnormal
RBC parameters, serum high-density lipoproteins (HDLs), WBCs: decreased
Drug-food. *High-fat meal:* increased peak plasma concentration and increased total drug exposure (with oral use)
Drug-herb. *Alfalfa, bergamot oil:* increased photosensitivity
St John's wort (with hormonal contraceptives): possible decreased contraceptive efficacy

Toxicity and overdose

• Overdose may cause vomiting, facial flushing, cheilosis, abdominal pain, headache, dizziness, and ataxia.
• All symptoms resolve quickly without apparent residual effects. Treat supportively, as needed.

Special considerations

• Each month of therapy, female patient must have negative urine or serum pregnancy test result. Repeat pregnancy test monthly before patient receives each prescription.
• Monitor WBC count for neutropenia.
• Obtain follow-up blood lipid levels under fasting conditions. If patient has consumed alcohol, wait at least 36 hours before testing lipids. Perform these tests at weekly or biweekly intervals until lipid response to drug is established.
• Obtain follow-up liver function tests at weekly or biweekly intervals until response to drug is established.
• Monitor patient carefully for vision problems. If these occur, stop drug and make sure patient receives ophthalmologic examination.

• Accutane may cause hearing impairment, which may persist even after therapy ends. If patient experiences tinnitus or hearing impairment, stop drug and provide specialist referral for further evaluation.
• Closely monitor blood glucose and serum CK levels.
• Acute pancreatitis may occur in patients with elevated or normal serum triglyceride levels. Rarely, fatal hemorrhagic pancreatitis has been reported with Accutane. Stop Accutane if hypertriglyceridemia cannot be controlled at acceptable level or if pancreatitis symptoms occur.
• Accutane has been associated with inflammatory bowel disease (including regional ileitis) in patients with no history of intestinal disorders. In some cases, symptoms persisted after drug withdrawal. Stop drug in patients experiencing abdominal pain, rectal bleeding, or severe diarrhea.

Patient education

• Instruct patient to read Medication Guide supplied (as required by law when drug is dispensed). For additional information, advise patient to read *Patient Product Information, Important Information Concerning Your Treatment with Accutane (isotretinoin)*. All patients must sign informed consent/patient agreement.
• Caution women with childbearing potential to avoid pregnancy when therapy begins and to use two effective contraceptive methods starting 1 month before initiation of therapy and continuing during treatment and for 1 month after therapy ends. Have patient read and sign consent form before starting therapy.
• Inform women with childbearing potential that frequent urine or serum pregnancy tests are mandatory during therapy.
• Advise patient not to share drug with others because of risk of birth defects and other serious adverse events.
• Caution patient not to donate blood during therapy and for 1 month afterward.
• Instruct patient to take drug with meal and to swallow capsule with full glass of liquid to

---

Only common or life-threatening adverse reactions are listed.

decrease risk of esophageal irritation.
• Tell patient to avoid wax epilation and skin resurfacing procedures (such as dermabrasion or laser) during therapy and for at least 6 months afterward because of scarring risk.
• Advise patient to avoid prolonged exposure to ultraviolet rays or sunlight during therapy.
• Inform patient that contact lens tolerance may decrease during and after therapy. Advise patient to report such problems, stop taking drug, and have ophthalmologic examination.
• Instruct breastfeeding patient not to take drug while breastfeeding.

kaolin and pectin
Kapectolin, K-P

Classification: Adsorbent, antidiarrheal
Pregnancy risk category C

Pharmacology
Kaolin adsorbs irritants, forms protective coating on intestinal mucosa, and enhances stool formation. (However, total water loss may be unchanged.) Pectin consolidates stool.

Pharmacokinetics
Drug is not absorbed. Roughly 90% of pectin decomposes in GI tract.

How supplied
Kaolin and pectin, Kapectolin oral suspension: 90 g kaolin and 2 g pectin/30 ml

Indications and dosages

FDA-APPROVED

➡ Symptomatic relief of diarrhea
Adults and children older than age 12: 60 to 120 ml P.O. after each bowel movement
Children ages 6 to 12: 30 to 60 ml P.O. after each bowel movement
Children ages 3 to 6: 15 to 30 ml P.O. after each bowel movement

➡ Mucositis after radiation therapy
Adults: As needed, various combinations of kaolin and pectin with diphenhydramine, kaolin and pectin with diphenhydramine and viscous lidocaine, or kaolin and pectin with diphenhydramine and sucralfate; usually in equal parts of components swished and expectorated or sometimes swallowed

Contraindications and precautions
Contraindicated in hypersensitivity to kaolin or pectin products and in diarrhea caused by pseudomembranous enterocolitis or toxigenic bacteria.

Use cautiously in diarrhea not controlled in 48 hours, fever, pregnancy, breastfeeding, *elderly patients,* and *children.*

Preparation and administration
• Give drug at least 2 hours before or after other medications.
• Force fluids during treatment period.
• Store drug at room temperature.

Adverse reactions
GI: constipation

Interactions
Drug-drug. *Anticholinergics, antidyskinetics, cardiac glycosides, lincomycins, loxapine, phenothiazines, thiothixenes:* decreased efficacy of these drugs
Other oral drugs: reduced absorption of these drugs

Toxicity and overdose
No information available

Special considerations
• Evaluate stools and monitor frequency and consistency of bowel movements.
• Monitor patient for dehydration.

Patient education
• Instruct patient to shake drug well before taking it.

K

• Advise patient to take drug at least 2 hours before or after other drugs.
• Instruct patient to drink large amounts of fluid during therapy.
• Urge patient to seek immediate medical attention or contact poison control center if accidental overdose occurs.
• Caution patient not to use drug for more than 2 days or if a high fever occurs, unless directed by physician.
• Inform parent or caregiver that drug should not be used in children younger than age 3 unless directed by physician.
• Caution patient not to exceed recommended dosage.
• Advise pregnant or breastfeeding patient to consult health care professional before using drug.

lenalidomide
Revlimid

Classification: Antineoplastic, immunomodulator
Pregnancy risk category X

Pharmacology
Lenalidomide inhibits secretion of proinflammatory cytokines and increases secretion of anti-inflammatory cytokines from peripheral mononuclear cells. It also inhibits proliferation of some cell lines (such as Namalwa cells) with chromosome 5 deletion and others without chromosome 5 deletions. Drug also may inhibit cyclooxygenase-2 (COX-2) expression.

Pharmacokinetics
Drug is absorbed rapidly and peaks in 0.6 to 1.5 hours. Elimination half-life is roughly 3 hours.

How supplied
Capsules: 5 mg, 10 mg

Indications and dosages

FDA-APPROVED

➥ Transfusion-dependent anemia resulting from low- or intermediate-1-risk myelodysplastic syndrome (MDS) associated with deletion 5q cytogenic abnormality (with or without additional cytogenic abnormalities)
Adults: 10 mg P.O. daily

DOSAGE MODIFICATIONS

• If thrombocytopenia develops within 4 weeks of starting treatment at 10 mg daily, adjust dosage as follows:
  Patients with baseline platelet count of 100,000/mm³ or higher: Interrupt treatment if platelet count falls below 50,000/mm³. Resume treatment at 5 mg daily when platelet count returns to 50,000/mm³ or higher.
  Patients with baseline platelet count below 100,000/mm³: Interrupt treatment if platelet count falls to 50% of baseline value. Resume treatment at 5 mg daily if baseline count was at or above 60,000/mm³ and returns to 50,000/mm³ or above, or if baseline count was below 60,000/mm³ and returns to 30,000/mm³ or above.
• If thrombocytopenia develops after 4 weeks of starting treatment at 10 mg daily, adjust dosage as follows: Interrupt treatment if platelet count drops below 30,000/mm³, or below 50,000/mm³ with platelet transfusion. Resume treatment at 5 mg daily when count returns to 30,000/mm³ or higher without hemostatic failure.
• If thrombocytopenia develops during treatment at 5 mg daily, interrupt treatment if platelet count is below 30,000/mm³, or above 50,000/mm³ with platelet transfusion. Resume treatment at 5 mg every other day when count returns to 30,000/mm³ or higher without hemostatic failure.
• If patient who started on 10-mg dosage experiences neutropenia within 4 weeks of starting treatment at 10 mg daily, adjust dosage as follows:

Only common or life-threatening adverse reactions are listed.

Patients with baseline absolute neutrophil count (ANC) of 1,000/mm^3 or higher: Interrupt treatment if neutrophil count falls below 750 mm^3; resume treatment at 5 mg daily when neutrophil count returns to 1,000/mm^3 or higher.

Patients with baseline ANC below 1,000/mm^3: Interrupt treatment if neutrophil count falls below 500/mm^3. Resume treatment at 5 mg daily when count returns to 500/mm^3 or higher.

- If neutropenia develops after 4 weeks of starting treatment at daily dosage of 10 mg, interrupt treatment if neutrophil count falls below 500/mm^3 for approximately 7 days, or falls below 500/mm^3 associated with fever of approximately 101.3° F (38.5° C). Resume treatment at 5 mg daily when neutrophil count returns to a level above 500/mm^3.
- If neutropenia develops during treatment at 5 mg daily, interrupt treatment if neutrophil count falls below 500/mm^3 for approximately 7 days or below 500/mm^3 associated with fever of approximately 101.3° F (38.5° C). Resume treatment at 5 mg every other day when count returns to a level above 500/mm^3.

⊠ WARNINGS

- Drug is analog of thalidomide, a known teratogen that causes severe, life-threatening birth defects. If taken during pregnancy, it may cause birth defects in or death of embryo or fetus. Female patients should be advised to avoid pregnancy during therapy.
- Drug is associated with significant neutropenia and thrombocytopenia in patients with deletion 5q MDS. Grade 3 or 4 hematologic toxicity occurred in 80% of patients, and dosage reduction was required; 34% required additional dosage reduction.
- Drug caused significantly increased risk of deep-vein thrombosis and pulmonary embolism in patients with multiple myeloma who received combination therapy.
- Drug may be prescribed only by licensed prescribers registered in RevAssist program

and may be obtained only through controlled distribution program through contracted pharmacy. It can be dispensed only to registered patients who meet all program conditions.

Contraindications and precautions

Contraindicated in hypersensitivity to drug or its components and in pregnancy.

Use cautiously in renal impairment, patients with childbearing potential, breastfeeding, and **elderly patients.** Safety and efficacy in **children** have not been established.

Preparation and administration

- Follow hazardous drug guidelines for handling, preparation, and administration. (See "Managing hazardous drugs," page 11.)
- Before drug is prescribed, female patient should have had two negative pregnancy tests with a sensitivity of at least 50 mIU/ml. First test should be done within 10 to 14 days before prescribing and second test within 24 hours before prescribing. Pregnancy test also should be done weekly during first 4 weeks of use, then every 4 weeks for patients with regular menses or every 2 weeks for those with irregular menses.
- Give drug with water.
- Store at controlled temperature of 77° F (25° C); excursions are permitted to 59° to 86° F (15° to 30° C).

Adverse reactions

CNS: dizziness, headache, hypoesthesia, peripheral neuropathy, insomnia, depression, rigors, fatigue

CV: hypertension, palpitations

EENT: epistaxis, rhinitis, pharyngitis, nasopharyngitis, sinusitis

GI: diarrhea, constipation, nausea, abdominal pain, vomiting, loose stools, anorexia, dry mouth, dysgeusia

GU: urinary tract infection, dysuria

Hematologic: thrombocytopenia, neutropenia, anemia, leukopenia, febrile neutropenia

Metabolic: hypokalemia, hypomagnesemia, hypothyroidism
Musculoskeletal: arthralgia, back pain, muscle cramp, limb pain, myalgia
Respiratory: cough, dyspnea, exertional dyspnea, bronchitis, upper respiratory tract infection, pneumonia
Skin: pruritus, rash, dry skin, contusion, ecchymosis, erythema
Other: fever, peripheral edema, pain, chest pain, cellulitis, night sweats, increased sweating

Interactions

Drug-diagnostic tests. *Magnesium, potassium, thyroid function tests*: decreased

Toxicity and overdose
• No known cases of overdose have occurred.
• To manage toxicity, reduce dosage sequentially or delay dose. Provide supportive care, including administration of blood products and growth factors, as indicated.

Special considerations
• Monitor CBC weekly for first 8 weeks, and then at least monthly.
• Observe carefully for signs and symptoms of thromboembolism.
• Patient must be able to reliably follow instructions to take drug and must be informed about conditions of RevAssist program.

Patient education
• Instruct patient to swallow capsules whole with water and not to open, chew, or crush them.
• Urge patient to seek immediate medical attention for shortness of breath, chest pain, or arm or leg swelling.
• Inform patient that burning may occur with first urination.
• Urge female patient to use two effective contraceptive methods simultaneously for at least 4 weeks before starting therapy, during therapy, during dosage interruptions, and for 4 weeks after therapy ends. Emphasize that she

must use contraception even if she has a history of infertility (unless she has had a hysterectomy).
• Instruct female patient to stop taking drug and notify prescriber if she misses a period, has unusual menstrual bleeding, suspects pregnancy, or stops using contraception.
• Advise patient to immediately report unprotected sexual contact or suspected pregnancy.
• Instruct male patient to use latex condom during any sexual contact with female of childbearing potential.
• Inform patients that they cannot donate blood during therapy.
• Advise male patients that they cannot donate sperm or semen during therapy.

letrozole
Femara

Classification: Antineoplastic, aromatase inhibitor
Pregnancy risk category D

Pharmacology
Letrozole inhibits conversion of androgens to estrogens through nonsteroidal competitive inhibition of aromatase enzyme system. This action reduces estrogen biosyntheses and decreases serum estrone, estradiol, and estrone sulfate, causing regression of estrogen-dependent tumors. Drug does not affect adrenocorticosteroid, aldosterone, or thyroid hormone synthesis.

Pharmacokinetics
Drug is absorbed from GI tract rapidly and completely; food does not affect absorption. It is metabolized slowly to inactive carbinol by CYP3A4 and CYP2A6, and shows weak protein-binding. It strongly inhibits CYP2A6 and moderately inhibits CYP2C19. Drug's metabolite (whose glucuronide conjugate is excreted renally) represents major clearance pathway.

About 90% of radiolabeled letrozole is recovered in urine.

How supplied
Tablets: 2.5 mg

Indications and dosages

FDA-APPROVED

➡ First-line treatment of hormone-receptor-positive or hormone-receptor-unknown locally advanced or metastatic breast cancer in postmenopausal women; treatment of advanced breast cancer in postmenopausal women with disease progression after anti-estrogen therapy; adjuvant treatment of postmenopausal women with hormone-receptor-positive early breast cancer; extended adjuvant treatment of early breast cancer in postmenopausal women who have received 5 years of adjuvant tamoxifen therapy
Adults: 2.5-mg tablet P.O. once daily without regard to meals

OFF-LABEL USES (SELECTED)

➡ Prevention of recurrence of early-stage breast cancer and prevention of new breast cancer (based on studies using anastrozole)
Adults: 2.5-mg tablet P.O. once daily

DOSAGE MODIFICATIONS

• In patients with cirrhosis or severe hepatic impairment, dosage should be reduced to 50% of usual dosage (2.5 mg every other day).
• Dosage reduction is recommended in patients with creatinine clearance of 10 ml/minute or less.

Contraindications and precautions
Contraindicated in hypersensitivity to drug or its components.
Use cautiously in hepatic and renal impairment, pregnancy, and breastfeeding. Safety and efficacy in *children* have not been established.

Preparation and administration
• Follow hazardous drug guidelines for handling, preparation, and administration. (See "Managing hazardous drugs," page 11.)
• Give drug without regard to meals.
• Continue therapy until tumor progression occurs.
• Store drug at 77° F (25° C); excursions are permitted from 59° to 86° F (15° to 30° C).

Adverse reactions
CNS: headache, insomnia, lethargy
GI: nausea, vomiting, anorexia, constipation, diarrhea
Hepatic: hepatotoxicity
Musculoskeletal: bone pain, back pain, arthralgia
Respiratory: dyspnea, cough
Skin: rash, pruritus
Other: hot flashes

Interactions
Drug-drug. *Tamoxifen:* 38% decrease in letrozole level
Drug-diagnostic tests. *Lymphocytes:* moderately decreased
Drug-food. *Grapefruit, pomegranates:* possible increased letrozole level
Drug-herb. *Alpha-lipoic acid, coenzyme Q10:* possible decreased chemotherapy efficacy
Cat's claw, echinacea, eucalyptus, feverfew, kava, licorice, peppermint oil, valerian: possible increased letrozole level
Glutamine: possible enhanced tumor growth

Toxicity and overdose
• No serious adverse events have been reported with overdose. In single-dose studies, highest dosage used (30 mg) was well tolerated; in multiple-dose trials, highest dosage of 10 mg was well tolerated.
• No firm recommendations exist for treatment of overdose. Induce emesis if patient is alert; provide supportive care and monitor vital signs frequently.

L

Special considerations

- Patients do not require glucocorticoid or mineralocorticoid replacement during therapy.
- Monitor hepatic and renal function.

Patient education

- Instruct patient to avoid driving and other hazardous activities during therapy because drug may cause dizziness and drowsiness.
- Advise patient to notify prescriber if she experiences yellowing of skin or eyes, respiratory difficulty, or other new symptoms.
- If pregnant patient is exposed to drug, inform her that drug may harm fetus and increase risk of pregnancy loss.

leucovorin calcium (citrovorum factor, folinic acid)

Classification: Antidote, vitamin
Pregnancy risk category C

Pharmacology

Leucovorin, a folic acid derivative, inhibits dihydrofolate reductase and counteracts therapeutic and toxic effects of folic acid antagonists (such as methotrexate). It enhances therapeutic and toxic effects of fluoropyrimidines used in cancer therapy, such as 5-fluorouracil (5-FU). It also stabilizes binding of fluorodeoxyuridylic acid to thymidylate synthase, increasing inhibition of this enzyme.

Pharmacokinetics

Drug has excellent bioavailability when given orally or parenterally. It is metabolized to its active metabolite by liver and intestinal mucosa. With oral use, absorption is rapid, onset occurs in 20 to 30 minutes, drug levels peak in 1.7 hours, and duration is 3 to 6 hours. With I.V. use, onset is less than 5 minutes and duration is 3 to 6 hours. With I.M. use, onset is 10 to 20 minutes, levels peak in 35 to 60 minutes, and duration is 3 to 6 hours. Drug is

eliminated in urine (80% to 90%) and feces (5% to 8%).

How supplied

Powder for injection: 50 mg/vial, 100 mg/vial, 350 mg/vial
Tablets: 5 mg, 10 mg, 15 mg, 25 mg

Indications and dosages

FDA-APPROVED

To prolong survival in palliative treatment of patients with advanced colorectal cancer (given with 5-FU)
Adults: May use either of two regimens. In one regimen, leucovorin is given as 200 mg/m^2 I.V. over at least 3 minutes, followed by 5-FU 370 mg/m^2 I.V; drugs are given daily for 5 days and repeated at 28-day intervals for two courses and then repeated at 28 to 35 days if patient has recovered from toxicity. Dosage of 5-FU is adjusted based on hematologic or GI toxicity.

In alternative regimen, leucovorin is given as 20 mg/m^2 I.V., followed by 5-FU 425 mg/m^2 I.V; drugs are given daily for 5 days and repeated at 28-day intervals for two courses and then repeated at 28 to 35 days if patient has recovered from toxicity. Dosage of 5-FU is adjusted based on hematologic or GI toxicity.

Leucovorin rescue after high-dose methotrexate therapy
Adults: Recommendations are based on methotrexate dosage of 12 to 15 g/m^2 given by I.V. infusion over 4 hours. Leucovorin rescue at 15 mg (about 10 mg/m^2) every 6 hours for 10 doses starts 24 hours after methotrexate infusion begins.

Impaired methotrexate elimination or inadvertent overdose
Adults: Begin leucovorin rescue promptly after inadvertent overdose and within 24 hours of methotrexate administration if excretion is delayed. Give leucovorin 10 mg/m^2 I.V., I.M., or P.O. every 6 hours until serum methotrexate level drops below 10^{-8} M. In GI toxicity, nausea, or vomiting, administer parenterally.

Only common or life-threatening adverse reactions are listed.

Obtain serum creatinine and methotrexate levels at 24-hour intervals. If 24-hour creatinine level rises 50% over baseline, 24-hour methotrexate level exceeds 5×10^{-6} M, or 48-hour methotrexate level exceeds 9×10^{-7} M, increase leucovorin dosage to 100 mg/m^2 I.V. every 3 hours until methotrexate level falls below 10^{-8} M. Maintain urine pH at 7 or above with hydration (3 L/day) and sodium bicarbonate solution.

DOSAGE MODIFICATIONS

• Leucovorin dosage does not need to be adjusted for 5-FU toxicity.
• Adjust leucovorin dosage or extend leucovorin rescue based on table below.

Guidelines for adjusting leucovorin dosage		
Clinical situation	Laboratory findings	Leucovorin dosage and duration
Normal methotrexate elimination	Serum methotrexate level approximately 10 µmol at 24 hours after administration, 1 µmol at 48 hours, and less than 0.2 µmol at 72 hours	15 mg P.O., I.M., or I.V. every 6 hours for 60 hours (10 doses starting 24 hours after methotrexate infusion begins)
Delayed late methotrexate elimination	Serum methotrexate level remaining above 0.2 µmol at 72 hours, and more than 0.05 µmol at 96 hours after administration	Continue 15 mg P.O., I.M., or I.V. every 6 hours until methotrexate level is below 0.05 µmol.
Delayed early methotrexate elimination and/or evidence of acute renal injury	Serum methotrexate level of 50 µmol or more at 24 hours, or 5 µmol or more at 48 hours after administration; or 100% or greater increase in serum creatinine level 24 hours after methotrexate administration (such as increase from 0.5 mg/dl to 1 mg/dl or more)	150 mg I.V. every 3 hours until methotrexate level is below 1 µmol; then 15 mg I.V. every 3 hours until methotrexate level is below 0.05 µmol

Contraindications and precautions

Contraindicated for intrathecal use and in pernicious anemia and other megaloblastic anemias secondary to lack of vitamin B_{12}.

Use cautiously in patients with GI symptoms, pregnancy, breastfeeding, *elderly* or debilitated patients, and *children.*

Preparation and administration

• Before each treatment, obtain CBC with differential and platelet count in patients treated with leucovorin/5-FU combination. During first two courses, repeat CBC with differential and platelet count weekly and thereafter once each cycle at time of anticipated WBC nadir. Obtain electrolyte levels and liver function tests before each treatment for first three cycles, and then before every other cycle.
• Do not administer drug intrathecally; doing so may be harmful or even fatal.
• Because leucovorin increases 5-FU toxicity, leucovorin and 5-FU combination therapy for advanced colorectal cancer should be given under supervision of physician experienced in use of antimetabolite cancer chemotherapy.
• Give I.V. leucovorin promptly when treating accidental methotrexate overdose. Monitor methotrexate level to determine leucovorin dosage and duration.
• Hydrate patient (3 L/day) and use sodium bicarbonate to alkalize urine when treating impaired methotrexate elimination or inadvertent overdose.
• Do not use oral doses above 25 mg because leucovorin absorption is saturable. Give drug I.V. if dosage exceeds that recommended for oral use.
• Defer treatment until WBC count rises to 4,000/mm^3 and platelet count rises to 130,000/mm^3. If counts do not reach these levels within 2 weeks, stop treatment. Follow patient with physical examination before each treatment course; arrange for appropriate radiologic examination as needed. Stop treatment if tumor progresses.
• Parenteral administration is preferable to

L

oral dosing if there is a chance that patient may vomit or not absorb drug.

- Do not mix in same infusion as 5-FU; precipitate may form.
- Dilute each 50-, 100-, and 350-mg vial to 10- to 20-mg/ml solution. For total doses less than 10 mg/m², dilute with bacteriostatic water for injection (contains benzyl alcohol as preservative). When giving doses above 10 mg/m², dilute with sterile water for injection and use immediately. Dilute further with 100 to 500 ml D_5W, $D_{10}W$, normal saline solution, Ringer's solution, or lactated Ringer's solution.
- Infuse slowly. Because of drug's calcium content, inject no more than 160 mg I.V. per minute (16 ml of 10-mg/ml or 8 ml of 20-mg/ml solution per minute).
- Store tablets at 59° to 77° F (15° to 25° C). Protect from light and moisture.
- Store dry powder and reconstituted solution for injection at controlled temperature of 59° to 86° F (15° to 30° C).

Adverse reactions
Respiratory: wheezing
Other: anaphylaxis

Interactions
Drug-drug. *5-FU:* increased 5-FU toxicity
Methotrexate: possible reduced efficacy of intrathecal methotrexate
Phenobarbital, phenytoin, primidone: possible counteraction of antiepileptic effect of these drugs; increased frequency of seizures in susceptible children
Trimethoprim-sulfamethoxazole: increased rates of *Pneumocystis carinii* pneumonia treatment failure and morbidity in HIV patients
Drug-herb. *Alpha-lipoic acid, coenzyme Q10:* possible decreased chemotherapy efficacy
Glutamine: possible enhanced tumor growth

Toxicity and overdose
- Excessive drug amounts may nullify chemotherapeutic effect of folic acid antagonists.
- No specific treatment for toxicity is indicated. Treat supportively.

Special considerations
- Monitor serum methotrexate levels to determine optimal dosage and duration of leucovorin treatment.
- Do not start or continue therapy with leucovorin and 5-FU in patients with symptoms of GI toxicity of any severity, until these resolve. Monitor patient with diarrhea until it resolves because rapid clinical deterioration and death can occur. In study using higher weekly leucovorin and 5-FU doses, elderly and debilitated patients were at greater risk for severe GI toxicity.

Patient education
- Advise patient to notify prescriber at once if hypersensitivity reactions occur.
- Emphasize importance of staying well hydrated during therapy.

leuprolide acetate
Eligard, Lupron, Lupron Depot, Viadur

Classification: Antineoplastic, hormone/hormone modifier, gonadotropin-releasing hormone (GnRH) analogue
Pregnancy risk category X

Pharmacology
Leuprolide, a luteinizing hormone-releasing hormone (LHRH) agonist, inhibits gonadotropin secretion when given continuously at therapeutic doses. It reversibly suppresses ovarian and testicular steroidogenesis, reduces testosterone to castrate levels in men, and reduces estrogens to postmenopausal levels in premenopausal women. It also inhibits growth of certain hormone-dependent tumors.

Pharmacokinetics
Drug is bioavailable only when given parenterally. Depot form is absorbed slowly over days; injectable solution, over several hours. Injectable solution has plasma half-life of about 3 hours.

Only common or life-threatening adverse reactions are listed.

How supplied

Leuprolide acetate depot, 1-month: 3.75-mg, 7.5-mg, and 11.25-mg single-dose vials with diluent
Leuprolide acetate depot, 3-month: 11.25-mg and 22.5-mg single-dose vials with diluent
Leuprolide acetate depot, 4-month: 30-mg single-dose vial with diluent
Leuprolide acetate for injection: 5 mg/ml multidose vial
Leuprolide acetate implant: 72 mg (65 mg free base)

Indications and dosages

FDA-APPROVED

➟ Advanced prostate cancer
Adults: Injection—1 mg daily subcutaneously. *Depot*—7.5 mg I.M. monthly, 22.5 mg I.M. every 3 months, or 30 mg I.M. every 4 months. *Implant*—72 mg subcutaneously once yearly.

OFF-LABEL USES (SELECTED)

➟ Treatment of breast cancer
Adults: Two dosage schedules are 3.75 mg I.M. every 4 weeks and 11.25 mg I.M. every 3 months.
➟ Treatment of endometrial cancer
Adults: One dosage schedule is 7.5 mg I.M. every 28 days.
➟ Treatment of ovarian cancer
Adults: Currently being studied; for dosage information, consult medical literature.

Contraindications and precautions

Contraindicated in hypersensitivity to GnRH, GnRH agonist analogues, or any excipient; undiagnosed abnormal vaginal bleeding; pregnancy; women with childbearing potential; and breastfeeding. Safety and efficacy of implant in *children* have not been established.

Use cautiously in known allergy to benzyl alcohol and in renal impairment.

Preparation and administration

• Follow hazardous drug guidelines for handling, preparation, and administration. (See "Managing hazardous drugs," page 11.)
• Patients with known allergies to benzyl alcohol (contained in drug's vehicle) may experience symptoms of hypersensitivity (usually local), such as erythema and induration at injection site.
• Use syringe and diluent supplied. If alternative syringe is needed, use insulin syringe.
• Shake vial well to achieve uniform suspension. Withdraw entire contents of single-use vial into syringe and inject immediately.
• Depot form does not contain preservative.
• Store below 77° F (25° C). Protect from light and freezing.

Adverse reactions

CNS: memory impairment, depression, spinal cord compression
CV: arrhythmias, heart failure, peripheral edema, hypertension, deep thrombophlebitis
GI: nausea, vomiting
GU: vaginal bleeding, breast tenderness, erectile dysfunction, decreased libido, ureteral obstruction
Hematologic: thrombocytopenia, thrombotic disorder
Musculoskeletal: bone pain
Respiratory: pulmonary embolism, dyspnea
Skin: alopecia
Other: anaphylaxis, hot flashes

Interactions

Drug-diagnostic tests. *Pituitary gonadotropin and gonadal function tests:* misleading results (depot suspension)

Toxicity and overdose

• In early clinical trials, dosages up to 20 mg daily for as long as 2 years caused no adverse effects other than those seen with 1-mg daily dosage.
• Treat symptomatically, if indicated.

Special considerations

• In several cases, preexisting hematuria and urinary tract obstruction temporarily worsened during first week of therapy. Also, a few cases of temporary weakness and paresthesia of lower limbs have been reported. Potential exacerbation of signs and symptoms during first few weeks of therapy is cause for concern in patients with vertebral metastases or urinary obstruction, because neurologic problems or increased urinary obstruction could occur. During first weeks of therapy, closely observe these patients.

• With implant, serum testosterone level increases transiently during first week. Patient may experience new or worsening symptoms, including bone pain, neuropathy, hematuria, or ureteral or bladder outlet obstruction.

• Bone density loss may be irreversible for 6 months or more. In patients with major risk factors for decreased bone mineral content (such as chronic alcohol or tobacco use, strong family history of osteoporosis, or chronic use of drugs that can reduce bone mass), depot may pose additional risk. In these patients, carefully weigh drug's risks against benefits.

• In patients with prostate cancer, monitor response by measuring serum testosterone and acid phosphatase levels.

• Monitor response 1 to 2 months after therapy begins with GnRH stimulation test and sex steroid levels.

• In therapeutic dosages, depot suppresses pituitary-gonadal system. Normal function usually resumes within 1 to 3 months after treatment ends.

• Diagnostic tests of pituitary gonadotropic and gonadal functions may be misleading during therapy and for up to 1 to 2 months afterward.

• When used monthly at recommended dosage, depot usually inhibits ovulation and stops menstruation. However, depot use does not ensure contraception.

• Magnetic resonance imaging does not affect implant's titanium alloy reservoir.

Patient education

• Inform patient that drug may cause or increase bone pain and may lead to difficulty urinating in first few weeks.

• Inform women with childbearing potential that drug may harm fetus. Urge them to use nonhormonal contraception during therapy and to seek medical advice for suspected pregnancy. If patient becomes pregnant during therapy, tell her to stop drug and contact prescriber.

• Tell female patient that menses or spotting may occur during first 2 months of therapy. Instruct her to notify physician if bleeding persists beyond second month.

levorphanol tartrate
Levo-Dromoran

Classification: Analgesic, opioid
Controlled substance schedule II
Pregnancy risk category C

Pharmacology

Levorphanol, an opioid agonist with activity at mu and kappa opioid receptors, inhibits release of pain neurotransmitters (including acetylcholine and dopamine). It produces analgesia at least equal to that of morphine and exceeding that of meperidine when used at far smaller doses.

Pharmacokinetics

Drug is metabolized in liver. Onset occurs in 30 to 90 minutes; drug levels peak in 30 to 60 minutes (depending on administration route). Duration is 6 to 8 hours; half-life, 11 to 16 hours. Drug is excreted in urine.

How supplied

Tablets: 2 mg

Indications and dosages

FDA-approved

➡ Moderate to severe pain
Adults: 2 mg P.O.every 6 to 8 hours (unless hypoventilation or excessive sedation occurs).

Only common or life-threatening adverse reactions are listed.

Increase to 3 mg every 6 to 8 hours if needed. Higher dosages may be appropriate for opioid-tolerant patients. Total daily dosage exceeding 12 mg is not recommended as starting dosage in opioid-intolerant patients.

DOSAGE MODIFICATIONS

• Decrease dosage in hepatic or renal insufficiency, Addison's disease, or hypothyroidism.
• Reduce dosage by at least 50% in patients who have respiratory disease and in those receiving drugs that may depress respiratory function. Adjust subsequent dosages according to response.
• Decrease dosage by at least 50% in elderly patients.
• Adjust dosage based on pain severity, age, weight, physical status, comorbidities, concomitant drugs, and other pertinent factors.

Contraindications and precautions

Contraindicated in opioid hypersensitivity, acute or severe bronchial asthma, upper airway obstruction, respiratory depression, anoxia, increased intracranial pressure, and acute alcoholism.

Use cautiously in cardiovascular, renal, or hepatic disease; pregnancy; breastfeeding; and *elderly* patients. Drug is not recommended for *children younger than age 18.*

Preparation and administration

• To counteract opioid-induced respiratory depression, keep opioid antagonist (such as naloxone) readily available when administering drug.
• When converting from P.O. morphine to P.O. levorphanol, start with total daily dosage of roughly one-fifteenth to one-twelfth of patient's total daily morphine dosage, and then adjust. Allow about 72 hours before making dosage changes if patient is on fixed-dose schedule.
• Keep patient supine immediately after administration to reduce risk of orthostatic hypotension, syncope, and other adverse effects.

• Store in tightly closed container at controlled temperature, protected from light.

Adverse reactions

CNS: dizziness, drowsiness, light-headedness, euphoria, sedation, confusion
CV: fainting, syncope, bradycardia, shock, peripheral circulatory collapse, cardiac arrest, vasodilation, orthostatic hypotension
EENT: blurred vision, miosis, diplopia
GI: nausea, vomiting, constipation, anorexia, dry mouth, cramps
GU: oliguria, urinary urgency or hesitancy, reduced libido
Hepatic: biliary tract spasm
Respiratory: respiratory depression, respiratory arrest
Skin: diaphoresis, pruritus
Other: physical or psychological dependence

Interactions

Drug-drug. *Agonist-antagonist analgesics (such as buprenorphine, butorphanol, dezocine, nalbuphine, pentazocine):* possible precipitation of withdrawal symptoms
Alfentanil, fentanyl, sufentanil, other CNS depressants: increased CNS and respiratory depression, increased risk of hypotension
Anticholinergics: increased risk of severe constipation
Antidiarrheals (such as atropine, difenoxin, kaolin, loperamide), antihypertensives: increased risk of hypotension
Metoclopramide: antagonism of metoclopramide's effects
Neuromuscular blockers: increased risk of prolonged CNS and respiratory depression
Drug-diagnostic tests. *Amylase, lipase:* increased
Drug-herb: *Ginkgo, thuja:* possible decreased seizure threshold
Gotu kola, kava, St. John's wort, valerian: possible additive sedation

Toxicity and overdose

• Serious overdose causes miosis, cold and clammy skin, respiratory depression, hypo-

tension, bradycardia, skeletal muscle flaccidity, pulmonary, and extreme somnolence progressing to stupor or coma. With less severe overdose, CNS depression, miosis, and respiratory depression may occur.
• For initial management, establish secure airway and support ventilation and perfusion. Monitor heart filling pressures; noncardiac pulmonary edema occurs in about 40% of patients. Evacuate stomach by emesis or gastric lavage if treatment can begin within 2 hours after ingestion. Naloxone may be used to antagonize opioid effects, but airway must be secured because vomiting may occur. Avoid giving narcotic antagonist to physically dependent patients, if possible; if antagonist must be used to treat serious respiratory depression, administer it with extreme care and titrate with smaller-than-usual dosages. Do not give antagonist in absence of clinically significant respiratory or cardiovascular depression. Administer I.V. fluids and vasopressors for hypotension, as indicated. Atropine may be useful for treatment of bradycardia. Forced diuresis, peritoneal dialysis, hemodialysis, and charcoal hemoperfusion have not proven beneficial.

Special considerations
• Monitor CNS and respiratory status frequently.
• Monitor renal function regularly.
• Prescribe and administer drug with same degree of caution as for morphine. Like other opioids, drug is subject to federal narcotics laws.
• Drug may obscure accurate diagnosis or clinical course in patients with acute abdominal conditions.

Patient education
• Instruct patient to avoid other CNS depressants (such as tranquilizers, sleeping pills, and alcohol).
• Advise patient to use caution when driving or performing other hazardous tasks because drug may cause drowsiness or dizziness.

• Tell patient to take drug exactly as prescribed.
• Caution patient not to use herbal remedies without consulting prescriber.
• Inform patient that drug may cause psychological and physical dependence. Advise patient to consult prescriber before increasing dosage or stopping drug abruptly.
• Advise patient to notify physician if pregnancy occurs, to discuss drug withdrawal.
• Provide counseling to help breastfeeding patient decide whether to discontinue breastfeeding or stop drug.

lomustine
CeeNU

Classification: Antineoplastic, alkylating agent, nitrosourea
Pregnancy risk category D

Pharmacology
Lomustine exerts cytotoxic action by alkylating DNA and RNA. It also may inhibit or modify several key enzymatic processes, including protein synthesis, RNA synthesis, messenger RNA processing, and DNA synthesis. It is cell cycle-nonspecific.

Pharmacokinetics
Drug is absorbed completely after oral administration and is metabolized extensively in liver to active metabolites. It is distributed widely (including cerebrospinal fluid). Serum half-life of metabolites ranges from 16 hours to 2 days. Metabolites are excreted in urine.

How supplied
Capsules: 10 mg, 40 mg, 100 mg
Dose pack: two 10-mg capsules, two 40-mg capsules, two 100-mg capsules

---

Only common or life-threatening adverse reactions are listed.

Indications and dosages

FDA-APPROVED

➥ Brain tumors (both primary and metastatic) in patients who have undergone appropriate surgical or radiotherapeutic procedures; secondary therapy with other approved drugs in patients with Hodgkin's disease who relapse during primary therapy or fail to respond to primary therapy

Adults and children: As single agent in previously untreated patients, 130 mg/m² P.O. as a single dose every 6 weeks. Do not give repeat course of capsules until circulating blood elements return to acceptable levels (platelet count above 100,000/mm³ and WBC count above 4,000/mm³), which usually occurs in 6 weeks. Peripheral blood smear should show adequate number of neutrophils.

OFF-LABEL USES (SELECTED)

➥ Melanoma, multiple myeloma, breast cancer, non-small-cell lung cancer, colorectal cancer

Adults: One dosage schedule is 100 mg/m² P.O. every 6 weeks.

➥ Non-Hodgkin's lymphoma

Adults: One regimen includes lomustine 60 mg/m² P.O. on day 1, ifosfamide 1.5 g/m² I.V. on days 1, 2 and 21, 22; bleomycin 5 mg/m² I.V. on days 1, 5 and 21, 25; vincristine 1.4 mg/m² I.V. on days 1, 8 and 21, 28; and cisplatin 25 mg/m² I.V. on days 3, 4, 5 and 23, 24, 25, every 42 days (CIBO-P regimen).

➥ Kidney cancer

Adults: One regimen includes lomustine 130 mg/m² P.O. every 6 weeks with vinblastine 5 to 10 mg/m² I.V. weekly.

➥ Mycosis fungoides

Adults: Lomustine has been compounded in various strengths and administered topically.

DOSAGE MODIFICATIONS

• In compromised bone marrow function, reduce dosage to 100 mg/m² every 6 weeks.
• Evaluate drug benefits against risks of toxic effects or adverse reactions. Most adverse reactions are reversible if detected early; if they occur, either reduce dosage or stop drug and take corrective measures. Reinstitute therapy with caution, considering patient's further need for drug; if reinstituting, stay alert for possible recurrence of toxicity.

• When giving capsules with other myelosuppressants, adjust dosage accordingly.
• After initial dose, adjust subsequent dosages based on hematologic response to preceding dose, as shown in the following table.

Nadir after previous dose

WBCs/mm³	Platelets/mm³	Percentage of previous dose to be given
Above 4,000	Above 100,000	100%
3,000 to 3,999	75,001 to 99,999	100%
2,000 to 2,999	25,000 to 74,999	70%
Below 2,000	Below 25,000	50%

⊠ WARNINGS

• Capsules should be given under supervision of qualified physician experienced in use of cancer chemotherapeutic agents.
• Most common and severe toxic effect is bone marrow depression—most notably thrombocytopenia and leukopenia, which may contribute to bleeding and overwhelming infections in already compromised patient.
• To detect delayed bone marrow depression, blood counts should be monitored weekly for at least 6 weeks after therapy. At recommended dosage, courses should not be given more often than every 6 weeks.
• Because bone marrow toxicity is cumulative, dosage adjustment must be considered on basis of nadir blood counts from previous dose.

Contraindications and precautions

Contraindicated in hypersensitivity to drug or its components.

Use cautiously in bone marrow depression, respiratory disorders, pregnancy, or breast-feeding. Select dosage carefully in *elderly patients* because drug is excreted substantially by kidneys. Use cautiously in *children*; delayed-onset pulmonary fibrosis may occur years after therapy or in patients who received related nitrosoureas in childhood and early adolescence.

Preparation and administration

≫ Follow hazardous drug guidelines for handling, preparation, and administration. (See "Managing hazardous drugs," page 11.)
• Obtain CBC and platelet counts before starting therapy.
• Give drug on empty stomach, preferably 2 to 4 hours after meal.
• Administer antiemetics as needed.
• Store at room temperature in well-closed container. Avoid exposure to temperatures above 104° F (40° C).

Adverse reactions

CNS: lethargy
GI: nausea, vomiting, anorexia, stomatitis, GI bleeding
GU: azotemia, nephrotoxicity, infertility
Hematologic: thrombocytopenia, leukopenia, myelosuppression, anemia
Hepatic: hepatotoxicity
Respiratory: pulmonary fibrosis, pulmonary infiltrate
Skin: alopecia
Other: secondary cancers

Interactions

Drug-drug. *Anticoagulants, nonsteroidal anti-inflammatory drugs:* increased risk of bleeding
Myelosuppressants: increased bone marrow depression
Drug-diagnostic tests. *BUN, creatinine, liver function tests, nitrogenous compounds:* increased
Hemoglobin, platelets, RBCs, WBCs: decreased

Drug-herb. *Alpha-lipoic acid, coenzyme Q10:* possible decreased chemotherapy efficacy
Glutamine: possible enhanced tumor growth

Toxicity and overdose

• Anticipated signs and symptoms of overdose are those of adverse reactions.
• No proven antidotes have been established. Treat supportively, as indicated.

Special considerations

• Myelosuppression usually occurs 4 to 6 weeks after therapy ends and is dose-related. Thrombocytopenia occurs about 4 weeks after therapy and lasts 1 to 2 weeks. Leukopenia arises 5 to 6 weeks after therapy and lasts 1 to 2 weeks. Cumulative myelosuppression may occur.
• Monitor blood counts weekly. Do not give repeat courses before 6 weeks because hematologic toxicity is delayed and cumulative.
• Although rare, pulmonary toxicity may occur with capsule use and appears to be dose-related. Onset may occur 6 months or more after drug initiation and with cumulative doses above 1,100 mg/m^2. Perform baseline pulmonary function studies, and repeat these frequently during treatment. At-risk patients are those with baseline below 70% of predicted forced vital capacity or carbon monoxide diffusing capacity.
• Monitor liver and renal function tests periodically.

Patient education

• Inform patient that capsules are given as single oral dose and will not be repeated for at least 6 weeks.
• Tell patient that nausea and vomiting usually last less than 24 hours, although appetite loss may last several days.
• Instruct patient to report signs and symptoms of serious adverse reactions, such as fever, chills, sore throat, unusual bleeding or bruising, shortness of breath, dry cough, swelling of feet or lower legs, mental confusion, and yellowing of eyes and skin.

Only common or life-threatening adverse reactions are listed.

• Advise women with childbearing potential to avoid pregnancy.
• Provide guidance to help breastfeeding patient decide whether to discontinue breastfeeding or stop drug.

loperamide hydrochloride
Imodium, Imodium A-D, Kaopectate II, Pepto Diarrhea Control

Classification: Antidiarrheal
Pregnancy risk category B

Pharmacology
Loperamide inhibits peristaltic activity by direct effect on circular and longitudinal muscles of intestinal wall. It prolongs intestinal transit time, reduces daily fecal volume, increases viscosity and bulk density, and diminishes fluid and electrolyte loss.

Pharmacokinetics
Drug is about 40% absorbed. It is metabolized in liver. Onset is 1 hour, peak is 2.5 to 5 hours, and half-life is approximately 10 hours. Drug is excreted primarily in feces, with small amount excreted in urine.

How supplied
Capsules: 2 mg
Solution: 1 mg/5 ml
Tablets: 2 mg

Indications and dosages

FDA-APPROVED

➥ Acute diarrhea
Adults: Initially, 4 mg P.O., followed by 2 mg after each unformed stool. Daily dosage should not exceed 16 mg. Clinical improvement usually occurs within 48 hours.
Children ages 8 to 12 weighing more than 30 kg (66 lb): 2 mg three times daily (6 mg/ 24 hours)

Children ages 6 to 8 weighing 20 to 30 kg (44 to 66 lb): 2 mg twice daily (4 mg/24 hours)
Children ages 2 to 5 weighing 13 to 20 kg (29 to 44 lb): 1 mg three times daily (3 mg/ 24 hours)
Note: In children ages 2 to 5 who weigh 20 kg or less, use nonprescription liquid form (loperamide 1 mg/5 ml). In children ages 6 to 12, either capsules or loperamide liquid may be used. After first treatment day, give subsequent doses (1 mg/10 kg) only after loose stool. Total daily dosage should not exceed recommended first-day dosage.

DOSAGE MODIFICATIONS

• Reduce dosage in children based on nutritional and dehydration status.

Contraindications and precautions
Contraindicated in hypersensitivity to drug, acute dysentery, and when constipation must be avoided.

Use cautiously in acute ulcerative colitis, concomitant use of drugs that inhibit intestinal motility, pseudomembranous colitis associated with broad-spectrum antibiotics, and pregnancy or breastfeeding. Use with extreme caution in young *children* because of their greater response variability. Dehydration (especially in younger children) may further affect child's response. Drug is not recommended in *children younger than age 2.*

Preparation and administration
• Stop drug promptly if abdominal distention, constipation, or ileus occurs.
• In acute diarrhea, stop drug if clinical improvement does not occur in 48 hours.
• Store drug at 59° to 77° F (15° to 25° C).

Adverse reactions
CNS: dizziness, somnolence, fatigue
GI: nausea, vomiting, dry mouth, constipation, abdominal pain
Other: hypersensitivity reaction

Interactions

Drug-drug. *Antidepressants, antihistamines, other anticholinergics:* additive anticholinergic effects

CNS depressants (including antihistamines, opioid analgesics, sedative-hypnotics): additive CNS effects

Drug-herb. *Angel's trumpet, belladonna:* increased anticholinergic effects

Chamomile, gotu kola, hops, kava, skullcap, St. John's wort, valerian: increased CNS effects

Toxicity and overdose

• Overdose may cause paralytic ileus and CNS depression.
• If vomiting occurs spontaneously after ingestion, administer slurry of 100 g activated charcoal P.O. as soon as patient can retain fluids. If vomiting does not occur, perform gastric lavage; then administer 100 g activated charcoal slurry through gastric tube. Monitor patient for CNS depression for at least 24 hours. If CNS depression occurs, give naloxone and repeat as needed. If patient responds to naloxone, monitor vital signs carefully for recurrence of overdose symptoms for at least 24 hours after last naloxone dose.

Special considerations

• In patients with hepatic dysfunction, monitor closely for signs and symptoms of CNS toxicity.
• Monitor patient closely for abdominal distention and other signs of toxic megacolon.
• Provide appropriate fluid and electrolyte replacement as needed.
• Evaluate number and consistency of bowel movements; monitor cultures as indicated.

Patient education

• Advise patient to contact physician if diarrhea does not improve after 48 hours, blood appears in stool, or fever develops.
• Instruct patient to increase fluid intake to prevent dehydration.
• Caution patient not to exceed prescribed dosage.

• Instruct patient to use caution when driving or performing hazardous activities because drug may cause drowsiness or dizziness.

lorazepam

Ativan, Lorazepam Intensol

Classification: Antianxiety agent, benzodiazepine
Controlled substance schedule IV
Pregnancy risk category D

Pharmacology

Lorazepam depresses CNS by potentiating effects of GABA at benzodiazepine receptor sites and disrupting neurotransmitters.

Pharmacokinetics

Drug is readily absorbed, with absolute bioavailability of 90%. It is metabolized in liver to inactive metabolites and peaks about 2 to 4 hours after dosing. About 85% is plasma protein-bound. Elimination half-life is 10 to 20 hours.

How supplied

Injectable solution: 2 mg/ml, 4 mg/ml
Solution (concentrated): 2 mg/ml
Tablets: 0.5 mg, 1 mg, 2 mg

Indications and dosages

> **FDA-APPROVED**

➡ Anxiety disorders, short-term relief of symptoms of anxiety or anxiety associated with depressive symptoms
Adults: Usual dosage is 2 to 6 mg daily P.O. in divided doses, not to exceed 10 mg daily. (Daily dosage may vary from 1 to 10 mg.)
Elderly adults: 1 to 2 mg daily P.O. in divided doses
Children: 0.05 mg/kg P.O. every 4 to 8 hours

➡ Chemotherapy-induced nausea and vomiting

Adults receiving chemotherapeutic agents with high emetogenic potential (level 5): 0.5 to 2 mg P.O., I.V., or sublingually every 4 to 6 hours on days 1 to 4

Adults receiving chemotherapeutic agents with moderate emetogenic potential (level 3 to 4): 0.5 to 2 mg P.O., I.V., or sublingually every 4 to 6 hours on day 1; may be given at same dosage on days 2 to 4

Adults receiving chemotherapeutic agents with low emetogenic potential (level 2): 0.5 to 2 mg P.O. or I.V. every 4 to 6 hours

Adults receiving emetogenic chemotherapy who experience breakthrough nausea and vomiting: 0.5 to 2 mg P.O. every 4 to 6 hours

• To avoid oversedation in elderly or debilitated patients, do not exceed initial daily dosage of 2 mg, and increase gradually according to patient's response.
• Drug should be tapered gradually; abrupt withdrawal may cause symptoms similar to those for which patient is being treated (such as anxiety, agitation, irritability, tension, insomnia, and occasional seizures).
• Monitor patient and adjust dosage in renal or hepatic impairment.

Contraindications and precautions

Contraindicated in hypersensitivity to benzodiazepines or to any component of formulation and in acute narrow-angle glaucoma.

Use with extreme caution in concurrent use of CNS depressants, *elderly patients,* very ill patients, and patients with limited pulmonary reserve (underventilation or hypoxic cardiac arrest may occur). Use cautiously in hepatic and renal impairment or compromised respiratory function (such as COPD or sleep apnea). Drug is not recommended in patients with primary depression (without adequate antidepressant therapy) or psychoses or in pregnant or breastfeeding patients. Safety and

efficacy in *children younger than age 12* have not been established.

Preparation and administration

• Administer largest dose at bedtime.
• When giving drug I.M., inject undiluted deep into muscle mass.
• Sublingual dose absorbs faster than P.O. dose, with effect comparable to that of I.M. dose.
• Immediately before I.V. administration, dilute injection form with equal volume of compatible solution. Inject directly into vein or tubing of existing I.V. infusion at a rate no faster than 2 mg/minute.
• Injection form can be diluted with sterile water for injection, normal saline solution injection, or D_5W injection.
• Store tablets in tightly closed container at controlled temperature of 59° to 86° F (15° to 30° C).
• Refrigerate solution for injection and protect from light.

L

Adverse reactions

CNS: dizziness, drowsiness, depression, lethargy
CV: orthostatic hypotension, ECG changes, tachycardia, bradycardia, cardiovascular collapse
EENT: blurred vision
GI: constipation, diarrhea, dry mouth
GU: urinary incontinence, urinary retention
Hematologic: blood dyscrasias, leukopenia
Respiratory: apnea
Skin: urticaria, pruritus, rash

Interactions

Drug-drug. *CNS depressants (such as barbiturates, MAO inhibitors, opioid analgesics, phenothiazines, and other antidepressants):* additive CNS effects (including CNS depression)
Hormonal contraceptives: increased lorazepam clearance
Scopolamine: increased sedation, hallucinations, and irrational behavior (injectable form)
Theophylline: decreased lorazepam effect

Drug-diagnostic tests. *ALP, ALT, AST, LDH:* increased
WBCs: decreased
Drug-herb. *Chamomile, gotu kola, kava, St. John's wort, valerian:* increased CNS effects

Toxicity and overdose

• Patients with overdose present with CNS depression ranging from drowsiness to coma. In mild cases, symptoms include drowsiness, mental confusion, and lethargy. In serious cases, patient may experience ataxia, hypotonia, hypotension, hypnosis, and stages 1 to 3 coma; death may occur (although rare).
• Provide supportive treatment until drug is removed from body. Monitor vital signs and fluid balance carefully. Maintain adequate airway, using assisted respiration if needed. With normally functioning kidneys, forced diuresis with I.V. fluids and electrolytes may speed drug elimination. Osmotic diuretics, such as mannitol, may be effective adjunctive measures. In more critical situations, patient may require renal dialysis and exchange blood transfusions. Flumazenil (benzodiazepine-receptor antagonist) is indicated for complete or partial reversal of drug's sedative effects and may be used in overdose; however, it may cause seizures, particularly in long-term lorazepam users and in cyclic antidepressant overdose.

Special considerations

• Drug may cause leukopenia or low-density lipoprotein elevations. Obtain periodic CBC with differential and liver function tests in patients on long-term therapy.
• Monitor vital signs and cardiovascular and respiratory function.
• Esophageal dilation occurred in studies. Although clinical significance is not known, patients should be monitored for signs and symptoms of upper GI disease when drug is used for prolonged periods or in elderly patients.
• Monitor for paradoxical reactions, especially in elderly patients and children.

• Drug efficacy for prolonged periods (more than 4 months) has not been established.
• Prolonged use may cause dependence. Withdrawal may occur after 4 to 6 weeks.

Patient education

• As appropriate, inform patient that drug produces sedation, relieves anxiety, and may cause lack of recall for certain events. Tell patient these effects may last 8 hours.
• Instruct patient to avoid alcohol and other CNS depressants during therapy. Caution him not to consume alcohol for at least 24 to 48 hours after receiving injectable form because of additive CNS depression.
• Advise patient not to drive, operate hazardous machinery, or engage in hazardous sports for 24 to 48 hours after injection.
• To ensure safe and effective use, instruct patient to consult physician before increasing dosage or stopping drug abruptly.
• Advise female patient to notify physician if pregnancy occurs; she may have to stop taking drug.
• Caution breastfeeding patient not to breastfeed during therapy.

mechlorethamine hydrochloride (HN₂, nitrogen mustard)
Mustargen

Classification: Antineoplastic, alkylating agent
Pregnancy risk category D

Pharmacology

Mechlorethamine inhibits rapidly proliferating cells by cross-linking and destroying DNA strands, resulting in cell death.

Pharmacokinetics

Drug is not bioavailable with oral use. With I.V. use, it rapidly deactivates in blood by re-

---

Only common or life-threatening adverse reactions are listed.

action with biomolecules. Drug has no significant organ metabolism. Elimination half-life is 15 minutes. Less than 0.01% of active drug appears in urine; more than 50% of inactive metabolites are excreted in urine within 24 hours.

How supplied
Powder: 10 mg/vial

Indications and dosages

FDA-APPROVED

➡ Palliative treatment of Hodgkin's disease (stages III and IV), lymphosarcoma, chronic myelocytic or chronic lymphocytic leukemia, polycythemia vera, mycosis fungoides, and bronchogenic carcinoma
Adults: Dosage varies with clinical situation, therapeutic response, and magnitude of hematologic depression. Total dosage of 0.4 mg/kg for each course usually is given either as single dose or in divided doses of 0.1 to 0.2 mg/kg daily I.V.
➡ Palliative treatment of metastatic carcinoma resulting in effusion
Adults: For intracavitary injection, usual dosage is 0.4 mg/kg. Dosage of 0.2 mg/kg (or 10 to 20 mg) has been given by intrapericardial route.

OFF-LABEL USES (SELECTED)

➡ Cutaneous T-cell lymphoma
Adults: 10 mg/dl in Aquaphor applied to total skin for a minimum of 6 hours daily

DOSAGE MODIFICATIONS

• Base dosage on ideal dry body weight. Take edema and ascites into account to ensure that dosage is based on actual weight unaugmented by these conditions.

⊠ WARNINGS

• Drug should be administered only under supervision of physician experienced in use of cancer chemotherapeutic agents.

• Drug is highly toxic; both powder and solution must be handled and administered with care. Avoid inhaling dust and vapors and avoid contact with skin, mucous membranes, and eyes. Avoid exposure during pregnancy. Before handling drug, review and follow special handling procedures necessitated by drug's toxic properties.
• Extravasation into subcutaneous tissues causes painful inflammation; affected area usually becomes indurated, and sloughing may occur. If drug leakage occurs, promptly infiltrate area with sterile isotonic sodium thiosulfate (1/6 M), and apply ice compresses for 6 to 12 hours to minimize local reaction. For 1/6 M sodium thiosulfate solution, use 4.14 g sodium thiosulfate per 100 ml sterile water for injection or 2.64 g anhydrous sodium thiosulfate per 100 ml, or dilute 4 ml sodium thiosulfate injection (10%) with 6 ml sterile water for injection.

M

Contraindications and precautions
Contraindicated in active infectious diseases and previous anaphylactic reactions to drug.
    Use cautiously in herpes zoster (do not give during acute phase), widely disseminated neoplasms, mechlorethamine and radiation therapy or other chemotherapy in alternating courses, hyperuricemia, chronic lymphatic leukemia (CLL), concurrent use of other alkylating agents, pregnancy, or breastfeeding. Safety and efficacy in *children* have not been established.

Preparation and administration
≫ Follow hazardous drug guidelines for handling, preparation, and administration. (See "Managing hazardous drugs," page 11.)
• Drug is a powerful vesicant intended mainly for I.V. use.
• Select patients carefully. Before giving drug, obtain accurate histologic diagnosis of patient's disease, knowledge of its natural course, and adequate clinical history; also evaluate

hematologic status. If indication for drug use is unclear, do not administer.

• Use care in dosing; drug has narrow margin of safety.

• Administer at night in case patient requires sedation for adverse effects.

• Administer with antiemetics.

• Concomitant use with sedatives may be beneficial.

• Ensure adequate fluid intake before treatment begins to help control hyperuricemia.

• Using sterile 10-ml syringe, inject 10 ml sterile water for injection or 10 ml sodium chloride injection into vial. With needle still in rubber stopper, shake vial several times to dissolve drug completely. Resulting solution contains 1 mg mechlorethamine per ml.

• To administer I.V., withdraw into syringe the calculated solution volume needed for a single injection. Discard remaining solution after neutralization. Although drug may be injected directly into any suitable vein, injecting it into rubber or plastic tubing of flowing I.V. infusion set is preferable and reduces risk of severe local reactions caused by extravasation or high drug concentration. Also, injecting drug into tubing rather than adding it to entire volume of infusion fluid minimizes chemical reaction between drug and solution.

• Give total dose I.V. over 3 to 5 minutes.

Intracavitary administration

• Technique and dosage for intracavitary route vary.

• To allow drug to more easily contact peritoneal and pleural linings, perform paracentesis first, removing most fluid from pleural or peritoneal cavity. For intrapleural or intrapericardial injection, introduce drug directly through thoracentesis needle. For intraperitoneal injection, administer through rubber catheter inserted into trocar used for paracentesis or through 18G needle inserted at another site. Inject drug slowly, with frequent aspiration to ensure free flow of fluid. Failure to aspirate fluid may cause pain and necrosis (due to injection of solution outside cavity). Free flow of fluid also helps to prevent injection into loculated pocket and to ensure adequate drug dissemination.

• Prepare solution as described for parenteral injection by adding 10 ml sterile water for injection or 10 ml sodium chloride injection to vial containing 10 mg of drug (50 to 100 ml normal saline solution also has been used). After injection, change patient's position every 5 to 10 minutes for 1 hour to obtain more uniform drug distribution throughout serous cavity; remaining fluid may be removed from pleural or peritoneal cavity by paracentesis 24 to 36 hours later. Follow patient carefully with clinical and X-ray examination to detect fluid reaccumulation.

Adverse reactions

CNS: headache, dizziness, drowsiness, paresthesia, coma, depression, weakness
EENT: tinnitus
GI: nausea, vomiting, diarrhea, stomatitis, anorexia
GU: impaired spermatogenesis, azoospermia, germinal aplasia, renal abnormalities
Hematologic: leukopenia, thrombocytopenia, lymphocytopenia, granulocytopenia, agranulocytopenia (rare), persistent pancytopenia, hyperheparinemia
Hepatic: hepatotoxicity, jaundice
Metabolic: hyperuricemia
Skin: alopecia, erythema multiforme
Other: weight loss, anaphylaxis, amyloidosis, secondary cancers

Interactions

Drug-drug. *Other antineoplastics:* bone marrow depression
Drug-diagnostic tests. *Granulocytes, lymphocytes, platelets, RBCs:* decreased
Liver function tests, uric acid: increased

Toxicity and overdose

• Total doses exceeding 0.4 mg/kg for a single course may lead to severe leukopenia, anemia, thrombocytopenia, and hemorrhagic diathesis with subsequent delayed bleeding. Death may result.

Only common or life-threatening adverse reactions are listed.

• Blood product transfusions, antibiotics given for complicating infections, and general supportive measures appear to be the only treatments for overdose.

Special considerations

• Lymphocytopenia usually occurs within 24 hours of administration. Granulocytopenia and thrombocytopenia usually occur 6 to 8 days after dose, and last 10 days to 3 weeks. Agranulocytopenia is rare. Leukopenia generally resolves by 2 weeks.

• Do not give subsequent courses until patient recovers hematologically from previous course, as shown by peripheral blood elements returning to normal levels. In some cases, repeated courses can be given as soon as 3 weeks after previous course.

• Observe precautions when alternating drug courses with radiation therapy or other chemotherapy (which typically depresses hematopoietic function). Do not give drug before or after radiation therapy until bone marrow function recovers. Irradiation of such areas as sternum, ribs, and vertebrae shortly after drug course may cause hematologic complications.

• Give drug with extreme caution to patients with CLL. Drug toxicity (especially sensitivity to bone marrow failure) seems to be more common in CLL patients.

• Bone and nervous tissue tumors respond poorly to drug. Results are unpredictable in disseminated and malignant tumors of different types.

• Drug should not be used routinely in patients with widely disseminated neoplasms.

• Drug has immunosuppressive activity and may predispose patient to bacterial, viral, or fungal infections.

• Hyperuricemia may develop during therapy. Anticipate urate precipitation (particularly in lymphoma patients). Institute adequate methods for controlling hyperuricemia.

• Drug has caused many hepatic and renal abnormalities in patients with neoplastic disease. Evaluate patient's renal and hepatic function frequently.

• Drug may be associated with increased incidence of secondary cancer, especially when given with other antineoplastic agents or radiation therapy.

• Drug has caused extensive and rapid development of amyloidosis.

• Nausea and vomiting typically begin 1 to 3 hours after dose. Vomiting may last 8 hours; nausea, 24 hours. Vomiting may be severe and cause vascular accidents in patients with hemorrhagic tendencies.

• Intracavitary route is indicated for patients with pleural, peritoneal, or pericardial effusion caused by metastatic tumors. Follow patient carefully with clinical and X-ray examinations to detect fluid reaccumulation.

• Pain rarely occurs with intrapleural use, but is common with intraperitoneal injections and often is associated with nausea, vomiting, and diarrhea lasting 2 to 3 days. Transient cardiac irregularities may follow intrapericardial injection.

• Death has been reported after intracavitary administration. Although drug probably is not absorbed completely with intracavitary administration, systemic effect is unpredictable. Acute adverse effects, such as nausea and vomiting, usually are mild. Bone marrow depression generally is milder than with I.V. administration. Avoid intracavitary route when patient is receiving systemic therapy with other agents that may suppress bone marrow function.

Patient education

• Instruct patient to recognize and immediately report signs and symptoms of hypersensitivity.

• Advise patient to report such adverse effects as nausea, vomiting, yellowing of eyes and skin, unusual bruising or bleeding, fever, chills, or sore throat.

• Inform patient that drug may impair fertility.

• Advise women with childbearing potential to avoid pregnancy during therapy because drug can harm fetus.

• Provide guidance to help breastfeeding patient decide whether to discontinue breastfeeding or stop drug.

medroxyprogesterone acetate

Amen, Curretab, Cycrin, Depo-Provera, Provera

Classification: Antineoplastic, hormone, progestin, contraceptive
Pregnancy risk category X

Pharmacology

Medroxyprogesterone, a progesterone derivative, has an unclear mechanism of action. However, it is thought to inhibit growth of progestin-sensitive cancer cells in endometrial and renal tissue.

Pharmacokinetics

Drug has good bioavailability and is metabolized in liver to inactive metabolites. Elimination half-life is up to 60 hours. Parent drug and metabolites are excreted in urine and bile.

How supplied

Injection: 150 mg/ml, 400 mg/ml
Tablets: 2.5 mg, 5 mg, 10 mg

Indications and dosages

FDA-APPROVED

➥ Adjunctive therapy and palliative treatment of inoperable, recurrent, or metastatic endometrial or renal carcinoma
Adults: Initially, 400 to 1,000 mg I.M. weekly; if improvement occurs and disease appears to be stabilized, it may be possible to maintain improvement with as little as 400 mg per month.

OFF-LABEL USES (SELECTED)

➥ Advanced breast cancer

Adults: Typical dosage is 400 mg P.O. daily or 500 mg I.M. daily for 28 days; then 500 mg I.M. twice weekly.

⊠ WARNINGS

• Use during first 4 months of pregnancy is not recommended.
• Starting in first trimester of pregnancy, drug has been used to prevent habitual spontaneous abortion. However, inadequate evidence exists to show that such use is effective when drug is given during first 4 months of pregnancy.
• Several reports suggest a link between intrauterine exposure to progestational drugs in first trimester and genital abnormalities in fetus.
• If patient is exposed to drug during first 4 months of pregnancy or if she becomes pregnant during therapy, she should be informed of potential risks to fetus.

Contraindications and precautions

Contraindicated in hypersensitivity to drug or its components, known or suspected breast carcinoma, active thrombophlebitis, current or history of thromboembolic disorders, cerebrovascular disease, hepatic dysfunction or disease, undiagnosed vaginal bleeding, as a diagnostic test for pregnancy, known or suspected pregnancy, and infants (if product contains benzyl alcohol).

Use cautiously in vision problems, diabetes mellitus, mental depression, and conditions that may be affected by fluid retention. Safety and efficacy in *children* have not been established.

Preparation and administration

• Perform breast and pelvic examination and Papanicolaou test as pretreatment evaluation.
• Inject drug deeply into deltoid or gluteal muscle. Rotate injection sites.
• Be alert to earliest manifestations of thrombotic disorders (thrombophlebitis, cerebrovas-

cular disorder, pulmonary embolism, and retinal thrombosis). Stop drug promptly if these occur or are suspected.

• Stop drug (pending examination) if patient experiences sudden partial or complete vision loss or sudden onset of proptosis, diplopia, or migraine. If examination shows papilledema or retinal vascular lesions, withdraw drug.

• Stop drug if signs or symptoms of hepatic impairment occur.

• Store tablets and injection at controlled temperature of 68° to 77° F (20° to 25° C).

Adverse reactions

CNS: nervousness, insomnia, somnolence
CV: thrombophlebitis, thromboembolism, cerebrovascular accident, myocardial infarction
EENT: papilledema
GI: nausea, cholestatic jaundice
GU: gynecomastia, testicular atrophy, erectile dysfunction, spontaneous abortion, infertility
Respiratory: pulmonary embolism
Skin: pruritus
Other: anaphylaxis, angioedema, hypersensitivity

Interactions

Drug-drug. *Aminoglutethimide:* decreased serum medroxyprogesterone level
Drug-diagnostic tests. *Butanol-extractable protein-bound iodine, protein-bound iodine, liver function tests:* possible increases
Factor II (prothrombin); factors VII, VIII, IX, and X: possible decreases
Gonadotropin, plasma and urinary steroids (such as cortisol, estradiol, pregnanediol, progesterone, testosterone), sex-hormone-binding globulin, triiodothyronine uptake: decreased
Low-density and high-density lipoproteins, total cholesterol, triglycerides: altered

Toxicity and overdose

No information available

Special considerations

• Monitor liver function tests, glucose and thyroid-stimulating hormone levels, and coagulation tests.

• Evaluate patient for signs and symptoms of thrombotic disorders.

• Drug may exacerbate signs and symptoms of depression.

• High doses impair fertility until drug therapy stops.

Patient education

• Inform patient about signs and symptoms of allergic reaction. Have patient repeat these to confirm understanding.

• Instruct patient to immediately report redness, pain, swelling of lower extremities, chest pain, sudden vision changes, or difficulty breathing.

• Advise patient to use caution when driving or performing other hazardous tasks until response to drug is known.

• Inform patient that drug may cause appetite changes, hot flashes, body hair growth, and decreased libido.

• Urge women with childbearing potential to use contraceptives during therapy.

• Tell patient to notify prescriber if she becomes pregnant during therapy.

megestrol acetate
Megace, Megace ES

Classification: Antineoplastic, hormone/hormone modifier, progestin, appetite stimulant
Pregnancy risk category D (tablets); **X** (suspension)

Pharmacology

Megestrol produces antineoplastic action in endometrial carcinoma through an unclear mechanism. Possible factors may include suppression of luteinizing hormone (through suppression of pituitary gonadotrophin production), which decreases estrogen secretion.

Pharmacokinetics

Drug is absorbed in GI tract, metabolized in liver, distributed and stored in fatty tissues, and excreted primarily by kidney.

How supplied

Oral suspension: 40 mg micronized megestrol acetate/ml, 625 mg megestrol acetate/ml
Tablets: 20 mg, 40 mg

Indications and dosages

FDA-APPROVED

➡ Palliative treatment of advanced breast carcinoma (recurrent, inoperable, or metastatic)
Adults: 40 mg P.O. four times daily (tablets) for at least 2 months
➡ Palliative treatment of endometrial carcinoma (recurrent, inoperable, or metastatic)
Adults: 40 to 320 mg P.O. daily (tablets) in divided doses for at least 2 months

OFF-LABEL USES (SELECTED)

➡ Ovarian adenocarcinoma and related gynecologic cancers (high-dose megestrol)
Adults: Typical dosage is 800 mg P.O. daily (tablets) for 1 month, then 400 mg daily (tablets) until disease progresses.
➡ Advanced breast cancer (high-dose megestrol)
Adults: Typical dosage is 800 or 1,600 mg P.O. daily (tablets).
➡ Prostate cancer
Adults: Typical dosage is 120 to 160 mg P.O. daily (tablets).
➡ Cancer-related anorexia and cachexia
Adults: Typical dosage is 800 mg P.O. daily (oral suspension) or 625 mg/ml Megace ES. (Megace 800 mg and Megace ES 625 mg are considered equivalent dosages.)

DOSAGE MODIFICATIONS

• Risk of toxic reactions may be greater in patients with renal impairment. Use care in selecting dosages for elderly patients, who are more likely to have decreased renal function.

⊠ WARNINGS

• Use of tablets during first 4 months of pregnancy is not recommended. If patient is exposed to drug during first 4 months of pregnancy or becomes pregnant during therapy, inform her of potential risks to fetus.

Contraindications and precautions

Contraindicated in hypersensitivity to drug or its components and in known or suspected pregnancy (suspension).

Use cautiously in history of thromboembolic disease, impaired renal function, diabetes mellitus, breastfeeding, and *elderly patients.* Safety and efficacy in *children* have not been established.

Preparation and administration

• Follow hazardous drug guidelines for handling, preparation, and administration. (See "Managing hazardous drugs," page 11.)
• Pretreatment evaluation in women should include breast and pelvic examinations and Papanicolaou test.
• Give drug with food to decrease adverse GI effects.

Adverse reactions

CNS: asthenia, insomnia
CV: thrombophlebitis, hypertension
GI: nausea, diarrhea, flatulence
GU: erectile dysfunction, decreased libido
Hematologic: anemia
Metabolic: diabetes mellitus exacerbation
Respiratory: pulmonary embolism
Skin: rash
Other: weight gain, fever

Interactions

Drug-diagnostic tests. *Coagulation tests, endocrine function tests, liver function tests, metyrapone test, pregnanediol, thyroid tests, serum glucose:* altered
Drug-herb. *Aloe (oral preparations):* possible decreased megestrol absorption

---

Only common or life-threatening adverse reactions are listed.

Toxicity and overdose

- No serious unexpected adverse effects have occurred in patients receiving up to 1,200 mg suspension daily and 1,600 mg tablets daily.
- Drug has not been tested for dialyzability. However, its low solubility suggests that dialysis is ineffective in treating overdose.

Special considerations

- Monitor hematologic tests, thyroid-stimulating hormone level, and coagulation tests.
- In elderly patients, monitor liver and kidney function tests.
- Drug may exacerbate diabetes mellitus and increase insulin requirements. Monitor serum glucose level.
- Closely monitor patients with history of thromboembolic disease.
- Consider risk of adrenal insufficiency during prolonged therapy or withdrawal from prolonged therapy in patients with signs or symptoms of hypoadrenalism (such as hypotension, nausea, vomiting, dizziness, or weakness) in either stressed or nonstressed state. Perform laboratory evaluation for adrenal insufficiency; consider replacement or stress doses of fast-acting glucocorticoid in such patients. Failure to recognize hypothalamic-pituitary-adrenal inhibition may result in death.

Patient education

- Instruct patient to report adverse reactions, particularly redness, pain, swollen feet or legs, chest pain, or difficulty breathing.
- Advise women with childbearing potential to use effective contraception during therapy and to notify physician if pregnancy occurs.
- Instruct breastfeeding patient to stop breastfeeding during therapy.

melphalan (L-PAM)
Alkeran, Alkeran I.V.

Classification: Antineoplastic, alkylating agent
Pregnancy risk category D

Pharmacology

Melphalan has cytotoxic action apparently related to the extent of its interstrand cross-linking with DNA (probably by binding at N7 position of guanine). It is active against both resting and rapidly dividing tumor cells.

Pharmacokinetics

Drug has unpredictable GI absorption, and is autometabolized rapidly in plasma by hydrolysis. It is 60% to 90% protein-bound, with elimination half-life of about 90 minutes. Roughly 10% to 15% is excreted unchanged in urine.

M

How supplied

Powder for injection: 50 mg/vial
Tablets: 2 mg

Indications and dosages

FDA-APPROVED

➥ Palliative treatment of multiple myeloma in patients for whom oral therapy is not appropriate
Adults: 16 mg/m² I.V. as single infusion over 15 to 20 minutes; given at 2-week intervals for four doses and then, after adequate recovery from toxicity, at 4-week intervals
➥ Palliative treatment of multiple myeloma
Adults: 6 mg (three tablets) P.O. daily. Entire daily dose may be given at one time. Adjust dosage, as needed, based on blood counts at intervals of approximately 1 week. After 2 to 3 weeks, stop drug for up to 4 weeks; during this hiatus, follow blood counts carefully. When WBC and platelets counts are rising, give maintenance dosage of 2 mg daily. Be-

➥ Orphan drug   ≫ Potentially carcinogenic

cause of patient variations in drug plasma levels with P.O. use, escalate dosage cautiously until some myelosuppression occurs, to ensure that potentially therapeutic drug levels have been reached.

Alternative regimens

1. *Adults:* 0.15 mg/kg P.O. daily for 7 consecutive days, followed by rest period of at least 2 weeks (up to 5 or 6 weeks). Maintenance therapy starts with 0.05 mg/kg daily or less when WBC and platelet counts are recovering; adjust dosage according to counts.

2. *Adults:* 0.25 mg/kg P.O. daily for 4 consecutive days or 0.2 mg/kg daily for 5 consecutive days, for total of 1 mg/kg per course. Repeat course every 4 to 6 weeks once WBC and platelet counts normalize.

3. *Adults:* 10 mg P.O. daily for 7 to 10 days. Start maintenance therapy with 2 mg daily when WBC count exceeds 4,000/mm³ and platelet count exceeds 100,000/mm³. Adjust dosage to 1 to 3 mg daily based on counts. Maintain bone marrow depression to keep WBC count within 3,000 to 3,500/mm³.

➥ Palliative treatment of nonresectable epithelial carcinoma of ovary

Adults: 0.2 mg/kg P.O. or I.V. daily for 5 days as single course. Repeat course every 4 to 5 weeks based on hematologic parameters.

OFF-LABEL USES (SELECTED)

➥ Bone marrow transplantation in non-Hodgkin's lymphoma

Adults: Dosages vary by facility. Several protocols exist; dosages are based on combination of drugs administered and whether radiation is used.

DOSAGE MODIFICATIONS

• Consider dosage reduction of up to 50% in patients with renal insufficiency (BUN at least 30 mg/dl) who are receiving drug I.V.

• Consider dosage adjustment based on blood counts at nadir and on treatment day.

• Repeated courses or continuous therapy should be given because improvement may continue slowly over many months, and max-

imum benefit may be missed if treatment ends too soon.

⚠ WARNINGS

• Drug should be given under supervision of qualified physician experienced in use of cancer chemotherapeutic agents.

• Severe bone marrow depression with resulting infection or bleeding may occur. Controlled trials comparing I.V. with P.O. use showed more myelosuppression with I.V. use.

• Hypersensitivity reactions (including anaphylaxis) have occurred in about 2% of patients who received drug I.V.

• Drug is leukemogenic and produces chromosomal aberrations *in vitro* and *in vivo*. It should be considered potentially mutagenic.

Contraindications and precautions

Contraindicated in hypersensitivity or previous resistance to drug.

Use with extreme caution in patients whose bone marrow reserve may have been compromised by previous irradiation or chemotherapy or whose marrow function is recovering from previous cytotoxic therapy; pregnancy; breastfeeding; and **elderly patients**. Safety and efficacy in **children** have not been established.

Preparation and administration

➤➤ Follow hazardous drug guidelines for handling, preparation, and administration. (See "Managing hazardous drugs," page 11.)

• Obtain at least one CBC with differential before each dose.

• Give oral dose on empty stomach to enhance absorption.

• Reconstitute drug for injection by rapidly injecting 10 ml of supplied diluent (yields 5 mg/ml solution) directly into vial of lyophilized powder using 20G or larger needle. Immediately shake vial vigorously until solution is clear.

• Immediately dilute dose in normal saline

solution injection to a concentration no greater than 0.45 mg/ml.
• Give diluted product over at least 15 minutes. Complete administration within 60 minutes of reconstitution.
• Solution is unstable; minimize interval between reconstitution or dilution and administration. If gap exceeds 30 minutes, drug's citrate derivative may appear in reconstituted material (from drug's reaction to sterile diluent). When diluted further with saline solution, nearly 1% of drug's labeled strength hydrolyzes every 10 minutes.
• Store refrigerated at 36° to 46° F (2° to 8° C) and protect from light.

Adverse reactions

GI: nausea, vomiting
Hematologic: bone marrow depression, leukopenia, thrombocytopenia, neutropenia
Hepatic: hepatotoxicity
Respiratory: interstitial pneumonitis, bronchospasm, pulmonary fibrosis, pulmonary dysplasia
Other: anaphylaxis, hypersensitivity

Interactions

Drug-drug. *Carmustine:* increased pulmonary toxicity
Cisplatin: renal dysfunction, leading to altered melphalan clearance
Cyclosporine: increased incidence of nephrotoxicity
Interferon alfa: decreased melphalan level
Nalidixic acid: increased incidence of severe hemorrhagic necrotic enterocolitis in children
Drug-herb. *Alpha-lipoic acid, coenzyme Q10:* possible decreased chemotherapy efficacy
Glutamine: possible enhanced tumor growth

Toxicity and overdose

• Overdoses resulting in death have occurred. Doses up to 290 mg/m^2 I.V. and 50 mg P.O. daily for 6 days have caused severe nausea and vomiting, decreased consciousness, seizures, muscle paralysis, venoocclusive disease, increased liver function test results, hypona-

tremia, cholinomimetic effects, severe mucositis, stomatitis, colitis, diarrhea, and GI hemorrhage. Primary toxic effect is bone marrow depression.
• Provide general supportive measures with appropriate blood transfusions and antibiotics. (Hemodialysis and hemoperfusion are ineffective in removing drug from plasma.) Follow hematologic indices for 3 to 6 weeks. Consider autologous bone marrow transplantation or hematopoietic growth factors.

Special considerations

• Monitor hematologic function with weekly CBC count with differential throughout therapy. Observe patient closely for signs and symptoms of bone marrow depression.
• If WBC count is below 3,000/mm^3 or platelet count is below 100,000/mm^3, stop drug until counts recover.
• Giving prednisone with drug may enhance palliation of multiple myeloma symptoms.
• Secondary cancers (including acute nonlymphocytic leukemia, myeloproliferative syndrome, and carcinoma) have occurred in cancer patients receiving drug.
• Drug suppresses ovarian function in premenopausal women, causing amenorrhea in many cases. Reversible and irreversible testicular suppression also have occurred.
• Use caution when selecting dosage for elderly patients, usually starting at low end of range. Elderly patients are more likely to have hepatic, renal, or cardiac impairment or other concomitant disease and are more likely to be receiving other drugs.

Patient education

• Advise patient to report rash, signs or symptoms of vasculitis, fever, persistent cough, nausea, vomiting, amenorrhea, weight loss, unusual lumps or masses, shortness of breath, yellowing of skin or eyes, unusual bruising or bleeding, black tarry stools, or flank or stomach pain.
• Inform patient that drug's major long-term toxicities are infertility and secondary cancers.

M

⊖ Orphan drug   ≫ Potentially carcinogenic

- Advise women with childbearing potential to avoid pregnancy during therapy.
- Caution breastfeeding patient not to breast-feed during therapy.

meperidine hydrochloride
Demerol Hydrochloride

Classification: Analgesic, opioid
Controlled substance schedule II
Pregnancy risk category C

Pharmacology
Meperidine acts on opioid receptors in CNS, altering response to pain and producing analgesia and sedation.

Pharmacokinetics
Drug is about 50% absorbed with oral use and is well absorbed with I.M. and subcutaneous use. It is metabolized by liver to active or inactive metabolites. Toxic byproduct can occur with regular use. With P.O. dose, onset is 15 minutes; peak, 20 minutes to 1 hour; and duration, 2 to 4 hours. With subcutaneous or I.M. dose, onset is 10 minutes; peak, 30 minutes to 1 hour; and duration, 2 to 4 hours. With I.V. use, onset is 5 minutes and duration is 2 hours. Drug has half-life of 3 to 4 hours; half-life of normeperidine (active metabolite) is 15 to 30 minutes. Drug is excreted by kidney.

How supplied
Solution: 10 mg/ml, 25 mg/ml, 50 mg/ml, 75 mg/ml, 100 mg/ml
Syrup: 50 mg/5 ml
Tablets: 50 mg, 100 mg

Indications and dosages

FDA-APPROVED

➥ Moderate to severe pain
Adults: 50 to 150 mg P.O., I.M., or subcutaneously every 3 or 4 hours as needed
Children: 1.1 to 1.8 mg/kg (0.5 to 0.8 mg/lb) P.O., I.M., or subcutaneously up to adult dosage, every 3 or 4 hours as needed

DOSAGE MODIFICATIONS

- Dosage should be decreased 25% to 50% when drug is given with phenothiazines or other tranquilizers.
- Dosage should be adjusted for renal impairment. Give 75% of usual dosage if creatinine clearance is 10 to 50 ml/minute; give 50% of usual dosage if creatinine clearance is below 10 ml/minute.

Contraindications and precautions
Contraindicated in hypersensitivity to drug and within 14 days of MAO inhibitor use.

Use cautiously in head injury, other intracranial lesions, or preexisting increased intracranial pressure (ICP). Use with extreme caution in chronic obstructive pulmonary disease or cor pulmonale; preexisting respiratory depression, upper airway obstruction, hypoxia, or hypercapnia; acute asthmatic attack; and substantially decreased respiratory reserve. Drug may cause severe hypotension in postoperative patients and in those who cannot maintain blood pressure adequately due to volume depletion or use of such drugs as phenothiazines or certain anesthetics.

Use with caution in debilitated patients; orthostatic hypotension; atrial flutter and other supraventricular tachycardias; acute abdominal conditions; sickle cell anemia; pheochromocytoma; adrenocortical insufficiency (such as Addison's disease); CNS depression or coma; history of seizure disorder; kyphoscoliosis associated with respiratory depression; myxedema or hypothyroidism; prostatic hypertrophy or urethral stricture; severe hepatic, pulmonary, or renal impairment; toxic psychosis; concurrent use of CNS depressants; acute alcoholism; delirium tremens; pregnancy; breastfeeding; *elderly patients; young infants;* and *neonates.*

Only common or life-threatening adverse reactions are listed.

Preparation and administration

- To counteract opioid-induced respiratory depression, keep opioid antagonist (such as naloxone) readily available when administering drug.
- For I.M. injection, inject well within body of large muscle.
- If necessary, give drug I.V. but inject very slowly (preferably as diluted solution). Rapid I.V. injection increases risk of serious adverse reactions (such as severe respiratory depression, apnea, hypotension, peripheral circulatory collapse, and cardiac arrest). Do not administer I.V. unless opioid antagonist and facilities for assisted or controlled respiration are immediately available. When giving drug parenterally (especially I.V.), ensure that patient is lying down.
- Administer each dose of syrup in half-glass of water. If taken undiluted, drug may have slight topical anesthetic effect on mucous membranes.
- Store at controlled temperature of 77° F (25° C); excursions are permitted to 59° to 86°F (15° to 30°C) for tablets.

Adverse reactions

CNS: dizziness, drowsiness, light-headedness, euphoria, confusion, sedation
CV: fainting, syncope, bradycardia, orthostatic hypotension, cardiac arrest, peripheral circulatory collapse, shock
EENT: blurred vision, miosis, diplopia
GI: dry mouth, nausea, vomiting, anorexia, constipation, cramps
GU: oliguria, urinary retention or hesitancy, reduced libido
Hepatic: biliary tract spasm
Respiratory: respiratory depression, respiratory arrest
Skin: diaphoresis, pruritus
Other: facial flushing, physical or psychological dependence, pain at injection site, hypersensitivity reaction

Interactions

Drug-drug. *Acyclovir:* increased meperidine level
Cimetidine: reduced clearance and volume of meperidine distribution
General anesthetics, other opioid analgesics or CNS depressants, phenothiazines, sedative-hypnotics (including barbiturates), tranquilizers, tricyclic antidepressants: possible respiratory depression, hypotension, and profound sedation or coma
MAO inhibitors: possible precipitation of unpredictable and potentially fatal reactions
Opioid agonist or antagonist analgesics (such as buprenorphine, butorphanol, nalbuphine, and pentazocine): reduced analgesic effect, possible precipitation of meperidine withdrawal symptoms
Phenytoin: enhanced hepatic metabolism of meperidine
Protease inhibitors: possible increase in normeperidine level
Skeletal muscle relaxants: enhanced neuromuscular blocking action, increased respiratory depression
Drug-herb. *Gotu kola, kava, St. John's wort, valerian:* increased CNS depression
L-tryptophan, SAM-e: increased risk of serotonin syndrome

Toxicity and overdose

- Serious overdose causes respiratory depression (decreased respiratory rate or tidal volume, Cheyne-Stokes respiration, cyanosis), extreme somnolence progressing to stupor or coma, skeletal muscle flaccidity, cold and clammy skin, and in some cases, bradycardia, hypotension, and pulmonary edema. Severe overdose (particularly with I.V. use) may cause apnea, circulatory collapse, and cardiac arrest, resulting in death.
- Maintain patent airway and institute assisted or controlled ventilation. Provide appropriate dosage of naloxone, preferably I.V., at same time as respiratory resuscitation efforts. If possible, avoid giving narcotic antagonist to physically dependent patient; if antagonist

M

must be used to treat serious respiratory depression, administer it with extreme care and titrate with smaller-than-usual dosages. Do not give antagonist in absence of clinically significant respiratory or cardiovascular depression. Implement oxygen, I.V. fluids, vasopressors, and other supportive measures, as indicated. Atropine may be useful in treating bradycardia. In tablet overdose, evacuate stomach by emesis or gastric lavage. Monitor heart filling pressures; noncardiac pulmonary edema occurs in about 40% of patients.

Special considerations
• Drug can cause morphine-type dependence and may be abused. Psychic and physical dependence and tolerance may occur with repeated use. Prescribe and administer drug with same degree of caution as for morphine. Like other opioids, drug is subject to federal narcotics laws.
• Monitor for CNS and respiratory depression.
• Monitor renal function regularly.
• Drug's potential vagolytic action may significantly increase ventricular response rate.
• Drug may obscure accurate diagnosis or clinical course in patients with acute abdominal conditions.
• Drug may have narrow therapeutic index in some patients, particularly when used with CNS depressants.

Patient education
• Advise patient not to adjust dosage without consulting prescriber.
• Caution patient not to use drug with alcohol or other CNS depressants (such as sleep aids or tranquilizers) unless directed by prescriber, because dangerous additive effects can cause serious injury or death.
• Instruct patient to consult physician if constipation occurs; laxatives may be indicated.
• Advise patient to use caution when driving and performing other hazardous tasks because drug may impair mental and physical abilities.
• Instruct patient to rise slowly when sitting

or standing up, to decrease risk of orthostatic hypotension.
• Advise patient to report pain and adverse experiences. Dosage must be individualized for optimal drug use.
• Inform patient who wishes to stop taking drug after several weeks that dosage must be tapered gradually. Caution him not to stop taking drug abruptly because withdrawal symptoms may occur.
• Tell patient that drug can be abused and must be protected from theft. Caution patient never to give it to anyone else.
• Instruct patient to keep drug in secure place out of reach of children. When drug is no longer needed, tell patient to destroy unused portion by flushing it down toilet.
• Caution women with childbearing potential not to use drug if pregnant because it may affect pregnancy and harm fetus.
• Provide guidance to help breastfeeding patient decide whether to discontinue breastfeeding or stop drug.

mercaptopurine
Purinethol

Classification: Antineoplastic, antimetabolite
Pregnancy risk category D

Pharmacology
Mercaptopurine, a purine analog, interferes with nucleic acid biosynthesis and acts against leukemias.

Pharmacokinetics
Drug absorption is incomplete and variable with oral use; on average, about 50% of dose is absorbed. Drug undergoes extensive first-pass metabolism in liver (dependent on xanthine oxidase). Elimination half-life is about 7 hours. Negligible amount enters cerebrospinal fluid. Intact drug and metabolites are excreted by kidney.

How supplied

Tablets: 50 mg

Indications and dosages

FDA-APPROVED

➡ Acute lymphatic (lymphocytic, lymphoblastic) leukemia (ALL), acute myelogenous and acute myelomonocytic leukemia
Adults and children: Dosage is calculated to nearest multiple of 25 mg. Total daily dosage may be given at one time. Therapy consists of two steps—induction and maintenance. *Induction:* Dosage is individualized. Initiate with 2.5 mg/kg P.O. daily (100 to 200 mg in average adult, 50 mg in average 5-year-old child). If no clinical improvement and no definite evidence of WBC or platelet depression occur after 4 weeks at this dosage, increase up to 5 mg/kg daily. *Maintenance:* Once complete hematologic remission occurs with monotherapy or other agents, maintenance therapy is essential. Dosage varies among patients. Usual maintenance dosage is 1.5 to 2.5 mg/kg P.O. daily as single dose.

DOSAGE MODIFICATIONS

• Consider dosage reduction in patients with renal or hepatic impairment. Start with smaller dosage in renal impairment because this condition slows drug elimination and leads to greater cumulative drug effect.
• Reduce dosage to one-third or one-quarter of usual dosage when giving drug concurrently with allopurinol.
• Unless deliberately attempting to induce bone marrow hypoplasia, stop drug temporarily at first sign of abnormally steep decrease in WBC count, platelet count, or hemoglobin. (Drug may have delayed action.) In many patients with drug-induced severe depression of formed blood elements, marrow appears hypoplastic on aspiration or biopsy; in other cases, it may appear normocellular. Drug does not cause qualitative changes in erythroid elements toward megaloblastic series. If WBC or

platelet count subsequently remains constant for 2 or 3 days or if it rises, resume therapy.
• Patients with inherited thiopurine methyltransferase (TPMT) deficiency may be unusually sensitive to drug's myelosuppressive effects and may develop rapid bone marrow suppression after initial therapy. To avoid life-threatening marrow suppression, dosage must be reduced substantially. This problem may be exacerbated by concurrent use of drugs that inhibit TPMT, such as aminosalicylates (including mesalamine, olsalazine, and sulfasalazine).
• Reduce dosage when drug is given concomitantly with xanthine oxidase inhibitor.

⊠ WARNINGS

• Drug is potent and should not be administered unless ALL diagnosis has been adequately established and physician knows how to evaluate response to chemotherapy.

M

Contraindications and precautions

Contraindicated in hypersensitivity to drug or its components and in previous resistance to drug or thioguanine.

Use cautiously in inherited TPMT deficiency; concurrent use of drugs that inhibit TPMT; concurrent use of xanthine oxidase inhibitors or hepatotoxic agents; jaundice, hepatomegaly, or anorexia with right hypochondrium tenderness; deteriorating liver function studies; toxic hepatitis; biliary stasis; myelosuppression; use of infectious agents or vaccines; pregnancy; and breastfeeding.

Preparation and administration

• Follow hazardous drug guidelines for handling, preparation, and administration. (See "Managing hazardous drugs," page 11.)
• Studies in children with ALL suggest that administering drug in evening (compared to morning) reduces risk of relapse.
• Store drug at 59° to 77° F (15° to 25° C) in a dry place.

◗ Orphan drug   ≫ Potentially carcinogenic

Adverse reactions

GI: nausea, vomiting, anorexia, diarrhea, stomatitis, pancreatitis, ulceration
GU: renal failure, oliguria, hematuria
Hematologic: leukopenia, thrombocytopenia, myelosuppression, anemia
Hepatic: hepatotoxicity
Skin: rash
Other: hyperuricemia, fever

Interactions

Drug-drug. *Aminosalicylate derivatives (such as mesalamine, olsalazine, and sulfasalazine), xanthine oxidase inhibitors (such as allopurinol):* increased mercaptopurine toxicity
Myelosuppressants, trimethoprim-sulfamethoxazole: increased bone marrow suppression
Warfarin: inhibited anticoagulant effect
Drug-diagnostic tests. *Hemoglobin, platelets, RBCs, uric acid, WBCs:* increased
Drug-herb. *Alpha-lipoic acid, coenzyme Q10:* possible decreased chemotherapy efficacy
Glutamine: possible enhanced tumor growth

Toxicity and overdose

• Overdose signs and symptoms may be immediate (such as anorexia, nausea, vomiting, and diarrhea) or delayed (such as myelosuppression, hepatic dysfunction, and gastroenteritis). Hematologic toxicity typically is more profound with prolonged overdose than single ingestion. Most frequent serious toxic effect is myelosuppression resulting in leukopenia, thrombocytopenia, and anemia.
• No known antagonist exists. Stop drug at once. If overdose was ingested within past 60 minutes, induce emesis; after that time, active measures (such as activated charcoal or gastric lavage) may be ineffective. Severe hematologic toxicity may warrant supportive therapy with platelet transfusions for bleeding, and antibiotics and granulocyte transfusions if sepsis occurs. Dialysis does not reliably clear drug; hemodialysis may be of marginal use.

Special considerations

• Evaluate hemoglobin or hematocrit, total WBC count with differential, and quantitative platelet count weekly during therapy.
• Monitor liver function tests (serum transaminases and bilirubin) to detect hepatotoxicity early. Monitor these tests weekly when therapy begins and monthly thereafter. More frequent testing may be needed in patients who are receiving other hepatotoxic drugs or have preexisting hepatic disease. If patient develops jaundice, hepatomegaly, or anorexia with right hypochondrium tenderness, withdraw drug immediately until exact cause is determined. If patient develops declining liver function test results, toxic hepatitis, or biliary stasis, stop drug and search for cause of hepatotoxicity.
• When given as single agent for induction, drug induces complete remission in about 25% of children and 10% of adults. However, do not rely on drug alone to induce initial remission of ALL. (Such remission is more likely to result from combination chemotherapy using vincristine, prednisone, and L-asparaginase than with mercaptopurine alone.)
• Drug is not effective in CNS leukemia, chronic lymphocytic leukemia, lymphomas (including Hodgkin's), and solid tumors.
• When giving drug concurrently with other hepatotoxic agents, monitor clinical and biochemical indicators of hepatic function. Approach combination therapy with other nonhepatotoxic drugs cautiously. Mercaptopurine/doxorubicin combination was hepatotoxic in 19 of 20 patients undergoing remission-induction therapy for leukemia resistant to previous therapy.
• Drug may cause subnormal response to infectious agents or vaccines.
• In children with ALL in remission, using drug with other agents (such as methotrexate) produced superior results in maintaining remission. Drug rarely should be relied on as single agent for maintaining remission in acute leukemia.

Only common or life-threatening adverse reactions are listed.

Patient education
- Advise patient to take drug on empty stomach (1 hour before or 2 hours after meal).
- Instruct patient to maintain adequate hydration during therapy.
- Tell patient to immediately report fever, sore throat, jaundice, nausea, vomiting, signs or symptoms of local infection, bleeding from any site, symptoms of anemia, swelling of feet or legs, abdominal pain, joint pain, or yellowing of skin or eyes.
- Caution women with childbearing potential to avoid pregnancy.
- Provide guidance to help breastfeeding patient decide whether to discontinue breastfeeding or stop drug.

mesna
Mesnex

Classification: Antineoplastic adjunct, detoxifying agent, cytoprotective, hemorrhagic cystitis inhibitor
Pregnancy risk category B

Pharmacology
Mesna reacts chemically in kidneys to detoxify urotoxic ifosfamide and cyclophosphamide metabolites and inhibit hemorrhagic cystitis. It also binds to double bonds of acrolein and to other urotoxic metabolites.

Pharmacokinetics
Drug is rapidly oxidized to major metabolite, mesna disulfide (dimesna). Mesna disulfide remains in intravascular compartment and is reduced to the free thiol compound, mesna, which is rapidly eliminated by kidney. With I.V. use, half-life is 0.37 hours for mesna and 1.17 hours for dimesna. With I.V. plus oral use (recommended regimen), half-life is 1.2 to 8.3 hours.

How supplied
Solution for injection: 1 g/10 ml in multidose vial
Tablets: 400 mg

Indications and dosages

➥ Prophylaxis to reduce incidence of ifosfamide-induced hemorrhagic cystitis
Adults: Mesna may be given on fractionated dosing schedule of three bolus I.V. injections or as single bolus injection followed by two oral administrations of mesna tablets as described below. If patient vomits within 2 hours of oral mesna dose, repeat dose or administer drug by I.V. route.
I.V. dosing schedule
Mesna is given as I.V. bolus injections in dosage equal to 20% of ifosfamide dosage (weight/weight) at time of ifosfamide administration and 4 and 8 hours after each ifosfamide dose. Total daily mesna dosage is 60% of ifosfamide dosage. See recommended dosing schedule below.

Drug	0 hours	4 hours	8 hours
ifosfamide	1.2 g/m²	None	None
mesna	240 mg/m²	240 mg/m²	240 mg/m²

I.V. and P.O. dosing schedule
Mesna injection is given as I.V. bolus injections in dosage equal to 20% of ifosfamide dosage (weight/weight) at time of ifosfamide administration. Mesna tablets are given P.O. in dosage equal to 40% of ifosfamide dosage 2 and 6 hours after each ifosfamide dose. Total daily mesna dosage is 100% of ifosfamide dosage. See the following recommended dosing schedule.

Drug	0 hours	2 hours	6 hours
ifosfamide	1.2 g/m²	None	None
mesna	240 mg/m²	480 mg/m²	480 mg/m²

➥ Prophylaxis to reduce incidence of cyclo-phosphamide-induced hemorrhagic cystitis
Adults: Mesna may be given I.V. in dosage equal to 20% of cyclophosphamide dosage every 3 hours for three to four doses, or in dosage equal to 40% of cyclophosphamide dosage P.O. every 4 hours for three doses.
➥ Cyclophosphamide-induced hemorrhagic cystitis in bone marrow transplant (BMT) recipients
Adults: Drug has been given by I.V. injection in daily dosage equivalent to 60% to 160% of cyclophosphamide daily dosage in three to five divided doses or by continuous I.V. infusion. In one study of BMT patients receiving cyclophosphamide (50 mg/kg I.V. daily for 3 to 4 days), mesna doses of 12 mg/kg were given by I.V. injection 30 minutes before each cyclophosphamide dose and at 3, 6, 9, and 12 hours after each dose. Alternatively, in BMT patients receiving cyclophosphamide (50 to 60 mg/kg I.V. daily for 2 to 4 days), mesna loading dose of 10 mg/kg has been given I.V. with cyclophosphamide dose, followed by mesna 60 mg/kg given by continuous I.V. infusion over 24 hours.

DOSAGE MODIFICATIONS

• Dosing schedule should be repeated on each day that ifosfamide is administered. When ifosfamide dosage is adjusted (either increased or decreased), mesna-to-ifosfamide ratio should be maintained.

Contraindications and precautions

Contraindicated in hypersensitivity to mesna or other thiol compounds.

Use cautiously in autoimmune disorders, impaired renal or hepatic function, pregnancy or breastfeeding, *elderly patients,* and *children.* Multidose vial contains benzyl alcohol; it should not be given to neonates or infants and should be used with caution in older children.

Preparation and administration

• For I.V. administration, drug can be diluted by adding mesna injection solution (for final concentration of 20 mg mesna/ml) to any of the following fluids: 5% dextrose injection, 5% dextrose and 0.2% sodium chloride injection, 5% dextrose and 0.33% sodium chloride injection, 5% dextrose and 0.45% sodium chloride injection, 0.92% sodium chloride injection, or lactated Ringer's injection.
• Give I.V. bolus over 1 minute.
• Diluted solutions are chemically and physically stable for 24 hours at 77° F (25° C).
• Store multidose vials at controlled temperature of 68° to 77° F (20° to 25° C); these vials may be used for up to 8 days.
• Store tablets at controlled temperature of 68° to 77° F.

Adverse reactions

CNS: fatigue, dizziness, headache, somnolence, anxiety, confusion, insomnia, asthenia
CV: chest pain, hypotension, tachycardia
GI: nausea, vomiting, constipation, anorexia, abdominal pain, diarrhea, dyspepsia
GU: hematuria
Hematologic: leukopenia, thrombocytopenia, anemia, granulocytopenia
Musculoskeletal: back pain, joint pain, myalgia
Respiratory: dyspnea, coughing, pneumonia
Skin: alopecia, sweating
Other: fever, injection site reaction, edema, pallor, dehydration, flushing, allergic reactions ranging from mild hypersensitivity to systemic anaphylactic reactions

Interactions

Drug-diagnostic tests. *Urinary ketones:* false positive

Toxicity and overdose

• Anticipated signs and symptoms of overdose include those of adverse reactions.
• No known antidote exists. Treat supportively, as indicated.

Special considerations

• Drug does not inhibit ifosfamide-induced adverse reactions other than hemorrhagic cystitis.

• Patients with autoimmune disorders who receive mesna and cyclophosphamide may have higher incidence of allergic reactions.

Patient education

• Instruct patient to drink at least 1 quart of fluid daily during therapy.

• Advise patient to contact prescriber if vomiting occurs within 2 hours of taking mesna tablets, if urine turns pink or red, or if he misses a dose.

• Provide guidance to help breastfeeding patient decide whether to discontinue breastfeeding or stop drug.

methadone hydrochloride
Dolophine

Classification: Opioid analgesic, opioid derivative
Controlled substance schedule II
Pregnancy risk category B

Pharmacology

Methadone acts on opioid receptors in CNS, altering response to pain and producing analgesia and sedation.

Pharmacokinetics

Drug is metabolized in liver and is highly protein-bound. With oral use, onset is 30 to 60 minutes; peak, 0.5 to 1 hour; and duration, 6 to 8 hours. With subcutaneous or I.M. use, onset is 10 to 20 minutes; peak, 1.5 to 2 hours; duration, 4 to 6 hours; and half-life, about 15 to 30 hours. Drug is excreted by kidney.

How supplied

Oral concentrate: 10 mg/ml

Oral solution: 5 mg/5 ml, 10 mg/5 ml
Oral tablets: 5 mg, 10 mg, 40 mg
Solution for injection: 10 mg/ml

Indications and dosages

FDA-APPROVED

➡ Severe pain
Adults: 2.5 to 10 mg P.O., I.M., or subcutaneously every 3 to 4 hours as needed

DOSAGE MODIFICATIONS

• Adjust dosage based on pain severity and response. Usual dosage may be exceeded for exceptionally severe pain or opioid-tolerant patients.

WARNINGS

• When used as analgesic, drug may be dispensed by any licensed pharmacy.
• Failure to abide by federal regulations may result in criminal prosecution and drug seizure.
• Elderly patients should receive initial dosages at lower end of recommended range.

Contraindications and precautions

Contraindicated in hypersensitivity to drug or its components.

Use cautiously in severe hepatic or renal failure, hypothyroidism, Addison's disease, prostatic hypertrophy, urethral stricture, acute abdominal conditions, pregnancy, breastfeeding, and *elderly* or debilitated patients. Methadone injection is not recommended in patients with respiratory depression (in absence of resuscitative equipment or in unmonitored settings), acute bronchial asthma, or hypercarbia.

Safety and efficacy in *children* have not been established.

Preparation and administration

• To counteract opioid-induced respiratory depression, keep opioid antagonist (such as

M

naloxone) readily available when administering drug.

- Oral administration is preferred (if tolerated). However, when given orally, drug is only about half as potent as when given parenterally. Oral administration results in delayed onset, lower peak level, and increased duration of analgesic effect.
- Mix dispersible tablets with 120 ml water or juice.
- When patient requires repeated doses, I.M. injection is preferred over subcutaneous route.
- In severe chronic pain, continuous around-the-clock dosing is preferred.

Adverse reactions

CNS: dizziness, drowsiness, light-headedness, euphoria, confusion, sedation
CV: fainting, syncope, bradycardia, orthostatic hypotension, cardiac arrest, peripheral circulatory collapse, shock
EENT: blurred vision, miosis, diplopia
GI: dry mouth, nausea, vomiting, anorexia, constipation, cramps
GU: oliguria, urinary retention or hesitancy, reduced libido
Hepatic: biliary tract spasm
Respiratory: respiratory depression, respiratory arrest
Skin: diaphoresis, pruritus
Other: facial flushing, physical or psychological dependence, pain at injection site, hypersensitivity reaction

Interactions

Drug-drug. *Desipramine:* increased serum desipramine level
Other CNS depressants (including antipsychotics, opioids, sedative-hypnotics, and skeletal muscle relaxants): increased CNS depression
Pentazocine: opioid withdrawal symptoms
Rifampin: reduced serum methadone level and subsequent withdrawal symptoms
Drug-diagnostic tests. *Amylase, lipase:* increased
Drug-food. *Grapefruit, pomegranate:* possible increased methadone levels

Drug-herb. *Cat's claw, echinacea, eucalyptus, feverfew, licorice, peppermint oil, valerian:* possible increased methadone levels
Chamomile, hops, Jamaican dogwood, kava, lavender, mistletoe, nettle, pokeweed, poppy, senega, skullcap, valerian: increased CNS depression
Corkwood: increased anticholinergic effects

Toxicity and overdose

- Major overdose manifestations include miosis, respiratory depression, somnolence, coma, cool and clammy skin, skeletal muscle flaccidity, hypotension, apnea, pulmonary edema, bradycardia, and death.
- Monitor heart filling pressures; noncardiac pulmonary edema occurs in about 40% of patients. For initial management, establish secure airway and support ventilation and perfusion. Evacuate stomach by emesis or gastric lavage if treatment can begin within 2 hours of oral ingestion. Naloxone may be used to antagonize opioid effects. Because methadone has a longer duration than naloxone, patient may require repeated doses or continuous I.V. infusion of naloxone. Avoid administering narcotic antagonist to physically dependent patients, if possible; if antagonist must be used to treat serious respiratory depression, administer with extreme care and titrate with smaller-than-usual dosages. Do not give antagonist in absence of clinically significant respiratory or cardiovascular depression. Administer I.V. fluids and vasopressors for hypotension, as indicated. Atropine may be useful in treating bradycardia. Forced diuresis, peritoneal dialysis, hemodialysis, and charcoal hemoperfusion have not proven beneficial.

Special considerations

- Drug can cause dependence of morphine type and may be abused. Psychic dependence, physical dependence, and tolerance may develop with repeated use. Prescribe and administer drug with same degree of caution as for morphine. Like other opioids, drug is subject to federal narcotics laws.

Only common or life-threatening adverse reactions are listed.

- Monitor for CNS and respiratory depression.
- Monitor renal function regularly.
- Drug use may obscure diagnosis or clinical course in patients with acute abdominal conditions.

Patient education

- Instruct patient to take drug with food or milk.
- Advise patient to seek immediate medical attention for confusion, difficulty swallowing or breathing, wheezing, light-headedness, or fainting.
- Instruct patient not to drink alcohol during therapy.
- Advise patient to consult physician or pharmacist before taking any new medication (including contraceptive).
- Caution patient not to share drug with anyone else.
- Inform patient that methadone may affect drug screening test results.
- Advise patient to use caution when driving or operating machinery on days when he takes drug.
- Tell female patient to notify physician or pharmacist if she becomes pregnant or is planning pregnancy.
- Caution breastfeeding patient not to breastfeed during therapy.

methotrexate sodium

Rheumatrex Dose Pack, Trexall

Classification: Antineoplastic, antimetabolite
Pregnancy risk category X

Pharmacology

Methotrexate inhibits dihydrofolic acid reductase, interfering with DNA, RNA, and protein synthesis, repair, and cellular replication. Actively proliferating tissues (such as malignant cells, bone marrow, fetal cells, buccal and intestinal mucosa, and urinary bladder cells) are more sensitive to this effect.

Pharmacokinetics

Drug is well absorbed when given orally (absorption is dose-dependent). It is metabolized primarily in liver, and is about 50% protein-bound. With oral use, levels peak in 1 to 2 hours; with I.M. use, in 30 to 60 minutes. Terminal half-life is about 3 to 10 hours (in high-dose therapy, 8 to 15 hours). Drug is excreted mainly by kidney.

How supplied

Isotonic liquid for injection: 25 mg/ml in 2- and 10-ml vials with preservative
Isotonic liquid for injection (preservative-free): 25 mg/ml in 2-, 4-, 8-, and 10-ml single-use vials
Powder for injection (preservative-free): 20 mg, 1 g
Tablets: 2.5 mg, 5 mg, 7.5 mg, 10 mg, 15 mg

Indications and dosages

M

FDA-APPROVED

➡ Gestational choriocarcinoma, chorioadenoma destruens, hydatidiform mole
Adults: 15 to 30 mg P.O. or I.M. daily for 5-day course; repeat three to five times as needed, with rest periods of 1 week or more interposed between courses until manifesting toxic symptoms subside
➡ Acute lymphoblastic leukemia
Adults and children: To induce remission, 3.3 mg/m² daily with 60 mg/m² prednisone. For maintenance, twice weekly P.O. or I.M. in total weekly doses of 30 mg/m², or 2.5 mg/kg I.V. every 14 days.
➡ Meningeal leukemia (therapeutic and preventive)
Children age 3 and older: 12 mg preservative-free form intrathecally every 2 to 5 days
Children age 2: 10 mg preservative-free form intrathecally every 2 to 5 days
Children age 1: 8 mg preservative-free form intrathecally every 2 to 5 days

Children younger than age 1: 6 mg preservative-free form intrathecally every 2 to 5 days
➡ Burkitt's lymphoma
Adults: For stages I and II, 10 to 25 mg P.O. daily for 4 to 8 days; for stage III, 0.625 to 2.5 mg/kg P.O. daily with other antitumor agents, interposed with 7- to 10-day rest periods
➡ Breast cancer, epidermoid cancers of head and neck, advanced mycosis fungoides (cutaneous T-cell lymphoma), lung cancer (especially squamous-cell and small-cell types)
Adults: Various regimens have been used.
➡ Mycosis fungoides (cutaneous T-cell lymphoma)
Adults: Methrotrexate 5 to 50 mg once weekly, or 15 to 37.5 mg twice weekly in patients who respond poorly to weekly therapy. Combination chemotherapy regimens that include methotrexate I.V. at higher doses with leucovorin rescue have been used in advanced disease stages.
➡ Lymphosarcoma (stage III)
Adults: 0.625 mg/kg to 2.5 mg/kg P.O. daily
⊖ Nonmetastatic osteosarcoma in patients who have undergone surgical resection or amputation for primary tumor
Adults: Methotrexate 12 g/m^2 I.V. as 4-hour infusion in weeks 4, 5, 6, 7, 11, 12, 15, 16, 29, 30, 44, and 44 after surgery. Give in combination with leucovorin 15 mg P.O. every 6 hours for 10 doses beginning 24 hours after start of methotrexate infusion, in addition to combinations of other chemotherapeutic agents (which may include doxorubicin, cisplatin, and bleomycin-cyclophosphamide-dactinomycin [BCD] regimen). If dosage does not produce peak serum methotrexate concentration of 1,000 μM (10^{-3} mol/L) at end of methotrexate infusion, dosage may be increased to 15 g/m^2 in subsequent treatments.

OFF-LABEL USES (SELECTED)

➡ Bladder cancer
Adults: Typically, methrotrexate 30 mg/m^2 I.V. on days 1, 15, and 22; given with vinblastine 3 mg/m^2 on days 2, 15, and 22; doxorubicin 30 mg/m^2 on day 2; and cisplatin 70 mg/m^2 on day 2
➡ Head and neck cancer
Adults: Typically, 40 to 60 mg/m^2 I.V. weekly

DOSAGE MODIFICATIONS

• Elderly patients may require dosage reduction because cerebrospinal fluid (CSF) volume and turnover may decrease with age.
• Drug is given until CSF cell count returns to normal, at which time additional dose is recommended.
• As appropriate, adjust, reduce, or discontinue systemic antileukemic therapy based on neurologic adverse reactions (such as seizures).
• Most adverse reactions (including vomiting, diarrhea, stomatitis, and drug-induced lung disease) are reversible if detected early. When these occur, reduce dosage or stop therapy and take appropriate corrective measures.
• Methotrexate should be continued only if potential benefit warrants risk of severe myelosuppression.
• In patients with renal impairment, ascites, or pleural effusions, reduce dosage or, in some cases, withdraw drug.

⊠ WARNINGS

• Drug should be used only by physicians who are knowledgeable and experienced in use of antimetabolite therapy.
• Use drug only in life-threatening neoplastic diseases or in patients with severe, recalcitrant, disabling psoriasis or rheumatoid arthritis that does not respond adequately to other therapies.
• Deaths have occurred when drug is used to treat malignancy, psoriasis, and rheumatoid arthritis.
• Monitor patient closely for bone marrow, liver, lung, and kidney toxicities. Explain risks involved, and follow patient during therapy.
• Use caution when administering high-dose regimen for osteosarcoma. (High-dose regimens for other neoplastic diseases are investi-

gational, with no established therapeutic advantage.)

• Do not use preserved forms and diluents for intrathecal or high-dose therapy.

• Do not use drug in pregnant women or women with childbearing potential unless medical evidence indicates that benefits may outweigh risks. (Drug has caused fetal death and congenital anomalies.)

• Patients with renal impairment, ascites, or pleural effusion have reduced drug elimination. Monitor them carefully for toxicity; dosage may need to be reduced or drug may need to be stopped.

• Unexpectedly severe (sometimes fatal) bone marrow depression, aplastic anemia, and GI toxicity have occurred in patients receiving drug (usually in high doses) concomitantly with nonsteroidal anti-inflammatory drugs (NSAIDs).

• Drug causes hepatotoxicity, fibrosis, and cirrhosis, but generally only after prolonged use. Acutely, liver enzyme elevations are common but usually transient and asymptomatic; they do not predict subsequent hepatic disease. Liver biopsy after sustained use typically shows histologic changes, and fibrosis and cirrhosis have occurred. The latter lesions may not be preceded by symptoms or abnormal liver function tests in psoriasis patients; perform periodic liver biopsies in psoriasis patients receiving long-term treatment.

• Potentially dangerous drug-induced lung disease may occur acutely at any time during therapy and is not always fully reversible. It has occurred at dosages as low as 7.5 mg weekly. For pulmonary symptoms (especially dry, nonproductive cough), therapy may need to be interrupted and careful investigation begun.

• Interrupt drug therapy for diarrhea and ulcerative stomatitis; otherwise, hemorrhagic enteritis and death from intestinal perforation may occur.

• Malignant lymphomas (which may regress after drug withdrawal) may occur in patients receiving low doses and may not require cytotoxic treatment. Discontinue drug first; if lymphoma does not regress, begin appropriate treatment.

• Drug may induce tumor lysis syndrome in patients with rapidly growing tumors. Use appropriate supportive measures to prevent or relieve this condition.

• Severe and occasionally fatal skin reactions have occurred after single or multiple doses within days of P.O., I.M., I.V., or intrathecal use. Drug withdrawal has resulted in recovery.

• Potentially fatal opportunistic infections (especially *Pneumocystis carinii* pneumonia) may occur.

• When given concomitantly with radiotherapy, drug may increase risk of soft-tissue necrosis and osteonecrosis.

Contraindications and precautions

Contraindicated in hypersensitivity to drug or its components; patients with psoriasis or rheumatoid arthritis who have alcoholism, alcoholic liver disease, or other chronic liver conditions; patients with psoriasis or rheumatoid arthritis who have overt or laboratory evidence of immunodeficiency syndromes; patients with psoriasis or rheumatoid arthritis who have preexisting blood dyscrasias, such as bone marrow hypoplasia, leukopenia, thrombocytopenia, or significant anemia; pregnant women with psoriasis or rheumatoid arthritis; and breastfeeding women.

Use with extreme caution in reduced hepatic or renal function, peptic ulcer disease, ulcerative colitis, active infection, decreased folate stores, preexisting hematopoietic impairment, and debilitated patients. Use in pregnant women with cancer only when benefit clearly outweighs risk to fetus. Safety and efficacy in *children* have been established only in cancer chemotherapy and polyarticular-course juvenile rheumatoid arthritis. Because injection form contains benzyl alcohol, do not use in neonates or for intrathecal or high-dose therapy.

M

Preparation and administration

• Follow hazardous drug guidelines for preparation, handling, and administration. (See "Managing hazardous drugs," page 11.)

• Perform baseline assessment, including CBC with differential and platelet count, hepatic enzyme levels, renal function tests, and chest X-ray.

• Oral administration of tablet form is often preferred when low dosages are given because of rapid absorption and effective serum levels.

• Methotrexate isotonic liquid for injection and powder for injection may be given by I.M., I.V., intra-arterial, or intrathecal route. However, preserved formulation contains benzyl alcohol and must not be used for intrathecal or high-dose therapy.

• Reconstitute each vial with preservative-free D_5W or normal saline solution; 25 mg/ml is maximum concentration that can be given I.V. Further dilute single dose with D_5W or normal saline solution immediately before infusing higher doses (100 mg or more).

• For I.V. injection, give each 10 mg over 1 minute. For I.V. infusion, give each dose over 30 minutes to 4 hours.

• Do not give drug I.M. if platelet count is below 50,000/mm^3.

• For intrathecal use, dilute preservative-free drug to concentration of 1 mg/ml in appropriate sterile, preservative-free medium (such as normal saline solution injection). CSF volume depends on age, not body surface area. (CSF is 40% of adult volume at birth and reaches adult volume in several years.)

• Store drug at controlled temperature of 68° to 77° F (20° to 25° C); excursions are permitted to 59° to 86° F (15° to 30° C). Protect from light.

Safety guidelines for high-dose therapy

• With high-dose therapy, follow safety guidelines for leucovorin rescue (see numbered list below). If patient vomits or cannot tolerate oral medication, give leucovorin I.V. or I.M. at same dosage and on same schedule.

1. Delay methotrexate administration until recovery if WBC count is below 1,500/

mm^3, neutrophil count is below 200/mm^3, platelet count is below 75,000/mm^3, serum bilirubin level exceeds 1.2 mg/dl, ALT exceeds 450 units/L, mucositis is present (until evidence of healing occurs), or persistent pleural effusion is present (this should be drained dry before infusion).

2. Adequate renal function must be documented. Serum creatinine level must be normal and creatinine clearance must exceed 60 ml/minute before therapy begins. Also, serum creatinine must be measured before each subsequent course. If it increases 50% or more over previous value, creatinine clearance must be measured and documented to be greater than 60 ml/minute (even if serum creatinine is within normal range).

3. Patient must be well hydrated, and must be treated with sodium bicarbonate for urinary alkalization. Administer 1,000 ml/m^2 of I.V. fluid over 6 hours before starting methotrexate infusion. Continue hydration at 125 ml/m^2/hour (3 L/m^2 daily) during infusion and for 2 days after infusion ends. Also, alkalize urine to maintain pH above 7.0 during methotrexate infusion and leucovorin therapy; this can be done with oral sodium bicarbonate administration or by incorporation into separate I.V. solution.

4. Obtain repeat serum creatinine and serum methotrexate levels 24 hours after starting methotrexate and at least once daily until methotrexate level is below 5×10^{-8} mol/L (0.05 μM).

5. Patients who experience delayed early methotrexate elimination are likely to develop nonreversible oliguric renal failure. Besides appropriate leucovorin therapy, these patients require continuing hydration and urinary alkalization with close monitoring of fluid and electrolyte status, until serum methotrexate level falls below 0.05 μM and renal failure resolves. If necessary, acute, intermittent hemodialysis with high-flux dialyzer may bring benefits in these patients.

Only common or life-threatening adverse reactions are listed.

6. Some patients have abnormal methotrexate elimination or abnormal renal function after methotrexate administration; although significant, these conditions are less severe than abnormalities described in established guidelines for leucovorin dosage. These abnormalities may or may not be associated with significant clinical toxicity. If significant clinical toxicity occurs, extend leucovorin rescue for additional 24 hours (total of 14 doses over 84 hours) in subsequent courses of therapy. Always reconsider possibility that patient is receiving other medications that interact with methotrexate (such as those that could interfere with methotrexate binding to serum albumin or with methotrexate elimination) when laboratory abnormalities or clinical toxicities occur.

7. Follow established guidelines for leucovorin dosage based on serum methotrexate levels. Do not administer leucovorin intrathecally. Also, infuse leucovorin slowly because of drug's calcium content.

Adverse reactions

CNS: acute chemical arachnoiditis (intrathecal use), leukoencephalopathy (intrathecal or I.V. use in patients who have had craniospinal irradiation), transient acute neurologic syndrome (with high-dose regimens), subacute myelopathy, malaise, fatigue, dizziness, headache, drowsiness, seizures

EENT: conjunctivitis, blurred vision

GI: nausea, vomiting, stomatitis, abdominal distress, GI ulceration and bleeding

GU: severe nephropathy or renal failure, azotemia, cystitis, hematuria, defective oogenesis or spermatogenesis, transient oligospermia, menstrual dysfunction, vaginal discharge, gynecomastia, infertility, spontaneous abortion, fetal defects

Hematologic: aplastic anemia, leukopenia, thrombocytopenia

Hepatic: hepatotoxicity (cirrhosis, hepatic fibrosis)

Musculoskeletal: stress fracture

Respiratory: dry nonproductive cough, respiratory fibrosis, respiratory failure, interstitial pneumonitis, chronic interstitial obstructive pulmonary disease, *Pneumocystis carinii* pneumonia

Skin: erythematous rashes, pruritus, urticaria, photosensitivity, pigmentary changes, alopecia, ecchymosis, telangiectasia, acne, furunculosis, erythema multiforme, toxic epidermal necrolysis, necrosis, ulceration, exfoliative dermatitis, Stevens-Johnson syndrome, rash, urticaria, pruritus, psoriasis, hyperpigmentation

Other: chills, fever, decreased resistance to infection, septicemia, tumor lysis syndrome, opportunistic infections (possibly fatal), anaphylactoid reactions, sudden death

Interactions

Drug-drug. *Cisplatin, other potentially nephrotoxic or hepatotoxic agents:* increased risk of toxicity

Folic acid: decreased response to systemic methotrexate

NSAIDs: elevated and prolonged serum methotrexate levels, possible death from severe hematologic and GI toxicity

Oral antibiotics (such as chloramphenicol, nonabsorbable broad-spectrum antibiotics, and tetracycline): decreased intestinal absorption or interference with enterohepatic circulation of methotrexate

Phenylbutazone, phenytoin, salicylates, sulfonamides: reduced renal tubular transport and increased toxicity of methotrexate

Sulfamethoxazole-trimethoprim: increased bone marrow depression

Theophylline: decreased theophylline clearance

Drug-diagnostic tests. *Iodine, transaminases, uric acid:* increased

Platelets, RBCs, WBCs: possible decreases

Drug-food. *Any food:* delayed absorption and decreased peak levels of drug

Drug-herb. *Alpha-lipoic acid, coenzyme Q10:* possible decreased chemotherapy efficacy

Black cohosh: increased risk of hepatic failure and autoimmune hepatitis

M

Comfrey, kava: additive adverse hepatic effects
Echinacea, melatonin: interference with immunosuppressive drug action
Glutamine: possible enhanced tumor growth
Thuja: increased risk of seizures

Toxicity and overdose

• Oral overdose commonly results from accidental daily use rather than weekly administration (single or divided doses). Symptoms include hematologic and GI reactions, sepsis or septic shock, renal failure, and aplastic anemia. Intrathecal overdose generally causes CNS symptoms, including headache, nausea and vomiting, seizures, and acute toxic encephalopathy.

• Give leucovorin to reduce toxicity and counteract effects of overdose. Monitor serum methotrexate level to determine optimal dosage and duration of leucovorin treatment. In massive overdose, use hydration and urine alkalization to prevent precipitation of drug or metabolites in renal tubules. Effective drug clearance has been reported with acute, intermittent hemodialysis using high-flux dialyzer. Accidental intrathecal overdose may warrant intensive systemic support, high-dose systemic leucovorin, alkaline diuresis, and rapid CSF drainage and ventriculolumbar perfusion.

Special considerations

• Drug clearance rate varies widely and generally decreases at higher doses.

• Monitor patient closely to allow prompt detection of toxic effects. Frequently monitor CBC with differential, platelet count, liver enzyme levels, renal function tests, and chest X-ray during initiation of therapy, after dosage changes, or during periods of increased risk of elevated methotrexate blood level (such as dehydration).

• Serum drug level monitoring may identify patients at high risk for toxicity and help guide leucovorin dosage adjustment.

• Promptly evaluate patient with profound granulocytopenia and fever. These effects usually warrant parenteral broad-spectrum antibiotic therapy.

• Monitor patient for acute chemical arachnoiditis, manifested by such symptoms as headache, back pain, nuchal rigidity, and fever.

• Chronic leukoencephalopathy manifests as confusion, irritability, somnolence, ataxia, dementia, seizures, and coma. This condition can be progressive and even fatal.

• Monitor for transient acute neurologic syndrome, which may occur with high-dose regimens. Manifestations may include confusion, hemiparesis, transient blindness, seizures, and coma.

• Monitor for subacute myelopathy characterized by paraparesis or paraplegia associated with involvement of one or more spinal nerve roots.

• Focal leukemic CNS involvement may not respond to intrathecal chemotherapy and is best treated with radiotherapy.

• Pulmonary symptoms (especially dry, nonproductive cough) or nonspecific pneumonitis may indicate potentially dangerous lesion and warrant therapy interruption and careful investigation.

• High doses used in osteosarcoma treatment may cause renal damage, leading to acute renal failure. Monitor renal function closely; use hydration and urine alkalization as necessary. Monitor serum drug and creatinine levels.

• Transient liver function test abnormalities are common after methotrexate administration and rarely necessitate modification of methotrexate therapy. However, persistent abnormalities or serum albumin depression may indicate serious hepatotoxicity and require evaluation.

• In women with childbearing potential, do not start methotrexate until pregnancy has been excluded. Provide thorough counseling on serious risk to fetus if pregnancy occurs during methotrexate therapy.

• If relapse occurs, repeating initial induction regimen usually reinduces remission.

Only common or life-threatening adverse reactions are listed.

Patient education

- Instruct patient to take drug at same time every day.
- Instruct patient who misses a dose to skip that dose and take next one at regular time.
- Advise patient to seek immediate medical attention for stomach pain; nausea; fever; sore throat; easy bruising or bleeding; weakness or lethargy; loose bowel movements; sores on cheeks, tongue, or lips; difficulty swallowing or breathing; wheezing; light-headedness; fainting; hives; itching; dizziness when standing or sitting up; or yellowing of eyes or skin.
- Advise women with childbearing potential to avoid pregnancy while either partner is receiving methotrexate and for at least 3 months afterward for males and at least one ovulatory cycle afterward for females.
- Caution breastfeeding patient not to breastfeed while taking this drug.

methylprednisolone
Medrol Dosepak, Methylpred DP

methylprednisolone acetate
Depo-Medrol

methylprednisolone sodium succinate
Solu-Medrol

Classification: Corticosteroid, glucocorticoid, anti-inflammatory, immunosuppressant
Pregnancy risk category B

Pharmacology

Methylprednisolone decreases inflammation by depressing polymorphonuclear leukocyte migration and activity of endogenous inflammation mediators. It suppresses immune system by interfering with macrophages and T cells.

Pharmacokinetics

Drug is well absorbed with oral use. It is metabolized in liver and peaks in 1 or 2 hours. Duration is 1.5 days; half-life, less than 3.5 hours. Drug is excreted unchanged by kidney.

How supplied

Powder for injection (sodium succinate): 40 mg/vial, 125 mg/vial, 500 mg/vial, 1 g/vial, 2 g/vial
Solution for injection (acetate): 20-mg/ml vial, 40-mg/ml vial, 80-mg/ml vial
Tablets: 2 mg, 4 mg, 8 mg, 16 mg, 24 mg, 32 mg

Indications and dosages

FDA-APPROVED

➡ Hypercalcemia associated with cancer; secondary thrombocytopenia in adults; acquired autoimmune hemolytic anemia; erythroblastopenia (RBC anemia); palliative management of leukemias and lymphomas in adults and acute leukemia of childhood
Adults: Initially, 4 to 48 mg daily P.O. in four divided doses, based on specific disease; adjust as needed. *Methylprednisolone acetate*— Dosage must be individualized based on disease severity and patient response. When used as temporary substitute for oral therapy, single injection during each 24-hour period is usually sufficient. When prolonged effect is desired, weekly dose may be calculated by multiplying daily dose by 7; that dose may be given as single weekly injection. *Methylprednisolone sodium succinate*—When high-dose therapy is required, recommended dosage is 30 mg/kg I.V. over 30 minutes. Dose may be repeated every 4 to 6 hours for 48 hours.

OFF-LABEL USES (SELECTED)

➡ Prevention of chemotherapy-induced nausea and vomiting
Adults: 40 to 500 mg P.O., I.M., or I.V. every 6 to 12 hours for up to 20 doses

M

DOSAGE MODIFICATIONS

• Dosage requirements vary and must be individualized based on disease and response. After favorable response, determine proper maintenance dosage by decreasing initial dosage in small decrements until reaching lowest dosage that maintains adequate clinical response.
• More severe disease states usually require daily divided high-dose therapy for initial disease control. Continue initial suppressive dosage level until clinical response is satisfactory.
• Increased dosage may be indicated before, during, and after unusually stressful situations.

Contraindications and precautions

Contraindicated in hypersensitivity to drug or its components, systemic fungal infections, intrathecal use (acetate), and *premature infants* (succinate and acetate).

Use cautiously in aspirin sensitivity, active or latent peptic ulcer disease, cirrhosis, diverticulitis, fresh intestinal anastomoses, hypertension, hypothyroidism, myasthenia gravis, nonspecific ulcerative colitis, ocular herpes simplex, osteoporosis, renal insufficiency, pregnancy, and breastfeeding. Live or live attenuated vaccines are not recommended in patients receiving immunosuppressive doses. (Killed or inactivated vaccines may be given, although response may be diminished.)

Preparation and administration

• With high-dose therapy, give antacids as needed to help prevent peptic ulcers.
• Acetate form is for I.M. use and must not be given I.V.
• Sodium succinate form may be given I.V. or I.M. It may be administered by direct I.V. injection after dilution with supplied diluent. For infusion, it may be diluted further with D_5W, dextrose 5% in normal saline solution, or normal saline solution. For I.V. injection, give each 500 mg over at least 2 or 3 minutes.

For I.V. infusion, administer over 10 to 20 minutes.
• After long-term therapy, withdraw drug gradually.
• After administration of desired dose, discard any drug remaining in single-dose vial.
• Store at controlled temperature of 68° to 77° F (20° to 25° C).

Adverse reactions

CNS: euphoria, insomnia, increased intracranial pressure, seizures
CV: arrhythmias, heart failure, circulatory collapse, thrombophlebitis, embolism, tachycardia
GI: peptic ulcer, pancreatitis, increased appetite
Hematologic: thrombocytopenia
Metabolic: adrenal insufficiency
Musculoskeletal: fractures, osteoporosis
Respiratory: bronchospasm

Interactions

Drug-drug. *Aspirin (long-term, high-dose therapy):* increased aspirin clearance with decreased salicylate level and increased risk of salicylate toxicity on methylprednisolone withdrawal
Cyclosporine: seizures, mutual inhibition of metabolism
Ketoconazole, troleandomycin: inhibited metabolism and decreased clearance of methylprednisolone
Oral anticoagulants: altered anticoagulant effect
Phenobarbital, phenytoin, rifampin: increased methylprednisolone clearance
Drug-food. *Grapefruit juice, pomegranate:* increased drug level
Drug-herb. *Aloe, buckthorn, cascara sagrada, Chinese rhubarb, senna:* hypokalemia
Aloe, licorice, perilla: possible increased methylprednisolone effects
Cat's claw, echinacea, eucalyptus, feverfew, kava, licorice, peppermint oil, valerian: possible increased methylprednisolone levels

---

Only common or life-threatening adverse reactions are listed.

Toxicity and overdose
No information available

Special considerations
• Prolonged use may cause posterior subcapsular cataracts and glaucoma with possible optic nerve damage, and may promote establishment of secondary ocular fungal or viral infections.
• If patient is exposed to chickenpox, prophylaxis with varicella zoster immune globulin may be indicated; for measles exposure, prophylaxis with pooled I.M. immunoglobulin may be indicated.
• Monitor patient closely for signs and symptoms of infection.

Patient education
• Advise patient to increase dietary potassium, calcium, and protein intake.
• Urge patient to carry emergency identification card that indicates steroid therapy.
• Instruct patient to notify prescriber if therapeutic response decreases; dosage may need to be adjusted.
• Caution patient not to stop drug abruptly after long-term use, because adrenal crisis could occur.
• Tell patient to avoid over-the-counter products (including salicylates and cough and cold products containing alcohol) and herbal products unless directed by prescriber.
• Advise patient to avoid live-virus vaccinations during therapy and to avoid persons with chickenpox, if possible.
• Ensure that patient can recognize cushingoid and adrenal insufficiency symptoms (such as nausea, anorexia, fatigue, dizziness, dyspnea, weakness, and joint pain). Instruct patient to report these symptoms at once.

metoclopramide hydrochloride
Reglan

Classification: Antiemetic, antivertigo agent, GI stimulant
Pregnancy risk category B

Pharmacology
Metoclopramide stimulates upper GI tract motility without stimulating gastric, biliary, or pancreatic secretions. It increases tone and amplitude of gastric (especially antral) contractions, relaxes pyloric sphincter and duodenal bulb, and increases peristalsis in duodenum and jejunum. These actions accelerate gastric emptying and intestinal transit. Drug also increases resting tone of lower esophageal sphincter.

Pharmacokinetics
Drug is absorbed rapidly through GI tract, metabolized by liver, and distributed to all body tissues. Onset with I.V. use is 1 to 3 minutes; with oral use, 30 minutes to 1 hour; with I.M. use, 10 to 15 minutes. With all routes, duration is 1 to 2 hours and half-life is about 4 hours. Drug is excreted in urine.

How supplied
Injection: 2-ml single-dose vials and ampules containing 5 mg/ml
Oral solution: 5 mg/5 ml
Tablets: 5 mg, 10 mg

Indications and dosages

FDA-approved

➡ Prevention of nausea and vomiting associated with emetogenic cancer chemotherapy
Adults: Initially, two doses of 2 mg/kg I.V. in patients receiving highly emetogenic drugs; or two doses of 1 mg/kg I.V. in patients receiving less emetogenic regimens

➥ Delayed nausea and vomiting
Adults: Typically, 20 to 40 mg P.O. every 4 to 6 hours
➥ Intractable hiccups
Adults: Typically, 10 to 20 mg (base) P.O. four times daily for 7 days. Initial dosage of 10 mg I.M. may be given if necessary.

DOSAGE MODIFICATIONS

• If symptoms are intermittent or occur only at specific times of day, single doses up to 20 mg before triggering situation may be preferred over continuous therapy.
• Patients more sensitive to therapeutic or adverse effects (such as elderly patients) usually require only 5 mg/dose.
• Use lowest effective dosage in elderly patients. If parkinsonian-like symptoms develop (usually within first 6 months), stop drug before initiating specific antiparkinsonian agents; symptoms usually subside within 2 or 3 months of drug withdrawal.
• For patients with creatinine clearance below 40 ml/minute, start therapy at roughly 50% of recommended dosage. Increase or decrease dosage, as needed, based on clinical efficacy.

Contraindications and precautions
Contraindicated in known drug sensitivity or intolerance; GI hemorrhage, mechanical obstruction, or perforation; pheochromocytoma; epilepsy; tardive dyskinesia; and concomitant use of drugs likely to cause extrapyramidal reactions.

Use cautiously in hypertension, cirrhosis, heart failure, Parkinson's disease, and depression. Safety and efficacy in *children* have not been established.

Preparation and administration
• For doses above 10 mg, dilute metoclopramide injectable in 50 ml D₅W, normal saline solution, dextrose 5% in half-normal saline solution, Ringer's solution, or lactated Ringer's solution.

• Infuse I.V. slowly over no less than 15 minutes (or no less than 30 minutes before starting cancer chemotherapy).
• Administer I.V. injection of undiluted drug slowly, allowing 1 or 2 minutes for 10-mg dose. (Rapid administration may cause transient but intense anxiety and restlessness, followed by drowsiness.)
• Watch for extrapyramidal symptoms, which usually occur within 24 to 48 hours of initiation. To treat symptoms, give diphenhydramine hydrochloride 50 mg I.M., as indicated.
• Store tablets at controlled temperature of 68° to 77° F (20° to 25° C). Dispense in tight, light-resistant container.
• Store oral solution at controlled temperature of 59° to 86° F (15° to 30° C). Protect from freezing. Dispense in tight, light-resistant container.
• Store solution for injection (vials, ampules) in carton until use. Do not store open single-dose vials or ampules for later use because they lack preservatives; instead, discard unused portion. Inspect before use and discard if discoloration or particulates appear. Store at controlled temperature of 59° to 86° F (15° to 30° C). Protect from light.

Adverse reactions
CNS: anxiety, fatigue, restlessness, sleeplessness, depression, drowsiness, suicidal ideation, seizures
CV: bradycardia, arrhythmias
GI: nausea, diarrhea, dry mouth
Hepatic: hepatotoxicity (rare)
Respiratory: bronchospasm

Interactions
Drug-drug. *Acetaminophen, tetracycline:* increased rate or extent of acetaminophen or tetracycline absorption from small intestine
Anticholinergics, opioids: antagonism of GI motility effect of metoclopramide
Bromocriptine: increased prolactin level, interference with bromocriptine effects
Cimetidine: decreased cimetidine effect

Cyclosporine: increased cyclosporine bioavailability

Digoxin: decreased digoxin absorption from stomach

Drugs that can cause extrapyramidal reactions: increased frequency and severity of extrapyramidal reactions

Hepatotoxic drugs: increased risk of hepatotoxicity

Levodopa, pergolide: decreased efficacy of these drugs

MAO inhibitors: hypertension

Mexiletine: accelerated mexiletine absorption

Opioids, sedative-hypnotics, tranquilizers: additive sedation

Succinylcholine: prolonged succinylcholine blockade

Drug-diagnostic tests. *Aldosterone, serum prolactin:* increased

Gonadorelin test: increased serum prolactin level

Liver function tests: altered

Drug-herb. *Aloe, barley, cascara:* possible decreased metoclopramide absorption

Toxicity and overdose
• Overdose symptoms may include drowsiness, disorientation, and extrapyramidal reactions.
• Provide supportive treatment. Anticholinergics, antiparkinsonians, or antihistamines with anticholinergic properties may help control extrapyramidal reactions. Dialysis is unlikely to remove drug effectively.

Special considerations
• Monitor patient's blood pressure.
• Observe for signs and symptoms of mental depression in all patients (even those with no history of depression). Manifestations range from mild to severe and may include suicidal ideation and suicide attempt.
• Monitor patient for signs and symptoms of tardive dyskinesia, which drug may suppress. Tardive dyskinesia may remit partially or completely within several weeks or months after drug withdrawal. However, because symptomatic suppression has unknown effect on long-term course of syndrome, using drug to control tardive dyskinesia symptoms is not recommended.
• Extrapyramidal effects (especially parkinsonism and tardive dyskinesia) are more likely to occur if elderly patients are given usual or high doses for prolonged periods.

Patient education
• Advise patient to seek immediate medical attention for muscle spasms, difficulty moving or controlling muscles, difficulty breathing or swallowing, wheezing, light-headedness, fainting, or dizziness when sitting or standing up.
• Advise patient not to drive or perform hazardous tasks until drug effects are known.
• Caution patient not to drink alcohol during therapy.
• Instruct breastfeeding patient not to breastfeed during therapy.

mitomycin
Mutamycin

Classification: Antineoplastic, antibiotic
Pregnancy risk category C

Pharmacology
Mitomycin selectively inhibits DNA synthesis and suppresses cellular RNA and protein synthesis.

Pharmacokinetics
Drug has poor bioavailability when given orally. It is rapidly metabolized to inactive form in liver, spleen, and kidney. With I.V. dose, elimination half-life is about 1 hour. Drug and inactive metabolites are excreted in urine.

How supplied
Powder for injection: 5-mg, 20-mg, and 40-mg vials

M

Indications and dosages

FDA-APPROVED

➡ Disseminated adenocarcinoma of stomach or pancreas in combination with other chemotherapeutic agents, or as palliative treatment when other modalities have failed
Adults or adolescents: After full hematologic recovery from previous chemotherapy, 20 mg/m^2 I.V. as single dose at 6- to 8-week intervals

OFF-LABEL USES (SELECTED)

➡ Bladder cancer
Adults: Typically, 40 mg instilled intravesically into bladder with indwelling catheter by gravity flow weekly and retained for 2 hours, with 1.3 g sodium bicarbonate given the night before, morning of, and 30 minutes before treatment. Administer for 6 weeks.
➡ Squamous-cell cancer of anus (combination therapy)
Adults: Common regimen is radiation at 1.8 Gy daily five times weekly for 5 weeks with 5-fluorouracil (5-FU) 1,000 mg/m^2/24 hours by continuous I.V. over 96 hours, given on day 1 and day 28 of radiation therapy with mitomycin 10 mg/m^2 (maximum, 20 mg per cycle) I.V. bolus on day 1 of each 5-FU course.

DOSAGE MODIFICATIONS

• For patients with WBC count below 2,000/mm^3 and platelet count below 25,000/mm^3, give 50% of previous dose.
• For patients with WBC count between 2,000 and 2,999/mm^3 and platelet count between 25,000 and 74,999/mm^3, give 70% of previous dose.
• For patients with WBC count of 3,000/mm^3 or higher and platelet count of 75,000/mm^3 or higher, give 100% of previous dose.
• Do not repeat dose until WBC count has risen to 4,000/mm^3 and platelet count has risen to 100,000/mm^3.
• When giving drug with other myelosuppressants, adjust dosage. If disease continues after two courses, stop drug because chance of response is minimal.

• Do not give drug to patients with serum creatinine above 1.7 mg/dl.

⊠ WARNINGS

• Bone marrow depression (notably thrombocytopenia and leukopenia) is most common and severe toxic effect.
• Systemic therapy may cause hemolytic uremic syndrome (HUS), marked by microangiopathic hemolytic anemia, thrombocytopenia, and irreversible renal failure. HUS may occur at any time when drug is used as single agent or in combination with other cytotoxic drugs. However, most cases occur at dosage of at least 60 mg. Blood transfusion may exacerbate HUS symptoms.

Contraindications and precautions

Contraindicated in hypersensitivity to drug or its components, previous idiosyncratic reaction to drug, thrombocytopenia, coagulation disorders, and increased bleeding tendencies.

Use cautiously in renal disease and bone marrow depression. Safety and efficacy in *children* have not been established.

Preparation and administration

≫ Follow hazardous drug guidelines for handling, preparation and administration. (See "Managing hazardous drugs," page 11.)
• Drug is not recommended as single-agent primary therapy and should not be used to replace appropriate surgery or radiotherapy.
• Drug may cause acute shortness of breath and severe bronchospasm, with symptom onset occurring within minutes to hours of injection. Use bronchodilators, corticosteroids, or oxygen for symptomatic relief.
• To dilute 5-mg, 20-mg, and 40-mg vials, add 10 ml, 40 ml, or 80 ml sterile water for injection respectively. Shake to dissolve. May dilute further for infusion with D$_5$W injection, normal saline solution, or sodium lactate injection.

Only common or life-threatening adverse reactions are listed.

- Give drug by I.V. route only, using care to avoid extravasation.
- Administer single dose by I.V. injection over 5 to 10 minutes; infusion rate depends on amount and type of solution.
- When reconstituted with sterile water for injection to concentration of 0.5 mg/ml, drug is stable for 14 days refrigerated or for 7 days at room temperature.
- With solutions using D_5W injection, drug is stable for 3 hours; with normal saline solution injection, for 12 hours; with sodium lactate injection, for 24 hours.
- Store unreconstituted drug at room temperature; drug remains stable for lot life indicated on package. Avoid exposure to temperatures above 72° F (22° C).

Adverse reactions
CNS: fever
GI: nausea, vomiting, diarrhea, anorexia
GU: renal failure
Hematologic: thrombocytopenia, leukopenia, anemia
Hepatic: hepatotoxicity
Respiratory: interstitial pneumonitis, pulmonary toxicity
Skin: rash, alopecia, extravasation
Other: septicemia, HUS

Interactions
Drug-drug. *Blood dyscrasia–causing drugs:* increased leukopenia or thrombocytopenia
Doxorubicin: increased cardiotoxicity
Other bone marrow depressants: additive bone marrow depression
Drug-diagnostic tests. *BUN, serum creatinine:* increased
Drug-herb. *Alpha-lipoic acid, coenzyme Q10:* possible decreased chemotherapy efficacy
Glutamine: possible enhanced tumor growth

Toxicity and overdose
- Toxicity signs and symptoms include nausea, vomiting, and myelosuppression.
- Provide supportive treatment with antiemet-ics, antibiotics, and blood components, as needed.

Special considerations
- Adult respiratory distress syndrome has occurred in several patients receiving drug with other chemotherapeutic agents who were maintained on fraction of inspired oxygen above 50% preoperatively. Administer only enough oxygen for adequate arterial saturation. Monitor fluid balance carefully, avoiding overhydration.
- Drug causes high incidence of bone marrow depression (notably thrombocytopenia and leukopenia). Obtain repeated studies of platelets, WBC with differential, and hemoglobin during therapy and for at least 8 weeks afterward.
- Observe patient for signs and symptoms of renal toxicity.

Patient education
- Instruct patient to report complaints or adverse reactions.
- Inform patient that drug may cause temporary hair loss and that new hair growth may differ in color and texture.
- Advise patients with low granulocyte counts to avoid crowds and people with infections.
- Instruct patient to avoid foods that contain citric acid, are spicy, or have a rough texture.

mitotane
Lysodren

Classification: Antineoplastic, miscellaneous
Pregnancy risk category C

Pharmacology
Mitotane, an adrenal cytotoxic agent, inhibits adrenal activity and decreases cortisol production without destroying cells. It also may modify peripheral metabolism of corticosteroids and directly suppress adrenal cortex.

Pharmacokinetics

Drug has moderate bioavailability and is metabolized in liver. It peaks about 4 hours after oral dose (although significant therapeutic effect does not occur until up to 4 weeks of continuous use). Elimination half-life varies but may be as long as 160 hours. Drug is eliminated in urine and bile.

How supplied

Tablets: 500 mg

Indications and dosages

FDA-APPROVED

➡ Inoperable adrenocortical carcinoma
Adults: 2 to 6 g P.O. daily in three to four divided doses, increased incrementally to 9 or 10 g daily P.O. in divided doses. Maximum daily dosage is 19 g.

DOSAGE MODIFICATIONS

• If severe side effects occur, reduce dosage to maximum tolerated amount. If patient can tolerate higher dosages and improved clinical response is possible, increase dosage until adverse reactions recur.
• Dosage should be decreased in patients with hepatic disease.

⊠ WARNINGS

• Drug therapy should be discontinued temporarily immediately if shock or severe trauma occurs (adrenal suppression is drug's main action). Exogenous steroids should be given because depressed adrenal gland may not start secreting steroids right away.

Contraindications and precautions

Contraindicated in hypersensitivity to drug or its components.

Use cautiously in hepatic disease, pregnancy, or breastfeeding. Safety and efficacy in *children* have not been established.

Preparation and administration

• Follow hazardous drug guidelines for handling preparation, and administration. (See "Managing hazardous drugs," page 11.)
• Start treatment in hospital until patient achieves stable dosage regimen.
• Some authorities recommend concomitant steroid replacement during therapy.
• Store tablets at room temperature.

Adverse reactions

CNS: depression, lethargy, dizziness, vertigo
GI: anorexia, nausea, vomiting, diarrhea
Skin: rash, flushing or redness
Other: fever

Interactions

Drug-drug. *CNS depressants:* additive CNS depression
Corticosteroids, glucocorticoids, mineralocorticoids: altered metabolism of these drugs
Corticotropin (ACTH): inhibited adrenal response to ACTH
Warfarin: increased warfarin metabolism
Drug-diagnostic tests. *Plasma cortisol, protein-bound iodine, serum uric acid, urinary 17-hydroxycorticosteroids:* decreased
Transaminases: increased
Drug-herb. *Alpha-lipoic acid, coenzyme Q10:* possible decreased chemotherapy efficacy
Glutamine: possible enhanced tumor growth

Toxicity and overdose

• Overdose signs and symptoms include diarrhea, vomiting, weakness, and numbness of extremities.
• Provide supportive treatment.

Special considerations

• If clinical benefits do not occur after 3 months at maximum tolerated dosage, consider therapy a clinical failure. However, 10% of patients require more than 3 months at maximum dosage to show measurable response.
• Long-term continuous, high-dose therapy may lead to brain damage and functional impairment. Perform behavioral and neurologic

Only common or life-threatening adverse reactions are listed.

assessments at regular intervals when continuous therapy extends beyond 2 years.

• Drug may accelerate warfarin metabolism, raising warfarin dosage requirement. Carefully monitor patient receiving warfarin or other coumarin-type anticoagulant for change in dosage requirements.

Patient education

• Instruct patient to use caution when driving or performing other tasks that require mental and physical alertness; drug may cause sedation, lethargy, vertigo, and other CNS side effects.

• Stress importance of taking only the dosage prescribed and consulting physician before stopping drug.

• Advise patient who misses a dose to take it promptly, unless it is nearly time for next dose.

• Instruct patient to wear or carry medical alert information indicating mitotane therapy.

• Caution patient to avoid alcohol and other CNS depressants during therapy.

• Tell patient to contact physician promptly if injury, infection, or other illness occurs.

• Inform patient of potential adverse effects, including depression, dizziness, appetite loss, nausea, vomiting, diarrhea, skin changes, and fever.

• Provide guidance to help breastfeeding patient decide whether to discontinue breastfeeding or stop drug.

mitoxantrone hydrochloride
Novantrone

Classification: Antineoplastic, antibiotic
Pregnancy risk category C

Pharmacology

Mitoxantrone, a DNA-reactive agent, intercalates into DNA through hydrogen bonding and interferes with RNA. It also strongly inhibits topoisomerase II (enzyme responsible for uncoiling and repairing damaged DNA). Cytocidal effect on both proliferating and nonproliferating cultured cells suggests it lacks cell-cycle-phase specificity. Drug also inhibits B-cell, T-cell, and macrophage proliferation and impairs antigen presentation and secretion of interferon gamma, tumor necrosis factor-alpha, and interleukin-2.

Pharmacokinetics

Drug has poor bioavailability. It is metabolized in liver and distributed extensively. Elimination half-life is 24 to 37 hours. Drug is eliminated in bile.

How supplied

Solution for injection: 2 mg/ml in 10-ml, 12.5-ml, and 15-ml vials

Indications and dosages

FDA-APPROVED

➔Pain related to advanced hormone-refractory prostate cancer (combination therapy with corticosteroids)
Adults: 12 to 14 mg/m² given as a short I.V. infusion every 21 days
➡ Initial treatment of acute nonlymphocytic leukemia (ANLL) in combination with other approved drugs
Adults: For induction, 12 mg/m² I.V. infusion daily on days 1 to 3, with 100 mg/m² cytarabine given as continuous 24-hour infusion daily on days 1 to 7. In incomplete antileukemic response to initial course, second induction course may be given for 2 days and cytarabine may be given for 5 days at same daily dosages after all signs or symptoms of severe or life-threatening nonhematologic toxicity have resolved.

OFF-LABEL USES (SELECTED)

➡ Breast cancer
Adults: Recommended dosage is 14 mg/m² given as single I.V. dose, which may be repeated at 21-day intervals. Lower initial dosage

(12 mg/m^2 or less) is recommended in patients with inadequate marrow reserves caused by previous therapy or poor general condition.

➡ Non-Hodgkin's lymphoma
Adults: Recommended dosage as part of CNOP regimen (cyclophosphamide, mitoxantrone [Novantrone], Oncovin [vincristine], and prednisone) is mitoxantrone 10 mg/m^2 I.V. on day 1 in combination with cyclophosphamide 750 mg/m^2 I.V. on day 1, vincristine 1.4 mg/m^2 I.V. on day 1 (maximum dosage, 2 mg), and prednisone 100 mg P.O. on days 1 to 5. Repeat cycle every 21 days.

➡ Chronic myelocytic leukemia in blast phase, nonlymphocytic leukemia
Adults: Recommended dosage for induction is 12 mg/m^2 given as single I.V. dose daily for 5 consecutive days (total of 60 mg/m^2). This dose is usually sufficient for complete remission. Reinduction on relapse may be attempted; recommended dosage is 12 mg/m^2 daily for 5 days.

⊠ WARNINGS

• Drug should be administered slowly into free-flowing I.V. infusion. It must never be given I.M., subcutaneously, intra-arterially, or intrathecally; severe local tissue damage may occur with extravasation.
• Except in ANLL treatment, drug generally should not be given to patients with baseline neutrophil counts below 1,500/mm^3. Frequent peripheral blood cell counts should be performed on all patients to monitor for bone marrow depression.
• Myocardial toxicity, whose severe form manifests as potentially fatal congestive heart failure (CHF), may occur during therapy or months to years afterward. Cardiotoxicity risk increases with cumulative dose. In cancer patients, risk of symptomatic CHF is about 2.6% for patients receiving cumulative dose of up to 140 mg/m^2. Monitor patient for evidence of cardiotoxicity and ask about CHF symptoms before starting therapy. In multiple sclerosis

patients who reach cumulative dose of 100 mg/m^2, monitor for evidence of cardiotoxicity before each subsequent dose; they should not receive cumulative dose above 140 mg/m^2.
• Active or dormant cardiovascular disease, previous or concomitant radiation to mediastinal or pericardial area, previous therapy with other anthracyclines or anthracenediones, or concomitant use of other cardiotoxic drugs may increase risk of cardiotoxicity.
• Secondary acute myelogenous leukemia (AML) has occurred in cancer patients and multiple sclerosis patients treated with drug. Refractory secondary leukemia is more common when anthracyclines are given with DNA-damaging antineoplastics, when patients have been heavily pretreated with cytotoxic drugs, or when anthracycline dosages have been escalated.

Contraindications and precautions
Contraindicated in hypersensitivity to drug or its components.

Use cautiously in hepatic insufficiency; CHF; preexisting myelosuppression or cardiovascular disease; previous mediastinal radiotherapy; previous therapy with daunorubicin, doxorubicin, or other anthracyclines; systemic infection; pregnancy; and breastfeeding. Safety and efficacy in *children* have not been established.

Preparation and administration
≫ Follow hazardous drug guidelines for handling, preparation, and administration. (See "Managing hazardous drugs," page 11.)
• Before each dose, left ventricular ejection fraction (LVEF) evaluation by echocardiogram or MUGA scan is recommended. Do not give drug if LVEF is below 50% or if significant reduction occurs.
• Monitor CBC with platelet count before each course and if signs or symptoms of infection develop. Monitor liver function tests before each course.

Only common or life-threatening adverse reactions are listed.

• Treat systemic infections concomitantly with or just before therapy begins.
• Dilute dose to at least 50 ml with normal saline solution injection or D_5W injection. Drug may be diluted further in D_5W, normal saline solution, or dextrose 5% with normal saline solution. Use immediately.
• Do not mix in same infusion with other drugs. Introduce diluted solution slowly into tubing as free-running I.V. infusion over 3 to 5 minutes. Discard unused infusion solution promptly and appropriately.
• Avoid extravasation at infusion site. Avoid drug contact with skin, mucous membranes, or eyes. If extravasation occurs (indicated by burning, pain, pruritus, erythema, swelling, bluish skin discoloration, or ulceration), stop injection or infusion and restart in another vein.
• In multidose use, after stopper penetration, store remaining portion of undiluted concentrate no longer than 7 days at 59° to 77° F (15° to 25° C) or 14 days if refrigerated.
• Store between 59° and 77° F. Do not freeze.

Adverse reactions

CNS: headache, seizures, fever
CV: arrhythmias, CHF
GI: bleeding, abdominal pain, nausea, vomiting, diarrhea, mucositis
GU: renal failure, bladder infection
Hematologic: thrombocytopenia, leukopenia, myelosuppression, anemia
Metabolic: hyperuricemia
Respiratory: cough, dyspnea
Skin: alopecia, petechiae, ecchymosis
Other: fever, sepsis

Interactions

Drug-drug. *Blood dyscrasia–causing drugs:* increased leukopenia or thrombocytopenia
Daunorubicin, doxorubicin: increased risk of cardiotoxicity
Oral quinolones (such as ciprofloxacin, gatifloxacin): decreased absorption of these drugs
Other bone marrow depressants: additive bone marrow depression

Drug-diagnostic tests. *Serum ALT, AST, and bilirubin:* increased
Serum or urine uric acid: increased
Drug-herb. *Alpha-lipoic acid, coenzyme Q10:* possible decreased chemotherapy efficacy
Glutamine: possible enhanced tumor growth

Toxicity and overdose

• Overdose signs and symptoms include infection and severe leukopenia.
• No specific antidote exists. Patients may require hematologic support and antimicrobial therapy during prolonged periods of severe myelosuppression. Peritoneal or hemodialysis are unlikely to be therapeutic.

Special considerations

• When given in high doses (above 14 mg/m² daily for 3 days), drug may cause severe myelosuppression. Make sure laboratory and supportive services for hematologic and chemistry monitoring and adjunctive therapies (including antibiotics) are available. Also ensure that blood and blood products are available to support patient during expected period of medullary hypoplasia and severe myelosuppression.
• Observe patient closely for signs and symptoms of infection and bleeding.
• Occasionally, acute CHF occurs in patients receiving drug for ANLL.
• Monitor uric acid level. Maintain hydration, provide hypouricemic therapy, and alkalize urine if necessary.

Patient education

• Stress importance of drinking adequate fluids to promote uric acid excretion.
• Inform patient that drug commonly causes nausea and vomiting. Stress importance of continuing therapy despite these side effects.
• Teach patient how to recognize other side effects—cough, shortness of breath, GI bleeding, leukopenia, infection, stomach pain, stomatitis, mucositis, arrhythmias, CHF, conjunctivitis, jaundice, renal failure, seizures, throm-

M

bocytopenia, allergic reaction, extravasation, local irritation, and phlebitis.
- Advise patient to contact physician promptly for unusual bleeding or bruising, black tarry stools, blood in urine or stools, or pinpoint red spots on skin.
- Instruct patient to avoid exposure to persons with infections, especially during periods of low blood counts.
- Tell patient to contact physician at once for fever or chills, cough or hoarseness, lower back or side pain, or painful or difficult urination.
- Instruct patient to consult physician before undergoing dental procedures.
- Tell patient to use care to avoid accidental cuts with sharp objects (such as safety razor or nail cutter).
- Advise patient that drug may turn urine blue-green and may turn whites of eyes blue.
- Inform patient that drug may cause hair loss but that normal hair should regrow after therapy ends.
- Counsel women with childbearing potential to avoid pregnancy during therapy. If patient is pregnant or becomes pregnant during therapy, inform her that drug may harm fetus.
- Instruct breastfeeding patient not to breastfeed during therapy.

modafinil
Provigil

Classification: Analeptic, CNS stimulant
Controlled substance schedule IV
Pregnancy risk category C

Pharmacology

Modafinil has an unclear mechanism of action. It has wake-promoting actions similar to some sympathomimetics, but is structurally distinct.

Pharmacokinetics

Drug is absorbed rapidly and metabolized in liver. Levels peak in 2 to 4 hours; half-life is 15 hours. It is excreted by kidney.

How supplied

Tablets: 100 mg, 200 mg

Indications and dosages

OFF-LABEL USES (SELECTED)

➡ Cancer patients with depression and lethargy
Adults: Initially, 50 to 100 mg P.O. daily in morning; may escalate to 200 mg P.O. daily in morning

DOSAGE MODIFICATIONS

- Reduce dosage in patients with severe hepatic impairment and elderly patients.

Contraindications and precautions

Contraindicated in hypersensitivity to drug.
 Use cautiously in cardiovascular disease; hypertension; severe hepatic or renal disease; history of emotional instability, psychosis, or drug abuse; pregnancy; breastfeeding; and *elderly patients.* Safety and efficacy in *children* have not been established.

Preparation and administration

- Give drug without food (food delays drug absorption).
- Monitor liver function before and during therapy.
- Store at controlled temperature of 68° to 77° F (20° to 25° C).

Adverse reactions

CNS: headache, nervousness, insomnia, anxiety, dizziness
CV: arrhythmias
EENT: rhinitis
GI: nausea, diarrhea, dyspepsia
Other: back pain

Only common or life-threatening adverse reactions are listed.

Interactions

Drug-drug. *Alpha-adrenergic blockers:* possible exaggeration of hypotensive reaction
Cyclosporines, theophylline: reduced levels of these drugs
CYP3A4 inducers and inhibitors: altered modafinil blood levels
Diazepam, phenytoin, propranolol: increased levels of these drugs
Hormonal contraceptives: decreased contraceptive efficacy
Potassium-sparing diuretics, trimethoprim: increased risk of hyperkalemia
Drug-diagnostic tests. *Glucose:* increased
Liver enzymes: altered
Drug-food. *Black tea, caffeine, coffee:* increased stimulation
Grapefruit, pomegranate: possible increased modafinil levels
Drug-herb. *Cat's claw, echinacea, eucalyptus, feverfew, kava, licorice, peppermint oil, valerian:* possible increased modafinil levels

Toxicity and overdose

• Overdose signs and symptoms include agitation, irritability, confusion, nervousness, tremors, palpitations, and increased pulse and blood pressure.
• Provide supportive treatment. Consider inducing emesis or gastric lavage (unless contraindicated by patient's condition). Institute cardiac monitoring.

Special considerations

• Monitor vital signs and ECG.
• Monitor patient for signs and symptoms of drug abuse.

Patient education

• Advise patient to take drug without food.
• Instruct patient to report chest pain, lightheadedness, shortness of breath, depression, and memory lapses.
• Instruct female with childbearing potential to inform prescriber if she becomes pregnant or intends to become pregnant during therapy.

• Advise female patient to notify prescriber if she is breastfeeding.

morphine sulfate

Astramorph PF, Avinza, Duramorph PF, Infumorph, Kadian, MS Contin, MSIR, MS/S, Oramorph SR, Rapi-Ject, RMS, Roxanol, Roxanol-T

Classification: Opioid analgesic
Controlled substance schedule II
Pregnancy risk category C

Pharmacology

Morphine, a potent centrally active analgesic, interacts with opioid receptors, causing respiratory depression, depression of cough center, antidiuretic hormone release, activation of vomiting center, pupillary constriction, reduced intestinal motility, increased biliary tract pressure, increased ureteral contraction amplitude, and decreased gastric, pancreatic, and biliary secretions.

Pharmacokinetics

Drug is metabolized in liver and is approximately 20% to 35% protein-bound. With oral use, onset, peak, and duration are variable. With I.M. use, onset is 30 minutes; peak, 30 minutes to 1 hour; and duration, 3 to 7 hours. With subcutaneous use, onset is 15 to 20 minutes; peak, 50 to 90 minutes; and duration, 3 to 5 hours. With I.V. use, peak is 20 minutes. With rectal use, peak is 30 minutes to 1 hour and duration is up to 24 hours. With intrathecal use, onset is rapid and duration is up to 24 hours. Drug has half-life of 1.5 to 2 hours. It is excreted in urine and bile.

How supplied

Capsules (extended-release): 30 mg, 60 mg, 90 mg, 120 mg
Capsules (immediate-release): 15 mg

M

Capsules (sustained-release): 20 mg, 30 mg, 50 mg, 60 mg, 100 mg

Injection: 1 mg/ml in 10-ml, 30-ml, 50-ml, and 60-ml prefilled syringes

Injection: 2 mg/ml in 1-ml ampules and 60 ml syringes

Injection: 4 mg/ml in 1-ml ampules

Injection: 5 mg/ml in 50-ml syringes, 30-ml ampules, and 1-ml vial

Injection: 8 mg/ml vials and syringes

Injection: 10 mg/ml in 1-ml ampules, vials, and syringes

Injection: 10 mg/ml in 10-ml, 20-ml, and 30-ml ampules

Injection: 15 mg/ml in 1-ml ampules and vials and in 20 ml-ampules

Injection (preservative-free): 0.5 mg/ml in 10-ml ampules and 10-ml vials

Injection (preservative-free): 1- and 2-mg/ml in prefilled syringes

Oral solution (immediate-release): 10 mg/5 ml, 20 mg/5 ml

Oral solution concentrate (immediate-release): 20-mg/ml strength in 30-ml and 120-ml sizes

Suppositories (foil-wrapped): 5 mg, 10 mg, 20 mg, 30 mg

Tablets (controlled-release): 15 mg, 30 mg, 60 mg, 100 mg, 200 mg

Tablets (extended-release): 15 mg, 30 mg, 60 mg, 100 mg

Tablets (immediate-release): 15 mg, 30 mg

Tablets (soluble): 10 mg, 15 mg, 30 mg

Indications and dosages

FDA-APPROVED

➥ Moderate to severe pain
Adults: Dosage is highly individualized. *I.V. formulations*—2.5 to 15 mg in 4 to 5 ml water for injection, injected I.V. slowly over 4 to 5 minutes. *Subcutaneous and I.M. forms*—10 mg/70 kg (range, 5 to 20 mg) subcutaneously or I.M., depending on patient and cause of pain. *Conventional P.O. forms*—5 to 30 mg P.O. every 4 hours (immediate-release oral solution, immediate-release tablets, or immediate-

release capsules). *Rectal forms*—10 to 20 mg P.R. every 4 hours.
Children: 0.1 to 0.2 mg/kg subcutaneously (maximum dosage, 15 mg)
➥ Moderate to severe pain in patients who require around-the-clock opioid analgesics for extended period
Adults: Dosage is highly individualized. For patients converting from parenteral morphine or other opioid therapy, opioid requirements during previous 24 hours should be calculated and converted to equianalgesic dose. Use conservative dosage conversion ratios to avoid toxicity.

DOSAGE MODIFICATIONS

• Adjust dosage based on pain severity and patient response, metabolism, age, and disease state. Maintain lowest dosage level that produces acceptable analgesia.

• For pain control in terminal illness, give appropriate dosage of oral morphine regularly every 4 hours at lowest dosage that produces acceptable analgesia. When converting patient to morphine from another opioid based on standard equivalence tables, use 1:3 ratio of parenteral:oral morphine equivalence. However, this ratio is conservative and may underestimate amount of morphine needed; if so, gradually increase oral morphine dosage to produce acceptable analgesia and tolerable adverse reactions.

• To convert from conventional oral to controlled-release oral morphine, establish patient's daily requirement using immediate-release morphine (dosing every 4 to 6 hours). Convert patient to controlled-release form by giving half of 24-hour requirement as controlled-release form on every-12-hour schedule (but do not give Kadian more often than every 12 hours); alternatively, give one-third of daily requirement as controlled-release form on every-8-hour schedule.

• If patient does not have proven tolerance to opioids, start with 20 mg and increase dosage by no more than 20 mg every other day.

• Elderly patients, very ill patients, and patients with respiratory problems may require lower dosages because drug may suppress respiration.

⊠ WARNINGS

• Avinza capsules (extended-release formulation) are indicated for once-daily administration for relief of moderate to severe pain requiring continuous, around-the-clock opioids for an extended period. Patients must either swallow Avinza capsules whole or sprinkle capsule contents onto applesauce to take. Capsule beads must not be chewed, crushed, or dissolved due to risk of rapid release and absorption of potentially fatal dose. Patients must not consume alcoholic beverages or use prescription or nonprescription drugs containing alcohol during Avinza therapy. Alcohol consumption during therapy may cause rapid release and absorption of potentially fatal morphine dose.

Contraindications and precautions

Contraindicated in hypersensitivity to drug or its components, respiratory depression, upper airway obstruction, acute or severe bronchial asthma, and paralytic ileus.

Use cautiously in sodium bisulfite sensitivity (some injection forms); atrial flutter and other supraventricular tachycardias; seizures; renal or hepatic dysfunction; severe hepatic, pulmonary, or renal impairment; myxedema or hypothyroidism; adrenocortical insufficiency (such as Addison's disease); CNS depression or coma; toxic psychosis; prostatic hypertrophy or urethral stricture; kyphoscoliosis; acute abdominal conditions; acute pancreatitis secondary to biliary tract disease; acute alcoholism; delirium tremens; inability to swallow; impending biliary tract surgery; pregnancy; breastfeeding; and *elderly* or debilitated patients.

Preparation and administration

• To counteract opioid-induced respiratory depression, keep opioid antagonist (such as naloxone) readily available when administering drug.

• Some morphine sulfate injections contain sodium bisulfite, which may cause allergic-type reactions (including anaphylactic symptoms and life-threatening or less severe asthmatic episodes in certain susceptible patients).

• If patient cannot swallow capsules, carefully open immediate-release capsules and add entire beaded contents to small amount of cool, soft food (such as applesauce or pudding) or liquid (such as water or orange juice). Have patient swallow mixture immediately. Do not store for future use.

• Avinza (extended-release) and Kadian (sustained-release) must be swallowed whole (not chewed, crushed, or dissolved), or may be opened and entire capsule contents sprinkled onto a small amount of applesauce (at room temperature) immediately before ingestion. Do not store for future use.

• Use controlled-release form in patients who need more than several days of continuous treatment with potent opioid analgesic.

• Use controlled-release 100-mg and 200-mg tablets only in opioid-tolerant patients who require daily morphine equivalent dosages of at least 400 mg. Reserve this strength for patients already titrated to stable analgesic regimen using lower strengths of controlled-release morphine or other opioid.

• No maximum dosage for morphine (except Avinza) is recommended as long as dosage is increased gradually. Avinza contains fumaric acid, which has not been demonstrated as safe in dosages above 1,600 mg daily and may cause serious renal toxicity.

• Store oral solution, tablets, and capsules at controlled temperature of 59° to 86° F (15° to 30° C); protect from light. Dispense in tight, light-resistant container with child-resistant closure.

• Discard opened bottle of oral solution after 90 days.

M

Adverse reactions

CNS: dizziness, drowsiness, light-headedness, euphoria, confusion, sedation
CV: fainting, syncope, bradycardia, orthostatic hypotension, cardiac arrest, peripheral circulatory collapse, shock
EENT: blurred vision, miosis, diplopia
GI: dry mouth, nausea, vomiting, anorexia, constipation, cramps
GU: oliguria, urinary retention or hesitancy, reduced libido
Hepatic: biliary tract spasm
Respiratory: respiratory depression, respiratory arrest
Skin: diaphoresis, pruritus
Other: facial flushing, physical or psychological dependence, pain at injection site, hypersensitivity reaction

Interactions

Drug-drug. *Cimetidine:* confusion, severe respiratory depression
Coumarin, other anticoagulants: increased anticoagulant activity
Diuretics: reduced diuretic efficacy or acute urinary retention (particularly in prostatism)
MAO inhibitors: possible precipitation of unpredictable and possibly fatal reactions
Mixed opioid agonist/antagonists (such as butorphanol, nalbuphine, and pentazocine): reduced analgesic effect, possible precipitation of withdrawal symptoms
Other CNS depressants: respiratory depression, hypotension, profound sedation or coma
Skeletal muscle relaxants: increased respiratory depression
Drug-food. *Cranberry juice (excessive amounts), oats:* possible decreased morphine effects
Drug-herb. *Chamomile, hops, Jamaican dogwood, kava, lavender, mistletoe, nettle, pokeweed, poppy, senega, skullcap, valerian:* increased CNS depression
Corkwood: increased anticholinergic effects

Toxicity and overdose

• Acute overdose manifests as respiratory depression, somnolence progressing to stupor or coma, skeletal muscle flaccidity, cold and clammy skin, constricted pupils, and in some cases pulmonary edema, bradycardia, hypotension, and mydriasis. Death may occur.
• For initial management, establish secure airway and support ventilation and perfusion. Monitor heart filling pressures; noncardiac pulmonary edema may occur. Evacuate stomach by emesis or gastric lavage—especially if patient took controlled-release capsules—if treatment can begin within 2 hours after oral ingestion. Naloxone may be used to antagonize opioid effects; however, its use in physically dependent patients should be avoided, if possible. If antagonist must be used to treat serious respiratory depression, administer with extreme care and titrate with smaller-than-usual dosages. Do not give antagonist in absence of clinically significant respiratory or cardiovascular depression. Administer I.V. fluids and vasopressors for hypotension, as indicated. Atropine may be useful for treatment of bradycardia. Forced diuresis, peritoneal dialysis, hemodialysis, and charcoal hemoperfusion have not proven beneficial.

Special considerations

• Drug can cause dependence and may be abused. Psychic dependence, physical dependence, and tolerance may develop with repeated use. Prescribe and administer drug with caution. Like other opioids, drug is subject to federal narcotics laws.
• Monitor for CNS and respiratory depression.
• Monitor renal function regularly.
• Severe hypotension may occur in patients who are volume-depleted, unable to maintain blood pressure, or receiving concurrent drugs such as phenothiazines or general anesthetics. Orthostatic hypotension may occur in ambulatory patients.
• Drug may obscure accurate diagnosis or clinical course in patients with acute abdominal conditions.
• In adults, analgesia duration increases progressively with age, although degree of analgesia is unchanged. Elderly patients may have

---

Only common or life-threatening adverse reactions are listed.

increased drug sensitivity and achieve higher and more variable serum levels.

• Infants younger than 1 month have decreased clearance and longer elimination half-life compared to older children; morphine clearance and elimination half-life begin to approach adult values by age 2 months. Children old enough to take capsules should have pharmacokinetic parameters similar to adults, dosed on per-kg basis.

Patient education

• Emphasize importance of swallowing controlled-release tablets whole without breaking, chewing, crushing, or dissolving them, to avoid rapid release and absorption of potentially toxic dose.

• Instruct patient who has trouble swallowing immediate-release capsules to open capsule carefully and sprinkle contents onto small amount of food or add to liquid. Contents of controlled-release Avinza or Kadian may be sprinkled onto small amount of soft food such as applesauce.

• Advise patient to measure liquid drug with measuring spoon or dropper, not with kitchen spoon.

• Instruct patient to seek immediate medical attention for difficulty breathing, swallowing, or urinating; shaking; chest pain or other signs of heart problems; sweating; cold skin; weakness or sleepiness; light-headedness or fainting; wheezing; or dizziness when sitting or standing up.

• Caution patient to avoid alcohol and alcohol-containing products and other CNS depressants (such as sleep aids or tranquilizers) before or after taking drug because of possible additive effects (including CNS depression). Tell patient to consult physician before taking other prescription medicines.

• Inform patient that drug may cause severe constipation. Discuss appropriate use of laxatives, stool softeners, or other treatments at start of therapy.

• Instruct patient to use extra caution when driving or performing other hazardous tasks

on days when he takes drug. Advise patient who uses extended-release tablets or changed dosage recently to refrain from these activities until drug effects are known.

• If patient is pregnant or plans to become pregnant, advise her to consult physician before using this or any other drug. Caution patient who is more than 6 months pregnant not to take drug.

• Advise breastfeeding patient to avoid breastfeeding while taking drug.

nilutamide
Nilandron

Classification: Antineoplastic, antiandrogen, hormone modifier
Pregnancy risk category C

Pharmacology

Nilutamine exerts antiandrogenic activity without other hormonal (estrogen, progesterone, mineralocorticoid, or glucocorticoid) effects. It blocks testosterone effects at androgen receptor level, preventing normal androgenic response that causes tumor growth.

Pharmacokinetics

Drug undergoes complete GI absorption and is metabolized in liver. Onset is rapid; levels peak within days. Drug has a duration of weeks and elimination half-life of about 45 hours. It is eliminated in urine.

How supplied
Tablets: 150 mg

Indications and dosages

FDA-APPROVED

➥ Metastatic prostate cancer
Adults: 300 mg P.O. once daily for 30 days; then 150 mg P.O. once daily

N

DOSAGE MODIFICATIONS

• At onset of dyspnea or worsening of preexisting dyspnea, interrupt drug therapy and determine if respiratory symptoms are drug-related. Obtain chest X-ray; if findings suggest interstitial pneumonitis, stop drug. Otherwise, restart drug and monitor pulmonary symptoms closely.

⊠ WARNINGS

• Interstitial pneumonitis has been reported in 2% of patients in controlled clinical trials. In one study, 17% developed interstitial pneumonitis. Postmarketing reports of interstitial changes (including pulmonary fibrosis) resulting in hospitalization and death have been rare. Signs and symptoms included exertional dyspnea, cough, chest pain, and fever. X-rays showed interstitial or alveolar-interstitial changes; pulmonary function tests revealed restrictive pattern with decreased lung diffusing capacity for carbon monoxide. Most cases occurred within first 3 months of treatment and reversed on drug withdrawal. Routine chest X-ray should be performed before treatment begins. Baseline pulmonary function tests may be considered. Patients should be instructed to report any new or worsening shortness of breath occurring during therapy. If symptoms occur, nilutamide should be discontinued immediately until it can be determined if symptoms are drug related.

Contraindications and precautions

Contraindicated in hypersensitivity to drug or its components and in severe hepatic impairment or severe respiratory insufficiency.

Drug is not indicated for use in women. Safety and efficacy in *children* have not been established.

Preparation and administration

• Follow hazardous drug guidelines for handling, preparation, and administration. (See "Managing hazardous drugs," page 11.)

• Before starting drug, obtain baseline liver enzyme levels and routine chest X-ray.

• Drug can be taken with or without food.

• For greatest benefit, start therapy on day of or after orchiectomy.

• Store between 59° F and 86° F (15° C and 30° C) protected from light.

Adverse reactions

CNS: drowsiness, insomnia, dizziness, hyperesthesia, depression
EENT: delayed visual adaptation to dark
GI: nausea, vomiting, diarrhea, constipation, abdominal pain
GU: decreased libido, erectile dysfunction, testicular atrophy, urinary tract infection, hematuria, nocturia, gynecomastia
Hematologic: anemia
Hepatic: hepatotoxicity
Respiratory: dyspnea
Other: hot flashes, edema

Interactions

Drug-drug. *Drugs with narrow therapeutic margins that are metabolized by CYP450 enzymes (such as phenytoin, theophylline, and vitamin K):* delayed elimination, increased elimination half-life, and increased risk of toxicity of these drugs
Warfarin, other coumarin anticoagulants: increased prothrombin time
Drug-diagnostic tests. *Hemoglobin, WBCs:* decreased
Serum ALP, ALT, AST, bilirubin, BUN, creatinine, estradiol, glucose, testosterone: increased
Drug-food. *Grapefruit:* possible increased drug levels
Drug-herb. *Echinacea, eucalyptus, feverfew, kava, peppermint:* possible increased drug levels

Toxicity and overdose

• Overdose signs and symptoms include nausea, vomiting, malaise, headache, and dizziness. Liver enzymes may be elevated.

• Because drug is protein-bound, dialysis may

---

prove ineffective in removing it. If patient does not vomit spontaneously, induce vomiting (if he is alert). Provide general supportive care, including frequent vital sign monitoring and close observation.

Special considerations
• Monitor liver enzymes at regular intervals (every 3 months); if transaminases increase more than 2 to 3 × ULN, stop drug.
• Perform appropriate laboratory tests at first sign or symptom of hepatic injury (such as jaundice, dark urine, fatigue, abdominal pain, and unexplained GI symptoms).

Patient education
• Caution patient to avoid alcoholic beverages during therapy because they may cause dizziness, malaise, or facial flushing.
• Instruct patient to seek immediate medical attention for vision or other eye problems; chest pain; fever; nausea or vomiting; dark urine; stomach swelling or pain; yellowing of eyes or skin; difficulty swallowing, wheezing, or breathing; or light-headedness or fainting.
• If patient reports delayed visual adaptation to dark (ranging from seconds to a few minutes), recommend wearing tinted glasses. Caution patient regarding driving at night or through tunnels. Mention that delayed adaptation may not abate during therapy.

octreotide acetate
Sandostatin, Sandostatin LAR Depot

Classification: Antidiarrheal, hormone modifier
Pregnancy risk category B

Pharmacology
Octreotide exerts actions similar to those of somatostatin (a natural hormone). It strongly inhibits growth hormone (GH), glucagon, and insulin. It also suppresses luteinizing hormone (LH) response to gonadotropin-releasing hormone (GnRH), decreases splanchnic blood flow, and inhibits release of serotonin, gastrin, vasoactive intestinal peptide, secretin, motilin, and pancreatic polypeptide.

Pharmacokinetics
Drug is absorbed rapidly and metabolized by hydrolysis throughout body. It is approximately 65% protein-bound. *Subcutaneous or I.V. use (Sandostatin injection):* Drug peaks within 1 hour. Duration is 12 hours (depending on tumor type) and elimination half-life is about 1.5 hours. It is eliminated in urine. *I.M. use (Sandostatin LAR Depot):* Transient initial peak of about 0.03 ng/ml/mg occurs within 1 hour, declines progressively over next 3 to 5 days, and then slowly increases and reaches its peak in about 2 weeks. Duration is approximately 4 weeks. Drug is eliminated in urine.

How supplied
Injection: 1-ml ampules containing 50, 100, and 500 mcg/ml; 5-ml multidose vials containing 200 and 1,000 mcg/ml
Injection (LAR Depot): 10 mg, 20 mg, and 30 mg in 5 ml-vials in single-use kits

Indications and dosages

FDA-approved

➥ Metastatic carcinoid tumor (symptomatic therapy)
Adults: 0.1 to 0.6 mg subcutaneously or I.V. (Sandostatin) daily in two to four doses for 2 weeks, titrated to patient response; or 20 mg I.M. (Sandostatin LAR) every 4 weeks for 2 months, adjusted for symptomatic control
➥ Vasoactive intestinal polypeptide tumors (VIPomas)
Adults: 0.2 to 0.3 mg subcutaneously or I.V. (Sandostatin) daily in two to four doses for 2 weeks, with dosage adjusted to achieve therapeutic response (dosages above 0.45 mg daily rarely are required); or 20 mg I.M (Sandostatin LAR Depot) every 2 weeks for 2 months, adjusted for symptomatic control

➥ Chemotherapy-induced diarrhea
Adults: Recommended dosage is 0.10 to 0.15 mg subcutaneously (Sandostatin) three times daily as a starting dose. Dosage may be increased up to 2.0 mg three times daily if needed. Treatment may last 3 to 5 days or until diarrhea resolves.

➥ Pancreatic cancer
Adults: Recommended initial dosage is 0.05 mg to 0.15 mg subcutaneously (Sandostatin) given twice daily 30 minutes before meals, with dosage increased gradually according to patient tolerance and response.

➥ Metastatic carcinoid syndrome
Adults: 10 mg to 30 mg I.M. (Sandostatin LAR Depot) once monthly. Or 0.3 to 0.9 mg (Sandostatin) subcutaneously daily has been used.

➥ Thyrotropin-secreting tumors
Adults: Recommended dosage is 20 mg I.M. (Sandostatin LAR Depot) every 4 weeks; or 0.25 to 0.30 mg (Sandostatin) subcutaneously or by continuous I.V. infusion daily.

➥ Gastroenteropancreatic endocrine tumors
Adults: Recommended initial dosage is 0.05 mg once or twice daily subcutaneously (Sandostatin), with dosage increased gradually to 0.1 to 0.2 mg three times daily based on clinical response.

DOSAGE MODIFICATIONS

• Because octreotide must reach therapeutically effective serum levels after initial injection of Sandostatin LAR Depot, patients with carcinoid tumors or VIPomas should continue to receive Sandostatin injection subcutaneously for at least 2 weeks in same dosage they were receiving before switch. Failure to continue subcutaneous injections for this period may lead to symptom exacerbation. (Some patients may require 3 or 4 weeks of subcutaneous therapy.)

• After 2 months of Sandostatin LAR Depot at 20-mg dose in patients with carcinoid tumors or VIPomas, increase to 30 mg every 4 weeks if symptoms are not adequately controlled. Reduce dosage to 10 mg for trial period in patients who achieve good control on 20-mg dose. Dosages above 30 mg are not recommended.

• Withdraw Sandostatin yearly for about 4 weeks in patients who have received irradiation, to evaluate disease activity. If GH or IGF-I (somatomedin C) levels increase and signs and symptoms recur, resume Sandostatin.

• Adjust dosage as needed in patients with renal failure requiring dialysis.

• In elderly patients, dosage adjustments may be necessary because of significant increase in drug's half-life (46%) and significant decrease in clearance (26%).

Contraindications and precautions

Contraindicated in hypersensitivity to drug or its components.

Use cautiously in pregnancy, breastfeeding, and **elderly patients**. Safety and efficacy in **children** have not been established.

Preparation and administration

• Obtain baseline 24-hour urine specimen for 5-HIAA.

• To reduce pain from subcutaneous administration, use smallest volume that will deliver desired dose and inject solution slowly. Avoid multiple subcutaneous injections at same site within short periods. Rotate injection sites.

• Sandostatin may be given subcutaneously (usual route) or I.V. However, I.V. administration is usually reserved for emergencies.

• Sandostatin is stable in sterile isotonic saline solution or sterile solution of D_5W for 24 hours. It may be diluted in volumes of 50 to 200 ml and infused I.V. over 15 to 30 minutes, or given by I.V. push over 3 minutes. In emergencies (such as carcinoid crisis), it may be given by rapid bolus.

• Sandostatin LAR Depot is available in single-use kits containing 5-ml vial of various strengths, 2-ml vial of diluent, 5-ml sterile plastic syringe, two sterile 1.5" 20G needles,

and three alcohol wipes. Kit also contains instruction booklet for preparation of drug suspension for injection. Follow dilution directions closely.
• Sandostatin LAR Depot is for I.M. use only; never give I.V. or subcutaneously. Inject slowly and deeply into gluteal muscle at 4-week intervals; using longer intervals is not recommended. Avoid deltoid injections, which may cause significant discomfort at injection site. Alternate gluteal injection sites to avoid irritation.
• For prolonged storage, refrigerate multidose vials at 36° to 46° F (2° to 8° C) and protect from light. At room temperature (70° to 86° F [20° to 30° C]), drug is stable for 14 days if protected from light. Let solution warm to room temperature before use; do not warm artificially. After initial use, discard multidose vials within 14 days.

Adverse reactions

CV: sinus bradycardia, conduction abnormalities, arrhythmias
GI: nausea, vomiting, diarrhea, abdominal pain, GI bleeding
Hepatic: hepatitis
Metabolic: hyperglycemia, hypoglycemia
Musculoskeletal: weakness
Skin: flushing, edema

Interactions

Drug-drug. *Antidiabetic agents (including sulfonylureas), diazoxide, GH, glucagon, insulin:* hypoglycemia or hyperglycemia
Beta-adrenergic blockers: increased bradycardic effect of octreotide
Cyclosporine: decreased cyclosporine blood level, possibly causing rejection episode
Drug-diagnostic tests. *ECG:* QT prolongation, axis shifts, early repolarization, low voltage, R/S transition, R-wave progression, nonspecific ST–T wave changes
Schilling test: abnormal
Serum ALP, ALT, AST, GGT : increased (if hyperbilirubinemia develops)
Serum glucose: possible alteration

Serum thyroxine, serum vitamin B_{12}: decreased
Serum zinc: excessive increase in patients receiving total parenteral nutrition when fluid loss is corrected
Drug-food. *Fatty foods:* altered drug absorption

Toxicity and overdose
• Overdose signs and symptoms include dizziness, blurred vision, hypoglycemia or hyperglycemia, drowsiness, and motor function loss.
• Provide supportive treatment.

Special considerations
• Evaluate 24-hour urinary 5-HIAA level periodically.
• Monitor liver function studies regularly.
• Single Sandostatin doses may inhibit gallbladder contractility and decrease bile secretion. Of patients who received drug for 12 months or longer, 52% experienced stones or sludge.
• Sandostatin alters balance among counter-regulatory hormones, insulin, glucagon, and GH, possibly causing hypoglycemia or hyperglycemia. It also suppresses secretion of thyroid-stimulating hormone (which may lead to hypothyroidism) and may cause cardiac conduction abnormalities. Monitor glycemic control, thyroid function, and ECG.
• Despite good overall symptom control, patients with carcinoid tumors and VIPomas commonly experience periodic symptom exacerbation during therapy.

Patient education
• Provide careful instructions in sterile subcutaneous injection technique to patient and others who may administer Sandostatin injection.
• Instruct patient to carefully select and rotate injection sites.
• Advise patient to let drug reach room temperature before administering if injection causes pain, stinging, tingling, or burning sensation.

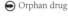

- Instruct patient in safe handling and disposal of needles and syringes. Caution against reusing needles and syringes.
- Stress importance of not missing dose of long-acting form.
- Instruct patient who misses a dose of immediate-release form to take dose promptly unless it is time for next dose, in which case he should follow regular dosing schedule. Caution him not to double the dose.
- Teach patient how to recognize potential side effects, especially arrhythmias, bradycardia, hyperglycemia, hypoglycemia, and acute pancreatitis.
- Instruct patient receiving drug for carcinoid tumor or VIPoma to record number of daily stools or flushing episodes.

ondansetron hydrochloride
Zofran, Zofran ODT

Classification: Antiemetic, antivertigo agent, selective 5-hydroxytryptamine₃ (5-HT)₃ receptor antagonist
Pregnancy risk category B

Pharmacology
Ondansetron exerts serotonin-blocking effect that appears to be associated with serotonin release from enterochromaffin cells of small intestine, which may stimulate vagal afferents through 5-HT₃ receptors and initiate vomiting reflex.

Pharmacokinetics
Drug is extensively metabolized. Levels peak immediately with I.V. use and in 1.7 to 2 hours with oral use. Elimination half-life is roughly 3.5 hours. Drug is excreted in urine and feces.

How supplied
Injection: 2 mg/ml in 2-ml single-dose and 20-ml multidose vials

Injection (premixed): 32 mg/50 ml in 5% dextrose
Oral solution: 4 mg/5 ml
Tablets: 4 mg, 8 mg, 24 mg
Tablets (orally disintegrating tablets [ODT]): 4 mg, 8 mg

Indications and dosages

FDA-APPROVED

➡ Prevention of nausea or vomiting associated with initial or repeat courses of emetogenic cancer chemotherapy (including high-dose cisplatin)
Adults and children ages 4 to 18: 0.15 mg/kg I.V. infused over 15 minutes, 30 minutes before chemotherapy begins; then 0.15 mg/kg I.V. 4 hours and 8 hours after first dose. Or 32 mg I.V. as single dose before start of emetogenic chemotherapy
➡ Prevention of nausea or vomiting associated with highly emetogenic cancer chemotherapy (including cisplatin at or above dosage of 50 mg/m²)
Adults: 24 mg P.O. (oral solution, conventional tablets, or ODT) 30 minutes before start of single-day highly emetogenic chemotherapy
➡ Prevention of nausea or vomiting associated with initial or repeat courses of moderately emetogenic cancer chemotherapy
Adults and children age 12 and older: One 8-mg conventional tablet or one 8-mg ODT or 10 ml (2 tsp equivalent to 8 mg ondansetron) oral solution twice daily. Administer first dose 30 minutes before emetogenic chemotherapy begins; give subsequent dose 8 hours after first dose. After chemotherapy ends, administer one 8-mg tablet or one 8-mg ODT or 10 ml (2 tsp equivalent to 8 mg ondansetron) oral solution twice daily (every 12 hours) for 1 to 2 days.
Children ages 4 to 11: One 4-mg tablet or one 4-mg ODT or 5 ml (1 tsp equivalent to 4 mg ondansetron) oral solution three times daily. Administer first dose 30 minutes before emetogenic chemotherapy begins; give subsequent doses 4 and 8 hours after first dose. Af-

---

Only common or life-threatening adverse reactions are listed.

ter chemotherapy ends, administer one 4-mg tablet or one 4-mg ODT or 5 ml (1 tsp equivalent to 4 mg ondansetron) oral solution three times daily (every 8 hours).

➥ Prevention of nausea and vomiting associated with radiotherapy in patients receiving total body irradiation, single high-dose fraction to abdomen, or daily fractions to abdomen

Adults: For total body irradiation, one 8-mg tablet or one 8-mg ODT or 10 ml (2 tsp equivalent to 8 mg ondansetron) oral solution 1 to 2 hours before each fraction of radiotherapy administered daily. For single high-dose fraction radiotherapy to abdomen, one 8-mg tablet or one 8-mg ODT or 10 ml (2 tsp equivalent to 8 mg ondansetron) oral solution 1 to 2 hours before radiotherapy; give subsequent doses every 8 hours after first dose for 1 to 2 days after radiotherapy ends. For daily fractionated radiotherapy to abdomen, one 8-mg tablet or one 8-mg ODT or 10 ml (2 tsp equivalent to 8 mg ondansetron) oral solution 1 to 2 hours before radiotherapy, with subsequent doses given every 8 hours after first dose for each day radiotherapy is given.

DOSAGE MODIFICATIONS

• In mild to moderate hepatic impairment, clearance is reduced twofold and mean half-life increases to 11.6 hours (compared with 5.7 hours in normal patients). In severe hepatic impairment (Child-Pugh score of 10 or higher), clearance is reduced two- to threefold and apparent distribution volume increases, causing half-life to increase to 20 hours. In patients with severe hepatic impairment, do not exceed total daily dosage of 8 mg. Infuse single maximal daily dose of 8 mg over 15 minutes, beginning 30 minutes before start of emetogenic chemotherapy.

Contraindications and precautions

Contraindicated in hypersensitivity to drug or its components.

Use cautiously in sensitivity to other selective 5-HT$_3$ receptor antagonists, pregnancy,

and breastfeeding. Closely monitor *infants younger than age 4 months.*

Preparation and administration

• Do not remove ODT from blister until just before dosing. Do not push tablet through foil. Instead, peel backing off blister with dry hands; gently remove tablet and immediately place it on patient's tongue to be dissolved and swallowed with saliva.

• For direct I.V. injection, give drug undiluted slowly over 2 to 5 minutes.

• For I.V. infusion, dilute in 50 ml normal saline solution injection, 5% dextrose injection, 5% dextrose and normal saline solution injection, 5% dextrose and half-normal saline solution injection, or 3% sodium chloride injection. Infuse over 15 minutes.

• After dilution, do not use beyond 24 hours.

• Injection form is stable at room temperature under normal lighting for 48 hours after dilution.

• Store Zofran injection and Zofran ODT between 36° and 86° F (2° and 30° C). Protect Zofran injection from light.

• Store premixed Zofran injection between 36° and 86° (2° and 30° C), protected from light. Avoid excessive heat and protect from freezing.

Adverse reactions

CNS: headache, dizziness, drowsiness, fatigue, extrapyramidal symptoms
GI: diarrhea, constipation, abdominal pain
Musculoskeletal: musculoskeletal pain
Respiratory: bronchospasm, hypoxia
Skin: rash
Other: shivering, fever, anaphylaxis

Interactions

Drug-drug. *Carbamazepine, phenytoin, rifampin:* significantly increased clearance and decreased blood level of ondansetron
CYP450 inducers and inhibitors: altered clearance and half-life of these agents
Tramadol: possible increase in patient-controlled tramadol administration

Drug-diagnostic tests. *Serum ALT, AST, and bilirubin:* increased

Drug-food. *Grapefruit, pomegranate:* possible increased ondansetron levels

Drug-herb. *Cat's claw, echinacea, eucalyptus, feverfew, kava, licorice, peppermint oil, valerian:* possible increased ondansetron levels

Toxicity and overdose

• Overdose signs and symptoms include sudden blindness, severe constipation, hypotension, and vasovagal episode with transient second-degree heart block.
• No specific antidote exists. Provide appropriate supportive therapy.

Special considerations

• Drug may mask progressive ileus or gastric distention.
• Monitor fluid intake and output.
• Evaluate vital signs.
• Monitor liver function tests in patients with hepatic impairment.

Patient education

• Instruct patient not to remove ODT from blister until just before dosing and not to push tablet through foil. Instead, instruct patient to peel backing off blister completely (using dry hands), remove tablet gently, and immediately place it on tongue to be dissolved and swallowed with saliva. (To promote proper use and handling, peelable illustrated stickers are affixed to product carton, which can be provided with prescription.)
• Emphasize importance of taking drug exactly as prescribed.
• Instruct patient who misses a dose to skip that dose and take next one at regular time.
• Advise patient to seek prompt medical attention for yellowing of eyes or skin, difficulty breathing or swallowing, wheezing, lightheadedness or fainting, dizziness when standing or sitting up, seizures, chest pain, or difficulty moving or controlling muscles.

oxaliplatin
Eloxatin

Classification: Antineoplastic, platinum agent
Pregnancy risk category D

Pharmacology

Oxaliplatin undergoes nonenzymatic conversion to form interstrand and intrastrand DNA cross-links, which inhibit DNA replication and transcription. Cytotoxicity is cell cycle phase-nonspecific.

Pharmacokinetics

Drug distributes rapidly into body tissues after spontaneous conversion through hydrolysis into active drug and metabolites. Terminal half-life exceeds 300 hours. It is excreted in urine.

How supplied

Powder for injection: 50 mg and 100 mg in single-use vials

Indications and dosages

FDA-APPROVED

➡ Advanced carcinoma of colon or rectum (combination therapy with infusional fluorouracil [5-FU]) and leucovorin in patients whose disease has recurred or progressed during or within 6 months after completing first-line therapy with combination of 5-FU/leucovorin and irinotecan

Adults: Day 1—oxaliplatin 85 mg/m^2 I.V. infusion in 250 to 500 ml D$_5$W and leucovorin 200 mg/m^2 I.V. infusion in D$_5$W, both given over 120 minutes at same time in separate bags using Y-line; followed by 5-FU 400 mg/m^2 I.V. bolus over 2 to 4 minutes; followed by 5-FU 600 mg/m^2 I.V. infusion in 500 ml D$_5$W (recommended) as 22-hour continuous infusion. *Day 2*—leucovorin 200 mg/m^2 I.V. infusion over 120 minutes; followed by 5-FU 400 mg/m^2 I.V. bolus over 2 to 4 minutes; followed by 5-FU 600 mg/m^2 I.V. infusion in 500 ml D$_5$W (recommended) as 22-hour continuous infusion. Repeat cycle every 2 weeks.

OFF-LABEL USES (SELECTED)

➥ Non-small-cell lung cancer
Adults: One regimen included oxaliplatin 130 mg/m^2 (2-hour I.V. infusion) on day 1 and vinorelbine on days 1 and 8 (I.V. infusion over 5 to 10 minutes), with dosages starting at 26 mg/m^2 daily. Treatment was repeated every 21 days.

➥ Esophageal cancer
Adults: One regimen included oxaliplatin 85 mg/m^2 on days 1, 15, and 29; protracted infusion of 5-FU 180 mg/m^2 for 24 hours for 35 days; and external-beam radiation therapy (XRT) 1.8 Gy in 28 fractions starting on day 8. At completion of cycle 1, eligible patients could undergo operation or begin cycle 2 without XRT. Postoperative patients were eligible for cycle 2. Stage IV patients were allowed three cycles in absence of disease progression.

➥ Ovarian cancer
Adults: One dosage schedule included oxaliplatin 130 mg/m^2 over 2 hours every 3 weeks.

➥ Head and neck cancer
Adults: One regimen included radiation therapy (dosage determined by tumor site and size) five times weekly for 6 weeks with oxaliplatin 70 mg/m^2 by I.V. infusion over 2 hours weekly, repeated six times.

DOSAGE MODIFICATIONS

For advanced carcinoma of colon or rectum (combination therapy with infusional 5-FU/ leucovorin)—

• Prolonging infusion time from 2 to 6 hours decreases peak concentration by estimated 32% and may mitigate acute toxicities. 5-FU and leucovorin infusion times do not need to be changed.

• For patients who experience persistent Grade 2 neurosensory events that do not resolve, consider reducing oxaliplatin dosage to 65 mg/m^2. For patients with persistent Grade

3 neurosensory events, consider stopping therapy. (5-FU/leucovorin regimen doses not need to be altered.)

• Reducing oxaliplatin dosage to 65 mg/m^2 and 5-FU by 20% (300 mg/m^2 bolus and 500 mg/m^2 as 22-hour infusion) is recommended for patients after recovery from Grade 3/4 GI toxicity (despite prophylactic treatment) or Grade 4 neutropenia or Grade 3/4 thrombocytopenia. Delay next dose until neutrophil count is at least 1.5×10^9/L and platelet count is at least 75×10^9/L.

⊠ WARNINGS

• Oxaliplatin injection should be administered under supervision of qualified physician experienced in use of cancer chemotherapeutic agents. Therapy and complications can be managed appropriately only when adequate diagnostic and treatment facilities are readily available.

• Anaphylactic-like reactions may occur within minutes of administration. Epinephrine, corticosteroids, and antihistamines have been used to relieve symptoms.

Contraindications and precautions

Contraindicated in known allergy to oxaliplatin or other platinum compounds.

Use cautiously in renal impairment, pregnancy, and breastfeeding. Safety and efficacy in *children* have not been established.

Preparation and administration

• Follow hazardous drug guidelines for handling, preparation, and administration. (See "Managing hazardous drugs," page 11.)

• Premedication with antiemetics (including 5-hydroxytryptamine$_3$ blockers with or without dexamethasone) is recommended.

• Do not reconstitute or dilute drug with sodium chloride solution or other chloride-containing solutions.

• Reconstitute lyophilized powder by adding 10 ml (50-mg vial) or 20 ml (100-mg vial) water for injection or D$_5$W injection. Further dilute with 250 to 500 ml 5% dextrose infusion solution.

• After reconstitution in original vial, refrigerate solution at 36° to 46° F (2° to 8° C) for up to 24 hours. After final dilution with 250 to 500 ml 5% dextrose injection, shelf life is 6 hours at room temperature (68° to 77° F [20° to 25° C]) or up to 24 hours refrigerated (36° to 46° F). Drug is not light-sensitive.

• Drug is incompatible in solution with alkaline drugs or media (such as basic 5-FU solutions) and must not be mixed with these or administered simultaneously through same infusion line. Flush infusion line with D$_5$W before administering any concomitant drug.

• Do not use needles or I.V. administration sets containing aluminum parts that may come in contact with oxaliplatin for preparation or mixing. Aluminum can degrade platinum compounds.

• Hypersensitivity and anaphylactic or anaphylactoid reactions (rash, urticaria, erythema, pruritus and, rarely, bronchospasm and hypotension) may occur within minutes of administration. These reactions usually are managed with standard epinephrine, corticosteroids, or antihistamine therapy and may require drug discontinuation.

• Monitor I.V. site closely to avoid extravasation.

• Store under normal lighting at 77° (25° C); excursions are permitted to 59° to 86° F (15° to 30° C).

Adverse reactions

CNS: fatigue, headache, dizziness, insomnia
CV: cardiac abnormalities
EENT: pharyngitis
GI: severe nausea, vomiting, diarrhea, weight loss, stomatitis, anorexia, gastroesophageal reflux, constipation, dyspepsia, mucositis, flatulence
GU: hematuria, dysuria
Hematologic: anemia, neutropenia, thrombocytopenia
Metabolic: hypokalemia

Respiratory: acute pharyngolaryngeal dysesthesia syndrome, pulmonary fibrosis, dyspnea, cough, rhinitis, upper respiratory tract infection
Skin: alopecia; rash; flushing; extravasation (resulting in local pain and inflammation that may be severe and lead to complications, including necrosis), redness, swelling, and pain at injection site; Stevens-Johnson syndrome
Other: anaphylaxis, angioedema, peripheral neuropathy, infection, fever

Interactions

Drug-drug. *Anticoagulants:* prolonged prothrombin time and INR
5-FU: increased 5-FU plasma level
Other bone marrow depressants: additive bone marrow depression, increased risk of adverse GI reactions
Other nephrotoxic or ototoxic drugs: increased risk of ototoxicity and nephrotoxicity
Drug-diagnostic tests. *Hemoglobin, platelets, neutrophils:* decreased
Serum ALT, AST, bilirubin, creatinine, liver function tests: increased
Drug-herb. *Alpha-lipoic acid, coenzyme Q10:* possible decreased chemotherapy efficacy
Glutamine: possible enhanced tumor growth

Toxicity and overdose

• Overdose may cause thrombocytopenia, myelosuppression, nausea, vomiting, diarrhea, and neurotoxicity.

• No known antidote exists. Monitor patient and provide supportive treatment.

Special considerations

• Monitor patient closely for signs and symptoms of acute pharyngolaryngeal dysesthesia syndrome, which occurs in 1% to 2% of patients previously untreated for advanced colorectal cancer. Syndrome is marked by subjective sensations of dysphagia or dyspnea without laryngospasm or bronchospasm (stridor or wheezing).

• Drug may cause persistent (longer than 14 days) and primarily peripheral sensory neu-

---

Only common or life-threatening adverse reactions are listed.

ropathy marked by paresthesia, dysesthesia, and hypoesthesia. Condition also may include proprioception deficits that interfere with daily activities (such as writing, buttoning, swallowing, and walking). Persistent neuropathy can occur without previous acute neuropathy event. Symptoms may improve in some patients when drug is stopped.

• Watch for unexplained respiratory signs and symptoms, such as nonproductive cough, dyspnea, crackles, or radiologic pulmonary infiltrates. Discontinue drug until further pulmonary investigation excludes interstitial lung disease or pulmonary fibrosis.

Patient education

• Inform patient and caregiver of drug's expected side effects. Tell them that acute neurosensory toxicity may occur or worsen with exposure to cold. Instruct patient to avoid cold beverages and ice, cover exposed skin before exposure to cold temperature or cold objects, avoid ice packs on body, and avoid deep inhalations of cold air. Also advise patient not to run air conditioner at high levels in home or car.

• Advise patient that drug may cause low blood counts. Instruct him to contact physician at once for fever (especially if associated with persistent diarrhea) or signs or symptoms of infection.

• Instruct patient to notify physician of persistent vomiting, diarrhea, signs of dehydration, cough, difficulty breathing, or allergic reaction.

• Instruct patient to avoid contact with persons with infections (especially if blood counts are low) and to contact physician at once for fever, chills, cough, hoarseness, lower back or side pain, or painful or difficult urination.

• Tell patient to promptly report unusual bleeding or bruising, black tarry stools, blood in urine or stools, or pinpoint red spots on skin.

• Advise women with childbearing potential to avoid becoming pregnant while receiving drug.

• Provide guidance to help breastfeeding patient decide whether to discontinue breastfeeding or stop drug.

oxycodone hydrochloride
Endocodone, M-Oxy, OxyContin, Oxydose, OxyFast, OxyIR, Percolone, Roxicodone

Classification: Opioid analgesic
Controlled substance schedule II
Pregnancy risk category C

Pharmacology
Oxycodone inhibits ascending pain pathways in CNS, increases pain threshold, and alters pain perception.

Pharmacokinetics
Drug is metabolized in liver and kidney. Onset is 15 to 30 minutes; peak, 1 hour; and duration, 4 to 6 hours. Drug is excreted in urine and breast milk.

How supplied
Capsules (immediate-release) 5 mg
Solution (oral): 5 mg/5 ml
Solution, concentrate: 20 mg/ml
Tablets (extended-release): 10 mg, 20 mg, 40 mg, 80 mg, 160 mg
Tablets (immediate-release): 5 mg, 15 mg, 30 mg

Indications and dosages

> **FDA-APPROVED**

➥ Moderate to severe pain when continuous, around-the-clock analgesic is needed for extended period
Adults: Dosage for extended-release tablets should be individualized based on patient's condition, previous analgesic use and dosage,

and previous opioid use and tolerance; reliability of conversion estimate used to calculate oxycodone dosage; safety of higher dosages of extended-release forms; and balance between pain control and adverse events. For patients receiving nonopioid analgesics, dosage is 10 mg P.O. every 12 hours; for patients who previously received opioid analgesics, use standard conversion ratio estimate to obtain equivalent total daily oxycodone dosage. Divide total daily dosage by two to obtain twice-daily dosage of extended-release oxycodone dose. Round down to dosage appropriate for available tablet strengths.

See table below for multiplication factors for converting daily dosage of previous opioids to daily dosage of oral oxycodone. However, this table is to be used only for conversion to *oral* oxycodone. For patients receiving high-dose parenteral opioids, a more conservative conversion is warranted; for example, for high-dose parenteral morphine, use 1.5 instead of 3 as multiplication factor.

Multiplication (×) factors for converting daily dosage of previous opioids to daily dosage of oral oxycodone

(mg/day previous opioid × factor = mg/day oral oxycodone)

Opioid	Previous oral opioid	Previous parenteral opioid
oxycodone	1	
codeine	0.15	
hydrocodone	0.9	
hydromorphone	4	20
levorphanol	7.5	15
meperidine	0.1	0.4
methadone	1.5	3
morphine	0.5	3

➡ Relief of moderate to moderately severe pain
Adults: 5 to 15 mg P.O. every 4 to 6 hours, or 5 mg OxyIR or OxyFast P.O. (immediate-release forms) every 6 hours

DOSAGE MODIFICATIONS

• Titrate dosage to adequate effect. Adjust dosage or give rescue drug to patients with breakthrough pain. Adjust dosage every 1 or 2 days (steady-state plasma levels are approximated within 24 to 36 hours). Increasing every-12-hour dosage is more appropriate than increasing dosing frequency.
• If excessive adverse effects occur, next dose should be reduced. If this adjustment leads to inadequate effect, supplemental dose of immediate-release form should be given.
• During chronic therapy (especially for non-cancer pain), reassess continued need for around-the-clock therapy periodically (such as every 6 to 12 months).
• When drug is not needed, taper dosage gradually to prevent withdrawal symptoms in physically dependent patients.
• Oxycodone can be used safely with usual doses of nonopioid analgesics and analgesic adjuvants, provided proper initial dosage is selected carefully.
• Oxycodone extended-release 160-mg tablet is comparable to two 80-mg tablets when taken on empty stomach. However, with high-fat meal, 160-mg tablet has 25% higher peak plasma level. Exert dietary caution when patient initially is titrated to 160-mg tablets.
• Reduce starting dosage to one-third to one-half of usual dosage in debilitated or nontolerant patients.

⊠ WARNINGS

• Drug is an opioid agonist and Schedule II controlled substance with abuse liability similar to that of morphine. When prescribing or dispensing, consider if increased risk of misuse, abuse, or diversion exists.

Only common or life-threatening adverse reactions are listed.

• Extended-release tablets are indicated for management of moderate to severe pain when patient requires continuous, around-the-clock analgesic for extended period. They are not intended for use on as-needed basis.
• Extended-release 80-mg and 160-mg tablets are for use in opioid-tolerant patients only. These tablet strengths may cause fatal respiratory depression when given to patients not previously exposed to opioids.
• Extended-release tablets must be swallowed whole and must not be broken, chewed, or crushed. Rapid release and absorption of potentially fatal dose may occur if patient ingests tablet that is broken, chewed, or crushed.

Contraindications and precautions

Contraindicated in hypersensitivity to drug or its components and in patients in whom opioids are contraindicated, including those with significant respiratory depression, acute or severe bronchial asthma, hypercarbia, or known or suspected paralytic ileus.

Use cautiously in acute abdominal conditions; acute alcoholism; adrenocortical insufficiency disorders (such as Addison's disease); biliary tract disease (including acute pancreatitis); CNS depression or coma; delirium tremens; hypothyroidism; kyphoscoliosis associated with respiratory depression; myxedema; seizure disorder; severe hepatic, pulmonary, or renal impairment; toxic psychosis; urethral stricture; pregnancy; breastfeeding; and *elderly* and debilitated patients. Safety and efficacy in *children* have not been established.

Preparation and administration

• Frequently evaluate pain relief and other opioid effects.
• Most patients receiving extended-release form around the clock need to have immediate-release form available for pain exacerbations or to prevent pain that occurs predictably during certain activities (incident pain).

• Oral concentrate solution is highly concentrated. To avoid acute overdose, use great care in prescribing, dispensing, and administering.
• Store at 77° F (25° C); excursions are permitted from 59° to 86° F (15° to 30° C). Dispense in tight, light-resistant container.

Adverse reactions

CNS: dizziness, drowsiness, light-headedness, euphoria, confusion, sedation
CV: fainting, syncope, bradycardia, orthostatic hypotension, cardiac arrest, peripheral circulatory collapse, shock
EENT: blurred vision, miosis, diplopia
GI: dry mouth, nausea, vomiting, anorexia, constipation, cramps
GU: oliguria, urinary retention or hesitancy, reduced libido
Hepatic: biliary-tract spasm
Respiratory: respiratory depression, respiratory arrest
Skin: diaphoresis, pruritus
Other: facial flushing, physical or psychological dependence, hypersensitivity reaction

Interactions

Drug-drug. *Amiodarone, polycyclic antidepressants, quinidine:* reduced oxycodone metabolism
Other CNS depressants (including centrally acting antiemetics, general anesthetics, phenothiazines, sedative-hypnotics, tranquilizers): respiratory depression, hypotension, profound sedation or coma
Other opioid analgesics: increased respiratory depression and skeletal muscle relaxation
Drug-diagnostic tests. *Amylase:* increased
Drug-food. *Pomegranates:* increased oxycodone levels
Drug-herb. *Corkwood:* possible increased anticholinergic effect
Goldenseal, Jamaican dogwood, kava, lavender, licorice, meadowsweet, mistletoe, nettle, pokeweed, poppy, senega, valerian: increased sedation
Thuja: possible decreased seizure threshold

Toxicity and overdose

• Signs and symptoms of acute overdose include respiratory depression, somnolence leading to stupor or coma, skeletal muscle flaccidity, cold and clammy skin, constricted pupils, bradycardia, and hypotension. Death may occur.

• Establish patent airway and institute assisted or controlled ventilation. Use supportive measures (including oxygen and vasopressors) to manage circulatory shock and pulmonary edema. Cardiac arrest or arrhythmias may warrant cardiac massage or defibrillation. Pure opioid antagonists (such as naloxone and nalmefene) are specific antidotes for respiratory depression; do not give these agents unless patient has clinically significant respiratory or circulatory depression secondary to oxycodone overdose.

Special considerations

• Drug reduces bowel motility. In postoperative patients, monitor for reduced bowel motility and provide standard supportive therapy as needed.

• Physical dependence and tolerance are not unusual during chronic opioid therapy.

• Opioid abstinence or withdrawal syndrome is characterized by restlessness, lacrimation, rhinorrhea, yawning, perspiration, chills, myalgia, and mydriasis. Other manifestations include irritability, anxiety, backache, joint pain, weakness, abdominal cramps, insomnia, nausea, vomiting, diarrhea, anorexia, and increases in blood pressure, respiratory rate, or heart rate.

• OxyContin consists of dual-polymer matrix intended for oral use only. Abuse of crushed tablet may lead to overdose and death (especially with concurrent abuse of alcohol and other substances). With parenteral abuse, tablet excipients (especially talc) can result in local tissue necrosis, infection, pulmonary granulomas, and increased risk of endocarditis and valvular heart injury. Parenteral drug abuse carries risk of transmitting infectious diseases, such as hepatitis and HIV.

• Anticipate such adverse events as constipation; treat with stimulant laxative or stool softener.

• Other opioid-related adverse reactions (such as sedation and nausea) commonly are self-limited and last only a few days. If nausea persists, consider antiemetics or other agents.

Patient education

• Emphasize that patient must swallow extended-release tablets whole. Stress that if broken, chewed, or crushed, tablets release all contents at once, resulting in possible fatal overdose.

• Clearly instruct patient on dosage for oral concentrate, to avoid acute overdose.

• Instruct patient to seek immediate medical attention for difficulty breathing, swallowing, or urinating; chest pain or other signs of heart problems; shaking; sweating; cold skin; weakness or sleepiness; wheezing; light-headedness or fainting; or dizziness when sitting or standing up.

• Advise patient to report breakthrough pain and adverse experiences.

• Instruct patient to consult prescriber before adjusting dosage.

• Inform patient that drug may impair mental and physical ability to perform potentially hazardous tasks (such as driving).

• Caution patient not to take drug with alcohol or other CNS depressants (such as sleep aids or tranquilizers) unless directed by prescriber. Doing so may lead to dangerous additive effects that can result in serious injury or death.

• Inform patient that drug may cause severe constipation. Discuss appropriate use of laxatives, stool softeners, or other treatments when starting therapy.

• Advise patient that oxycodone is a potential drug of abuse. Stress importance of protecting it from theft and not giving it to anyone else.

• Tell patient not to be alarmed when empty matrix "ghosts" (tablets) appear in colostomy or stool. Explain that drug already has been absorbed.

Only common or life-threatening adverse reactions are listed.

• Inform patient that when discontinuing extended-release oxycodone after continued use, dosage must be tapered. Tell him that stopping drug abruptly may cause withdrawal symptoms. Tell patient to consult physician for dosage schedule for gradual discontinuation.

• Instruct patient to keep drug in secure place away from children. When he no longer needs to take drug, tell him to flush unused tablets down toilet.

• Advise female patient who becomes pregnant or is planning pregnancy to consult physician about effects of drug on pregnancy and fetus.

• Advise breastfeeding patient to avoid breastfeeding while taking drug.

paclitaxel
Onxol, Taxol

Classification: Antineoplastic, antimicrotubule agent, antimitotic
Pregnancy risk category D

Pharmacology

Paclitaxel stabilizes microtubules by preventing depolymerization. This action inhibits normal dynamic reorganization of microtubule network essential for vital interphase and mitotic cellular functions. Drug also induces abnormal microtubule bundles throughout cell cycle and multiple asters of microtubules during mitosis.

Pharmacokinetics

Drug is metabolized in liver and widely distributed. Elimination half-life is about 15 to 50 hours. Drug and metabolites are excreted predominantly in bile.

How supplied

Injection: 30-mg/5 ml, 100-mg/16.7 ml, and 300-mg/50 ml multidose vials

Indications and dosages

⊖Advanced carcinoma of ovary
Adults: For previously untreated patients, paclitaxel 175 mg/m² I.V. over 3 hours followed by 75 mg/m² cisplatin I.V. every 3 weeks; or paclitaxel 135 mg/m² I.V. over 24 hours followed by 75 mg/m² cisplatin I.V. every 3 weeks. For previously treated patients, paclitaxel 135 or 175 mg/m² I.V. over 3 hours every 3 weeks.

⊖Adjuvant treatment of node-positive breast cancer
Adults: 175 mg/m² I.V. over 3 hours every 3 weeks for four courses, given sequentially with combination chemotherapy that includes doxorubicin

⊖Breast cancer after failure of combination chemotherapy for metastatic disease or relapse within 6 months of adjuvant chemotherapy
Adults: 175 mg/m² I.V. over 3 hours every 3 weeks

➡ Non-small-cell lung cancer in patients ineligible for potentially curative surgery or radiation therapy
Adults: 135 mg/m² I.V. over 24 hours followed by 75 mg/m² cisplatin I.V. every 3 weeks

⊖AIDS-related Kaposi's sarcoma
Adults: 135 mg/m² I.V. over 3 hours every 3 weeks, or 100 mg/m² I.V. over 3 hours every 2 weeks

➡ Head and neck cancer
Adults: One regimen includes paclitaxel 175 mg/m² I.V. over 3 hours on day 1; ifosfamide 1,000 mg/m² I.V. over 2 hours on days 1 to 3; mesna 400 mg/m² I.V. before ifosfamide and 200 mg/m² I.V. 4 hours after ifosfamide; and cisplatin 60 mg/m² IV on day 1. Cycle repeats every 21 to 28 days.

➡ Metastatic esophageal cancer
Adults: Some dosage schedules include paclitaxel 250 mg/m² I.V. over 24 hours every 21

P

days or 200 mg/m² I.V. over 24 hours every 3 weeks, with cisplatin 75 mg/m² I.V. on day 1. Cycle repeats every 21 days.

➡ Prostate cancer

Adults: One regimen includes paclitaxel 120 mg/m² I.V. by continuous infusion on days 1 to 4, with estramustine 600 mg/m² P.O. daily starting 24 hours before paclitaxel; cycle repeats every 21 days.

➡ Advanced gastric cancer

Adults: One regimen includes paclitaxel 175 mg/m² I.V. on day 1 with 5-fluorouracil 500 mg/m² by continuous I.V. on days 1 to 5; repeat every 3 weeks.

DOSAGE MODIFICATIONS

• In patients with advanced HIV, the following dosage modifications are recommended: Reduce dosage of dexamethasone (as one of three premedication drugs) to 10 mg P.O. (instead of 20 mg P.O.); initiate or repeat paclitaxel therapy only if neutrophil count is at least 1,000/mm³; reduce paclitaxel dosage in subsequent courses by 20% for patients with severe neutropenia (neutrophil count below 500/mm³ for 1 week or more); and initiate concomitant hematopoietic growth factor (G-CSF), as clinically indicated.

• For patients with solid tumors (of ovary, breast, and non-small-cell lung cancer), do not repeat paclitaxel course until neutrophil count is at least 1,500/mm³ and platelet count is at least 100,000/mm³.

• In patients who develop severe neutropenia (neutrophil count below 500/mm³ for 1 week or more) or severe peripheral neuropathy during therapy, reduce dosage by 20% in subsequent courses.

• Patients with hepatic impairment may be at increased risk for toxicity, particularly Grade 3-4 myelosuppression. Recommendations for dosage adjustment for first course are shown in the following table for both 3-hour and 24-hour infusions.

Dosage recommendations for patients with hepatic impairment*

Trans-aminase levels		Bilirubin levels†	Recomended paclitaxel dosage‡
24-hour infusion			
Less than 2 × ULN	and	1.5 mg/dl or less	135 mg/m²
2 to less than 10 × ULN	and	1.5 mg/dl or less	100 mg/m²
Less than 10 × ULN	and	1.6 to 7.5 mg/dl	50 mg/m²
10 or higher × ULN	or	More than 7.5 mg/dl	Not recommended
3-hour infusion			
Less than 10 × ULN	and	1.25 or lower × ULN	175 mg/m²
Less than 10 × ULN	and	1.26 to 2 × ULN	135 mg/m²
Less than 10 × ULN	and	2.01 to 5 × ULN	90 mg/m²
10 or higher × ULN	or	5 or higher × ULN	Not recommended

* Based on clinical trial data. Recommendations are based on dosages for patients without hepatic impairment of 135 mg/m² over 24 hours or 175 mg/m² over 3 hours; data not available to make adjustment recommendations for other regimens (such as for AIDS-related Kaposi's sarcoma).

† Differences in criteria for bilirubin levels between 3- and 24-hour infusion result from differences in clinical trial design.

‡ Dosage recommendations are for first course of therapy. Base further dosage reduction in subsequent courses on individual tolerance.

⊠ WARNINGS

• In clinical trials, 2% to 4% of patients experienced anaphylaxis and severe hypersensitivity reactions (characterized by dyspnea and hypotension that necessitated treatment), angioedema, and generalized urticaria. Fatal reactions have occurred despite premedication.

Only common or life-threatening adverse reactions are listed.

All patients should be pretreated with corticosteroids, diphenhydramine, and histamine$_2$ antagonists. Patients who experience severe hypersensitivity reactions should not be rechallenged with drug.

• To monitor for bone marrow depression (primarily neutropenia, which may be severe and cause infection), perform frequent peripheral blood cell counts on all patients.

Contraindications and precautions

Contraindicated in hypersensitivity to paclitaxel or other drugs formulated in Cremophor EL (polyoxyethylated castor oil) and in patients with solid tumors and baseline neutrophil counts below 1,500/mm^3 or AIDS-related Kaposi's sarcoma with baseline neutrophil counts below 1,000/mm^3.

Use cautiously in increased serum bilirubin level, hepatic impairment, cardiovascular disease, CNS disorders, pregnancy, breastfeeding, and *elderly* patients. Safety and efficacy in *children* have not been established.

Preparation and administration

• Follow hazardous drug guidelines for handling, preparation, and administration. (See "Managing hazardous drugs," page 11.)
• Premedicate all patients to prevent severe hypersensitivity reactions. Premedication may consist of dexamethasone 20 mg P.O. given 12 and 6 hours before paclitaxel, diphenhydramine (or its equivalent) 50 mg I.V. given 30 to 60 minutes before paclitaxel, and cimetidine (300 mg) or ranitidine (50 mg) I.V. given 30 to 60 minutes before paclitaxel.
• Before infusion, dilute drug in normal saline solution injection, D$_5$W injection, 5% dextrose and normal saline solution injection, or 5% dextrose in Ringer's injection to final concentration of 0.3 to 1.2 mg/ml.
• Do not use PVC containers or administration sets. Prepare drug solution and store in glass, polypropylene, or polyolefin containers. Use non-PVC administration sets, such as polyethylene-lined sets.

• Administer through in-line filter with microporous membrane not exceeding 0.22 micron. Filter devices that incorporate short inlet and outlet PVC-coated tubing (such as IVEX-2 filters) have not caused significant DEHP leaching.
• Monitor infusion site closely for infiltration because of extravasation risk.
• Unopened vials are stable until date indicated on package if kept between 68° and 77° F (20° and 25° C) and stored in original package. Solutions for infusion prepared as recommended are stable at ambient temperature (about 77° F) and lighting for up to 27 hours.

Adverse reactions

CV: bradycardia, hypotension, abnormal ECG
GI: nausea, vomiting, diarrhea, mucositis
Hematologic: neutropenia, leukopenia, thrombocytopenia, anemia, bleeding
Hepatic: hepatic impairment
Musculoskeletal: arthralgia, myalgia
Skin: alopecia
Other: infection, peripheral neuropathy, hypersensitivity reactions, anaphylaxis, cellulitis at injection site

Interactions

Drug-drug. *Blood dyscrasia–causing drugs:* increased leukopenia and thrombocytopenia
Other bone marrow depressants: additive bone marrow depression
Drug-diagnostic tests. *Serum ALP, AST, bilirubin, and triglycerides:* increased
Drug-food. *Grapefruit, pomegranates:* possible increased drug levels
Drug-herb. *Cat's claw, echinacea, eucalyptus, feverfew, kava, licorice, peppermint oil, valerian:* possible increased drug level

Toxicity and overdose

• Overdose signs and symptoms include bone marrow depression, peripheral neurotoxicity, and mucositis. Overdose in children may be associated with acute ethanol toxicity (drug contains dehydrated alcohol).

P

• No known antidote exists. Treat supportively.

Special considerations
• Monitor blood counts frequently. Do not retreat patient with subsequent cycles until neutrophil count recovers to above 1,500/mm³ (above 1,000/mm³ for patients with Kaposi's sarcoma) and platelet count recovers to above 100,000/mm³.
• Perform continuous cardiac monitoring during subsequent therapy if patient develops significant conduction abnormalities during drug infusion.
• Monitor blood pressure and heart rate frequently.
• Drug contains dehydrated alcohol (396 mg/ml); consider possible CNS and other effects of alcohol.

Patient education
• Urge patient to immediately report difficulty swallowing or breathing, chest pain, irregular heart beat, wheezing, light-headedness or fainting, or dizziness when sitting or standing up.
• Advise women with childbearing potential to avoid becoming pregnant.
• Instruct breastfeeding patient to discontinue breastfeeding during therapy.

paclitaxel protein-bound particles
Abraxane

Classification: Antineoplastic, antimicrotubule agent
Pregnancy risk category D

Pharmacology
Paclitaxel protein-bound particles is an antimicrotubule agent that promotes assembly of microtubules from tubulin dimers and stabilizes microtubules by preventing depolymerization. This stability inhibits normal dynamic reorganization of microtubule network that is essential for vital interphase and mitotic cellular functions. Paclitaxel induces abnormal arrays or bundles of microtubules throughout cell cycle and multiple microtubule asters during mitosis.

Pharmacokinetics
Drug is metabolized in liver and widely distributed. Elimination half-life is 27 hours. Approximately 20% of drug is excreted in feces.

How supplied
Powder for injectable suspension (lyophilized): 100 mg in single-use vial

Indications and dosages
FDA-APPROVED
➥ Treatment of breast cancer after failure of combination chemotherapy for metastatic disease or relapse within 6 months of adjuvant therapy; previous therapy should have included an anthracycline (unless clinically contraindicated).
Adults: 260 mg/m² I.V. over 30 minutes every 3 weeks

DOSAGE MODIFICATIONS
• If patient experiences severe neutropenia (neutrophil count of 500/mm³ for 1 week or longer) or severe sensory neuropathy, reduce dosage in subsequent courses to 220 mg/m². If severe neutropenia or severe sensory neuropathy recurs, make additional dosage reductions to 180 mg/m².
• For Grade 3 sensory neuropathy, withhold drug until condition resolves to Grade 1 or 2, followed by dosage reduction for all subsequent courses.

WARNINGS
• Drug should be administered under supervision of physician experienced in use of cancer chemotherapeutic agents. Appropriate

management of complications is possible only when adequate diagnostic and treatment facilities are readily available.

• Drug should not be administered to metastatic breast cancer patients with baseline neutrophil counts below 1,500/mm³.

• To monitor for bone marrow suppression (primarily neutropenia, which may be severe and cause infection), monitor frequent peripheral blood cell counts in all patients.

• This albumin form of paclitaxel may substantially affect drug's functional properties (compared to drug in solution). Do not substitute for or with other paclitaxel formulations.

Contraindications and precautions

Contraindicated in patients with baseline neutrophil counts below 1,500/mm³.

Use cautiously in patients with increased serum bilirubin levels, hepatic impairment, cardiovascular disease, CNS disorder, pregnancy or breastfeeding, and in *elderly patients*. Safety and efficacy in *children* have not been established.

Preparation and administration

• Follow hazardous drug guidelines for handling, preparation, and administration. (See "Managing hazardous drugs," page 11.)

• Drug is supplied as sterile lyophilized powder for reconstitution before use. To avoid errors, read entire preparation instructions before reconstitution.

• Each milliliter of reconstituted formulation contains 5 mg/ml paclitaxel.

• To calculate exact total dosing volume of 5 mg/ml suspension required for patient, use this formula:

Dosing volume (ml) = total dose (mg)/5 (mg/ml)

• To reconstitute each vial, slowly inject 20 ml normal saline solution injection over at least 1 minute; direct solution flow onto inside wall of vial. Do not inject normal saline solution injection directly onto lyophilized cake because this causes foaming. Once injection is complete, let vial sit for at least 5 minutes to ensure proper wetting of lyophilized cake or powder. Then gently swirl or invert vial slowly for at least 2 minutes until cake or powder dissolves completely. Avoid generating foam. If foaming or clumping occurs, let solution stand for at least 15 minutes until foam subsides. Do not filter.

• Unopened vials are stable until date indicated on package when stored between 68° and 77° F (20° and 25° C) in original package. Reconstituted drug should be used immediately, but may be stored at 36° to 46° F (2° to 8° C) for up to 8 hours if necessary.

Adverse reactions

CNS: sensory neuropathy, asthenia
CV: bradycardia, hypotension, severe cardiovascular events, abnormal ECG
EENT: vision disturbances
GI: nausea, vomiting, diarrhea, mucositis
Hematologic: neutropenia, thrombocytopenia, anemia, bleeding, febrile neutropenia
Musculoskeletal: myalgia, arthralgia
Respiratory: cough, dyspnea
Skin: alopecia
Other: infection, fluid retention, edema, injection site reaction, hypersensitivity reaction

Interactions

Drug-diagnostic tests. *Serum ALT, AST, and bilirubin:* increased
Drug-food. *Grapefruit, pomegranates:* possible increased drug levels
Drug-herb. *Cat's claw, echinacea, eucalyptus, feverfew, kava, licorice, peppermint oil, valerian:* possible increased drug levels

Toxicity and overdose

• Primary anticipated complications of overdose are bone marrow depression, sensory neurotoxicity, and mucositis.

• No known antidote exists. Treat supportively.

Special considerations
• Obtain frequent peripheral blood counts to monitor for neutropenia and thrombocytopenia. Patient should not be retreated in subsequent cycles until neutrophil count recovers to above 1,500/mm³ and platelet count recovers to above 100,000/mm³.

Patient education
• Instruct patient to report sensory neuropathy (numbness, tingling, or burning in hands and feet).
• Inform patient that drug causes increased susceptibility to infection and fever.
• Advise patient that drug may cause such side effects as low blood pressure, asthenia, arthralgia, and myalgia. Inform patient taking high dosages that vision disturbances may occur.
• Instruct patient to immediately reports signs and symptoms of hypersensitivity reaction, such as difficulty breathing, flushing, chest pain, or irregular heartbeats.

palonosetron hydrochloride
Aloxi

Classification: Antiemetic, antivertigo agent, serotonin-receptor antagonist
Pregnancy risk category B

Pharmacology
Palonosetron selectively blocks serotonin action at 5-hydroxytryptamine₃ (5-HT)₃ receptor sites on vagus nerve terminals and centrally in chemoreceptor trigger zone. Serotonin is thought to initiate vomiting reflex after release from enterochromaffin cells of small intestine.

Pharmacokinetics
After I.V. dose, plasma level initially declines, followed by slow elimination. Drug is mostly bound to plasma proteins. Elimination half-life is about 40 hours. It is excreted primarily in urine.

How supplied
Solution: 0.25 mg in 5-ml vials

Indications and dosages

➡ Prevention of acute nausea and vomiting associated with initial and repeat courses of moderately or highly emetogenic cancer chemotherapy; prevention of delayed nausea and vomiting associated with initial and repeat courses of moderately emetogenic chemotherapy
Adults: 0.25 mg I.V. about 30 minutes before chemotherapy starts. Do not repeat sooner than 7 days.

Contraindications and precautions
Contraindicated in hypersensitivity to drug or its components.

Use cautiously in hypokalemia; hypomagnesemia; congenital QT syndrome; cumulative high-dose anthracycline therapy; or concomitant use of other 5-HT₃ receptor antagonists, diuretics that can cause electrolyte abnormalities, or antiarrhythmics or other agents that cause QT prolongation. Safety and efficacy in *children* have not been established.

Preparation and administration
• Give drug undiluted; infuse I.V. over 30 seconds. Do not mix with other drugs. Flush infusion line with normal saline solution before and after administration.
• Store at controlled temperature of 68° to 77° F (20° to 25° C); excursions are permitted to 59° to 86° F (15° to 30° C). Protect from freezing and light.

Adverse reactions
CNS: headache, anxiety, dizziness
CV: arrhythmia, hypertension, myocardial ischemia, tachycardia
GI: constipation
Metabolic: hyperglycemia
Respiratory: bronchospasm

Only common or life-threatening adverse reactions are listed.

Skin: pruritus
Other: fatigue, fever

Interactions

Drug-diagnostic tests. *AST, bilirubin, blood glucose, potassium:* increased

Toxicity and overdose

• Major signs and symptoms of toxicity are seizures, gasping, pallor, cyanosis, and collapse.
• No known antidote exists. Manage overdose with supportive care. Dialysis is unlikely to be effective.

Special considerations

• Monitor vital signs and ECG.
• Monitor electrolyte and blood glucose levels.

Patient education

• Advise patient to seek medical attention at once for chest pain or pressure.
• Instruct patient to keep physician appointments to monitor progress and drug effects.
• Instruct female patient to tell prescriber if she becomes pregnant, is planning pregnancy, or is breastfeeding.

pegaspargase
Oncaspar

Classification: Antineoplastic, enzyme
Pregnancy risk category C

Pharmacology

Pegaspargase, a modified version of L-asparaginase, breaks down extracellular asparagine, an amino acid necessary for leukemic cell survival. It interferes with DNA and RNA protein synthesis in leukemic cells. (Normal cells are less affected because they cannot produce their own asparagines.) Activity is specific for G_1 phase of cell division.

Pharmacokinetics

Drug is metabolized in reticuloendothelial system and has a rapid onset. Duration is 2 weeks; half-life, 5.5 days. Drug is not detected in urine.

How supplied

Injection: 750 international units/ml in 5-ml vials

Indications and dosages

FDA-APPROVED

➡ Acute lymphoblastic leukemia in patients who require L-asparaginase but have developed hypersensitivity to native L-asparaginase forms; given in combination with other chemotherapy drugs
Adults and children with body surface area (BSA) 0.6 m² or more: 2,500 international units/m² I.M. or I.V. every 14 days
Children with BSA under 0.6 m²: 82.5 international units/kg I.M. or I.V. every 14 days

DOSAGE MODIFICATIONS

• Drug should not be used as sole induction agent except in unusual situation in which combined regimen is inappropriate because of toxicity or other specific patient-related factors or in patients refractory to other therapy. As sole induction agent, recommended adult dosage is also 2,500 international units/m² every 14 days.

Contraindications and precautions

Contraindicated in previous serious allergic reactions to drug, pancreatitis or history of pancreatitis, and significant hemorrhagic events associated with previous L-asparaginase therapy.

Use cautiously in hepatic, renal, or CNS disease; infection; patients receiving concurrent hepatotoxic agents; pregnancy or breastfeeding; and *elderly patients.*

P

Preparation and administration
- Follow hazardous drug guidelines for handling, preparation. and administration. (See "Managing hazardous drugs," page 11.)
- Avoid excessive agitation of vial. Do not shake.
- I.M. route is preferred. Limit volume at single injection site to 2 ml. If volume to be given exceeds 2 ml, use multiple injection sites.
- For I.V. use, administer over 1 to 2 hours in 100 ml sodium chloride or dextrose injection 5% through already-running infusion.
- Use only one dose per vial; do not re-enter vial. Discard unused portions.
- Observe patient for 1 hour after administration. Keep resuscitation equipment and appropriate drugs on hand to treat anaphylaxis.
- Refrigerate at 36° to 46° F (2° to 8° C). Do not use drug if stored at room temperature for more than 48 hours. Do not freeze (freezing inactivates drug); do not administer if there are indications that drug has been frozen.

Adverse reactions
CNS: dizziness, headache, coma, fatigue, confusion, seizures, paresthesia, mood changes
CV: chest pain, hypertension
GI: nausea, vomiting, anorexia, cramps, stomatitis, diarrhea, pancreatitis
GU: urinary frequency, renal failure, glycosuria, polyuria
Hematologic: thrombocytopenia, leukopenia, anemia, thromboembolic events, disseminated intravascular coagulation
Hepatic: hepatotoxicity
Metabolic: hyperglycemia
Musculoskeletal: musculoskeletal pain, arthralgia
Respiratory: severe bronchospasm, upper respiratory tract infection
Skin: petechial rash, itching
Other: chills, fever, hypersensitivity, anaphylaxis

Interactions
Drug-drug. *Aspirin, dipyridamole, heparin, NSAIDs, warfarin:* potential imbalance in coagulation factors, leading to bleeding or thrombosis
Methotrexate: decreased methotrexate action
Protein-bound drugs: possible increased toxicity of these drugs
Some antitumor agents: possible unfavorable reactions, including interference with enzymatic hepatic detoxification of these agents
Drug-diagnostic tests. *Blood glucose, liver function tests, serum amylase and lipase, uric acid:* increased
Fibrinogen, partial thromboplastin time (PTT), plasma proteins, prothrombin time (PT): altered
Lymphoblasts: decreased
Drug-herb. *Alpha-lipoic acid, coenzyme Q10, glucosamine, glutamine:* possible decreased chemotherapy efficacy

Toxicity and overdose
- Anticipated overdose symptoms include liver enzyme elevation and rash.
- Treat supportively. Monitor liver enzymes levels and administer antihistamine, as indicated.

Special considerations
- Obtain frequent serum amylase levels to detect early evidence of pancreatitis.
- Monitor blood glucose, fibrinogen, PT, and PTT frequently.
- When using with hepatotoxic chemotherapy, monitor patient for hepatic dysfunction.
- Observe patient closely for signs and symptoms of infection.

Patient education
- Instruct patient to immediately report signs and symptoms of serious adverse reactions, such as fever, chills, sore throat, mental confusion, unusual thirst, unusual bleeding or bruising, rash, difficulty breathing, or yellowing of eyes and skin.
- Caution patient to avoid using drug simultaneously with other drugs that may increase risk of bleeding (including aspirin).
- Advise patient to maintain fastidious oral hygiene and to contact prescriber for symp-

---

Only common or life-threatening adverse reactions are listed.

toms of stomatitis, including painful redness, swelling, or mouth sores.

• Provide guidance to help breastfeeding patient decide whether to discontinue breastfeeding or stop drug.

pegfilgrastim
Neulasta

Classification: Colony-stimulating factor (CSF), hematopoietic agent
Pregnancy risk category C

Pharmacology

Pegfilgrastim is an amino acid protein and covalent conjugate of recombinant methionyl human G-CSF (filgrastim) and monomethoxypolyethylene glycol. It acts on hematopoietic cells by binding to specific cell-surface receptors, stimulating proliferation, differentiation, commitment, and end-cell functional activation.

Pharmacokinetics

Drug has half-life of 15 to 80 hours when given subcutaneously, with biological activity lasting much longer. Neutrophil-receptor binding is an important component in clearance, and serum clearance directly relates to neutrophil count. Heavy patients may experience higher systemic exposure to drug. Compared to filgrastim, pegfilgrastim has prolonged in vivo persistence and reduced renal clearance.

How supplied

Injection: 6 mg/0.6 ml (10 mg/ml) in prefilled, single-dose syringe with UltraSafe Needle Guard

Indications and dosages

FDA-APPROVED

➡ To reduce incidence of infection in patients with nonmyeloid malignancies who are receiving myelosuppressive anticancer drugs

associated with clinically significant incidence of febrile neutropenia

Adults and children weighing more than 45 kg (99 lb): 6 mg subcutaneously once per chemotherapy cycle

DOSAGE MODIFICATIONS

• Drug should be discontinued or withheld until adult respiratory distress syndrome (ARDS) resolves.

Contraindications and precautions

Contraindicated in hypersensitivity to drug, *Escherichia coli*–derived proteins, filgrastim, or other components of product.

Use cautiously in myeloid malignancies, sickle cell disease, ARDS, left upper abdominal pain, shoulder tip pain, concurrent chemotherapy, pregnancy or breastfeeding, and *elderly patients.* Safety and efficacy in *children weighing less than 99 lb (45 kg)* have not been established.

Preparation and administration

• Obtain CBC and platelet count before chemotherapy begins to evaluate patient's hematologic status and ability to tolerate myelosuppressive chemotherapy.
• Do not give drug 14 days before or 24 hours after cytotoxic chemotherapy because rapidly dividing myeloid cells may have increased sensitivity to cytotoxic chemotherapy.
• Do not use 6-mg, fixed-dose, single-use syringe form in infants, children, or smaller adolescents weighing less than 99 lb (45 kg).
• Withdraw drug if allergic reaction occurs.
• To activate UltraSafe Needle Guard, place hands behind needle, grasp guard with one hand, and slide guard forward until needle is completely covered and guard clicks into place. Avoid shaking syringe.
• Before injection, drug may be allowed to reach room temperature for up to 48 hours but should be protected from light. Discard if left at room temperature for more than 48 hours.

• Store drug in refrigerator at 36° to 46° F (2° to 8° C). Avoid freezing. If drug is accidentally frozen, allow it to thaw in refrigerator; if frozen a second time, discard.

Adverse reactions

CNS: headache, fatigue, dizziness, generalized weakness, insomnia
GI: nausea, vomiting, diarrhea, constipation, abdominal pain, anorexia, taste perversion, dyspepsia, mucositis, stomatitis, splenic rupture
Hematologic: leukocytosis, granulocytopenia, neutropenic fever, aggravation of sickle cell disease, splenic rupture
Musculoskeletal: skeletal pain, myalgia, arthralgia
Respiratory: ARDS in neutropenic patients
Skin: alopecia, urticaria, rash
Other: pyrexia, peripheral edema, allergic reactions including anaphylaxis

Interactions

Drug-drug. *Lithium:* increased neutrophil release
Drug-diagnostic tests. *Serum ALP, lactate dehydrogenase, uric acid:* increased (reversible)

Toxicity and overdose

• Maximum amount that can be given safely in single or multiple doses has not been determined. In overdose, expect leukocytosis.
• Consider leukapheresis in management of symptomatic patient.

Special considerations

• Regularly monitor patient's hematocrit and platelet count.
• Keep patients with sickle cell disease well hydrated, and monitor for sickle cell crisis.
• If patient has left upper abdominal or shoulder tip pain, evaluate for enlarged spleen or splenic rupture. Rare cases of splenic rupture have been reported.
• ARDS has occurred in neutropenic patients with sepsis who have received filgrastim (possibly from neutrophil influx to inflammatory

lung sites). If neutropenic patient develops fever, lung infiltrates, or respiratory distress, evaluate for ARDS. Provide appropriate medical management for this condition.

Patient education

• Inform patient of possible adverse effects, including signs and symptoms of allergic reaction. Advise him to report these right away.
• Stress importance of regular physician visits and compliance with treatment, including regular blood count monitoring.
• If patient or caregiver will administer drug at home, provide appropriate instructions on proper use of drug and proper handling and disposal of drug, needles, and syringes.

pemetrexed
Alimta

Classification: Antineoplastic, antimetabolite
Pregnancy risk category D

Pharmacology

Pemetrexed disrupts folate-dependent metabolic processes essential for cell replication. In vitro studies show that it inhibits thymidylate synthase (TS), dihydrofolate reductase, and glycinamide ribonucleotide formyltransferase (GARFT). Drug is converted inside cell to polyglutamate forms by folyl-polyglutamate synthetase. Polyglutamate forms are retained in cells and inhibit TS and GARFT.

Pharmacokinetics

Drug is not appreciably metabolized. Approximately 81% is plasma–protein bound. Elimination half-life is 3.5 hours in patients with normal renal function. Total systemic clearance is 91.8 ml/minute. Impaired renal function reduces drug clearance and increases AUC. Total AUC and maximum plasma concentration increase proportionally with dose. Pharmacokinetics do not change over multiple treatment cycles. Drug is eliminated mainly in urine, with 70% to 90% of dose recovered unchanged within first 24 hours.

How supplied
Powder for infusion: 500 mg sterile lyophilized powder in single-use vials

Indications and dosages

FDA-APPROVED
➡ Malignant pleural mesothelioma in patients whose disease is unresectable or who are not otherwise candidates for curative surgery
Adults: Pemetrexed 500 mg/m² I.V. infusion over 10 minutes on day 1 of each 21-day cycle, in combination with cisplatin 75 mg/m² infused over 2 hours starting approximately 30 minutes after pemetrexed administration ends
➡ Locally advanced or metastatic non-small-cell lung cancer after previous chemotherapy
Adults: 500 mg/m² I.V. infusion over 10 minutes on day 1 of each 21-day cycle

DOSAGE MODIFICATIONS
• For pemetrexed and cisplatin therapy–induced hematologic toxicities with nadir absolute neutrophil count (ANC) below 500/mm³ and nadir platelet count of 50,000/mm³ or more, give 75% of previous dosages of both drugs. For such toxicities in which nadir ANC is below 50,000/mm³ (regardless of nadir platelet count), give 50% of previous dosages of both drugs.
• If patient develops nonhematologic toxicity (excluding neurotoxicity) at or greater than Grade 3 (except Grade 3 transaminase elevation), withhold pemetrexed until toxicity resolves to less than or equal to pretherapy value. Except in mucositis, resume therapy at 75% reduction of previous pemetrexed and cisplatin dosages. For Grade 3 or 4 mucositis, resume therapy at 50% of previous pemetrexed dosage and 100% of previous cisplatin dosage.

• For common toxicity criteria (CTC) Grades 0 to 1 neurotoxicity, give 100% of previous dosages of both drugs. For CTC Grade 2 neurotoxicity, give 100% of previous pemetrexed dosage and 50% of previous cisplatin dosage.
• Discontinue therapy if patient experiences hematologic or nonhematologic Grade 3 or 4 toxicity (except Grade 3 transaminase elevations) after two dosage reductions. Discontinue therapy immediately if Grade 3 or 4 neurotoxicity occurs.
• Do not administer when creatinine clearance is below 45 ml/minute. Use caution when administering drug concurrently with NSAIDs to patients with creatinine clearance below 80 ml/minute.

Contraindications and precautions
Contraindicated in severe hypersensitivity reaction to drug or its components.
  Use cautiously in hepatic or renal impairment, neurotoxicity, and pregnancy or breastfeeding. Safety and efficacy in *children* have not been established.

Preparation and administration
• Drug is intended for I.V. use only.
• Pretreatment with dexamethasone (or equivalent) reduces incidence and severity of cutaneous reactions.
• Hydrate patient consistent with local practice (usually 1 to 2 L of fluid infused over 8 to 12 hours) before and after cisplatin administration. Maintain adequate hydration and urine output during next 24 hours.
• For patients with clinically significant third-space fluid, consider draining effusion before administering drug.
• To reduce toxicity, patient must take at least five daily doses of low-dose folic acid preparation or multivitamin with folic acid within 7 days before first pemetrexed dose. Folic acid therapy should continue during full course of therapy and for 21 days after final dose. Patient also must receive one I.M. injection of vitamin B₁₂ during week before first pemetrexed dose and every three cycles thereafter.

P

(Patients in clinical trials received vitamin B_{12} 1,000 mcg I.M. and, most commonly, folic acid 400 mcg P.O.)

• Reconstitute 500-mg vial with 20 ml preservative-free normal saline solution injection, yielding 25 mg/ml. Gently swirl vial until powder completely dissolves. Resulting solution is clear and ranges from colorless to yellow or greenish yellow. Further dilute appropriate volume of reconstituted solution to 100 ml with preservative-free normal saline injection, and administer I.V. over 10 minutes.

• Drug is physically incompatible with diluents containing calcium, including Ringer's and lactated Ringer's solutions. Coadministration of pemetrexed with other drugs and diluents is not recommended.

• Patients with mild to moderate renal insufficiency should avoid taking NSAIDs with short elimination half-lives for 5 days before, on day of, and for 2 days after pemetrexed administration. If concomitant NSAID use is necessary, monitor patient closely for toxicities (especially myelosuppression and renal and GI toxicity).

• Store at 77° F (25° C); excursions are permitted to 59° to 86° F (15° to 30° C). Discard unused portion. Drug is not light sensitive.

Adverse reactions

CNS: fatigue, mood alteration, depression, sensory neuropathy
CV: thromboembolism, chest pain
EENT: pharyngitis
GI: stomatitis, nausea, vomiting, constipation, anorexia, diarrhea, dysphagia, esophagitis, odynophagia
GU: renal failure
Hematologic: neutropenia, leukopenia, thrombocytopenia, anemia
Respiratory: dyspnea
Skin: rash, desquamation
Other: fever, dehydration, infection, hypersensitivity reaction

Interactions

Drug-drug. *Ibuprofen:* approximately 20% reduction in pemetrexed clearance and AUC in patients with normal renal function
Nephrotoxic drugs, tubularly secreted drugs (such as probenecid): possible delay in pemetrexed clearance
Drug-diagnostic tests. *ALT, AST, creatinine:* increased
CBC, platelets: decreased
Drug-herb. *Alpha-lipoic acid, coenzyme Q10, glucosamine, glutamine:* possible decreased chemotherapy efficacy

Toxicity and overdose

• Few cases of overdose have occurred. Anticipated complications include bone marrow depression (neutropenia, thrombocytopenia, and anemia), infection with or without fever, diarrhea, and mucositis.

• If overdose occurs, provide general supportive measures. For some Grade 3 or 4 toxicities, I.V. leucovorin may be indicated.

Special considerations

• Monitor CBC and platelet count and periodic chemistry tests in all patients. Monitor for nadir and recovery before each dose and on days 8 and 15 of each treatment cycle. Do not start new cycle unless ANC is 1,500/mm³ or higher, platelet count is 100,000/mm³ or higher, and creatinine clearance is 45 ml/minute or higher.

Patient education

• Instruct patient to take folic acid and vitamin B_{12} as prescribed to reduce risk of treatment-related hematologic and GI toxicity.

• Instruct patient to drink ten 8-oz glasses of fluids and urinate frequently during first 24 hours after therapy that includes cisplatin.

• Advise women with childbearing potential to avoid pregnancy. If patient becomes pregnant during therapy, inform her that drug may harm fetus.

• Instruct breastfeeding patient to stop breastfeeding during therapy.

Only common or life-threatening adverse reactions are listed.

pentostatin
Nipent

Classification: Antineoplastic, antimetabolite
Pregnancy risk category D

Pharmacology
Pentostatin, which is isolated from fermentation cultures of *Streptomyces antibioticus,* strongly inhibits adenosine deaminase (ADA). Greatest ADA activity occurs in lymphoid cells. T cells have higher ADA activity than B cells, and T-cell cancers have higher ADA activity than B-cell cancers. ADA inhibition leads to cytotoxicity, particularly in presence of adenosine or deoxyadenosine. Drug also inhibits RNA synthesis and causes increased DNA damage. Precise mechanism of antitumor action in hairy cell leukemia is unknown.

Pharmacokinetics
Drug undergoes little metabolism and has low plasma protein–binding (approximately 4%). Elimination half-life is 2.6 to 15 hours. Most of dose is eliminated in urine unchanged.

How supplied
Powder for injection: 10 mg in single-dose vial

Indications and dosages

FDA-approved

➥ Interferon alfa–refractory hairy cell leukemia
Adults: 4 mg/m² by I.V. bolus over 1 minute or diluted in larger volume and given over 20 to 30 minutes, every other week

Off-label uses (selected)

➲ Cutaneous T-cell lymphoma, including Sézary syndrome and mycosis fungoides
Adults: One dosage schedule specifies 5 mg/m² I.V. daily for 3 days, repeated every 3 weeks.

➲ Relapsed or refractory chronic lymphocytic leukemia
Adults: One dosage schedule specifies 4 mg/m² I.V. weekly for 3 weeks, then 4 mg/m² every other week for 6 weeks and once monthly for 6 months.

Dosage modifications

- Withhold dose in patients with elevated serum creatinine level. In patients with impaired renal function (creatinine clearance below 60 ml/minute), give drug only if potential benefit justifies potential risk.
- Withhold drug temporarily if absolute neutrophil count (ANC) decreases from pretreatment baseline value above 500/mm³ to below 200/mm³ during therapy. Therapy can resume when ANC returns to pretreatment level.
- Interrupt therapy temporarily if active infection occurs. Resume therapy when infection is controlled.
- Withhold dose or discontinue therapy if patient experiences severe adverse reactions or signs and symptoms of neurotoxicity. Withhold dose in patients with severe rash.

WARNINGS

- Do not give dosages above those specified. Dose-limiting renal, hepatic, pulmonary, and CNS toxicities may occur.
- Using drug in combination with fludarabine phosphate in patients with refractory chronic lymphocytic leukemia is not recommended due to high risk of severe or fatal pulmonary toxicity. In clinical investigations using drug at recommended dosages in combination with fludarabine, four of six patients experienced severe or fatal pulmonary toxicity.

Contraindications and precautions
Contraindicated in hypersensitivity to drug.
  Use cautiously in infection; renal or hepatic impairment; bone marrow depression; administration with fludarabine; combination treatment with carmustine and high-dose cyclo-

P

phosphamide; and pregnancy or breastfeeding. Safety and efficacy in *children* have not been established.

Preparation and administration

• Follow hazardous drug guidelines for handling, preparation, and administration. (See "Managing hazardous drugs," page 11.)

• Before initiating therapy, obtain serum creatinine or creatinine clearance assay.

• Hydrate patient with 500 to 1,000 ml 5% dextrose in half-normal saline solution or equivalent before drug is given. Administer additional 500 ml 5% dextrose solution or equivalent after drug is given.

• Inject 5 ml sterile water for injection into vial and mix thoroughly; yields 2 mg/ml solution.

• Give drug by I.V. bolus injection or dilute in larger volume (25 to 50 ml) with 5% dextrose injection or normal saline solution injection. Diluting entire contents of reconstituted vial with 25 or 50 ml yields concentration of 0.33 mg/ml or 0.18 mg/ml, respectively.

• Solution does not interact with PVC infusion containers or administration sets at concentrations of 0.18 to 0.33 mg/ml.

• Refrigerate vial at 36° to 46° F (2° to 8° C). Store reconstituted vials, or reconstituted and further diluted vials, at room temperature under ambient light. Use within 8 hours; drug contains no preservatives.

Adverse reactions

CNS: fatigue, headache
CV: peripheral edema, ECG abnormalities, hypotension
GI: nausea, vomiting, diarrhea, anorexia
GU: severe renal toxicity, GU disorder
Hematologic: leukopenia, anemia, thrombocytopenia
Hepatic: hepatic disorder
Musculoskeletal: myalgia
Respiratory: increased cough, upper respiratory tract infection
Skin: rash, skin disorder

Other: chills, fever, infection, pain, allergic reaction

Interactions

Drug-drug. *Carmustine, cyclophosphamide (high doses):* pulmonary edema, hypotension
Fludarabine: increased risk of fatal pulmonary toxicity
Drug-diagnostic tests. *Creatinine, liver function tests, uric acid:* increased
Granulocytes, platelets, WBCs: decreased
Drug-herb. *Alpha-lipoic acid, coenzyme Q10, glucosamine, glutamine:* possible decreased chemotherapy efficacy

Toxicity and overdose

• Administration at dosages higher than recommended (20 to 50 mg/m^2 in divided doses over 5 days) may cause death from severe renal, hepatic, pulmonary, or CNS toxicity.

• No specific antidote exists. In overdose, provide general supportive measures.

Special considerations

• Monitor serum creatinine level before each dose and at other appropriate times during therapy.

• Monitor hematologic parameters with CBCs before each dose and at other appropriate times during therapy. If severe neutropenia continues after initial cycles, evaluate patient for overall disease status (including bone marrow examination).

• Periodically monitor peripheral blood for hairy cells to evaluate response to treatment.

• Bone marrow aspirates and biopsies may be needed at 2- to 3-month intervals to evaluate response to treatment.

• Monitor blood chemistry values regularly.

• Evaluate response to therapy after 6 months. If patient has not responded, discontinue drug. If partial response occurs, continue therapy in attempt to obtain complete response. If complete response occurs, give two additional doses and then stop therapy. If best response at end of 12 months is partial response, stop therapy.

Only common or life-threatening adverse reactions are listed.

Patient education

- Inform patient of signs and symptoms of side effects.
- Caution women with childbearing potential to avoid pregnancy.
- Provide guidance to help breastfeeding patient decide whether to discontinue breastfeeding or stop drug.

plicamycin (mithramycin)
Mithracin

Classification: Antineoplastic, antibiotic
Pregnancy risk category X

Pharmacology

Plicamycin, produced by *Streptomyces plicatus,* has an unclear mechanism of action. It forms complexes with DNA, inhibits DNA-directed RNA synthesis, and shows potent cytotoxicity against malignant cells of human origin (Hela cells) growing in tissue culture. It may inhibit effects of parathyroid hormone on osteoclasts and inhibit bone resorption, thereby lowering serum calcium and phosphate levels and blocking hypercalcemic actions of vitamin D.

Pharmacokinetics

Drug is metabolized in liver. Onset is 1 to 2 days; peak, 2 to 3 days; and duration, 3 to 15 days. Drug may localize in areas of active bone resorption. Elimination half-life is approximately 2 hours. Parent drug and metabolites are eliminated by kidney.

How supplied

Powder for injection: 2,500 mcg plicamycin with 100 mg mannitol and disodium phosphate as freeze-dried, sterile preparation in each vial

Indications and dosages

FDA-APPROVED

➥ Testicular cancer in patients for whom successful treatment with surgery or radiation is impossible
Adults: Initially, 25 to 30 mcg/kg I.V. daily over 4 to 6 hours for 8 to 10 days, not to exceed 30 mcg/kg daily; may be repeated at monthly intervals if tumor mass remains unchanged. If significant testicular tumor regression occurs, give additional courses at monthly intervals until tumor masses regress completely or new tumor masses show definite progression despite continued therapy.
➥ Reversal of hypercalcemia and hypercalciuria associated with advanced malignancy
Adults: 25 mcg/kg I.V. over 4 to 6 hours daily for 3 to 4 days; may be repeated weekly or on schedule of two or three doses weekly until adequate response occurs

DOSAGE MODIFICATIONS

- Daily dosage is based on body weight. In abnormal fluid retention (such as edema, hydrothorax, or ascites), use patient's ideal rather than actual weight.

P

⊠ WARNINGS

- Drug is for I.V. use only.
- Due to possibility of severe reactions, drug should be given only to hospitalized patients by or under supervision of qualified physician experienced in use of cancer chemotherapeutic agents. Facilities for necessary laboratory studies must be available.
- Severe thrombocytopenia, hemorrhagic tendency, and even death may occur. Although severe toxicity is more likely in patients who have far-advanced disease or otherwise are considered poor risks for therapy, serious toxicity also may occur in patients in relatively good condition.
- Before therapy begins, carefully weigh potential therapeutic benefit against risk of toxicity. Also thoroughly review data regarding

drug use in treatment of testicular tumors and hypercalcemic or hypercalciuric conditions associated with various advanced cancers.

Contraindications and precautions

Contraindicated in thrombocytopenia, thrombocytopathy, coagulation disorders, increased risk of bleeding, impaired bone marrow function, and women with childbearing potential.

Use cautiously in significant renal or hepatic impairment, electrolyte imbalance, concurrent radiation therapy, and breastfeeding.

Preparation and administration

• Follow hazardous drug guidelines for handling, preparation, and administration. (See "Managing hazardous drugs," page 11.)
• Before therapy, correct electrolyte imbalances (especially hypocalcemia, hypokalemia, and hypophosphatemia).
• Obtain renal function studies before therapy.
• Give antiemetic before and during therapy to relieve nausea and vomiting.
• Before reconstitution, store at 36° to 46° F (2° to 8° C) in light-resistant container.
• To reconstitute, add 4.9 ml sterile water for injection to vial, to yield solution of 500 mcg/ml. After removing appropriate dose, discard remaining solution. Dilute calculated dose in 1 L 5% dextrose injection or normal saline solution injection.
• Give by slow I.V. infusion over 4 to 6 hours. Avoid rapid, direct I.V. injection because it may be associated with higher incidence and greater severity of GI adverse effects.
• Drug is a vesicant. Extravasation may cause local irritation and cellulitis at injection site. If thrombophlebitis or perivascular cellulitis occurs, stop infusion and reinstitute at another site. Applying moderate heat to extravasation site may help disperse drug and minimize discomfort and local tissue irritation.

Adverse reactions

CNS: drowsiness, weakness, lethargy, headache, depression

EENT: epistaxis
GI: nausea, vomiting, anorexia, diarrhea, stomatitis, hematemesis
GU: proteinuria
Hematologic: hemorrhagic syndrome, thrombocytopenia, clot retraction
Metabolic: hypocalcemia, hypophosphatemia, hypokalemia
Skin: rash, cellulitis
Other: facial flushing

Interactions

Drug-drug. *Other antineoplastics:* increased toxicity
Drug-diagnostic tests. *BUN, liver enzymes, prothrombin time, serum creatinine:* increased
Serum calcium, phosphate, and potassium: decreased
Drug-herb. *Alpha-lipoic acid, coenzyme Q10, glucosamine, glutamine:* possible decreased chemotherapy efficacy
Anise, arnica, chamomile, clove, dong quai, fenugreek, garlic, ginger, ginkgo, ginseng (Panax), *licorice:* possible increased risk of bleeding

Toxicity and overdose

• Anticipated effects of overdose are exaggeration of usual adverse effects.
• No specific antidote exists. Provide general supportive measures and close monitoring of hematologic function, including clotting factors, liver and kidney function test results, and serum electrolyte levels.

Special considerations

• Closely monitor hematologic function and observe patient for signs and symptoms of hemorrhagic syndrome, which may begin with epistaxis or hematemesis.
• Continue to monitor renal and hepatic function and serum electrolytes closely during and after therapy.

Patient education

• Instruct patient to immediately report nosebleed or GI bleeding.

Only common or life-threatening adverse reactions are listed.

- Instruct patient to inspect mouth daily and report white spots and ulcerations.
- Advise patient to report leg cramps, tingling of fingertips, and weakness.
- If patient uses drug while pregnant or becomes pregnant while taking it, inform her of potential hazard to fetus.
- Provide guidance to help breastfeeding patient decide whether to discontinue either breastfeeding or drug.

porfimer sodium
Photofrin

Classification: Antineoplastic, miscellaneous
Pregnancy risk category C

Pharmacology

Porfimer, a mixture of oligomers composed of up to eight porphyrin units, is a photosensitizing agent that causes cellular damage and tumor death when combined with light. Cellular damage caused by photodynamic therapy (PDT) with drug results from propagation of radical reactions.

Pharmacokinetics

Drug is 90% protein-bound. It peaks in 1.5 hours in women and in 0.17 hours in men. Half-life is 250 hours. It is eliminated primarily through biliary system.

How supplied

Powder for injection: 75 mg as freeze-dried cake or powder in vial

Indications and dosages

FDA-approved

➡ Palliation in completely obstructing esophageal cancer or in partially obstructing esophageal cancer in patients who cannot be satisfactorily treated with Nd:YAG laser therapy; reduction of obstruction and symptom palliation in completely or partially obstructing endobronchial non-small-cell lung cancer; ablation of high-grade dysplasia in Barrett's esophagus in patients who do not undergo esophagectomy

Adults: Initially, 2 mg/kg as single, slow I.V. injection over 3 to 5 minutes; then, 40 to 50 hours later, laser light illumination at 630-nm wavelength; then residual tumor debridement followed by second laser light application 96 to 120 hours after initial drug injection. Patient may receive second PDT course no sooner than 30 days (90 days for dysplasia in Barrett's esophagus) after initial therapy. Up to three courses, each separated by at least 30 days (90 days for dysplasia in Barrett's esophagus), can be given.

➡ Microinvasive endobronchial non-small-cell lung cancer in patients for whom surgery and radiotherapy are not indicated

Adults: Initially, 2 mg/kg as single, slow I.V. injection over 3 to 5 minutes; then, 40 to 50 hours later, laser light illumination at 630-nm wavelength; then residual tumor debridement followed by second laser light application 96 to 120 hours after initial drug injection. Patient may receive second PDT course no sooner than 30 days after initial therapy. Up to three courses, each separated by at least 30 days, can be given.

Off-label uses (selected)

➡ Transitional-cell carcinoma in situ of bladder

Adults: 2 mg/kg I.V. injection followed 40 to 50 hours later by whole-bladder intravesical laser light treatment at 630 nm

Contraindications and precautions

Contraindicated in porphyria, porphyrin allergy, tracheoesophageal or bronchoesophageal fistula, and tumor eroding into major vessel.

Use cautiously in esophageal varices, endobronchial tumors at sites where treatment-induced inflammation could obstruct main airway, and pregnancy or breastfeeding. Safety

P

and efficacy in *children* have not been established.

Preparation and administration
- Give drug as single, slow I.V. injection over 3 to 5 minutes.
- Reconstitute each vial with 31.8 ml 5% dextrose injection or normal saline solution injection, yielding 2.5 mg/ml. Shake well until dissolved. Do not mix with other drugs in same solution. Use reconstituted product immediately; protect from bright light.
- Inspect vial for particles and discoloration before administration.
- Take precautions to prevent extravasation at injection site. If extravasation occurs, guard area against light. (Injecting extravasation site with another substance achieves no known benefit.)
- Before second laser light treatment, residual tumor should be debrided. Vigorous debridement may cause tumor bleeding. For endobronchial tumors, necrotic tissue debridement should be discontinued when bleeding volume increases (which may indicate that debridement has gone beyond zone of PDT treatment effect).
- Store at controlled temperature of 68° to 77° F (20° to 25° C).

Adverse reactions
CNS: anxiety, confusion, insomnia
CV: hypotension, hypertension, atrial fibrillation, cardiac failure, tachycardia
GI: abdominal pain, constipation, diarrhea, dyspepsia, dysphagia, eructation, esophageal edema, hematemesis, melena, nausea, vomiting, anorexia, esophageal strictures
GU: nocturia, bladder spasm, pain on urination
Hematologic: anemia
Metabolic: hyperthermia
Musculoskeletal: substernal chest pain
Respiratory: pleural effusion, pneumonia, dyspnea, respiratory insufficiency, tracheo-esophageal fistula
Other: photosensitivity reaction

Interactions
Drug-drug. *Fluoroquinolones, griseofulvin, phenothiazines, sulfonamides, sulfonylureas, tetracyclines, thiazides:* increased photosensitivity
Drug-diagnostic tests. *Hemoglobin:* decreased
Liver function tests: increased
Drug-herb. *Alfalfa, bergamot oil, bishop's weed, St. John's wort:* possible potentiation of photosensitivity
Alpha-lipoic acid, coenzyme Q10, glucosamine, glutamine: possible decreased chemotherapy efficacy

Toxicity and overdose
- No information exists on overdose or its effects on photosensitivity duration.
- If overdose occurs, patient must protect eyes and skin from direct sunlight or bright indoor light for 30 days. After overdose, patient should not receive laser treatment.

Special considerations
- PDT with porfimer is a two-stage process. Stage 1 is I.V. injection of drug. Tissue clearance occurs over 40 to 72 hours, but tumors, skin, and reticuloendothelial organs (including liver and spleen) retain drug for longer period. Stage 2 is illumination with 630-nm wavelength laser light. Tumor selectivity occurs through combination of selective porfimer retention and selective light delivery.
- PDT is not suitable for emergency treatment of patients with severe acute respiratory distress caused by obstructing endobronchial lesion, because 40 to 50 hours must elapse between drug injection and laser light treatment.
- PDT is not suitable for patients with esophageal or gastric varices or esophageal ulcers larger than 1 cm in diameter.
- If PDT will precede radiotherapy, allow sufficient interval to ensure that inflammatory response from first treatment has subsided before radiotherapy; allow 2 to 4 weeks after PDT before starting radiotherapy. Similarly, if radiotherapy will precede PDT, allow 4 weeks

---

Only common or life-threatening adverse reactions are listed.

for acute inflammatory reaction from radio-therapy to subside before administering PDT.
• Closely monitor patients with endobronchial lesions for respiratory distress between laser light therapy and mandatory debridement bronchoscopy. Inflammation, mucositis, and necrotic debris may cause airway obstruction. If respiratory distress occurs, bronchoscopy must be performed immediately to remove secretions and debris and allow airway to open.

Patient education

• Instruct patient to wear sunglasses with average white light transmittance below 4% and to avoid exposure to sunlight or bright light for 30 days after treatment.
• Inform patient that conventional UV sunscreens do not protect against photosensitivity reactions caused by drug.
• Tell patient that substernal chest pain may occur after PDT due to inflammatory response within treatment area. Pain may be sufficiently intense to warrant short-term opioid analgesic use.
• Advise women with childbearing potential that drug's effect on fetus is unknown.
• Caution breastfeeding patient not to breastfeed during therapy.

prednisone
Deltasone, Liquid Pred, Meticorten, Orasone, Sterapred, Winpred

Classification: Corticosteroid
Pregnancy risk category B

Pharmacology

Prednisone causes profound and varied metabolic effects, including modification of immune responses to diverse stimuli and reduction of the inflammation that causes cancer pain. In hormone-sensitive disease stimulated by weak adrenal androgens, it may suppress androgens through negative feedback on secretion of adrenocorticotropic hormone, in turn reducing pain.

Pharmacokinetics

Drug has good oral bioavailability. It is metabolized in liver, primarily to its active form, prednisolone. Peak is 1.3 hours; elimination half-life, 2.6 to 3 hours. Excretion routes are not well defined.

How supplied

Oral solution: 5 mg/5 ml
Oral solution (concentrate): 5 mg/ml
Tablets: 1 mg, 2.5 mg, 5 mg, 10 mg, 20 mg, 50 mg

Indications and dosages

FDA-APPROVED

➡ Metastatic, androgen-independent (hormone-refractory) prostate cancer
Adults: Prednisone 5 mg P.O. twice daily on days 1 to 21 with docetaxel 75 mg/m² I.V. as 1-hour infusion on day 1; repeat cycle every 21 days.
➡ Stage III and IV Hodgkin's lymphoma (MOPP regimen)
Adults: 40 mg/m² P.O. daily on days 1 to 14 during cycles 1 and 4
➡ Acute leukemia
Children: When used in combination with other chemotherapy drugs for induction, consolidation, and intensification, usual dosage is 40 mg/m² P.O. daily given in various schedules depending on regimen.
➡ Non-Hodgkin's lymphoma
Adults: In combination with cyclophosphamide, doxorubicin, and vincristine (CHOP), prednisone 50 mg/m² P.O. daily on days 1 to 5; cycle repeated every 21 days
Adults: In combination with rituximab, cyclophosphamide, doxorubicin, and vincristine (CHOP plus rituximab), prednisone 40 mg/m² P.O. daily on days 1 to 5 or 100 mg/m² P.O. daily on days 1 to 5; cycle repeated every 21 days

P

Adults: In combination with cyclophosphamide, mitoxantrone, and vincristine (CNOP), prednisone 50 mg/m^2 P.O. daily on days 1 to 5; cycle repeated every 21 days

Adults: In combination with cyclophosphamide and vincristine (COP), prednisone 60 mg/m^2 P.O. daily on days 1 to 5, then tapered over 3 days; cycle repeated every 14 days

Adults: In combination with cyclophosphamide and vincristine (CVP), prednisone 40 mg/m^2 P.O. daily on days 1 to 5; cycle repeated every 21 days for 8 cycles

Off-label uses (selected)

➥ Pain relief in patients with metastatic prostate cancer

Adults: Various dosage schedules, including use as monotherapy, 7.5 to 10 mg P.O. daily; as combination therapy, 5 mg P.O. four times daily with flutamide 250 mg P.O. three times daily

➥ Chronic lymphocytic leukemia

Adults: Various dosage schedules, including use as single agent in symptomatic patients with autoimmune hemolytic anemia and immune thrombocytopenia, 60 to 100 mg/m^2 P.O. daily for 3 to 6 weeks

Dosage modifications

• Dosage requirements vary and must be individualized based on disease being treated and patient's response. After favorable response, determine proper maintenance by reducing initial dosage in small decrements at appropriate intervals until reaching lowest dosage that maintains adequate clinical response.

• Children's dosages should be determined more on basis of severity of condition and patient response than on age or weight. Determining dosage in terms of mg/kg increases risk of overdose, especially in very young, short, or heavy children.

• To minimize drug's potential effects on growth, titrate dosage in children to lowest effective level.

Contraindications and precautions

Contraindicated in hypersensitivity to drug and systemic fungal infections.

Use cautiously in diabetes mellitus, glaucoma, osteoporosis, seizure disorders, ulcerative colitis, peptic ulcer disease, heart failure, myasthenia gravis, renal disease, esophagitis, hypothyroidism, cirrhosis, pregnancy, breastfeeding, *elderly patients,* and *children*.

Preparation and administration

• Administering drug with food may minimize indigestion or mild GI irritation.

• Store at controlled temperature of 68° to 77° F (20° to 25° C).

Adverse reactions

CNS: euphoria, insomnia, mood changes, seizures, headache

CV: hypertension

EENT: increased intraocular pressure, glaucoma, cataracts

GI: GI hemorrhage, increased appetite, pancreatitis, peptic ulcer disease, abdominal distention

GU: menstrual irregularities

Metabolic: hyperglycemia, negative nitrogen balance, hypokalemia

Musculoskeletal: fractures, osteoporosis, weakness, myopathy, slowed bone growth (children)

Skin: acne, poor wound healing, ecchymosis, petechiae

Other: infection, fluid retention

Interactions

Drug-drug. *Aspirin, NSAIDs:* increased risk of GI ulceration

Cyclosporine: increased cyclosporine concentration

CYP450 3A4 inducers (such as barbiturates, ephedrine, phenytoin, rifampin): decreased prednisone concentration

CYP450 3A4 inhibitors (such as ketoconazole), estrogens: increased prednisone concentration

Oral anticoagulants: altered anticoagulant efficacy

Only common or life-threatening adverse reactions are listed.

Potassium-depleting drugs (such as amphotericin B, thiazide diuretics): increased risk of hypokalemia

Drug-diagnostic tests. *Blood glucose; liver function tests; serum cholesterol, sodium, and uric acid; urine glucose:* increased

Calcium, ¹³¹I uptake, potassium, protein-bound iodine: decreased

Nitroblue tetrazolium test: false negative

Skin tests: possible suppressed reaction

Drug-food. *Grapefruit, pomegranate, wild cherry:* possible increased prednisone levels

Drug-herb. *Aloe, buckthorn, cascara, rhubarb, senna:* possible increased risk of potassium deficiency

Cat's claw, devil's claw, feverfew, garlic, ginkgo, goldenseal, kava, milk thistle, red yeast, valerian: possible increased prednisone levels

Licorice: possible increased prednisone levels and duration of activity, possible increased potassium loss

Pycnogenol: possible decreased immunosuppressive activity

Toxicity and overdose

• Overdose is rare. When drug is used for less than 3 weeks, toxicity rarely occurs even with large doses. However, chronic use may cause muscle weakness, hypothalamic-pituitary-adrenal suppression, cushingoid appearance, and osteoporosis.

• Provide supportive treatment for toxicity.

Special considerations

• Patients receiving immunosuppressive doses are more susceptible to infection. Chickenpox and measles, for example, can have a more serious or even fatal course in adults.

• Alternate-day therapy minimizes growth suppression and should be used if such suppression occurs.

• Hepatic disease may decrease prednisone conversion to active form, requiring use of prednisolone instead.

Patient education

• Instruct patient receiving immunosuppressive doses to avoid exposure to chickenpox and measles. If exposure occurs, tell patient to seek medical advice without delay.

• Advise patient to avoid alcohol, products containing aspirin, and other over-the-counter drugs that may increase risk of GI bleeding (such as indomethacin).

procarbazine hydrochloride
Matulane

Classification: Antineoplastic, miscellaneous
Pregnancy risk category D

Pharmacology

Procarbazine may act by inhibiting protein, RNA, and DNA synthesis. It also may inhibit transmethylation of methyl groups of methionine into t-RNA. Absence of functional t-RNA may cause cessation of protein synthesis and, consequently, DNA and RNA synthesis. In addition, drug may directly damage DNA. Hydrogen peroxide, formed during drug's autooxidation, may attack protein sulfhydryl groups in residual protein (which is tightly bound to DNA). Drug is a weak MAO inhibitor.

Pharmacokinetics

Drug is well absorbed, metabolized in liver, and well distributed to cerebrospinal fluid. Peak occurs in approximately 1 hour; elimination half-life is also approximately 1 hour. Drug is excreted mainly in urine.

How supplied

Capsules: 50 mg

Indications and dosages

FDA-APPROVED

➡ Stage III or IV Hodgkin's lymphoma

Adults: As single agent, single or divided doses of 2 to 4 mg/kg P.O. daily for first week; then 4 to 6 mg/kg P.O. daily until maximum response occurs, WBC count decreases below 4,000/mm³, or platelet count drops below 100,000/mm³. When maximum response occurs, dosage may be maintained at 1 to 2 mg/kg/daily. In combination with nitrogen mustard, vincristine, procarbazine, and prednisone (MOPP regimen), procarbazine dosage is 100 mg/m² P.O. daily for 14 days.

Children: As single agent, 50 mg/m² P.O. daily for 7 days, followed by 100 mg/m² P.O. daily until desired response, leukopenia, or thrombocytopenia occurs. When response is maximal, 50 mg/m² P.O. daily as maintenance. As part of bleomycin, etoposide, doxorubicin, cyclophosphamide, vincristine, procarbazine, and prednisone (BEACOPP) regimen, procarbazine 100 mg/m² P.O. daily on days 1 to 7. Repeat cycle every 21 days.

OFF-LABEL USES (SELECTED)

➤ Non-Hodgkin's lymphoma
Adults: One regimen includes procarbazine in combination with methotrexate, teniposide, and dexamethasone, 100 mg/m² P.O. on days 2 through 15 of regimen cycle.
➤ Progressive or recurrent nonresectable glioblastoma
Adults: One dosage schedule is 130 to 150 mg/m² P.O. daily.
➤ Small- and large-cell lung carcinomas, bronchogenic carcinoma, brain tumor, myeloma, melanoma, mycosis fungoides
Adults: Various dosage schedules

DOSAGE MODIFICATIONS

• When maximum response occurs in therapy for Stage III or IV Hodgkin's lymphoma, maintain dosage at 1 to 2 mg/kg P.O. daily. If signs and symptoms of hematologic or other toxicity occur, discontinue drug until recovery. After toxic adverse effects subside, therapy may resume at 1 to 2 mg/kg P.O. daily.
• In children with Stage III or IV Hodgkin's lymphoma who have evidence of hematologic

or other toxicity, discontinue drug until recovery. After toxic adverse effects subside, therapy may resume.
• When used in combination with other anticancer drugs (as in MOPP regimen), dosage should be reduced appropriately.
• Dosages should be reduced in hepatic or renal failure.
• Therapy should be discontinued immediately if any of the following occur: CNS symptoms, such as paresthesia, neuropathies, or confusion; leukopenia (WBC count below 4,000/mm³); thrombocytopenia (platelet count below 100,000/mm³); hypersensitivity reaction; stomatitis (drug should be withdrawn at first small ulceration or persistent spot soreness in oral cavity); diarrhea; hemorrhage; or bleeding tendency.
• All dosages are based on actual weight. Estimated lean body mass (dry weight) may be used if patient is obese or has had spurious weight gain from edema, ascites, or other form of abnormal fluid retention.

☒ WARNINGS

• Drug should be given only by or under supervision of physician experienced in use of potent antineoplastic drugs. Adequate clinical and laboratory facilities should be available for proper monitoring of treatment.

Contraindications and precautions

Contraindicated in hypersensitivity to drug or inadequate marrow reserve (as shown by bone marrow aspiration). Consider inadequate marrow reserve in patients with leukopenia, thrombocytopenia, or anemia.

Use cautiously in renal or hepatic disease, recent therapy with chemotherapeutic agents with known marrow-depressant activity, recent radiation therapy, pregnancy, breastfeeding, and *elderly patients.* Use with extreme caution in *children.*

Preparation and administration

>> Follow hazardous drug guidelines for handling, preparation, and administration. (See "Managing hazardous drugs," page 11.)

• To decrease nausea, dose may be given at bedtime or in divided doses throughout day at beginning of therapy.

• Store in tight, light-resistant container below 104° F (40° C), preferably between 59° and 86° F (15° and 30° C), unless otherwise specified by manufacturer.

Adverse reactions

CNS: tremors, coma, seizures, paresthesia, neuropathy, insomnia, hallucinations, confusion

CV: hypotension

EENT: retinal hemorrhage, nystagmus, photophobia, diplopia, epistaxis

GI: nausea, vomiting, anorexia, diarrhea, constipation, dry mouth, stomatitis

GU: urinary tract infection, azoospermia, menses cessation

Hematologic: thrombocytopenia, anemia, leukopenia, bleeding tendencies

Hepatic: hepatic dysfunction

Musculoskeletal: arthralgias, myalgias

Respiratory: cough, pneumonitis, pleural effusion

Skin: rash, pruritus, dermatitis, alopecia, herpes, hyperpigmentation

Other: secondary nonlymphoid malignancies, allergic reactions

Interactions

Drug-drug. *Antihistamines, barbiturates, opioids, phenothiazines, other CNS depressants:* increased CNS depression

Guanethidine, levodopa, MAO inhibitors, methyldopa, reserpine, sympathomimetics: hypertension

Insulin, oral antidiabetic drugs: increased hypoglycemia

Tricyclic antidepressants: increased risk of neurotoxicity

Drug-diagnostic tests. *Hematocrit, hemoglobin, platelets, WBCs:* decreased

Drug-food. *Caffeine-containing foods:* hypertension, arrhythmia

Foods with high tyramine content (such as cheese and bananas): hypertension

Drug-herb. *Alpha-lipoic acid, coenzyme Q10, glucosamine, glutamine:* possible decreased chemotherapy efficacy

Toxicity and overdose

• Overdose signs and symptoms may include nausea, vomiting, enteritis, diarrhea, hypotension, tremors, seizures, and coma. Also expect hematologic and hepatic manifestations (because drug's major toxicities are hematologic and hepatic).

• Administer emetic or perform gastric lavage to treat overdose. Provide general supportive measures, such as I.V. fluids. Monitor CBC and liver function tests throughout recovery and for at least 2 weeks afterward; if abnormalities appear, immediately take appropriate measures for correction and stabilization.

Special considerations

• In patients who have received radiation therapy or chemotherapeutic agents that depress bone marrow, wait at least 1 month before starting procarbazine. Interval length also may be determined by evidence of bone marrow recovery based on successive bone marrow studies.

• Monitor hematologic, renal, and hepatic function frequently.

• To avoid toxicity in children, maintain close clinical monitoring.

Patient education

• Instruct patient to take drug with plenty of water.

• At beginning of therapy, advise patient to take drug either in two or three divided doses or at bedtime all at once (unless otherwise instructed).

• Caution patient to avoid foods and beverages with high tyramine content, such as ripe cheese, bananas, wine, and yogurt. Provide list of such foods and beverages.

P

⊖ Orphan drug

>> Potentially carcinogenic

• Instruct patient not to consume alcohol during therapy; disulfiram (Antabuse)-like reaction, (flushing, headache, and sweating) may occur.

• Instruct patient to avoid over-the-counter preparations unless approved by physician.

• Urge patient to stop taking drug and notify prescriber immediately if he experiences temperature above 100° F (38° C), chills, cough, pain or burning on urination, blood in urine, black or tarry stools, pinpoint red spots on skin, or signs and symptoms of serious high blood pressure (such as severe chest pain, fast or slow heartbeat, severe headache, or clammy skin).

• Instruct patient to avoid people with active infections.

prochlorperazine
Compazine, Compazine Spansule, Compro, Procot

Classification: Phenothiazine antiemetic, antivertigo agent
Pregnancy risk category C

Pharmacology
Prochlorperazine centrally inhibits dopamine receptors in medullary chemoreceptor trigger zone, which in turn acts on vomiting center. It also peripherally blocks vagus nerve in GI tract.

Pharmacokinetics
Drug is metabolized in liver and excreted in urine.

How supplied
Injection: 5 mg/ml

Indications and dosages

OFF-LABEL USES (SELECTED)

➥ Nausea and vomiting associated with emetogenic chemotherapy

Adults: Suggested dosages include 10 to 20 mg I.V., or 30 to 40 mg I.V., or 0.8 mg/kg I.V. 30 minutes before and 3 hours after chemotherapy.

➥ Nausea and vomiting associated with highly emetogenic chemotherapy
Adults: Suggested dosages include 2 mg/kg I.V. 30 minutes before chemotherapy and repeated every 2 hours for two doses, then every 3 hours for three doses.

Contraindications and precautions
Contraindicated in hypersensitivity to phenothiazines, CNS depression, coma, bone marrow depression, severe hypotension, history of blood dyscrasias, and in *children* weighing less than 9 kg (20 lb), younger than age 2, or undergoing surgery.

Use cautiously in sulfite allergy, cardiovascular disease, glaucoma, tardive dyskinesia, history of neuroleptic malignant syndrome, seizures, prostatic hypertrophy, stenosing peptic ulcer disease, pregnancy, breastfeeding, and *elderly patients*. Use cautiously in *children* with acute illness, dehydration, electrolyte imbalance, or signs and symptoms that suggest Reye's syndrome.

Preparation and administration
• Off-label I.V. dosages exceed manufacturer's recommended maximum dosage of 40 mg daily. Give I.V. only when absolutely necessary. Newer agents, such as serotonin (5-HT₃) receptor antagonists, may be more effective. Expect extrapyramidal symptoms and treat with diphenhydramine I.M.

• I.V. use is not recommended in children.

• Some formulations contain sulfites; use caution when giving to patients with allergies, especially asthmatic patients.

• Keep patient in supine position and monitor blood pressure and pulse before administration.

• Do not mix injection form with other agents in same syringe.

• Slight yellowish discoloration of solution for

Only common or life-threatening adverse reactions are listed.

injection does not alter potency. If markedly discolored, discard.

• Give undiluted, or dilute each 5 mg (1 ml) with 9 ml normal saline solution (1 ml equals 0.5 mg). Add dosages above 10 mg to 50 ml to 1 L D_5W, normal saline solution, dextrose 5% in half-normal saline injection, Ringer's solution, or Ringer's lactate solution, and give as intermittent or prolonged infusion.

• Administer by slow I.V. injection at a rate not exceeding 5 mg/minute. Do not use bolus injection because hypotension can occur.

• Avoid subcutaneous administration; it may cause local irritation.

• Store below 104° F (40° C). Protect from light and freezing.

Adverse reactions

CNS: neuroleptic malignant syndrome, extrapyramidal reactions, tardive dyskinesia, euphoria, depression, drowsiness, restlessness, tremor, dizziness, seizures
CV: hypotension
EENT: blurred vision
GI: nausea, vomiting, constipation, cholestatic jaundice
GU: urine discoloration
Hematologic: agranulocytosis, leukopenia
Skin: contact dermatitis, photosensitivity
Other: weight gain

Interactions

Drug-drug. *Barbiturates, opioids, sedative-hypnotics:* increased CNS depression
Gatifloxacin, moxifloxacin, tricyclic antidepressants: increased risk of QT prolongation
Guanethidine, thiazide diuretics: increased hypotension
Lithium: possible encephalopathic syndrome
Oral anticoagulants: decreased anticoagulant effect
Phenytoin: increased phenytoin toxicity
Propranolol: increased plasma levels of both drugs
Drug-diagnostic tests. *Phenylketonuria test:* false positive

Urine pregnancy test: false positive or false negative
Drug-herb. *Alfalfa, bergamot oil, bishop's weed, St. John's wort:* increased risk of photosensitivity
Evening primrose, ginkgo, thuja: increased seizure risk
L-tryptophan: possible increased sexual disinhibition, reversible dyskinesias, reversible parkinsonian-like rigidity

Toxicity and overdose

• Overdose causes primarily dystonic reactions and CNS depression to point of somnolence or coma. Agitation and restlessness also may occur. Other possible manifestations include seizure, ECG changes, arrhythmias, fever, and autonomic reactions (such as hypotension, dry mouth, and ileus).

• Determine if patient has taken other drugs (multiple-dose therapy is common in overdose). Provide symptomatic and supportive treatment. Keep patient under observation, and maintain open airway. In severe overdose, extrapyramidal involvement may cause dysphagia and respiratory difficulty. Do not try to induce emesis because dystonic head or neck reaction may occur, causing aspiration. Treat extrapyramidal symptoms with antiparkinsonians, barbiturates, or diphenhydramine. Avoid giving stimulants that can cause seizures. If hypotension occurs, initiate standard measures for managing circulatory shock. If patient requires vasoconstrictor, norepinephrine and phenylephrine are most suitable. Other pressor agents (including epinephrine) are not recommended because phenothiazine derivatives may reverse usual elevating action of these drug and cause further blood pressure reduction. Limited experience shows that phenothiazines are not dialyzable.

Special considerations

• Monitor neurologic and hematologic status frequently.
• Expect extrapyramidal symptoms and hypotension with large I.V. doses; be prepared to

manage these adverse reactions appropriately.
• Continue to monitor blood pressure and pulse between doses.
• Drug may suppress cough reflex; monitor closely if patient vomits.

Patient education
• Advise patient to rise slowly from a sitting or lying position after receiving a dose.
• Advise patient to avoid hazardous activities or activities requiring alertness; drug may cause dizziness.
• Instruct patient to avoid alcohol, sedative-hypnotics, barbiturates, opioids, and tranquilizers.
• Instruct patient to report involuntary muscle movements.
• Inform patient that drug may turn urine pink to reddish brown.
• Caution patient to avoid prolonged sun exposure.

promethazine hydrochloride
Anergan, Pentazine, Phenergan, Phenoject-50, Promethegan

Classification: Phenothiazine antiemetic, antivertigo agent, histamine$_1$ (H$_1$)-receptor antagonist
Pregnancy risk category C

Pharmacology
Promethazine exerts antihistaminic, sedative, anti–motion sickness, antiemetic, and anticholinergic actions. Although it is a competitive H$_1$-receptor antagonist, it does not block histamine release. It has central anticholinergic effects on vestibular apparatus, integrative vomiting center, and medullary chemoreceptive trigger zone of midbrain. Unlike neuroleptic phenothiazines, drug has minimal dopamine-antagonist properties. It can produce either CNS stimulation or depression, but at therapeutic doses, it more commonly causes CNS depression, manifested by sedation.

Pharmacokinetics
Drug is metabolized in liver and is highly protein-bound. Onset is 3 to 5 minutes with I.V. use and 20 minutes with I.M., P.O., and P.R. use. Duration is 4 to 6 hours. Parent compound has elimination half-life of 7 to 15 hours. Drug is excreted by kidney.

How supplied
Injection: 25 mg/ml, 50 mg/ml
Suppositories: 12.5 mg, 25 mg, 50 mg
Syrup: 6.25 mg/5 ml, 25 mg/5 ml
Tablets: 12.5 mg, 25 mg, 50 mg

Indications and dosages

> **FDA-APPROVED**

➥ Nausea
Adults: 12.5 to 25 mg P.O., I.M., I.V., or P.R. every 4 to 6 hours as needed
Children older than age 2: 0.25 to 0.5 mg/kg P.O., I.M., I.V., or P.R. every 4 to 6 hours as needed, not to exceed half of adult dosage

Contraindications and precautions
Contraindicated in hypersensitivity to drug, its components, or other H$_1$-receptor antagonists or phenothiazines; subcutaneous administration; acute asthma attack; lower respiratory tract symptoms; coma; and *children* who are acutely ill or dehydrated.
Use cautiously in sulfite allergy, increased intraocular pressure, cardiac disease, bronchial asthma, seizure disorder, stenosing peptic ulcer disease, prostatic hypertrophy, bladder neck obstruction, bone marrow depression, hepatic impairment, pregnancy, breastfeeding, and *elderly patients.* Drug is not recommended in *children* who are younger than age 2; have acute infection, hepatic disease, uncomplicated vomiting, or signs and symptoms of Reye's syndrome; or who are receiving other CNS depressants.

Only common or life-threatening adverse reactions are listed.

Preparation and administration

- Do not give subcutaneously (may cause tissue necrosis). Preferred parenteral route is deep I.M. injection.
- Slightly yellow color of injection form does not alter potency. Discard if significantly discolored.
- Keep patient in supine position and monitor blood pressure and pulse before parenteral administration.
- When administering I.M., inject deeply into large muscle mass.
- For I.V. use, make sure ampule indicates "For I.V. use"; may be given undiluted, or dilute 1 ml (25 or 50 mg) with 9 ml normal saline solution to equal 2.5 to 5 mg/ml, respectively. Concentration should not exceed 25 mg/ml. Administer I.V. through Y-tube or three-way stopcock of free-flowing I.V. line at a rate of 25 mg over 1 minute. Drug may form precipitate with heparin; flush heparinized infusion sets with sterile water for injection or normal saline solution before and after administration.
- Inadvertent intra-arterial injection or extravasation may cause gangrene of affected extremity. Injection into or near a nerve may cause permanent tissue damage.
- Store syrup at controlled temperature of 59° to 77° F (15° to 25° C) in tightly closed bottle protected from light.
- Store tablets at 68° to 77° F (20° to 25° C) in tightly closed container protected from light.
- Store suppositories at 36° to 46° F (2° to 8° C); suppositories are stable for 2 weeks at room temperature and 36 months when refrigerated.
- Store injection at controlled temperature at 59° to 86° F (15° to 30° C). Protect from light. Keep covered in carton until time of use.

Adverse reactions

CNS: dizziness, drowsiness, poor coordination, confusion, extrapyramidal symptoms, neuroleptic malignant syndrome, hallucinations, euphoria, seizures

CV: hypotension
EENT: blurred vision, diplopia
GI: constipation, dry mouth, nausea, vomiting, ileus
Hematologic: thrombocytopenia, agranulocytosis, leukopenia
Hepatic: jaundice
Respiratory: respiratory depression; apnea in young children, infants, and neonates
Skin: rash, urticaria, photosensitivity

Interactions

Drug-drug. *Barbiturates, opioids, sedative-hypnotics:* increased CNS depression
Epinephrine: possible reversal of epinephrine's vasopressor effect
Gatifloxacin, moxifloxacin, tricyclic antidepressants: increased risk of QT prolongation
MAO inhibitors: increased risk of extrapyramidal effects
Drug-diagnostic tests. *Urine pregnancy test:* false positive or false negative
Drug-herb. *Alfalfa, bergamot oil, bishop's weed, St. John's wort:* increased risk of photosensitivity
Evening primrose, ginkgo, thuja: increased seizure risk
L-tryptophan: possible sexual disinhibition, reversible dyskinesias, reversible parkinsonian-like rigidity

Toxicity and overdose

- Overdose signs and symptoms range from mild CNS and cardiovascular depression to profound hypotension, respiratory depression, and unconsciousness. Stimulation may occur, especially in elderly patients and children. Overdose also may cause atropine-like signs and symptoms (dry mouth, fixed dilated pupils, flushing) and GI effects.
- Provide symptomatic and supportive treatment. Naloxone does not reverse depressant effects of promethazine injection. Avoid analeptics, which may cause seizure. Preferred treatment for hypotension is administration of I.V. fluids, accompanied by patient repositioning if indicated. If vasopressors are needed to

manage severe hypotension unresponsive to I.V. fluids and repositioning, consider norepinephrine or phenylephrine. Do not give epinephrine; in patients with partial adrenergic blockade, it may further decrease blood pressure. For extrapyramidal reactions, give anticholinergic antiparkinsonians, diphenhydramine, or barbiturates. Administer oxygen if needed; diazepam may be used to control seizures. Correct acidosis and electrolyte losses. Limited experience indicates that dialysis is not helpful.

Special considerations

- Avoid sedatives and other CNS depressants in patients with history of sleep apnea.
- With parenteral use, monitor patient for extrapyramidal symptoms and hypotension; be prepared to manage these adverse reactions appropriately.
- Continue to monitor blood pressure and pulse between doses.
- Drug may suppress cough reflex; monitor closely if patient vomits.
- Children with dehydration are at increased risk for dystonic reactions.

Patient education

- Instruct patient to immediately report persistent pain or burning at injection site.
- Caution patient to avoid driving and other hazardous activities until drug's effects are known.
- Advise parents of child receiving drug to closely supervise child to avoid potential injury during bike riding and other hazardous activities.
- Advise patient to rise slowly from a sitting or lying position after receiving dose.
- Instruct patient to avoid sedative-hypnotics (including barbiturates) and alcohol.
- Instruct patient to report involuntary muscle movements.
- Caution patient to avoid prolonged sun exposure.

raloxifene hydrochloride
Evista

Classification: Selective estrogen-receptor modulator, hormone/hormone modifier
Pregnancy risk category X

Pharmacology

Raloxifene binds to estrogen receptors, activating certain estrogenic pathways and blocking others. It decreases bone resorption and reduces biochemical markers of bone turnover to premenopausal range. It also decreases total and low-density lipoprotein (LDL) levels but does not affect triglyceride or high-density lipoprotein levels.

Pharmacokinetics

Drug undergoes extensive first-pass glucuronidation. It is highly plasma protein–bound. Parent drug peaks in 6 hours; glucuronides, in 1 hour. Mean elimination half-life is 32.5 hours. Drug is excreted in feces and breast milk.

How supplied

Tablets: 60 mg

Indications and dosages

OFF-LABEL USES (SELECTED)

➡ Reduction of incidence of estrogen-receptor-positive breast cancer
Adults: Chemopreventive use in high-risk women is under clinical evaluation.

Contraindications and precautions

Contraindicated in hypersensitivity to drug or its components, active or past history of venous thromboembolic events, premenopausal women, and pregnancy or breastfeeding.

Use cautiously in prolonged immobilization, severe hepatic insufficiency, and concomitant use of systemic estrogens. Drug should not be used in *children.*

Only common or life-threatening adverse reactions are listed.

Preparation and administration

- Follow hazardous drug guidelines for handling, preparation, and administration. (See "Managing hazardous drugs," page 11.)
- Drug may be given any time of day without regard to meals.
- Administer cautiously with other highly protein-bound drugs.
- Store at controlled temperature of 68° to 77° F (20° to 25° C).

Adverse reactions

CNS: insomnia, migraine, depression
EENT: sinusitis, pharyngitis, laryngitis
GI: nausea, vomiting, diarrhea, anorexia, cramps
Musculoskeletal: arthralgia, myalgia, leg cramps, arthritis
Respiratory: increased cough, pneumonia
Skin: rash
Other: hot flashes, sweating, flulike syndrome

Interactions

Drug-drug. *Ampicillin, cholestyramine:* decreased raloxifene action
Anticoagulants: decreased anticoagulant action
Highly protein-bound drugs (such as diazepam, diazoxide, lidocaine): possible effect on protein binding of these drugs
Levothyroxine: decreased levothyroxine action
Drug-diagnostic tests. *Apolipoprotein A_1, calcium, fibrinogen, inorganic phosphates, total protein:* increased
Apolipoprotein B_1, hormone-binding globulin, LDLs, platelets, serum albumin, total serum cholesterol: decreased
Drug-herb. *Aloe, cascara, rhubarb:* possible decreased absorption due to reduced GI transit time

Toxicity and overdose

- No cases of overdose have been reported. Dosages of 600 mg daily have been well tolerated.
- No specific antidote exists.

Special considerations

- Efficacy as chemopreventative measure for breast cancer in high-risk women has not been proven and is not approved for use in premenopausal women. Monitor these patients carefully.
- Monitor cholesterol, calcium, total protein, and platelet levels.

Patient education

- Instruct patient to discontinue drug 72 hours before anticipated period of prolonged bed rest.
- Advise patient not to stay in one position for long periods.
- Instruct patient to immediately report swelling, warmth, or pain in calf.
- Advise patient to take calcium and vitamin D supplements if her dietary intake of these elements is inadequate.

rituximab
Rituxan

Classification: Antineoplastic, monoclonal antibody
Pregnancy risk category C

Pharmacology

Rituximab binds specifically to CD20 antigen (human B-lymphocyte-restricted differentiation antigen, Bp35), a protein on pre-B and mature B lymphocytes. This antigen also is expressed on more than 90% of B-cell non-Hodgkin's lymphomas but is not found on hematopoietic stem cells, pre-B cells, normal plasma cells, or other normal tissues. CD20 regulates early step in activation process for cell-cycle initiation and differentiation, and possibly functions as calcium ion channel. CD20 is not shed from cell surface and does not internalize on antibody binding. Rituximab's immunoglobulin structure binds to antigen CD20 on lymphocytes, causing host immune response that results in lysis of normal and malignant B cells. Exact cell lysis mechanism is unclear but may involve complement-dependent cytotoxicity and antibody-dependent cell-mediated cytotoxicity.

Pharmacokinetics

Drug is not bioavailable with oral use. With I.V. use, it is taken up by B lymphocytes and degraded throughout body by proteolysis. Elimination half-life is 3.2 to 8.5 days. No appreciable excretion occurs.

How supplied

Solution for injection: 10 mg/ml in 10-ml (100-mg) and 50-ml (500-mg) vials

Indications and dosages

FDA-APPROVED

➲ Relapsed or refractory low-grade or follicular, CD20+, B-cell non-Hodgkin's lymphoma
Adults: Initially, 375 mg/m^2 I.V. infusion once weekly for four or eight doses; in patients who subsequently develop progressive disease, 375 mg/m^2 I.V. infusion once weekly for four doses

OFF-LABEL USES (SELECTED)

➡ Chronic lymphocytic leukemia
Adults: Typical dosage is 375 mg/m^2 I.V. infusion each week during 4-week cycle.

⊠ WARNINGS

• Deaths have occurred within 24 hours of infusion. These fatal reactions followed infusion reaction complex that included hypoxia, pulmonary infiltrates, adult respiratory distress syndrome (ARDS), myocardial infarction, ventricular fibrillation, and cardiogenic shock. Approximately 80% of fatal infusion reactions occur with first infusion.
• If patient develops severe infusion reaction, infusion should be stopped and patient should receive medical treatment.
• Acute renal failure requiring dialysis has been reported, in some cases leading to death from tumor lysis syndrome.

• Severe, life-threatening mucocutaneous reactions have been reported.
• Patients with hematologic malignancies may experience hepatitis B virus (HBV) reactivation with fulminant hepatitis, hepatic failure, and death. Patients at high risk for HBV infection should be screened before rituximab therapy begins. HBV carriers should be monitored closely for clinical and laboratory signs of active HBV infection and for signs and symptoms of hepatitis during therapy and for up to several months afterward. In patients who develop viral hepatitis, rituximab and any concomitant chemotherapy should be discontinued and appropriate treatment (including antiviral therapy) initiated.

Contraindications and precautions

Contraindicated in hypersensitivity to drug or murine proteins.
Use cautiously in pregnancy and breastfeeding. Safety and efficacy in *children* have not been established.

Preparation and administration

• Drug may be administered in outpatient settings.
• To administer, withdraw required amount and dilute to final concentration of 1 to 4 mg/ml into infusion bag containing normal saline solution or D$_5$W. Gently invert bag to mix solution. Discard unused portion. Inspect for particulates and discoloration before administration.
• Do not mix or dilute with other drugs.
• Do not administer as I.V. push or bolus.
• During first infusion, administer I.V. at initial rate of 50 mg/hour.
• Stay alert for severe infusion reaction, which may be fatal. Severe reactions typically occur during first infusion, starting 30 to 120 minutes after infusion begins. Signs and symptoms include hypotension, angioedema, hypoxia, and bronchospasm. Condition may warrant interruption of therapy.

Only common or life-threatening adverse reactions are listed.

• Unless hypersensitivity or infusion reaction occurs, increase infusion rate in 50-mg/hour increments every 30 minutes, to maximum of 400 mg/hour. If hypersensitivity (non-IgE-mediated) reaction or infusion reaction occurs, temporarily slow or interrupt infusion. When symptoms improve, infusion can resume at 50% of previous rate.

• For severe infusion reaction, in addition to interrupting infusion, provide supportive care as indicated (such as I.V. fluids, vasopressors, oxygen, diphenhydramine, acetaminophen, and bronchodilators).

• If patient tolerates first infusion well, subsequent infusions can be given at initial rate of 100 mg/hour and increased by 100-mg/hour increments at 30-minute intervals, to maximum of 400 mg/hour, as tolerated. If patient did not tolerate first infusion well, administer as for first infusion.

• Solution contains no preservative. Store diluted solution at 36° to 46° F (2° to 8° C) for 24 hours. Solution remains stable for an additional 24 hours at room temperature. Protect vial from direct sunlight.

Adverse reactions

CNS: headache, dizziness
CV: hypotension, heart failure, arrhythmias, angina
EENT: rhinitis
GI: nausea, vomiting, anorexia, diarrhea
GU: renal failure
Hematologic: lymphopenia, leukopenia, neutropenia, thrombocytopenia
Musculoskeletal: myalgia
Respiratory: cough, bronchospasm
Skin: irritation at injection site, rash, fatal mucocutaneous infections, Stevens-Johnson syndrome
Other: angioedema, tumor lysis syndrome, infusion reactions, hypersensitivity reactions

Interactions

Drug-drug. *Cisplatin:* increased risk of renal failure

Drug-diagnostic tests. *Calcium, hemoglobin, platelets, WBCs:* decreased
Drug-herb. *Alpha-lipoic acid, coenzyme Q10, glucosamine, glutamine:* possible decreased chemotherapy efficacy

Toxicity and overdose

• No experience with overdose has occurred. Single doses up to 500 mg/m^2 have been given. Anticipated signs and symptoms of overdose are those of the most commonly occurring adverse reactions (fever, infusions reactions, and lymphopenia).

• If overdose occurs, discontinue infusion and treat symptomatically.

Special considerations

• Monitor CBC with differential and platelet counts at regular intervals during therapy, and more frequently in patients who develop cytopenias. Duration of cytopenias caused by rituximab may extend well beyond treatment period.

• Continue to observe patient closely for signs of infusion reactions.

• Monitor for mucocutaneous reactions, arrhythmias, angina, renal dysfunction, and hypersensitivity reactions. Be prepared to intervene appropriately.

• Monitor potassium and uric acid levels and observe for signs of tumor lysis syndrome, which can be fatal (irregular heartbeat, shortness of breath, high potassium levels, high uric acid levels, impaired mental ability, kidney failure).

Patient education

• Instruct patient to immediately report such adverse reactions as difficulty breathing, unusual bleeding or bruising, or rash.

• Advise breastfeeding patient to stop breastfeeding until blood tests show that drug is no longer detectable.

R

sargramostim (GM-CSF)
Leukine

Classification: Recombinant human granulocyte-macrophage colony stimulating factor (GM-CSF)
Pregnancy risk category C

Pharmacology
Sargramostim stimulates proliferation and differentiation of granulocytes and macrophages (hematopoietic progenitor cells) and can activate mature granulocytes and macrophages. It induces various cellular responses by binding to specific receptors expressed on surface of target cells.

Pharmacokinetics
Drug peaks during or immediately after I.V. infusion and 1 to 4 hours after subcutaneous injection. It is degraded throughout body, predominantly in liver and kidneys. Elimination half-life is 1.5 to 2.7 hours with I.V. or subcutaneous use. No appreciable excretion occurs.

How supplied
Powder for injection (lyophilized): 250 mcg, 500 mcg
Solution for injection: 500 mcg/ml

Indications and dosages

FDA-APPROVED

➡ Neutrophil recovery after induction chemotherapy in acute myelogenous leukemia (AML)
Adults age 55 and older: 250 mcg/m² daily I.V. over 4 hours starting on day 11 or 4 days after completion of chemotherapy induction
➡ Mobilization of autologous peripheral blood progenitor cells (PBPCs)
Adults: 250 mcg/m² daily either I.V. over 24 hours or subcutaneously once daily, continued at same dosage throughout PBPC collection period

➡ Post-PBPC transplantation
Adults: 250 mcg/m² daily I.V. over 24 hours or subcutaneously once daily, starting immediately after progenitor cell infusion and continuing until absolute neutrophil count (ANC) is above 1,500/mm³ for 3 consecutive days
➡ Myeloid reconstitution after autologous or allogeneic bone marrow transplantation
Adults: If post–marrow infusion ANC is below 500/mm³, give 250 mcg/m² daily I.V. over 2 hours, starting 2 to 4 hours after marrow infusion and no less than 24 hours after last chemotherapy or radiotherapy dose; continue until ANC is above 1,500 cells/mm³ for 3 consecutive days.
➡ Bone marrow transplantation failure or engraftment delay
Adults: 250 mcg/m² I.V. infusion over 2 hours daily for 14 days; repeat after 7 days of therapy if engraftment has not occurred.

DOSAGE MODIFICATIONS

• When drug is used for neutrophil recovery after induction chemotherapy in AML, day-10 bone marrow should be hypoplastic with fewer than 5% blasts. Repeat sargramostim daily until ANC exceeds 1,500/mm³ for 3 consecutive days or maximum of 42 days. Use same criteria if second cycle of induction chemotherapy is indicated. Discontinue drug immediately if leukemic regrowth occurs. If severe adverse reaction occurs, dosage can be reduced by 50% or drug can be discontinued temporarily until reaction abates.
• When drug is used for mobilization of autologous PBPCs, if WBC is above 50,000 cells/mm³, reduce sargramostim dosage by 50%. If adequate numbers of progenitor cells are not collected, consider other mobilization therapy.
• When drug is used for myeloid reconstitution after autologous or allogeneic bone marrow transplantation, if severe adverse reaction occurs, dosage can be reduced by 50% or drug can be discontinued temporarily until reaction abates. Discontinue drug immediately if blast cells appear or disease progresses.

Only common or life-threatening adverse reactions are listed.

• When drug is used for engraftment delay, if engraftment does not occur after two courses, third course of 500 mcg/m² daily for 14 days may be given 7 days after previous therapy. If there is still no improvement, further dosage escalation is not likely to be beneficial. If severe adverse reaction occurs, dosage can be reduced by 50% or drug can be discontinued temporarily until reaction abates. Discontinue drug immediately if blast cells appear or disease progresses.

• If dyspnea occurs during administration, reduce infusion rate by 50%. If respiratory symptoms worsen despite reduced infusion rate, discontinue infusion. Subsequent I.V. infusions may be given using standard dosing schedule and careful monitoring.

• Interrupt therapy or decrease dosage by 50% if ANC exceeds 20,000/mm³ or if platelet count exceeds 500,000/mm³.

Contraindications and precautions

Contraindicated in hypersensitivity to drug, yeast-derived products, or product components; concomitant use with chemotherapy and radiotherapy; and excessive leukemic myeloid blasts in bone marrow or peripheral blood (10% or more).

Use cautiously in edema, capillary leak syndrome (CLS), pleural effusion, pericardial effusion, preexisting cardiac or lung disease, hypoxia, pulmonary infiltrate, heart failure, malignancy with myeloid characteristics, and pregnancy or breastfeeding. Safety and efficacy in AML patients younger than age 55 have not been evaluated. Safety and efficacy in *children* have not been established.

Preparation and administration

• Do not administer within 12 hours before or after radiation therapy or within 24 hours before or after administration of myelosuppressive antineoplastics.

• Reconstitute lyophilized powder for injection with 1 ml sterile water for injection or bacteriostatic water for injection. Do not mix together contents of vials reconstituted with different diluents.

• Lyophilized vials contain no antibacterial preservative. Give solutions prepared with sterile water for injection as soon as possible and within 6 hours after reconstitution or dilution for I.V. infusion. Do not reenter or reuse vial. Do not save unused portion for administration more than 6 hours after reconstitution.

• When reconstituting, direct diluent at side of vial and swirl contents gently to avoid foaming. Avoid excessive or vigorous agitation. Do not shake vial.

• For subcutaneous use, do not further dilute drug.

• For I.V. infusion, dilute with normal saline solution injection. If final drug concentration is less is than 10 mcg/ml, add albumin (human) to saline solution before adding drug, to prevent adsorption to components of drug delivery system. To obtain final concentration of 1 mg/ml (0.1%), add 1 mg albumin (human) per 1 ml normal saline solution injection. For instance, use 1 ml 5% albumin (human) in 50 ml normal saline solution injection.

• Do not use in-line membrane filter for I.V. infusion.

• To ensure correct concentration after reconstitution, make sure to eliminate air bubbles from needle hub of syringe used to prepare diluent.

• For parenteral administration, use precautions appropriate for recombinant proteins in case allergic or untoward reaction occurs. Serious allergic reactions have been reported. If such a reaction occurs, discontinue drug immediately and initiate appropriate therapy.

• Rarely, hypotension with flushing and syncope have been reported after first sargramostim dose. These signs resolved with symptomatic treatment and rarely recurred with subsequent doses in same treatment cycle.

• Reconstituted solutions prepared with bacteriostatic water for injection (0.9% benzyl alcohol) may be stored up to 20 days at 36° to 46° F (2° to 8° C) before use. Discard reconstituted solution after 20 days. Previously reconstituted solutions mixed with freshly re-constituted solutions must be administered within 6 hours of mixing.

• Do not give liquid solutions containing benzyl alcohol—including sargramostim liquid or lyophilized sargramostim reconstituted with bacteriostatic water for injection (0.9% benzyl alcohol)—to neonates.

• Store liquid form and reconstituted lyophilized solution at 36° to 46° F. Do not freeze.

Adverse reactions
CNS: asthenia, malaise
CV: transient supraventricular arrhythmia, peripheral edema, pericardial effusion
GI: nausea, vomiting, diarrhea, anorexia, GI hemorrhage, stomatitis
GU: urinary tract disorder, abnormal renal function
Hematologic: blood dyscrasia, hemorrhage
Hepatic: hepatic damage
Musculoskeletal: bone pain
Respiratory: dyspnea, pleural effusion
Skin: alopecia, rash
Other: fever, flulike syndrome, CLS, hypersensitivity reaction including anaphylaxis

Interactions
Drug-drug. *Antineoplastics, myelosuppressants:* prolonged myelosuppression
Corticosteroids, lithium: increased myeloproliferation

Toxicity and overdose
• Maximum amount that can be given safely in single or multiple doses has not been determined. Expected overdose signs and symptoms include increased WBC count and respiratory symptoms.

• If overdose occurs, discontinue drug and monitor patient carefully.

Special considerations
• Continue to monitor patient for hypersensitivity reactions.

• To avoid potential complications of excessive leukocytosis (WBC count above 50,000/

mm^3 and ANC above 20,000/mm^3), obtain CBC with differential twice weekly during therapy.

• Granulocyte sequestration in pulmonary circulation and dyspnea may follow drug infusion. Pay special attention to respiratory symptoms during and immediately after infusion, especially in patients with preexisting lung disease.

• Drug can act as growth factor for any tumor type, particularly myeloid malignancies. Exercise caution when administering to patients who have malignancies with myeloid characteristics.

• If disease progresses during treatment, discontinue drug.

• Carefully monitor patient's weight and hydration status.

Patient education
• Advise patient to immediately report new symptoms, including difficulty breathing, easy bruising, swelling, change in urination, irregular heartbeat, or rash.

• Advise patient to avoid crowds and persons with infections.

sodium phosphate P 32
Classification: Antineoplastic, radiopharmaceutical
Pregnancy risk category C

Pharmacology
Sodium phosphate P 32 concentrates in areas of rapid bone formation associated with metastatic tumors localized to bone. Beta emissions of drug cause localized therapeutic radiation and destruction of tumor cells localized to bone matrix. Phosphorus (as phosphate) incorporates into DNA and concentrates to a high degree in rapidly proliferating hematopoietic cells. Subsequent radiation damage to these cells halts their reproduction.

Only common or life-threatening adverse reactions are listed.

Pharmacokinetics

Drug diffuses rapidly into extra- and intracellular fluids after I.V. dose, concentrating mostly in bone marrow, liver, and spleen. Half-life is 14.3 days. Elimination is primarily renal, with small percentage in feces. In healthy patients, 5% to 10% is eliminated in urine within 24 hours and about 20% is eliminated within 1 week.

How supplied

Solution: 185 MBq (5 mCi) in single-dose vial; radioactive concentration is 0.67 mCi/ml (24.8 MBq/ml).

Indications and dosages

FDA-APPROVED

➡ Chronic myeloid and chronic lymphocytic leukemia
Adults: 222 to 555 MBq (6 to 15 millicuries) I.V., usually given with hormone manipulation
➡ Palliative treatment of selected patients with multiple areas of skeletal metastasis
Adults: One regimen is 370 to 777 MBq (10 to 21 mCi) I.V. given over 3 to 4 weeks as 111 MBq (3 mCi) on day 1, followed by two doses of 74 MBq (2 mCi) every other day during first week, then two doses of 74 MBq (2 mCi) during second and third weeks, and then 37 MBq (1 mCi) twice weekly until total of 777 MBq (21 mCi) has been given.

Contraindications and precautions

Contraindicated in sensitivity to radiopharmaceutical preparation, polycythemia vera with WBC count below 5,000/mm³ and platelet count below 150,000/mm³, chronic myelocytic leukemia with WBC count below 20,000/mm³, and bone metastases with WBC count below 5,000/mm³ and platelet count below 100,000/mm³.

Use cautiously in women with childbearing potential, breastfeeding patients, and *elderly patients.* Safety and efficacy in *children* have not been established.

Preparation and administration

• Follow hazardous drug guidelines for handling, preparation, and administration. (See "Managing hazardous drugs," page 11.)
• This radiopharmaceutical should not be administered for intracavitary use.
• Measure dosage by suitable radioactivity calibration immediately before use.
• Carefully ensure minimum radiation exposure to patient, consistent with proper patient management. Also ensure minimum radiation exposure to occupational workers.
• Visually inspect injection to avoid accidental I.V. administration of *chromic* phosphate P 32. Sodium phosphate P 32 is a clear, colorless solution; chromic phosphate P 32 is a green, cloudy liquid intended for intracavitary therapy.
• In women with childbearing potential, examinations using radiopharmaceuticals (especially if elective) should be performed during first few (approximately 10) days after menses onset.
• Oral administration of high-specific-activity sodium phosphate P 32 in fasting state may equal I.V. administration.
• Store at room temperature below 86° F (30° C).

Adverse reactions

None known

Interactions

Drug-drug. *Bone marrow depressants:* increased bone marrow depression
Drug-diagnostic tests. *BUN, serum calcium:* increased

Toxicity and overdose

• Overdose may cause serious hematopoietic effects.
• Provide supportive treatment. Monitor blood and bone marrow carefully at regular intervals.

S

Special considerations
• Monitor CBC and differential and bone marrow results frequently.

Patient education
• Advise breastfeeding patient to stop breastfeeding during therapy.

sorafenib
Nexavar

Classification: Antineoplastic, multikinase inhibitor
Pregnancy risk category D

Pharmacology
Sorafenib decreases tumor cell proliferation *in vitro* and inhibits tumor growth of murine renal-cell carcinoma. It interacts with multiple intracellular and cell surface kinases, several of which are thought to be involved with angiogenesis.

Pharmacokinetics
Drug is 29% less bioavailable when given with high-fat meal; when given with moderate-fat meal, bioavailability resembles that of fasting state. Drug is metabolized primarily in liver, undergoing oxidative metabolism mediated by CYP3A4 as well as glucuronidation. It is 99.5% protein-bound, and reaches peak plasma level in approximately 3 hours. Mean elimination half-life is approximately 25 to 48 hours. Drug is eliminated through urine and feces.

How supplied
Tablets: 200 mg

Indications and dosages

➡ Advanced renal-cell carcinoma
Adults: 400 mg P.O. twice daily given without food. Treatment should continue until no clinical benefit occurs or until unacceptable toxicity occurs.

➡ Recurrent epithelial ovarian cancer, advanced pancreatic cancer
Adults: 400 mg P.O. twice daily given continuously in combination with gemcitabine 1,000 mg/m² I.V. weekly. Cycle 1 consists of gemcitabine for 7 weeks followed by 1-week break; then weekly administration for first 3 weeks of each subsequent 4-week cycle.

• If severe or persistent hypertension occurs despite antihypertensive therapy or if cardiac ischemia occurs, consider temporary or permanent discontinuation of drug.
• Temporarily interrupt sorafenib therapy in patients undergoing major surgical procedures.
• Discontinue drug if bleeding event occurs.
• If skin toxicity occurs, modify dosage as shown in table below.

Skin toxicity grade	Occurrence	Suggested modification
Grade 1: Numbness, dysesthesia, paresthesia, tingling, painless swelling, erythema, or discomfort of hands or feet that does not disrupt normal activities	Any occurrence	Continue treatment; consider topical therapy for symptomatic relief.
Grade 2: Painful erythema and swelling of hands or feet, or discomfort that affects normal activities	First occurrence	Continue treatment; consider topical therapy for symptomatic relief.

(continued)

Skin toxicity grade	Occurrence	Suggested modification
Grade 2: *(continued)*	No improvement within 7 days of first occurrence; second or third occurrence	Interrupt treatment until toxicity resolves to Grade 0 to 1. When resuming treatment, decrease dosage by one dose level (400 mg daily). If additional dosage reduction is needed, reduce dosage to 400 mg every other day.
	Fourth occurrence	Discontinue treatment.
Grade 3: Moist desquamation, ulceration, blistering or severe pain of hands or feet, or severe discomfort that renders patient unable to work or perform activities of daily living	First or second occurrence	Interrupt treatment until toxicity resolves to Grade 0 to 1. When resuming treatment, decrease dosage by one dose level (400 mg daily). If additional dosage reduction is needed, reduce dosage to 400 mg every other day.
	Third occurrence	Discontinue treatment.

Contraindications and precautions

Contraindicated in hypersensitivity to drug or its components.

Use cautiously in dermatologic toxicities; hypertension; bleeding; cardiac ischemia; myocardial infarction; concurrent use of CYP3A4 inducers, irinotecan, doxorubicin, or CYP2B6 and CYP2C8 substrates; patients undergoing surgical procedures; and pregnancy or breast-feeding. Safety and efficacy in *children* have not been established.

Preparation and administration

• Administer without food (1 hour before or 2 hours after eating).

• Store in dry place at 77° F (25° C). Excursions are permitted to 59° F to 86° F (15° C to 30° C).

Adverse reactions

CNS: fatigue, sensory neuropathy, headache, asthenia, depression
CV: hypertension, myocardial ischemia or infarction
GI: nausea, vomiting, diarrhea, anorexia, constipation, abdominal pain, mouth pain, mucositis, stomatitis, dyspepsia, dysphagia
GU: erectile dysfunction
Hematologic: hemorrhage, leukopenia, lymphopenia, anemia, thrombocytopenia
Musculoskeletal: arthralgia, myalgia
Respiratory: cough, dyspnea, hoarseness
Skin: rash, desquamation, hand-foot skin reaction, alopecia, pruritus, dry skin, erythema, exfoliative dermatitis, acne, flushing
Other: weight loss, flulike syndrome, fever

Interactions

Drug-drug. *CYP3A4 inducers (such as carbamazepine, dexamethasone, phenytoin, phenobarbital, and rifampin):* possible increased sorafenib metabolism and decreased concentration
Doxorubicin, irinotecan: increased AUC of these drugs
Warfarin: increased risk of bleeding and elevated INR
Drug-diagnostic tests. *Amylase, lipase:* elevated
Hemoglobin, phosphates, platelets, WBCs: decreased
Serum transaminases: transient increases
Drug-herb. *St. John's wort:* decreased sorafenib concentration

Toxicity and overdose

• With high doses (800 mg twice daily), adverse reactions were primarily diarrhea and dermatologic events.

• No specific treatment exists. In suspected overdose, withhold drug and provide supportive care. Management of dermatologic toxicity may include topical therapies for symptomatic relief, temporary treatment interruption or dosage modification or, in severe or persistent cases, permanent discontinuation of drug.

Special considerations

- Monitor CBC with differential, platelets, hemoglobin, serum phosphate, INR, amylase, lipase, and hepatic enzyme levels.
- Monitor blood pressure weekly during first 6 weeks of therapy and thereafter as needed.
- Monitor patient closely for hand-foot skin reactions.

Patient education

- Instruct patient to take drug 1 hour before or 2 hours after eating.
- Tell patient to immediately report rash, bleeding, or chest pain.
- Instruct patient to report hand-foot skin reactions (redness, pain, swelling, or blisters). Inform him that dosage may need to be decreased if any of these reactions occur.
- Stress importance of weekly blood pressure checks during first 6 weeks of therapy.
- Advise women with childbearing potential to avoid pregnancy during therapy and for at least 2 weeks after treatment ends. Men and women should use effective birth control during this time.
- Advise breastfeeding patient to discontinue breastfeeding during therapy.

streptozocin
Zanosar

Classification: Alkylating antineoplastic, nitrosourea
Pregnancy risk category D

Pharmacology

Streptozocin, produced by *Streptomyces achromogenes,* has an unclear mechanism of antineoplastic action. In vivo, drug undergoes spontaneous decomposition to produce reactive methylcarbonium ions that alkylate DNA and cause interstrand cross-linking. It inhibits DNA synthesis in bacterial and mammalian cells. Although drug inhibits cell progression into mitosis, no specific cell-cycle phase is particularly sensitive to its lethal effects.

Pharmacokinetics

Drug is bioavailable only with I.V. administration. It is metabolized primarily in liver; metabolites readily distribute into cerebrospinal fluid. Elimination half-life is less than 1 hour. Parent drug and metabolites are excreted in urine.

How supplied

Powder for injection: 1-g vial

Indications and dosages

FDA-APPROVED

➡ Metastatic islet-cell carcinoma of pancreas
Adults: 500 mg/m^2 I.V. daily for 5 consecutive days every 6 weeks until maximum benefit or treatment-limiting toxicity occurs (dosage increase not recommended). Weekly regimen is 1,000 mg/m^2 I.V. once weekly for 2 weeks; dosage may be increased in patients who did not achieve therapeutic response and did not experience significant toxicity during previous course, not to exceed single dose of 1,500 mg/m^2.

DOSAGE MODIFICATIONS

- Dosages above 1,500 mg/m^2 may cause azotemia.
- Effects of renal impairment on drug elimination have not been evaluated. However, some clinicians recommend giving 75% of usual dosage to patients with creatinine clearance of 10 to 50 ml/minute, and 50% of usual dosage to those with creatinine clearance below 10 ml/minute.

WARNINGS

- Sterile powder should be administered under supervision of physician experienced in use of cancer chemotherapeutic agents.
- Although patients do not need be hospitalized to receive drug, they should have access

---

Only common or life-threatening adverse reactions are listed.

to facility with laboratory and supportive resources sufficient to monitor drug tolerance and protect and maintain patient who becomes compromised by drug toxicity.

• Renal toxicity is dose-related and cumulative, and may be severe or fatal. Other major toxicities include nausea and vomiting, which may be severe and at times treatment-limiting. Hepatic dysfunction, diarrhea, and hematologic changes also may occur.

• Drug is mutagenic. When given parenterally, it may be tumorigenic or carcinogenic.

• Before prescribing drug, weigh potential benefits against known toxic effects.

Contraindications and precautions

Contraindicated in hypersensitivity to drug and in combination with other potential nephrotoxins.

Use cautiously in impaired renal function and pregnancy or breastfeeding. Safety and efficacy in *children* have not been established.

Preparation and administration

>> Follow hazardous drug guidelines for handling, preparation, and administration. (See "Managing hazardous drugs," page 11.)

• Obtain baseline and serial urinalysis, BUN, serum creatinine and electrolyte levels, and creatinine clearance before therapy, at least weekly during therapy, and for 4 weeks afterward. Serial urinalysis is particularly important for early detection of proteinuria, and should be quantitated with 24-hour collection if proteinuria occurs. Mild proteinuria is one of first signs of renal toxicity and may herald further deterioration of renal function.

• Keep patient adequately hydrated to help reduce risk of nephrotoxicity.

• Drug irritates tissues. Extravasation may cause severe tissue lesions and necrosis. If extravasation occurs, discontinue infusion immediately and administer in another site. Elevate affected extremity and apply warm, moist compresses; consider injection of long-acting

dexamethasone throughout extravasated tissue.

• Administer by short I.V. infusion (over 10 to 15 minutes) or prolonged I.V. infusion (over 6 hours).

• Reconstitute with 9.5 ml dextrose injection or normal saline solution injection. Resulting pale-gold solution contains 100 mg streptozocin and 22 mg citric acid per ml. When more dilute infusion solution is desirable, dilute further with same diluent. Total storage time for reconstituted solution should not exceed 12 hours. Vial contains no preservatives and is not intended for use as multidose vial.

• When given on weekly schedule, median time to onset of response is about 17 days; median time to maximum response is about 35 days. Median total dose to onset of response is about 2,000 mg/m^2, and median total dose to maximum response is about 4,000 mg/m^2.

• Store unopened vial between 36° and 46° F (2° and 8° C), protected from light.

Adverse reactions

CNS: confusion, lethargy, depression (with continuous I.V. infusion)
GI: nausea, vomiting, diarrhea
GU: renal toxicity
Hematologic: fatal hematologic toxicity with substantially reduced WBC and platelet counts, anemia
Hepatic: hypoalbuminemia
Metabolic: hypoglycemia, insulin shock
Skin: necrosis

Interactions

Drug-drug. *Doxorubicin:* prolonged elimination half-life of doxorubicin, which may lead to severe bone marrow depression
Myelosuppressive nitrosoureas (such as carmustine): increased hematologic toxicity of both drugs
Nephrotoxic agents: increased renal toxicity
Phenytoin: decreased cytotoxic effects of streptozocin on pancreatic beta cells

S

Drug-diagnostic tests. *Albumin, blood glucose:* decreased
AST, lactate dehydrogenase: increased

Toxicity and overdose
• Anticipated signs and symptoms of overdose are nausea, vomiting, hematologic changes, and renal toxicity.
• No specific antidote exists. Monitor renal function and WBC and platelet counts. Decrease dosage or stop drug as indicated. Provide supportive care, such as whole blood products or blood modifiers (such as darbepoetin alfa, epoetin alfa, or filgrastim) to treat bone marrow toxicity.

Special considerations
• For patients with functional tumors, serial monitoring of fasting insulin level helps determine biochemical response to therapy. For patients with functional or nonfunctional tumors, measurable reductions in tumor size (including reduction of organomegaly, masses, or lymph nodes) help determine response.
• Drug commonly causes renal toxicity, which manifests as azotemia, anuria, hypophosphatemia, glycosuria, and renal tubular acidosis. Such toxicity is dose-related and cumulative, and may be severe or fatal. Monitor renal function before and after each course. Adequate hydration may help reduce risk of nephrotoxicity to renal tubular epithelium by decreasing renal and urinary concentration of drug and metabolites.

Patient education
• Advise patient to avoid tasks that require alertness until effects of continuous I.V. drug infusion are known.
• Instruct patient to immediately report redness, pain, or swelling at injection site.
• Advise breastfeeding patient not to breastfeed during therapy.

strontium chloride Sr 89
Metastron

Classification: Antineoplastic, radiopharmaceutical
Pregnancy risk category D

Pharmacology
Strontium chloride Sr 89, a calcium analogue, follows same biochemical pathways as calcium in vivo. It concentrates in areas of increased osteogenesis (such as increased mineral turnover), not in marrow cells. Reactive osteoid at primary bone tumor and metastatic sites accumulate more strontium than surrounding normal bone. Retained strontium delivers radiation dose large enough to produce palliative effect (relief of bone pain). Due to short range of beta particles, cells near regions containing strontium are preferentially irradiated.

Pharmacokinetics
Drug has fairly rapid clearance and localizes selectively in bone hydroxyapatite. Pain relief may begin 7 to 21 days after administration, with maximum relief by 6 weeks. Duration of pain relief averages 6 months, with range of 4 to 12 months. Elimination half-life is 14 days for normal bone and more than 50 days for metastatic sites. Excretion is primarily renal by glomerular filtration and secondarily fecal in patients with bone metastasis. Renal excretion is greatest in first 2 days after treatment.

How supplied
Solution for injection: 10-ml single-use vial containing 148 MBq, 4 mCi

Indications and dosages

FDA-APPROVED

➡ Bone pain in patients with metastatic bone lesions

Only common or life-threatening adverse reactions are listed.

Adults: 148 MBq, 4 mCi, by slow I.V. injection over 1 or 2 minutes

Contraindications and precautions

Contraindicated in sensitivity to radiopharmaceutical preparation.

Use cautiously in patients with platelet counts below 60,000/mm³ and WBC counts below 2,400/mm³, cancer not involving bone, renal dysfunction, and pregnancy or breast-feeding. Safety and efficacy in *children* have not been established.

Preparation and administration

• Follow hazardous drug guidelines for handling, preparation, and administration. (See "Managing hazardous drugs," page 11.)
• Before therapy begins, bone metastases must be confirmed (such as with skeletal imaging using technetium Tc 99m–labeled phosphate or phosphonate radiopharmaceutical).
• Dose should be measured by suitable radioactivity calibration system immediately before administration.
• Base repeated administration on patient's response, current symptoms, and hematologic status. Generally, repeated administration is not recommended at intervals of less than 90 days.
• Because of drug's delayed onset of pain relief, administration to patients with very short life expectancy is not recommended.
• Metastron is a sterile, nonpyrogenic, aqueous solution for I.V. use. Solution contains no preservative. Each ml contains strontium chloride 10.9 to 22.6 mg and water for injection. Radioactive concentration is 37 MBq/ml, 1 mCi/ml, and specific activity is 2.96 to 6.17 MBq/mg, 80 to 167 Ci/mg at calibration.
• After administration, take special precautions in incontinent patients (such as urinary catheterization) to minimize risk of radioactive contamination of clothing, bed linen, and other items.
• Keep vial inside its transportation shield whenever possible.

• Calibration date for radioactivity content and expiration date are printed on vial label. Expiration date is 28 days after calibration.

Adverse reactions

Hematologic: thrombocytopenia, leukopenia
Musculoskeletal: bone pain
Other: chills, fever, flushing

Interactions

Drug-drug. *Blood dyscrasia–causing drugs:* increased leukopenia and thrombocytopenia
Calcium-containing drugs: decreased bone uptake of drug (from saturation of bone-binding sites by calcium)
Drug-diagnostic tests. *ALP:* decreased
Serum tumor markers: decreased concentration

Toxicity and overdose

No information available

Special considerations

• Monitor CBC with differential frequently.
• Closely monitor renal function.

Patient education

• Urge patient to inform health care professional of incontinence before administration. Catheterization may be required to prevent radiation contamination.
• Instruct male patient to use normal toilet instead of urinal for first week after administration. Advise him to double-flush toilet, wipe spilled urine with tissue and then flush, and wash hands after using or cleaning toilet.
• Tell patient or family to immediately launder clothes and linens soiled with patient's urine or blood, washing them separately from other clothes. Instruct them to wash away spilled blood.
• Caution patient to avoid exposure to persons with bacterial infections.

S

sucralfate
Carafate

Classification: GI cytoprotective agent
Pregnancy risk category B

Pharmacology
Sucralfate forms complex that adheres to peptic ulcer site and absorbs pepsin. It reacts with gastric acid to form protective coating on ulcer surface, inhibiting gastric acid secretion, pepsin, and bile salts.

Pharmacokinetics
Drug is minimally absorbed from GI tract. It binds to ulcer site up to 6 hours after oral administration. It is excreted primarily in urine.

How supplied
Oral suspension: 500 mg/5 ml
Tablets: 1 g

Indications and dosages

OFF-LABEL USES (SELECTED)

➡ Chemotherapy- and radiation-induced mucositis and stomatitis
Adults: Typical dosage is 1 g sucralfate suspension (swished and swallowed) four times daily for 14 days starting on day 1 of therapy.

Contraindications and precautions
No known contraindications.

Use cautiously in chronic renal failure, patients on dialysis, and pregnancy or breastfeeding. Safety and efficacy in *children* have not been established.

Preparation and administration
• Inadvertent injection of insoluble sucralfate and its insoluble excipients may cause fatal complications, including pulmonary and cerebral emboli. Drug is not intended for I.V. use.
• When bioavailability alterations are critical, administer separately from other drugs (due to its potential to alter absorption of certain drugs). Monitor patient appropriately.
• Despite conflicting efficacy results in mucositis and stomatitis, some clinicians use drug for these conditions.
• For mucositis treatment, suspension may be prepared by dissolving eight 1-g sucralfate tablets in 40 ml sterile water for irrigation, then adding 40 ml sorbitol 70% and shaking solution well. Suspension of two flavor packets dissolved in 10 ml sterile water for irrigation may be added to drug mixture, along with sufficient sterile water for irrigation to bring total volume to 120 ml.
• For stomatitis treatment, suspension (1 g/ 15 ml) may be prepared using sucralfate 12 g dissolved in 60 ml water, followed by addition of Benylin syrup 60 ml and Maalox suspension up to a total of 180 ml.
• Patient should swish suspension thoroughly before swallowing it.
• Store at controlled temperature of 59° to 86° F (15° to 30° C). Avoid freezing. Suspensions prepared for mucositis and stomatitis are stable for 14 days in refrigerator and should be labeled "Shake well."

Adverse reactions
CNS: drowsiness, dizziness
GI: dry mouth, constipation, nausea, gastric pain, vomiting, bezoars
Skin: urticaria, rash, pruritus

Interactions
Drug-drug. *Aluminum-containing antacids:* decreased binding of sucralfate to GI mucosa, causing reduced sucralfate efficacy
Cimetidine, digoxin, fat-soluble vitamins, ketoconazole, phenytoin, ranitidine, tetracyclines, theophylline: decreased actions of these drugs
Ciprofloxacin: decreased ciprofloxacin absorption

Toxicity and overdose
• Risks associated with acute overdose should be minimal because drug is minimally absorbed from GI tract. Most patients with sus-

---

pected overdose are asymptomatic. Possible adverse events include dyspepsia, abdominal pain, nausea, and vomiting.
• Due to limited experience, no specific treatment for overdose is recommended.

Special considerations
• Bezoars are more likely in patients with underlying medical conditions that may predispose them to bezoar formation (such as delayed gastric emptying) and in those receiving concomitant enteral tube feedings.

Patient education
• Instruct patient to shake suspension well before using.
• Instruct patient to separate sucralfate administration from other drugs by 2 hours when possible.

tamoxifen citrate
Nolvadex

Classification: Antineoplastic, antiestrogen agent, selective estrogen-receptor modulator, hormone/hormone modifier
Pregnancy risk category D

Pharmacology
Tamoxifen, a nonsteroidal agent, has antiestrogenic effects that may relate to its ability to compete with estrogen for binding sites in target tissues (such as breast). In cytosols derived from human breast adenocarcinomas, it competes with estradiol for estrogen-receptor protein.

Pharmacokinetics
Drug has good oral bioavailability and is metabolized in liver. It peaks 3 to 6 hours after single dose. Elimination half-life is approximately 5 to 7 days. Neither drug nor its major metabolite appears in bile or urine.

How supplied
Tablets: 10 mg, 20 mg

Indications and dosages

FDA-APPROVED
➡ Metastatic breast cancer in women and men, adjuvant treatment of breast cancer (treatment of axillary node–positive breast cancer in postmenopausal women after total or segmental mastectomy, axillary dissection, and breast irradiation; treatment of axillary node–negative breast cancer in women after total or segmental mastectomy, axillary dissection, and breast irradiation)
Adults: 20 to 40 mg P.O. daily; may be divided into two doses (morning and evening)
➡ To reduce risk of breast cancer in high-risk women; to reduce risk of invasive breast cancer in ductal carcinoma in situ (DCIS) after breast surgery and radiation
Adults: 20 mg P.O. daily for 5 years

OFF-LABEL USES (SELECTED)
➡ Hepatocellular carcinoma, other cancers with estrogen receptors
Adults: Various dosage schedules have been studied.

WARNINGS

• Serious and life-threatening events associated with drug in risk-reduction setting (women at high risk for cancer and women with DCIS) include uterine cancers, stroke, and pulmonary embolism. These events may be fatal.
• Health care professionals should discuss potential benefits and risks with women at high risk for breast cancer and with women who have DCIS to determine whether to use drug to reduce breast cancer risk.
• In women already diagnosed with breast cancer, drug's benefits outweigh risks.

T

Contraindications and precautions

Contraindicated in hypersensitivity to drug or its components, women who require concomitant coumarin-type anticoagulant therapy, and women with history of deep vein thrombosis or pulmonary embolus.

Use cautiously in hypocalcemia, leukopenia, thrombocytopenia, ocular disturbances, hepatic impairment, and pregnancy or breastfeeding. Long-term effects in *children* have not been established. Safety and efficacy in girls ages 2 to 10 with Albright's syndrome and precocious puberty have not been studied beyond 1 year of treatment.

Preparation and administration

▶▶ Follow hazardous drug guidelines for handling, preparation, and administration. (See "Managing hazardous drugs," page 11.)
• Store at controlled temperature of 68° to 77° F (20° to 25° C) in tightly closed, light-resistant container.

Adverse reactions

CNS: headache, light-headedness, depression, fatigue
CV: chest pain
EENT: ocular lesion, retinopathy, corneal opacity, blurred vision (high doses)
GI: nausea, vomiting, altered taste, anorexia
GU: vaginal discharge, menstrual irregularities, uterine fibroid
Hematologic: thrombocytopenia, leukopenia, thromboembolic event
Metabolic: hyperlipidemia, hypertriglyceridemia, hypercalcemia
Musculoskeletal: bone pain
Skin: rash
Other: fluid retention, hot flashes

Interactions

Drug-drug. *Aminoglutethimide, rifampin:* decreased tamoxifen level
Anticoagulants: increased risk of bleeding
Cytotoxic agents: increased thromboembolic events
Letrozole: decreased letrozole level

Drug-diagnostic tests. *Lipids, liver function tests, serum calcium and thyroxine (T₄):* increased

Drug-food. *Grapefruit, pomegranate:* possible increased tamoxifen levels
Soy: possible antagonism of tamoxifen
Drug-herb. *Cat's claw, devil's claw, feverfew, garlic, ginkgo, goldenseal, kava, milk thistle, valerian:* possible increased tamoxifen levels
St. John's wort: reduced tamoxifen efficacy

Toxicity and overdose

• Acute overdose has not been reported. In a study of patients with advanced metastatic cancer to determine maximum tolerated dose (in evaluating use of high doses to reverse multidrug resistance), acute neurotoxicity manifested by tremor, hyperreflexia, unsteady gait, and dizziness arose within 3 to 5 days of drug initiation and cleared within 2 to 5 days after drug withdrawal. No permanent neurologic toxicity occurred.
• No specific treatment for overdose exists. Provide symptomatic treatment.

Special considerations

• Monitor CBC and differential, liver function tests, and serum calcium and T₄ levels.
• Within a few weeks of starting drug, breast cancer patients with metastases may develop hypercalcemia. In this event, take appropriate measures; if severe, discontinue therapy.
• Ocular disturbances (such as reduced color-vision perception, corneal changes, retinal vein thrombosis, retinopathy, and cataracts) may occur.
• Drug has been associated with changes in liver enzyme levels and, in rare cases, more severe hepatic abnormalities (including fatty liver, cholestasis, hepatitis, and hepatic necrosis), which may prove fatal.
• In sexually active women with childbearing potential, tamoxifen citrate therapy should be initiated during menstruation. In women with menstrual irregularity, negative B-HCG test immediately before therapy begins is sufficient.

Only common or life-threatening adverse reactions are listed.

Patient education

- Instruct patient to immediately report pain, swelling, or tenderness in legs or calves; sudden chest pain or shortness of breath; coughing up blood; new breast lumps; vaginal bleeding; menstrual irregularities; change in vaginal discharge; pelvic pain or pressure; and vision changes.
- Emphasize importance of having regular gynecologic exams, mammograms, and blood tests to identify early signs of adverse reactions.
- Advise women with childbearing potential to avoid pregnancy during therapy.
- Provide guidance to help breastfeeding patient decide whether to discontinue breastfeeding or stop drug.

temozolomide

Temodar

Classification: Antineoplastic, alkylating agent
Pregnancy risk category D

Pharmacology

Temozolomide is not directly active, but undergoes rapid nonenzymatic conversion at physiologic pH to the reactive compound monomethyl triazeno imidazole carboxamide (MTIC). Cytotoxicity of MTIC may result primarily from DNA alkylation, which occurs mainly at O6 and N7 positions of guanine.

Pharmacokinetics

Drug has good bioavailability (enhanced by empty stomach). It is converted to MTIC spontaneously in bloodstream, and peaks in approximately 1 hour. Elimination half-life is approximately 1.8 hours. Parent drug, MTIC, and other metabolites are eliminated in urine.

How supplied

Capsules: 5 mg, 20 mg, 100 mg, 250 mg

Indications and dosages

FDA-APPROVED

➡ Newly diagnosed glioblastoma multiforme treated concomitantly with radiotherapy
Adults: Initially, 75 mg/m^2 P.O. daily for 42 days. Then, 4 weeks after completion of temozolomide and radiotherapy phase, 150 mg/m^2 P.O. daily for 5 days followed by 23 days without treatment (maintenance phase cycle 1). Then, at start of cycle 2, 200 mg/m^2 P.O. daily for first 5 days. Given for total of 6 cycles.
➡ Refractory anaplastic astrocytoma
Adults: 150 mg/m^2 P.O. daily for 5 days during 28-day cycle

OFF-LABEL USES (SELECTED)

⊜ Malignant glioma, metastatic melanoma
Adults: 150 to 200 mg/m^2 P.O. for 5 days every 4 weeks

DOSAGE MODIFICATIONS

- Dosage adjustment is based on nadir neutrophil and platelet counts.
- During treatment, obtain CBC on day 22 (21 days after first dose) or within 48 hours of that day, and weekly until absolute neutrophil count (ANC) exceeds 1.5×10^9/L (1,500/mm^3) and platelet count exceeds 100×10^9/L (100,000/mm^3). Do not begin next cycle until ANC and platelet count exceed these levels. If ANC falls below 1.0×10^9/L (1,000/mm^3) or platelet count falls below 50×10^9/L (50,000/mm^3) during any cycle, reduce dosage in next cycle by 50 mg/m^2, but not below 100 mg/m^2 (lowest recommended dosage).

Contraindications and precautions

Contraindicated in hypersensitivity to drug, its components, or dacarbazine.

Use cautiously in patients receiving radiation therapy, renal or hepatic disease, pregnancy or breastfeeding, and *elderly patients.* Safety and efficacy in *children* have not been established.

T

Preparation and administration

- Follow hazardous drug guidelines for handling, preparation, and administration. (See "Managing hazardous drugs," page 11.)
- Administer consistently (for instance, always on empty stomach). Although food reduces drug absorption, no dietary restrictions apply.
- To reduce nausea and vomiting, administer on empty stomach. Bedtime administration may be advisable. Antiemetic may be given before or after drug.
- Therapy can continue until disease progresses.
- Store at 77° F (25° C). Excursions are permitted to 59° to 86° F (15° to 30° C).

Adverse reactions

CNS: seizures, hemiparesis, dizziness, poor coordination, amnesia, insomnia, somnolence, ataxia, anxiety, depression, confusion, fatigue, headache
EENT: blurred vision, diplopia, pharyngitis, sinusitis
GI: nausea, anorexia, vomiting
Hematologic: thrombocytopenia, leukopenia, anemia
Musculoskeletal: back pain
Respiratory: coughing
Skin: rash, pruritus
Other: fever, edema

Interactions

Drug-drug. *Other antineoplastics:* increased myelosuppression
Valproic acid: decreased temozolomide clearance
Drug-food. *Any food:* reduced drug absorption
Drug-herb. *Alpha-lipoic acid, coenzyme Q10, glucosamine, glutamine:* possible decreased chemotherapy efficacy

Toxicity and overdose

- Dose-limiting toxicity is hematologic and can occur at any dosage, but is more severe at higher dosages. Potential adverse reactions after at least 5 days of therapy include infection and bone marrow depression, which may be severe, prolonged, and fatal.
- If overdose occurs, perform hematologic evaluation. Provide supportive measures as necessary.

Special considerations

- Monitor CBC and differential frequently.
- Higher incidence of *Pneumocystis carinii* pneumonia (PCP) may occur when drug is given for prolonged period. For patients with newly diagnosed glioblastoma multiforme, administer prophylaxis against PCP if patient is receiving temozolomide concomitantly with radiotherapy.

Patient education

- Instruct patient to swallow capsules whole with a glass of water. Caution against opening or chewing them.
- If capsules are accidentally opened or damaged, caution patient to avoid inhaling capsule contents or letting contents contact skin or mucous membranes.
- Instruct patient to immediately report unusual bruising or bleeding.
- Tell patient to report signs or symptoms of infection (such as fever, sore throat, and flu-like symptoms).
- Advise patient to avoid driving and other hazardous activities until drug's effects on concentration, alertness, and vision are known.
- Caution women with childbearing potential to avoid pregnancy during therapy. If patient is pregnant or becomes pregnant while taking drug, inform her of potential hazards to fetus.
- Instruct breastfeeding patient to discontinue breastfeeding during therapy.

Only common or life-threatening adverse reactions are listed.

teniposide
Vumon

Classification: Antineoplastic, epipodophyllotoxin
Pregnancy risk category D

Pharmacology
Teniposide acts in late S or early G_2 phase, preventing cells from entering mitosis. It causes dose-dependent single- and double-stranded breaks in DNA and DNA:protein cross-links. Mechanism of action appears to relate to inhibition of type II topoisomerase activity; drug does not intercalate into or bind strongly to DNA. Cytotoxic effects relate to relative number of double-stranded DNA breaks produced in cells, which reflects stabilization of topoisomerase II-DNA intermediate. Drug has broad spectrum of in vivo antitumor activity against murine tumors, including hematologic cancers and various solid tumors. It is notably active against sublines of certain murine leukemias with acquired resistance to cisplatin, doxorubicin, amsacrine, daunorubicin, mitoxantrone, or vincristine.

Pharmacokinetics
Drug is bioavailable only with I.V. administration. It is almost completely metabolized in liver and is more than 99% protein-bound. Drug peaks at 1 to 2 hours. Elimination half-life is 5 hours. Metabolites are excreted in bile and urine.

How supplied
Solution for injection: 50-mg (5-ml) ampules

Indications and dosages

FDA-APPROVED
➲ Refractory childhood acute lymphoblastic leukemia
Children: Teniposide 165 mg/m² I.V. infusion in combination with cytarabine 300 mg/m²
I.V. infusion twice weekly for eight or nine doses; or in combination with vincristine and prednisone, teniposide 250 mg/m² I.V. infusion with vincristine 1.5 mg/m² I.V. infusion weekly for 4 to 8 weeks and prednisone 40 mg/m² P.O. daily for 28 days

OFF-LABEL USES (SELECTED)
➡ Refractory non-Hodgkin's lymphoma
Adults: Typical dosage schedules include 30 mg/m² I.V. infusion daily for 10 days; or as single agent, 50 to 100 mg/m² I.V. infusion weekly; or in combination with other chemotherapy agents, 60 to 70 mg/m² I.V. infusion weekly.
➡ Neuroblastoma
Adults: Dosage schedules have included teniposide as single agent, 130 to 180 mg/m² I.V. infusion weekly; or in combination with other chemotherapy agents, 100 mg/m² I.V. infusion every 21 days.
Children: One chemotherapy regimen included cyclophosphamide 750 mg/m² on day 1, vincristine 1.5 mg/m² on day 1 and Adriamycin (doxorubicin) 50 mg/m² on day 1 (CAV), alternating with teniposide or etoposide 60 mg/m² on days 1 to 5 and cisplatin 20 mg/m² on days 1 to 5 (EP regimen) by I.V. infusion.
➡ Small-cell lung cancer
Adults: Teniposide 60 mg/m² I.V. on days 1 through 5 in combination with carboplatin

DOSAGE MODIFICATIONS
• Patients with both Down syndrome and leukemia may be especially sensitive to drug. Therefore, initial dosage should be reduced, with first course given at half of usual dosage. Higher dosages may be given in subsequent courses, depending on degree of myelosuppression and mucositis in earlier courses.
• Patients receiving two or more bone marrow–depressant therapies (including radiation) concurrently or consecutively may require dosage reductions.

T

⊠ WARNINGS

Contraindications and precautions

Contraindicated in hypersensitivity to drug, etoposide, or Cremophor EL (polyoxyethylated castor oil).

Use cautiously in bone marrow depression, severe hepatic or renal disease, bacterial infection, CNS depression, hypotension, hypoalbuminemia, infection, chickenpox (current, recent, or recent exposure to), herpes zoster, pregnancy or breastfeeding, and in *children with Down syndrome.*

Preparation and administration

≫ Follow hazardous drug guidelines for handling, preparation, and administration. (See "Managing hazardous drugs," page 11.)
• Evaluate CBC and differential, platelet count, hemoglobin, and kidney and liver function tests carefully before therapy starts.
• If undiluted injection concentrate comes in contact with plastic equipment or devices used to prepare solutions for infusion, plastic may soften or crack and product leakage may occur. (This effect has not been reported with diluted solutions.) To prevent extraction of plasticizer DEHP, solutions for injection concentrate should be prepared in non-DEHP-containing LVP container, such as glass or polyolefin plastic bags or containers. Solutions should be administered with I.V. administration sets that do not contain DEHP.
• Dilute with 5% dextrose injection or normal saline solution injection for final concentration of 0.1 mg/ml, 0.2 mg/ml, 0.4 mg/ml, or 1 mg/ml. Solutions prepared in 5% dextrose injection or normal saline solution injection at concentrations of 0.1 mg/ml, 0.2 mg/ml, or 0.4 mg/ml are stable at room temperature for up to 24 hours. Give solutions prepared at final concentration of 1 mg/ml within 4 hours to reduce risk of precipitation. Refrigeration of solutions is not recommended.
• Precipitation may occur during 24-hour infusions diluted to concentrations of 0.1 to 0.2 mg/ml, causing occlusion of central venous access catheter. Heparin solutions can cause drug precipitation. To prevent these problems, flush administration apparatus thoroughly with 5% dextrose injection or normal saline solution injection before and after drug administration.
• Give drug only by slow I.V. infusion lasting at least 30 to 60 minutes. Hypotension may occur with rapid I.V. injection (possibly from direct effect of Cremophor EL).
• Improper administration may cause extravasation, leading to local tissue necrosis and thrombophlebitis. If extravasation occurs, discontinue infusion immediately and administer in another site. Elevate affected extremity and apply warm, moist compresses; consider injection of long-acting dexamethasone throughout extravasated tissue.
• With first dose, hypersensitivity reaction (variably manifested by chills, fever, urticaria, tachycardia, bronchospasm, dyspnea, hypertension or hypotension, and facial flushing) may occur. Reaction may be life-threatening if not treated promptly with antihistamines, corticosteroids, epinephrine, I.V. fluids, and other supportive measures.
• Store at 36° to 46° F (2° to 8° C) in original package. Protect from light.

Adverse reactions

CNS: CNS depression
CV: hypotension
EENT: mucositis
GI: nausea, vomiting, diarrhea
Hematologic: myelosuppression, bleeding
Metabolic: hypoalbuminemia
Skin: alopecia, rash
Other: secondary malignancy (risk is up to 12

Only common or life-threatening adverse reactions are listed.

times higher in patients treated on weekly or twice-weekly schedule), infection, fever, hypersensitivity

Interactions

Drug-drug. *Antiemetics:* possible increased risk of additive CNS depression (from alcohol content of teniposide)
Bone marrow depressants: increased bone marrow depression
Methotrexate: altered methotrexate level
Phenobarbital, phenytoin: increased clearance and decreased efficacy of teniposide
Sodium salicylate, sulfamethizole, tolbutamide: teniposide displacement from protein-binding sites, leading to increased risk of toxicity
Drug-diagnostic tests. *CBC and differential, hemoglobin, platelets:* decreased
Plasma albumin: increased steady-state volume of teniposide distribution, decreased plasma albumin concentration
Drug-herb. *Alpha-lipoic acid, coenzyme Q10, glucosamine, glutamine:* possible decreased chemotherapy efficacy
Devil's claw, feverfew, ginkgo, kava: possible increased teniposide levels

Toxicity and overdose

• Anticipated complications of overdose result from bone marrow depression.
• No known antidote exists. Provide supportive treatment, including blood products and antibiotics as indicated.

Special considerations

• Evaluate patient frequently for myelosuppression during and after therapy. Dose-limiting bone marrow depression is most significant toxicity.
• At start of therapy and before each subsequent dose, monitor hemoglobin, WBC count and differential, and platelet count. If necessary, repeat bone marrow examination before decision to continue therapy in face of severe myelosuppression.
• Monitor plasma albumin level, platelet count, hemoglobin, and kidney and liver

function tests carefully throughout therapy.
• Observe for acute CNS depression and hypotension in patients receiving high doses who have been pretreated with antiemetics. Depressant effects of antiemetics and alcohol content of teniposide may increase risk of CNS depression.
• Observe patient; be prepared for possible hypersensitivity reaction throughout therapy.

Patient education

• Instruct patient to immediately report redness, pain, swelling, or lump under skin at injection site.
• Instruct patient or caregiver to contact physician immediately if patient experiences symptoms of hypersensitivity reaction, such as, fever, chills, rapid heartbeat, flushing, difficulty breathing, or rash.
• Advise patient or caregiver to immediately report signs or symptoms of bone marrow depression, including fever, chills, cough or hoarseness, lower back or side pain, unusual bleeding or bruising, black tarry stools, blood in urine or stools, and pinpoint red spots on skin.
• Inform patient or caregiver that drug contains alcohol.
• Advise women with childbearing potential to avoid pregnancy during therapy.
• Provide guidance to help breastfeeding patient decide whether to discontinue breastfeeding or stop drug.

testolactone
Teslac

Classification: Antineoplastic, aromatase inhibitor, hormone/hormone modifier
Controlled substance schedule III
Pregnancy risk category C

Pharmacology

Testolactone exerts antineoplastic activity through an unknown mechanism. It may inhibit steroid aromatase activity and reduce estrone synthesis from adrenal androstenedione (a major estrogen source in postmenopausal women). Aromatase inhibition may be noncompetitive and irreversible, explaining persistence of drug's effect on estrogen synthesis after withdrawal.

Pharmacokinetics
Drug is well absorbed from GI tract and metabolized in liver. Parent drug and metabolites are eliminated through kidney.

How supplied
Tablets: 50 mg

Indications and dosages

FDA-APPROVED

➡ Adjunctive therapy in palliative treatment of advanced or disseminated breast cancer in postmenopausal women when hormonal therapy is indicated
Adults: 250 mg P.O. four times daily

Contraindications and precautions
Contraindicated in hypersensitivity to drug and in males with breast carcinoma.

Use cautiously in hypercalcemia, premenopausal women, and ***elderly patients.*** Safety and efficacy in ***children*** have not been established.

Preparation and administration
• Follow hazardous drug guidelines for handling, preparation, and administration. (See "Managing hazardous drugs," page 11.)
• Store at 77° F (25° C).

Adverse reactions
CNS: paresthesia, dizziness
CV: hypertension, edema
GI: nausea, vomiting, anorexia, glossitis
GU: urinary retention, renal failure
Musculoskeletal: muscle ache
Skin: alopecia, rash, nail changes, facial hair growth

Other: deepening voice

Interactions
Drug-drug. *Oral anticoagulants:* increased anticoagulant effect
Drug-diagnostic tests. *Estradiol:* decreased *Serum calcium, urinary 17-hydroxycorticosteroids:* increased
Drug-herb. *Aloe, cascara, rhubarb:* possible decreased testolactone absorption due to reduced GI transit time

Toxicity and overdose
• No reports of acute overdose have been reported.
• If overdose occurs, provide supportive treatment.

Special considerations
• Monitor patient routinely for hypercalcemia.
• Monitor renal function in elderly patients.
• Discontinue therapy for at least 3 months to evaluate response unless active disease progression occurs.

Patient education
• Instruct patient to notify prescriber if side effects occur or become more pronounced.
• Tell patient to consult prescriber if she misses a dose.

thalidomide
Thalomid

Classification: Immunomodulator, tumor necrosis factor modulator
Pregnancy risk category X

Pharmacology
Thalidomide has an incompletely characterized spectrum of activity. Its immunologic effects can vary substantially under different conditions, but may relate to suppression of excessive tumor necrosis factor-alpha (TNF-α)

production and down-modulation of selected cell-surface adhesion molecules involved in leukocyte migration. For example, drug decreases circulating TNF-α levels in patients with erythema nodosum leprosum and increases plasma TNF-α levels in HIV-positive patients.

Pharmacokinetics

Drug is absorbed slowly and incompletely from GI tract. It is metabolized by spontaneous hydrolysis and is well distributed. Elimination half-life is 5 to 7 hours.

How supplied

Capsules: 50 mg, 100 mg, 200 mg

Indications and dosages

OFF-LABEL USES (SELECTED)

➡ Advanced refractory multiple myeloma
Adults: Typical dosages range from 200 mg to 800 mg P.O. daily.
➡ Prostate cancer
Adults: Docetaxel-thalidomide study showed that addition of thalidomide to docetaxel therapy is a promising therapeutic approach to metastatic prostate cancer. However, this combination requires subsequent confirmation due to size and intent of trial.
➡ Clinical manifestations of Kaposi's sarcoma or primary brain malignancies
Adults: Typical dosages range from 400 to 1,000 mg P.O. daily.
➡ Recurrent glioblastoma multiforme of CNS
Adults: Typical dosages are 800 mg P.O. daily for first 2 weeks, followed by dosage increase of 200 mg P.O. daily every 2 weeks, to maximum dosage of 1,200 mg P.O. daily, if tolerated.

⊠ WARNINGS

• If taken during pregnancy, drug can cause severe birth defects or fetal death. It should never be used by women who are pregnant or could become pregnant during therapy. Even a single dose taken by a pregnant woman can cause severe birth defects.
• To reduce chance of fetal exposure, drug is approved only under special restricted distribution program approved by FDA (System for Thalidomide Education and Prescribing Safety, or STEPS). Under this program, only prescribers and pharmacists registered with program are allowed to prescribe and dispense drug. Patients must be advised of, agree to, and comply with STEPS program requirements to receive product.
• Drug may be prescribed only by licensed prescribers registered in STEPS program. Before dispensing drug, pharmacist must activate authorization number on every prescription by calling Celgene Customer Care Center at 1-888-4-Celgene and obtaining confirmation number. Confirmation number must be written on prescription. Prescription should be accepted only if it has been issued within previous 7 days. No telephone prescriptions are permitted. Drug can be dispensed in no more than a 4-week (28-day) supply; new prescription is required for further dispensing. Subsequent prescriptions may be dispensed only if fewer than 7 days of therapy remain on previous prescription. Prescriber must not issue prescription until written report of negative pregnancy test has been obtained.
• Drug is contraindicated in females with childbearing potential and in sexually mature males unless alternative therapies are considered inappropriate and patient meets all of the following conditions: (1) understands and can carry out instructions reliably; (2) is capable of complying with mandatory contraceptive measures, pregnancy testing, patient registration, and patient survey as described in STEPS program; (3) has received oral and written warnings of hazards of taking drug during pregnancy and of exposing fetus to drug; (4) has received oral and written warnings of risk of possible contraception failure and of need to use two reliable contraceptive methods simultaneously (except in female patient who has chosen continuous abstinence from het-

T

erosexual sexual contact); (5) acknowledges in writing that he or she understands these warnings and the need to use two reliable contraceptive methods for 4 weeks before starting therapy, during therapy, and for 4 weeks after therapy ends. In addition, female patient must have had a negative pregnancy test within 24 hours before therapy begins; male patient must have been informed of drug's presence in semen and of the need to always use latex condom during sexual contact with women of childbearing potential, even if he has had successful vasectomy.

• Reliable contraception is required even if patient has a history of infertility, unless she has had a hysterectomy or has been postmenopausal for at least 24 months.

• Use in women with childbearing potential hinges on initial and continued confirmed negative pregnancy tests. Obtain pregnancy test within 24 hours before therapy starts and weekly during first month of therapy, then monthly thereafter in patient with regular menstrual cycles or every 2 weeks in patient with irregular cycles.

• If pregnancy occurs during therapy, drug must be discontinued immediately. Suspected fetal exposure must be reported to FDA immediately by calling MedWATCH (1-800-FDA-1088). It must also be reported to Celgene Corporation.

Contraindications and precautions

Contraindicated in hypersensitivity to drug or its components and in pregnancy.

Use cautiously in bradycardia, women with childbearing potential (as described in "Warnings"), and breastfeeding. Safety and efficacy in **children younger than age 12** have not been established.

Preparation and administration

• Follow hazardous drug guidelines for handling, preparation, and administration. (See "Managing hazardous drugs," page 11.)

• In women with childbearing potential, use

hinges on initial and continued confirmed negative pregnancy tests (as described in "Warnings").

• Store between 59° and 86° F (15° and 30° C). Protect from light.

Adverse reactions

CNS: drowsiness, peripheral neuropathy, dizziness, vertigo, sedation, tremor, asthenia, seizures

CV: bradycardia, orthostatic hypotension, peripheral edema, thrombotic event

EENT: rhinitis, sinusitis, pharyngitis, tooth pain

GI: nausea, constipation, diarrhea, oral candidiasis, abdominal pain

Hematologic: neutropenia

Musculoskeletal: back pain

Respiratory: pulmonary embolism

Skin: exfoliative, purpuric, bullous, or maculopapular rash; pruritus; fungal dermatitis; nail disorder; photosensitivity; toxic epidermal necrolysis, Stevens-Johnson syndrome

Other: chills, accidental injury, hypersensitivity reactions, increased HIV viral load, severe birth defects, fetal death

Interactions

Drug-drug. *Barbiturates, chlorpromazine, reserpine, sedative-hypnotics, other CNS depressants:* increased sedation

Drugs linked to peripheral neuropathy (such as isoniazid, metronidazole, and vincristine): increased risk of peripheral neuropathy

Drug-diagnostic tests. *Lactate dehydrogenase, lipids, liver function tests:* increased

Neutrophils, WBCs: decreased

Drug-food. *High-fat meal:* delayed drug absorption

Drug-herb. *Aloe, cascara, rhubarb:* possible decreased thalidomide absorption due to reduced GI transit time

Toxicity and overdose

• Three cases of overdose (all attempted suicides) have been reported. No reported deaths have occurred with dosages up to 14.4 g. All

---

Only common or life-threatening adverse reactions are listed.

patients recovered without reported sequelae. Anticipated signs and symptoms are those of adverse reactions.
• If overdose occurs, treat supportively.

Special considerations
• Monitor WBC with differential frequently.
• Observe closely for hypersensitivity reactions.

Patient education
• Instruct patient to take drug with 8 oz of water just before bedtime or at least 1 hour after dinner.
• Tell patient not to take drug with high-fat meal.
• Caution patient not to handle capsules extensively and not to open them. Instruct him to store them in blister packs until ingestion.
• Advise patient to immediately report signs and symptoms of hypersensitivity reaction (especially rash) or peripheral neuropathy (including numbness, tingling, and pain or burning sensation in feet or hands).
• Instruct patient to avoid driving or performing other hazardous tasks during therapy because drug causes drowsiness.
• Caution patient not to consume alcohol or take other drugs that may cause drowsiness.
• Inform patient that drug may cause low blood pressure with position changes. Advise him to sit upright for a few minutes before standing up.
• Instruct patient to use sunscreen and wear protective clothing when outdoors and to avoid prolonged exposure to sunlight or ultraviolet light.
• To minimize constipation (especially in patients with multiple myeloma), advise patient to increase fluid intake, perform physical activity (if possible), and increase dietary fiber intake.
• Make sure females with childbearing potential and their partners have received oral and written instructions according to STEPS program guidelines.
• Explain risks of fetal exposure to drug.

• Caution females with childbearing potential to use two highly effective birth control methods simultaneously, from 1 month before first dose until 1 month after last dose.
• Make sure male patients know that they need to use latex condoms.
• Provide guidance to help breastfeeding patient decide whether to discontinue breastfeeding or stop drug.
• Caution patient not to donate blood or sperm during therapy.

thioguanine
Tabloid

Classification: Antineoplastic, antimetabolite
Pregnancy risk category D

Pharmacology
Thioguanine has multiple metabolic effects. Tumor inhibitory properties may stem from its effects on feedback inhibition of de novo purine synthesis, inhibition of purine nucleotide interconversions, or incorporation into DNA and RNA. Net effect of actions is sequential blockade of synthesis and utilization of purine nucleotides.

Pharmacokinetics
Drug is absorbed slowly and modestly when taken orally. It is metabolized almost completely in liver and peaks in approximately 8 hours. Elimination half-life is approximately 80 minutes (range is 25 to 240 minutes). Metabolites are excreted in urine.

How supplied
Tablets: 40 mg

Indications and dosages

> **FDA-APPROVED**

➡ Acute nonlymphocytic leukemia
Adults and children age 3 and older: 2 mg/kg P.O. daily; if no clinical improvement occurs

after 4 weeks, increase dosage slowly to 3 mg/kg daily.

Off-label uses (selected)

➡ Chronic myelogenous leukemia (CML)
Adults: Although thioguanine is one of several drugs with activity in treatment of chronic phase of CML, more objective responses occur with busulfan. Therefore, busulfan usually is considered the preferred drug. Thioguanine dosage is 100 mg/m² P.O. every 12 hours on days 1 through 5, given in combination with cytarabine and daunorubicin.

Dosage modifications

• When drug is given for acute nonlymphocytic leukemia, total daily dosage may be rounded to nearest 20 mg and given at one time.
• Unlike mercaptopurine and azathioprine, thioguanine dosage does not depend on whether patient is receiving allopurinol.
• Dosage may need to be reduced when drug is combined with other agents whose primary toxicity is myelosuppression.
• Because drug may have delayed effect, it should be discontinued temporarily at first sign of abnormally steep fall in any formed blood element.
• Decision to increase, decrease, continue, or discontinue a given dosage must be based not only on absolute hematologic values but also on how fast these values are changing.

⊠ WARNINGS

• Thioguanine is a potent drug and should not be used unless diagnosis of acute nonlymphocytic leukemia has been adequately established and responsible physician knows how to assess patient's response to chemotherapy.

Contraindications and precautions

Contraindicated in previous drug resistance.
Use cautiously in bone marrow depression (WBC count below 2,500/mm³, platelet count below 100,000/mm³, and anemia), inherited deficiency of thiopurine methyltransferase (TPMT), radiation therapy, concomitant use of bone marrow depressants or aminosalicylate derivatives, pregnancy, and *elderly patients.*

Preparation and administration

• Follow hazardous drug guidelines for handling, preparation, and administration. (See "Managing hazardous drugs," page 11.)
• Only physicians experienced with drug's risks and knowledgeable in natural history of acute nonlymphocytic leukemias should administer drug.
• Effective tolerated dosage varies with stage and type of patient's neoplastic process.
• Store between 59° and 77° F (15° and 25° C) in dry place.

Adverse reactions

CNS: unsteady gait
GI: ulceration, nausea, vomiting, anorexia, diarrhea, appetite loss
GU: uric acid nephropathy
Hematologic: thrombocytopenia, leukopenia, granulocytopenia, bone marrow depression
Hepatic: hepatotoxicity, hepatic fibrosis, toxic hepatitis, hepatic veno-occlusive disease
Metabolic: hyperuricemia
Skin: rash, itching
Other: immunosuppression, infection

Interactions

Drug-drug. *Blood dyscrasia–causing drugs:* increased leukopenia or thrombocytopenia
Bone marrow depressants: increased bone marrow depression
Mesalamine, olsalazine, sulfasalazine: TPMT inhibition, causing exacerbated bone marrow depression
Drug-diagnostic tests. *Liver function tests:* abnormal
Platelets, WBCs: decreased
Serum and urinary uric acid: increased
Drug-herb. *Alpha-lipoic acid, coenzyme Q10, glucosamine, glutamine:* possible decreased chemotherapy efficacy

Only common or life-threatening adverse reactions are listed.

Toxicity and overdose

• Some signs and symptoms of overdose (such as nausea, vomiting, malaise, hypotension, and diaphoresis) may be immediate. Others (such as myelosuppression and azotemia) may be delayed. Most consistent dose-related toxicity is bone marrow depression, which manifests as anemia, leukopenia, thrombocytopenia, or any combination. (Any of these findings also may reflect underlying disease progression.) Overdose symptoms may occur after a single dose of as little as 2 to 3 mg/kg. Up to 35 mg/kg has been given as a single oral dose and has caused reversible myelosuppression.

• No known antagonist exists. Because drug may have delayed effect, therapy must be interrupted at first sign of abnormally steep fall in any formed element of blood. Drug rapidly metabolizes to active intracellular derivatives with long persistence; therefore, hemodialysis does not appreciably reduce toxicity. Severe hematologic toxicity may necessitate supportive therapy with platelet transfusions to treat bleeding and granulocyte transfusions and antibiotics if sepsis occurs. Inducing emesis may be helpful in patients seen immediately after accidental overdose.

Special considerations

• Monitor hemoglobin, hematocrit, WBC and differential counts, and quantitative platelet counts frequently during therapy. If cause of fluctuation in formed elements of peripheral blood is obscure, bone marrow examination may be useful to evaluate marrow status. In many cases (especially during induction phase for acute leukemia), CBCs must be obtained more frequently to evaluate effect of therapy. For remission induction to succeed, myelosuppression may be unavoidable during induction phase of adult acute nonlymphocytic leukemia. Whether this warrants dosage modification or therapy cessation depends on response of underlying disease and careful consideration of supportive treatment (such as platelet transfusions). Thioguanine-induced granulocytopenia and thrombocytopenia may cause life-threatening infection and bleeding.

• Monitor liver function studies weekly when therapy begins and monthly thereafter. Deteriorating liver function warrants drug withdrawal and further exploration of cause of hepatotoxicity.

• Drug plasma level monitoring has questionable value. Drug rapidly enters into anabolic and catabolic pathways for purines, and active intracellular metabolites have longer half-lives than parent drug. Biochemical effects of single dose appear long after parent drug has disappeared from plasma.

Patient education

• Inform patient about signs and symptoms of myelosuppression, hepatotoxicity, and GI toxicity.

• Instruct patient to immediately report fever, sore throat, local infection, bleeding from any site, yellowing of skin or eyes, nausea, and vomiting.

• Caution female patient to avoid pregnancy during therapy.

• Provide guidance to help breastfeeding patient decide whether to discontinue breastfeeding or stop drug.

thiotepa

Classification: Antineoplastic, alkylating agent
Pregnancy risk category D

Pharmacology

Thiotepa, a polyfunctional cytotoxic drug, is related chemically and pharmacologically to nitrogen mustard. Its radiomimetic action may occur through release of ethylenimine radicals that disrupt DNA bonds. A principal bond disruption is initiated by guanine alkylation at N7 position, which severs linkage between purine base and sugar and liberates alkylated guanines.

Pharmacokinetics

Drug is bioavailable by parenteral route only and is metabolized extensively in liver. Elimination half-life is 2 to 3 hours. Metabolites are excreted in urine.

How supplied

Solution for injection: 15 mg

Indications and dosages

FDA-APPROVED

➥ Adenocarcinoma of breast or ovary, Hodgkin's lymphoma, other lymphomas
Adults: 0.3 to 0.4 mg/kg by rapid I.V. administration at 1- to 4-week intervals
➥ Intracavitary effusion secondary to diffuse or localized neoplastic disease
Adults: 0.6 to 0.8 mg/kg intracavitary (usually a one-time infusion)
➥ Superficial papillary urinary bladder carcinoma
Adults: 60 mg in 60 ml sodium chloride injection (normal saline solution) instilled in bladder by catheter and retained for 2 hours, once weekly for 4 weeks; repeated monthly if necessary

OFF-LABEL USES (SELECTED)

➥ Autologous bone marrow transplantation
Adults: In combination with other drugs as part of cytoreductive conditioning regimen before bone marrow transplantation (BMT), 500 mg/m² I.V.; or as single agent, 1,125 mg/m² I.V. (maximum tolerated dosage)
Children: In combination with other drug as part of cytoreductive conditioning regimen before BMT, 300 mg /m² I.V. daily for 3 days (total dose, 900 mg/m²)
➥ Carcinomatous meningitis
Adults: 1 to 10 mg/m² intrathecally once or twice weekly

DOSAGE MODIFICATIONS

• If patient with papillary bladder carcinoma cannot retain 60 ml for 2 hours, dose may be given in volume of 30 ml.

• Initially, administer higher dosage in given range. Adjust maintenance dosage weekly based on pretreatment control blood counts and subsequent blood counts.
• Lower dosage is recommended if benefits outweigh risks in patients with hepatic, renal, or bone marrow damage. Discontinue therapy if WBC count falls to 3,000/mm³ or lower or platelet count falls to 150,000/mm³.
• Elderly patients may require lower dosages.

Contraindications and precautions

Contraindicated in hypersensitivity to drug.

Use cautiously in hepatic or renal disorders, myelosuppression, intravesical administration, pregnancy or breastfeeding, and *elderly patients.* Safety and efficacy in *children* have not been established; however, drug is used in children before autologous BMT.

Preparation and administration

⟫ Follow hazardous drug guidelines for handling, preparation, and administration. (See "Managing hazardous drugs," page 11.)
• Do not give drug orally because absorption from GI tract varies.
• Dosage must be individualized carefully. Slow response to drug does not necessarily signify lack of effect; therefore, increasing dosing frequency may only increase toxicity risk. After maximum benefit occurs with initial therapy, continue patient on maintenance therapy (at 1- to 4-week intervals). To continue optimal effect, do not give maintenance doses more often than weekly to preserve correlation between dose and blood counts.
• For I.V. use, reconstitute each 15 mg with 1.5 ml sterile water for injection to yield 10 mg/ml. Shake gently and allow to stand until clear.
• In papillary bladder carcinoma, dehydrate patient for 8 to 12 hours before treatment. Instill diluted drug into bladder by catheter. For maximum effect, patient should retain intravesical solution for 2 hours. If desired, patient may be repositioned every 15 minutes for maximum area contact. Give second and third

---

Only common or life-threatening adverse reactions are listed.

courses with caution due to increased risk of bone marrow depression. After intravesical administration, deaths have occurred from bone marrow depression caused by systemic drug absorption.

• Reconstituted solution is hypotonic; dilute further with normal saline solution before I.V. use. When solution is reconstituted with sterile water for injection, store in refrigerator and use within 8 hours. If reconstituted solution has been further diluted with normal saline solution, use immediately.

• To eliminate haze, filter solution through 0.22-micron filter before administration. (Filtering does not alter solution potency.) Reconstituted solution should be clear. Do not use solution that is opaque or precipitates after filtration.

• Administer at a rate of 60 mg (or fraction thereof) by I.V. injection over 1 minute.

• Store in refrigerator between 36° and 46° F (2° and 8° C). Protect from light.

Adverse reactions

CNS: confusion and somnolence (high doses), dizziness, headache, fatigue, weakness
EENT: conjunctivitis, blurred vision
GI: nausea, vomiting, abdominal pain, anorexia, mucositis
GU: cystitis (intravesical use), dysuria, urinary retention
Hematologic: myelosuppression
Respiratory: prolonged apnea (with preoperative succinylcholine administration after combined use of thiotepa and other anticancer agents)
Skin: contact dermatitis, dermatitis, alopecia
Other:. secondary malignancies and myelodysplastic syndrome (with long-term intravesical use), pain at injection site

Interactions

Drug-drug. *Cyclophosphamide, nitrogen mustard:* additive toxicity
Drug-diagnostic tests. *Blood-forming elements:* decreased
Liver function tests: increased

Drug-herb. *Alpha-lipoic acid, coenzyme Q10, glucosamine, glutamine:* possible decreased chemotherapy efficacy

Toxicity and overdose

• Hematopoietic toxicity may follow overdose and manifests as decreased WBC or platelet count. (RBC count is less accurate indicator of toxicity.) Bleeding may occur. Patient may become more vulnerable to infection and less able to combat infection. Dosages within and minimally above recommended therapeutic dosages have been associated with potentially life-threatening hematopoietic toxicity. Drug has toxic, dose-related effect on hematopoietic system.

• No known antidote exists. Drug is dialyzable. Transfusions of whole blood or platelets have proven beneficial against hematopoietic toxicity.

Special considerations

• Obtain weekly WBC with differential and platelet counts during therapy and for at least 3 weeks afterward.

• Carefully monitor patients with hepatic or renal impairment.

Patient education

• Instruct patient not to drink fluids for 8 to 12 hours before each bladder instillation.

• Encourage patient to retain dose in bladder for 2 hours and to change position every 15 minutes to ensure maximum area contact.

• Advise patient to inform prescriber of signs or symptoms of bleeding (such as epistaxis, easy bruising, change in urine color, or black stool) or infection (including fever and chills).

• Caution patients with childbearing potential or partners of such patients to use effective contraception during therapy. If patient uses drug during pregnancy or becomes pregnant during therapy, inform her and her partner of potential hazard to fetus.

• Provide guidance to help breastfeeding patient decide whether to discontinue breastfeeding or stop drug.

T

topotecan hydrochloride
Hycamtin

Classification: Antineoplastic, topoisomerase inhibitor
Pregnancy risk category D

Pharmacology
Topotecan binds to topoisomerase I–DNA complex and prevents religation of single-strand breaks. (Topoisomerase I relieves torsional strain in DNA by inducing reversible single-strand breaks.) Cytotoxicity may relate to double-strand DNA damage produced during DNA synthesis, when replication enzymes interact with ternary complex formed by topotecan, topoisomerase I, and DNA.

Pharmacokinetics
Drug is not extensively metabolized after I.V. administration. Elimination half-life is approximately 2 to 3 hours. Significant portion is excreted unchanged in urine.

How supplied
Powder for injection: 4 mg in single-dose vial

Indications and dosages

➡ Metastatic ovarian carcinoma and small-cell lung cancer after chemotherapy failure
Adults: 1.5 mg/m^2 I.V. infusion given over 30 minutes for 5 consecutive days, starting on day 1 of 21-day course and given for at least four courses unless tumor progresses; reduced by 0.25 mg/m^2 for subsequent courses if severe neutropenia occurs or if platelet count falls below 25,000/mm^3

➡ Non-small-cell lung cancer (evidence rating IIIA)
Adults: Various dosage schedules include topotecan 1 mg/m^2 I.V. for 5 consecutive days every 21 or 28 days.
➡ Myelodysplastic syndrome (evidence rating II/IIID)
Adults: Various dosage schedules include topotecan 1.25 mg/m^2 I.V. over 30 minutes daily for 5 days every 3 weeks, given alone or in combination regimens containing topotecan, thalidomide, and cytarabine; topotecan and amifostine; or both regimens.
➡ Chronic myelomonocytic leukemia (evidence rating IIID)
Adults: Various dosages given alone or in combination with cytarabine

DOSAGE MODIFICATIONS

• Drug is not recommended as first-line therapy for non-small-cell lung cancer (evidence rating IIIA), but may be considered for later use in management of this disease.
• Dosage adjustment to 0.75 mg/m^2 is recommended for patients with moderate renal impairment (creatinine clearance of 20 to 39 ml/minute).
• Patients should not receive subsequent courses until neutrophil count recovers to above 1,000/mm^3, platelet count to above 100,000/mm^3, and hemoglobin to or above 9 g/dl (with transfusion if necessary).
• Drug is likely to cause greater myelosuppression when given with other cytotoxic agents, necessitating dosage reduction.

⊠ WARNINGS

• Drug should be given under supervision of physician experienced in use of chemotherapeutic agents. Complications can be managed appropriately only when adequate diagnostic and treatment facilities are readily available.
• Drug should not be given when baseline neutrophil count is below 1,500/mm^3. To monitor for bone marrow depression (primarily neutropenia, which may be severe and result in infection and death), obtain frequent peripheral blood cell counts for all patients.

Only common or life-threatening adverse reactions are listed.

Contraindications and precautions

Contraindicated in hypersensitivity to drug or its components, severe bone marrow depression, and pregnancy or breastfeeding.

Use cautiously in bone marrow depression, impaired renal function, and **elderly patients.** Safety and efficacy in **children** have not been established.

Preparation and administration

• Follow hazardous drug guidelines for handling, preparation, and administration. (See "Managing hazardous drugs," page 11.)
• Before first course, patients must have baseline neutrophil count above 1,500/mm^3 and platelet count above 100,000/mm^3.
• Reconstitute each 4-mg vial with 4 ml sterile water for injection. Then dilute appropriate volume of reconstituted solution in normal saline solution for I.V. infusion or 5% dextrose for I.V. infusion.
• Lyophilized form contains no antibacterial preservative; reconstituted product should be used immediately.
• If granulocyte colony-stimulating factor (G-CSF) is used, administer it 24 hours after topotecan administration ends. For instance, start G-CSF on day 6 of 21-day cycle.
• Extravasation has been associated with mild erythema and bruising.
• Store in original carton at controlled temperature of 68° to 77° F (20° to 25° C). Protect from light.

Adverse reactions

CNS: asthenia, headache, pain, paresthesia
GI: abdominal pain, constipation, diarrhea, obstruction, nausea, stomatitis, vomiting, anorexia
Hematologic: anemia, neutropenia, leukopenia, thrombocytopenia
Musculoskeletal: arthralgia, myalgia
Respiratory: dyspnea, cough
Skin: total alopecia, rash
Other: sepsis

Interactions

Drug-drug. *Cisplatin:* increased myelosuppression
G-CSF: prolonged neutropenia duration
Drug-diagnostic tests. *Neutrophils, platelets, RBCs, WBCs:* decreased
Serum ALT, AST, bilirubin: increased
Drug-herb. *Alpha-lipoic acid, coenzyme Q10, glucosamine, glutamine:* possible decreased chemotherapy efficacy

Toxicity and overdose

• Primary anticipated complication of overdose is bone marrow depression.
• No known antidote exists. Provide supportive treatment and withhold topotecan until myelosuppression improves sufficiently. Neutropenia recovery may be aided by filgrastim or pegfilgrastim administration after day 6 and at least 24 hours after last topotecan dose. Patient also may require platelets and RBC or whole blood transfusions.

Special considerations

• Neutropenia is dose-limiting toxicity and is not cumulative over time. Monitor CBC with differential frequently.
• Monitor renal and hepatic function, especially in elderly patients.

Patient education

• Instruct patient to use caution when driving or performing other hazardous activities.
• Caution women with childbearing potential to avoid pregnancy during therapy because drug may harm fetus. Advise them to use effective contraception. If patient becomes pregnant during therapy, inform her of potential hazard to fetus.
• Caution breastfeeding patient to stop breastfeeding because drug may harm infant.

T

toremifene citrate
Fareston

Classification: Antineoplastic, antiestrogen, selective estrogen-receptor modulator, hormone/hormone modifier
Pregnancy risk category D

Pharmacology
Toremifene binds to estrogen receptors and may exert estrogenic or antiestrogenic activities, depending on treatment duration, patient gender, target organ, or endpoint selected. Antitumor effect in breast cancer may result primarily from drug's ability to compete with estrogen for binding sites in tumor, blocking growth-stimulating effects of estrogen. Drug decreases estradiol-induced vaginal cornification index in some postmenopausal women, reflecting antiestrogenic activity.

Pharmacokinetics
Drug has good oral bioavailability and is metabolized in liver to active metabolites, principally by CYP3A4 pathway. It is bound extensively to plasma proteins. Elimination half-life is approximately 5 days. Parent drug and metabolites are excreted mainly in feces, with about 10% excreted in urine.

How supplied
Tablets: 60 mg

Indications and dosages

FDA-APPROVED

➡ Metastatic breast cancer in postmenopausal women with estrogen-receptor positive or unknown tumors
Adults: 60 mg P.O. daily

DOSAGE MODIFICATIONS

• Because of drug's extensive hepatic transformation, dosage adjustments may be needed in

patients with hepatic impairment. However, no specific recommendations are available.

Contraindications and precautions
Contraindicated in hypersensitivity to drug.
    Use cautiously in hypercalcemia, tumor flare, hepatic impairment, endometrial hyperplasia, history of thromboembolic disease, and pregnancy or breastfeeding. No indication exists for use in *children*.

Preparation and administration
• Follow hazardous drug guidelines for handling, preparation, and administration. (See "Managing hazardous drugs," page 11.)
• Store at 77° F (25° C); excursions are permitted to 59° to 86° F (15° to 30° C). Protect from heat and light.

Adverse reactions
CNS: headache, light-headedness, dizziness, depression
CV: heart failure, myocardial infarction, chest pain
EENT: cataract, ocular lesion, retinopathy, corneal opacity, dry eyes, blurred vision (high doses)
GI: nausea, altered taste, anorexia
GU: vaginal discharge, pruritus vulvae, endometrial hyperplasia
Hematologic: thrombocytopenia, leukopenia
Metabolic: hypercalcemia
Respiratory: pulmonary embolism
Other: hot flashes; sweating; tumor flare (syndrome of diffuse musculoskeletal pain and erythema with increased tumor size that later regresses)

Interactions
Drug-drug. *CYP450 3A4 inducers (such as carbamazepine, phenobarbital, and phenytoin):* increased rate of toremifene metabolism
CYP450 3A4 inhibitors (such as erythromycin and ketoconazole): decreased rate of toremifene metabolism
Thiazide diuretics, other drugs that decrease renal

Only common or life-threatening adverse reactions are listed.

calcium excretion: increased risk of hypercalcemia

Warfarin: increased prothrombin time

Drug-diagnostic tests. *ALP, AST, bilirubin, calcium:* increased

Drug-food. *Grapefruit, pomegranate:* possible increased toremifene levels

Drug-herb. *Cat's claw, devil's claw, feverfew, garlic, ginkgo, goldenseal, kava, milk thistle, licorice, valerian:* possible increased toremifene levels

St. John's wort: possible decreased toremifene levels

Toxicity and overdose

• Theoretically, overdose may manifest as increased antiestrogenic effects (such as hot flashes), estrogenic effects (such as vaginal bleeding), or nervous system disorders (such as vertigo, dizziness, ataxia, and nausea).

• No specific antidote exists. Provide symptomatic treatment.

Special considerations

• Monitor CBC, calcium level, and liver function tests periodically.

• Tumor flare may occur in breast cancer patients with bone metastases during first weeks of therapy. This syndrome is often associated with hypercalcemia and does not imply therapeutic failure or tumor progression. In severe hypercalcemia, discontinue drug.

Patient education

• Instruct patient to contact prescriber if vaginal bleeding occurs.

• If patient has bone metastases, describe typical signs and symptoms of hypercalcemia and tell her to contact prescriber if these occur.

tositumomab and iodine ^{131}I tositumomab

Bexxar Dosimetric, Bexxar ^{131}I Dosimetric, Bexxar ^{131}I Therapeutic, Bexxar Therapeutic

Classification: Antineoplastic, monoclonal antibody

Pregnancy risk category X

Pharmacology

Tositumomab binds to CD20 antigen expressed on pre-B and mature B lymphocytes and in more than 90% of B-cell non-Hodgkin's lymphomas. Possible mechanisms of action include apoptosis induction, complement-dependent cytotoxicity, and antibody-dependent cellular cytotoxicity. Also, cell death is associated with ionizing radiation from radioisotope. Drug causes sustained reduction in circulating CD20+ cells.

Pharmacokinetics

Drug has median blood clearance of 68.2 mg/hour (with 485-mg dosage) in patients with non-Hodgkin's lymphoma. With high tumor burden, splenomegaly, or bone marrow involvement, clearance is faster, distribution volume is larger, and terminal half-life is shorter. Mean total-body effective half-life is 67 hours. ^{131}I is eliminated by decay and excretion in urine.

How supplied

Dosimetric package: Tositumomab—two single-use 225-mg vials (16.1 ml) and one single-use 35-mg vial (2.5 ml) at protein concentration of 14 mg/ml. ^{131}I tositumomab—single-use vial within lead pot; each vial contains no less than 20 ml iodine ^{131}I tositumomab at nominal protein and activity concentrations of 0.1 mg/ml and 0.61 mCi/ml (at calibration), respectively.

T

Therapeutic package: Tositumomab—two single-use 225-mg vials (16.1 ml) and one single-use 35-mg vial (2.5 ml) at protein concentration of 14 mg/ml. Iodine ^{131}I tositumomab—one or two single-use vials within lead pot; each vial contains no less than 20 ml ^{131}I tositumomab at nominal protein and activity concentrations of 1.1 mg/ml and 5.6 mCi/ml (at calibration), respectively.

Indications and dosages

FDA-APPROVED

➡ CD20+ follicular non-Hodgkin's lymphoma, with and without transformation, when disease is refractory to rituximab and has relapsed after chemotherapy
Adults: Bexxar therapeutic regimen has four components in two steps—dosimetric step, followed 7 to 14 days later by therapeutic step.
Dosimetric step: (1) Tositumomab 450 mg I.V. in 50 ml normal saline solution over 60 minutes. (2) Iodine ^{131}I tositumomab (containing 5.0 mCi ^{131}I and 35 mg tositumomab) I.V. in 30 ml normal saline solution over 20 minutes.
Therapeutic step: (Do not administer this step if biodistribution is altered. For assessment information regarding biodistribution, see manufacturer's prescribing information.)
(1) Tositumomab 450 mg I.V. in 50 ml normal saline solution over 60 minutes. (2) ^{131}I tositumomab: See manufacturer's prescribing information for calculating iodine ^{131}I activity.

DOSAGE MODIFICATIONS

• *Patients with infusion reactions:* Reduce infusion rate 50% for mild to moderate infusional toxicity; interrupt infusion for severe infusional toxicity. After toxicity resolves completely, resume infusion with rate reduced 50%.
• *Patients with platelet count of 150,000/mm³ or higher:* Recommended dosage is ^{131}I activity calculated to deliver 75 cGy total body irradiation and 35 mg tositumomab, given I.V. over 20 minutes.

• *Patients with NCI Grade 1 thrombocytopenia (platelet count above 100,000/mm³ but below 150,000/mm³):* Recommended dosage is ^{131}I activity calculated to deliver 65 cGy total body irradiation and 35 mg tositumomab, given I.V. over 20 minutes.

⊠ WARNINGS

• Keep appropriate drugs available for immediate use in case severe hypersensitivity reaction occurs.
• Most patients who receive Bexxar therapeutic regimen experienced severe thrombocytopenia and neutropenia. Regimen should not be given to patients with more than 25% lymphoma marrow involvement and/or impaired bone marrow reserve.
• Bexxar therapeutic regimen can cause fetal harm when given to pregnant patients.
• Bexxar therapeutic regimen contains a radioactive component and should be administered only by physicians and other health care professionals qualified by training in safe use and handling of therapeutic radionuclides. Drug should be given only by physicians who are certified (or in process of being certified) by GlaxoSmithKline in dosage calculation and administration of Bexxar therapeutic regimen.

Contraindications and precautions

Contraindicated in hypersensitivity to murine proteins or other components of Bexxar therapeutic regimen, patients unable to tolerate thyroid-blocking agents, women with childbearing potential, and pregnancy.
Use cautiously in handling radioactive material and in cytopenia or impaired renal function; breastfeeding; and *elderly patients.* Safety and efficacy in *children* have not been established.

Preparation and administration

• Follow hazardous drug guidelines for handling, preparation, and administration. (See "Managing hazardous drugs," page 11.)

Note: Specific guidelines exist for preparation and administration of Bexxar therapeutic regimen. See manufacturer's prescribing information for more guidelines on qualifications to administer, radiation precautions, preparation, and dose calibrations. Regimen components are shipped only to individuals who are participating in certification program or have been certified in preparation and administration of Bexxar therapeutic regimen. Components are shipped separately. When ordering, make sure components are scheduled to arrive on same day.

• Obtain CBC with differential and platelet count before administering Bexxar therapeutic regimen.

• Administer Bexxar therapeutic regimen through I.V. tubing set with inline 0.22-micron filter.

• Use same I.V. tubing set and filter during entire dosimetric or therapeutic step. Filter change could cause drug loss.

• Patients should not receive dosimetric dose unless they have received the following medications:

(1) *Thyroid-protective agents:* Saturated solution of potassium iodide (SSKI) 4 drops P.O. three times daily; Lugol's solution 20 drops P.O. three times daily; or potassium iodide tablets 130 mg P.O. daily. Initiate therapy at least 24 hours before iodine ^{131}I tositumomab dosimetric dose and continue until 2 weeks after therapeutic dose.

(2) *Acetaminophen* 650 mg P.O. and (3) *diphenhydramine* 50 mg P.O. 30 minutes before tositumomab in dosimetric and therapeutic steps.

Iodine ^{131}I tositumomab

• Store drug frozen in original lead pot in freezer at −36° F (−20° C) or below until removal for thawing before administration. Do not use beyond expiration date on lead pot label.

• Thawed dosimetric and therapeutic doses are stable for up to 8 hours at 36° to 46° F (2° to 8° C). Solutions diluted for infusion contain no preservatives. Store refrigerated at 36°

to 46° F before use; do not freeze. Discard unused portion according to federal and state laws.

Tositumomab

• Store vials (35 and 225 mg) refrigerated at 36° to 46° F (2° to 8° C) before dilution. Do not use beyond expiration date. Discard unused portions left in vial. Do not shake or freeze.

• Solutions of diluted tositumomab are stable for up to 24 hours when refrigerated at 36° to 46° F (2° to 8° C) and for up to 8 hours at room temperature. Refrigerate diluted solution at 36° to 46° F before use (it lacks preservatives); do not freeze. Protect from strong light. Discard unused portion.

Adverse reactions

CNS: asthenia, headache
CV: hypotension
EENT: rhinitis, pharyngitis
GI: nausea, vomiting, abdominal pain, diarrhea, decreased appetite
Hematologic: thrombocytopenia, neutropenia, anemia
Metabolic: hypothyroidism
Respiratory: cough, dyspnea, pleural effusion, pneumonia
Skin: herpes
Other: sepsis, flulike symptoms, hypersensitivity reactions including anaphylaxis, secondary malignancies, shivering, antibody development, dehydration

Interactions

Drug-diagnostic tests. *Platelets, RBCs, thyroid-stimulating hormone (TSH), WBC count with differential:* altered
Tests using murine antibody technology: possible alterations, if human anti-mouse antibodies immune response develops

Toxicity and overdose

• Overdose has caused Grade 3 hematologic toxicity.

• In accidental overdose, monitor patient closely for cytopenias and radiation-related toxicity. Efficacy of hematopoietic stem-cell transplantation as supportive care measure for marrow injury has not been studied.

Special considerations

• Safety of Bexxar therapeutic regimen was established only in patients receiving thyroid-blocking agents and premedication to reduce or prevent infusion reactions. After therapy, screen for biochemical evidence of hypothyroidism annually. Evaluate patient for hypothyroidism symptoms.

• Safety of Bexxar therapeutic regimen has not been established in patients with more than 25% lymphoma marrow involvement, platelet count below 100,000/mm^3, or neutrophil count below 1,500/mm^3.

• Continue weekly monitoring of CBC with differential for at least 10 weeks after Bexxar therapeutic regimen (or until persistent cytopenias resolve completely). Patients with evidence of moderate or more severe cytopenias require more frequent monitoring.

• [131]I is excreted primarily by kidney. Impaired renal function may decrease ^{131}I excretion rate and increase patient exposure to radioactive component. No data exist on safety of Bexxar therapeutic regimen in patients with impaired renal function.

Patient education

• Before administering Bexxar therapeutic regimen, advise patient that radioactive material will remain in body for several days after discharge. Provide oral and written instructions for minimizing exposure of family, friends, and general public.

• Inform patient of hypothyroidism risk; stress importance of complying with thyroid-blocking therapy and need for life-long thyroid monitoring.

• Explain risks of cytopenias and associated symptoms, need for frequent monitoring for up to 12 weeks after treatment, and risk of cytopenias lasting beyond 12 weeks.

• Inform patient of risk of secondary cancers.

• Caution women with childbearing potential to avoid pregnancy during therapy. If patient becomes pregnant while receiving Bexxar therapeutic regimen, inform her of potential risk to fetus.

• Caution breastfeeding patient to stop breast-feeding because drug may harm infant.

tramadol hydrochloride
Ultram

Classification: Opioid-like analgesic
Pregnancy risk category C

Pharmacology

Tramadol, a centrally acting synthetic analgesic, has an unclear mechanism of action. However, at least two complementary mechanisms seem applicable: binding of parent and M1 metabolite to µ-opioid receptors and weak inhibition of norepinephrine and serotonin reuptake. Opioid activity results from low-affinity binding of parent compound and higher-affinity binding of O-demethylated metabolite M1 to µ-opioid receptors. Drug inhibits norepinephrine and serotonin reuptake in vitro. These mechanisms may contribute independently to overall analgesic effects.

Pharmacokinetics

Drug is absorbed rapidly and almost completely, and undergoes extensive metabolism. It reaches steady state in 2 days. Approximately 30% is excreted in urine as unchanged drug.

How supplied

Tablets: 50 mg

Indications and dosages

OFF-LABEL USES (SELECTED)

➡ Cancer pain
Adults: Cancer patients usually respond to

---

dosages of 150 to 300 mg P.O. daily. Maximum recommended daily dosage is 400 mg.

Contraindications and precautions

Contraindicated in hypersensitivity to drug or its components, acute alcohol intoxication, or when opioids are contraindicated (such as in acute intoxication with alcohol, hypnotics, opioids, centrally acting analgesics, or psychotropic drugs).

Use cautiously in epilepsy; history of seizures; risk of seizures (as in head trauma, metabolic disorders, alcohol or drug withdrawal, or CNS infection); risk of respiratory depression; increased intracranial pressure; acute abdominal conditions; renal or hepatic disease; opioid dependency; concurrent use of CNS depressants, MAO inhibitors, SSRIs, or tricyclic antidepressants; pregnancy or breast-feeding; and *elderly patients.* Safety and efficacy in *children younger than age 16* have not been established.

Preparation and administration

• Anaphylactoid reactions may follow first dose. Be prepared to treat appropriately.
• Withdrawal symptoms may occur with abrupt discontinuation.
• Store in tightly closed container at controlled temperature up to 77° F (25° C).

Adverse reactions

CNS: dizziness, CNS stimulation, somnolence, sleep disorder, headache, nervousness, anxiety, confusion, euphoria, coordination disturbance, seizures, hallucinations
CV: vasodilation
EENT: visual disturbances
GI: nausea, constipation, vomiting, dry mouth, diarrhea, abdominal pain, anorexia, flatulence
GU: urinary retention, urinary frequency, menopausal symptoms
Skin: rash, itching, urticaria, vesicles
Other: angioedema, allergic reactions including anaphylactoid reactions

Interactions

Drug-drug. *Carbamazepine:* decreased tramadol level
MAO inhibitors: inhibited norepinephrine and serotonin reuptake
MAO inhibitors, neuroleptics, opioids, other drugs that reduce seizure threshold, SSRI antidepressants or anorectics, tricyclic antidepressants and other tricyclic compounds (such as cyclobenzaprine, promethazine): increased seizure risk
Opioids, sedative-hypnotics: increased CNS depression
Quinidine: increased tramadol level
Drug-diagnostic tests. *Creatinine, hepatic enzymes:* increased
Hemoglobin: decreased
Drug-food. *Grapefruit, pomegranate:* possible increased tramadol levels
Drug-herb. *Aloe, cascara, rhubarb:* possible decreased tramadol absorption due to reduced GI transit time
Cat's claw, devil's claw, feverfew, garlic, ginkgo, goldenseal, kava, licorice, milk thistle, valerian: possible increased tramadol levels
Chamomile, hops, kava, skullcap, valerian: increased CNS depression
L-tryptophan, St. John's wort, SAM-e: possible additive serotonin effects and increased risk of serotonin syndrome

Toxicity and overdose

• Potential consequences of overdose include respiratory depression and seizures. Estimates of ingested dosage in deaths have ranged from 3 to 5 g.
• In overdose, maintain adequate ventilation and provide general supportive treatment. Naloxone can reverse some, but not all, overdose symptoms, but also increases risk of seizures. Hemodialysis is not helpful, removing less than 7% of dose over 4-hour dialysis period.

Special considerations

• Monitor patient for anaphylactoid reaction and seizures.

Patient education

• Inform patient of signs and symptoms of allergic reactions to drug.

• Caution patient not to stop drug abruptly after high-dose or long-term use because withdrawal symptoms could occur.

• Advise patient not to take drug with alcoholic beverages, tranquilizers, sedative-hypnotics, or other opioids.

• Inform patient that drug may impair ability to drive or perform other hazardous activities.

• Instruct female patient to tell prescriber if she is pregnant, thinks she might be pregnant, or is trying to become pregnant.

trastuzumab
Herceptin

Classification: Antineoplastic, recombinant DNA-derived monoclonal antibody
Pregnancy risk category B

Pharmacology

Herceptin selectively binds with high affinity in cell-based assay to extracellular domain of human epidermal growth factor receptor 2 protein (HER2). It inhibits cancer cell proliferation.

Pharmacokinetics

Drug binds strongly to cells that overexpress HER2/neu molecules. Distribution outside vascular compartment is minimal. Half-life is probably very short. Drug is minimally cleared by kidney and liver.

How supplied

Powder for injection: 440 mg in multidose vial

Indications and dosages

FDA-APPROVED

Metastatic breast cancer in patients with tumors that overexpress HER2 and who have received one or more chemotherapy regimens; in combination with paclitaxel for treatment of patients with metastatic breast cancer whose tumors overexpress HER2 and who have not received chemotherapy for metastatic disease
Adults: As single agent and in combination therapy, trastuzumab 4 mg/kg I.V. infusion over 90 minutes, followed by 2 mg/kg I.V. infusion over 30 minutes once weekly as maintenance; in combination therapy, paclitaxel dosage is 175 mg/m² I.V. over 3 hours every 21 days for at least six cycles.

OFF-LABEL USES (SELECTED)

➡ Metastatic breast cancer in patients with tumors that overexpress HER2 and who have received one or more chemotherapy regimens
Adults: May be given as single agent or in combination; 8 mg/kg I.V. infusion over 90 minutes, followed by 6 mg/kg I.V. over 90 minutes every 3 weeks

➡ Adjuvant treatment in patients with surgically removed HER2-positive breast cancer
Adults: Typical regimens include trastuzumab 4 mg/kg I.V. infusion, followed by 2 mg/kg I.V. infusion for 51 weeks in combination with paclitaxel 175 mg/m² every 3 weeks for four cycles; or trastuzumab 4 mg/kg I.V. infusion, followed by 2 mg/kg I.V. infusion for 51 weeks in combination with paclitaxel 80 mg/m² I.V. weekly for 12 weeks after four cycles of doxorubicin and cyclophosphamide.

⊠ WARNINGS

• Drug can cause ventricular dysfunction and heart failure. Left ventricular function should be evaluated in all patients before and during therapy. Strongly consider drug discontinuation in patients who develop clinically significant decrease in left ventricular function. Incidence and severity of cardiac dysfunction is particularly high in patients who receive drug in combination with anthracyclines and cyclophosphamide.

• Drug can cause severe hypersensitivity reactions (including anaphylaxis), infusion reac-

Level 1: Minimal emetic risk (less than 10% emesis frequency)

No routine emesis prophylaxis is required. If the patient experiences nausea and vomiting at any time up to 24 hours after the first chemotherapy dose, consider using the regimen recommended for low emetic risk.

Delayed-onset emesis

Delayed-onset emesis occurs after the first 24 hours of chemotherapy administration. Continue recommended antiemetic therapy for at least 4 days before adding a delayed-onset regimen, except in patients receiving palonosetron, which is given only on day 1 of therapy.

For patients receiving high-emetic-risk chemotherapy drugs, add one of the following to the regimen:
- dexamethasone 8 mg P.O. or I.V. daily or 4 mg P.O. or I.V. b.i.d.
- metoclopramide 20 to 40 mg P.O. every 6 hours and diphenhydramine 25 to 50 mg P.O. or I.V. every 4 to 6 hours as needed, plus dexamethasone 8 mg P.O. or I.V. daily or 4 mg P.O. or I.V. b.i.d.

In addition to either regimen above, add *one* of the following 5-HT$_3$ antagonists:
- dolasetron 100 mg P.O. daily or 1.8 mg/kg I.V. or 100 mg I.V.
- granisetron 1 to 2 mg P.O. daily or 1 mg P.O. b.i.d. or 0.01 mg/kg (maximum, 1 mg) I.V.
- ondansetron 8 mg P.O. twice daily, or 16 mg P.O. daily or 8 mg I.V.

For patients receiving cisplatin, dexamethasone with metoclopramide or a 5-HT$_3$ antagonist alone is recommended.

For patients receiving low- to intermediate-emetic-risk drugs, no regular antiemetic prophylaxis is recommended for delayed-onset emesis.

Breakthrough emesis

Breakthrough emesis occurs during the course of chemotherapy when an antiemetic regimen is not effective. If the patient has nausea and vomiting, add *one* of the following antiemetic regimens to the acute-onset regimen:
- dexamethasone 12 mg P.O. or I.V. daily (if not given previously)
- dolasetron 100 mg P.O. daily or 1.8 mg/kg I.V. or 100 mg I.V.
- granisetron 1 to 2 mg P.O. once daily or 1 mg P.O. twice daily or 0.01 mg/kg (maximum, 1 mg) I.V.
- haloperidol 1 to 2 mg P.O. every 4 to 6 hours or 1 to 3 mg I.V. every 4 to 6 hours
- lorazepam 0.5 to 2 mg P.O. every 4 to 6 hours
- metoclopramide 20 to 40 mg P.O. every 4 to 6 hours as needed or 1 to 2 mg/kg I.V. every 3 to 4 hours, plus diphenhydramine 25 to 50 mg P.O. or I.V. every 4 to 6 hours
- olanzapine 2.5 to 5 mg P.O. twice daily as needed
- ondansetron 8 mg P.O. or I.V. daily
- prochlorperazine 10 mg P.O. every 4 to 6 hours or 25 mg P.R. every 12 hours or spansules 15 mg P.O. every 8 to 12 hours
- promethazine 25 to 50 mg P.O. or P.R. every 6 hours as needed

Anticipatory emesis

Anticipatory emesis occurs before chemotherapy begins. Add *one* of the following single-agent antiemetic regimens, starting the night before chemotherapy:
- alprazolam 0.5 mg P.O. three times daily
- lorazepam 0.5 to 2 mg P.O., I.V., or sublingually every 6 hours

The ELSEVIER *Guide to*

ONCOLOGY DRUGS & REGIMENS

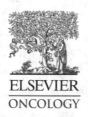

D0167588

ELSEVIER
ONCOLOGY

www.oncologydrugguide.com

ELSEVIER
ONCOLOGY

46 Green Street, 2nd floor
Huntington, NY 11743

PRESIDENT AND PUBLISHER: Anthony J. Cutrone

Production Director: Wendy McGullam

Editorial Manager: Gail M. VanKoot

Senior Editors: Randi Londer Gould, Conor Lynch

Design Director: Edwin S. Geffner

Director, Sales and Marketing: Joseph T. Schuldner

Group Sales Director: Timothy Wolfinger

National Sales Representative: David Horowitz

Sales Administrator: Devin Gregorie

PROJECT DIRECTED AND MANAGED BY
MEDVANTAGE PUBLISHING

Director: Patricia Dwyer Schull, RN, MSN

Clinical Manager: Minnie Bowen Rose, BSN, MEd

Editorial Manager: Karen C. Comerford

Design Manager: Stephanie Peters

Website Development Manager: Joseph J. Clark

Research Coordinator and Analyst: Lois Piano, RN, MSN, EdD

Clinical Editors: Julie M. Gerhart, MS, RPh; Cheryl A. Grandinetti, PharmD; Cynthia Saver, RN, MS

Editors: Naina Chohan, Kathy E. Goldberg, Andy McPhee, Doris Weinstock

Copy Editor: Denise Martini

Designers: Joseph J. Clark, Jan Greenberg

Editorial Assistant: Julia S. Knipe

Indexer: Karen C. Comerford

Cover Design: John Hubbard

Table of contents

Foreword   v
Advisors   vii
Contributors and reviewers   viii
Preface and user's guide   xi

Part 1

Chemotherapy principles and practice   3
Managing hazardous drugs   11

Part 2

Drugs A to Z   25

Part 3

Chemotherapy regimens and supportive therapy   369

Appendices
Appendix A: Common oncology abbreviations   459
Appendix B: Calculating body surface area   461
Appendix C: Chemotherapy admixture compatibilities   462
Appendix D: Normal laboratory values and calculations   466
Appendix E: Performance scales   469
Appendix F: Supportive therapy for cancer patients   470
Appendix G: Oncology drug codes   484
Appendix H: Oncology drugs in the pipeline   489
Appendix I: Online resources for oncology practitioners
        and patients   492

References   495
Index   517

www.oncologydrugguide.com

Foreword

JUST TWO DECADES AGO, the oncologist's arsenal of chemotherapy drugs contained just a handful of active antineoplastic agents. Few combination chemotherapy options existed, and even fewer supportive care drugs were available for disease management.

But recent research advances—and the pharmacotherapeutic innovations that evolved from them—have ushered in an extremely exciting era in medical oncology. Many new antineoplastic drugs have entered the arena—some of them streamlined to zero in on specific biological pathways or alter the behavior of the disease. What's more, entirely new drug categories have been introduced.

Some researchers are taking a pharmacogenomic approach to antineoplastic therapy, attempting to predict which patients might benefit (or suffer serious adverse effects) from specific therapies. Other current directions in cancer therapy include refinements in specific treatment programs and drug delivery methods, variations in the timing and dosing of antineoplastic drugs, and innovative combinations of chemotherapy strategies in both advanced and adjuvant settings. Future oncology research is sure to add even more new drugs and treatment strategies.

For many cancer patients, these advances have improved both survival and quality of life. For one thing, the newer agents tend to be more effective and gentler on normal cells compared to older cytotoxic drugs. Also, greater emphasis on supportive care has enabled cancer patients to better tolerate the short-term toxic effects of antineoplastic drugs. Thanks to supportive drugs, many patients can lead normal or near-normal lives even during periods of intensive therapy. Also, a growing number of cancer patients are receiving multiple therapeutic regimens—such as neoadjuvant, adjuvant, primary metastatic, and second-line therapy—during the course of illness.

With these important advances comes a corresponding need for oncology professionals to stay thoroughly up-to-date on the drugs, regimens, and supportive care agents used for a wide range of neoplastic diseases. In particular, questions about how to modify drug dosages for certain patient populations arise often among oncology practitioners. Dosage modification is especially critical for patients with preexisting comorbidities. In the past, for instance, many diabetics with mild renal insufficiency were ineligible for certain antineoplastic drugs or regimens. Today, thanks to a wealth of dosage modification data obtained largely from clinical trials, patients who would not have been candidates for potentially life-saving drugs even 10 years ago are now able to receive them.

How can busy oncology practitioners and nurses obtain current, reliable information on antineoplastic and supportive care drugs, including optimal dosages, schedules, combinations, toxicities, adverse effects, and interactions? To meet this challenge, Elsevier has created an exciting new multidimensional oncology drug information program. It provides the practical information needed to prescribe, dispense, or administer oncology drugs safely and effectively.

Elsevier developed this drug information program after conducting extensive research on the information needs of practicing oncology physicians and nurses. With the aid of an internationally recognized advisory board, an experienced development staff, and physicians, nurses, and cancer pharmacists with specialized knowledge, the publisher has created a unique, user-friendly system with integrated components. Each component is designed to suit a particular situation, time, and place.

- *The Elsevier Guide to Oncology Drugs & Regimens* provides complete coverage of more than 150 commonly used oncology drugs, including 40 supportive therapy drugs, more than 180 regimens related to 30 cancer-specific disease types, as well as guidelines for safe handling of hazardous drugs. It also offers additional supplementary information in the appendices. As the centerpiece of Elsevier's drug information program, this book is ideal for use in the office or clinic, at the bedside, or at home.

- The companion website, *www.oncologydrugguide.com*, offers many of the same outstanding features as the comprehensive reference—and more. It gives you instant access to oncology codes, new oncology drug news updates (including new FDA approvals, drug warnings, and indications), patient teaching aids to download and give to patients, and links to other relevant oncology sites.

- A PDA version includes all full monographs and regimens from the comprehensive reference, as well as other selected features. You can download it from the companion website or the Elsevier Oncology website.

- *The Elsevier Pocket Guide to Oncology Drugs & Regimens,* a condensed version of the comprehensive reference, fits in your lab pocket for maximum portability. It includes selected and abbreviated monographs, regimens, and features.

Today's challenges demand that oncology professionals have fast access to reliable and current drug information in virtually any setting. Elsevier's multidimensional oncology drug information program delivers this resource. Use it with the assurance that it will keep you current on every facet of the exciting and rapidly changing world of cancer drug therapy.

Maurie Markman, MD
Vice President for Clinical Research
MD Anderson Cancer Center
University of Texas
Houston

Advisors

Advisory board members

Martin Abeloff, MD
Professor & Chair
Department of Oncology
Director, Sidney Kimmel Comprehensive
    Cancer Center at Johns Hopkins
Baltimore, Md.

David Henry, MD
Vice Chairman, Department of Medicine
Clinical Professor of Medicine
Joan Karnell Cancer Center at Pennsylvania
    Hospital
Philadelphia, Pa.

William McGivney, PhD
Chief Executive Officer
National Comprehensive Center Network
Jenkintown, Pa.

Christine Miaskowski, RN, PhD, FAAN
Professor & Chair
Department of Physiological Nursing
University of San Francisco
San Francisco, Calif.

Steven Rosen, MD
Director
Robert H. Lurie Comprehensive Cancer
    Center of Northwestern University
Chicago, Ill.

Neal Slatkin, MD, DABPM
Director
Department of Supportive Care, Pain &
    Palliative Medicine
City of Hope National Medical Center
Duarte, Calif.

Foreword author

Maurie Markman, MD
Vice President for Clinical Research
MD Anderson Cancer Center
Univeristy of Texas
Houston

Contributors and reviewers

Helena Joy Altizer, RN, BSN, OCN
Kootenai Medical Center
North Idaho College
Coeur d'Alene, Idaho

Lisa M. Barbarotta, RN, MSN
Oncology RN
Hospital of St. Raphael's
New Haven, Conn.

Ronald H. Blum
Professor, Department of Medicine
Albert Einstein College of Medicine
Director, Cancer Center
Beth Israel Medical Center
New York, N.Y.

Joseph Bubalo, PharmD, BCPS, BCOP
Assistant Professor of Medicine
Oregon Health and Science University
   Hospital & Clinics
Portland, Ore.

Katherine L. Byar, MSN, APRN, BC
Hematological Malignancy Nurse Practitioner
University of Nebraska Medical Center
Omaha, Nebr.

Joanna E. Cain, RN, BSN
President
Auctorial Pursuits, Inc.
Wilmington, N.C.

Gregory T. Clark, BS, BCOP
Clinical Oncology Pharmacist
Rochester General Hospital
Rochester, N.Y.

Julene A. Diedrich, RN, APNP, OCN
Nurse Practioner, Oncology/Hematology
Marshfield Clinic
Marshfield, Wis.

Robert Dreicer, MD, FACP
Professor of Medicine
Cleveland Clinic Lerner College of Medicine
Director Genitourinary Medical Oncology
Taussig Cancer Center
Cleveland Clinic Foundation
Cleveland, Ohio

Matthew E. Eckley, PharmD
Clinical Pharmacy Specialist—Oncology
Huntsville Hospital
Huntsville, Ala.

Karen M. Fancher, PharmD, BCOP
Clinical Pharmacist
Blood & Marrow Transplantation
H. Lee Moffitt Cancer Center & Research
   Institute
Tampa, Fla.

Julie M. Gerhart, MS, RPh
Manager, Pharmacy Affairs
Merck & Co., Inc.
West Point, Pa.

Dawn Goetz, PharmD, BCOP
Clinical Pharmacist
Medical Oncology
H. Lee Moffitt Cancer Center & Research
   Institute
Tampa, Fla.

Janet Gordils-Perez, RN, MA, OCN, APN-C
Advance Practice Nurse
Cancer Institute of New Jersey
New Brunswick, N.J.

Cheryl A. Grandinetti, PharmD
Senior Clinical Research Pharmacist
Cancer Therapy Evaluation Program
Division of Cancer Treatment and Diagnosis
National Cancer Institute
Rockville, Md.

Myke Green, PharmD, BCOP
Clinical Oncology Pharmacist
H. Lee Moffitt Cancer Center and Research
Institute
Tampa, Fla.

Karen Groth, MSN, CNS, ARNP
Cancer Care Northwest
Spokane, Wash.

Heidi D. Gunderson, PharmD, BCOP
Hematology/Oncology Pharmacist
Mayo Clinic
Rochester, Minn.

David H. Henry, MD
Vice Chairman, Department of Medicine
Clinical Professor of Medicine
Joan Karnell Cancer Center at Pennsylvania
Hospital
Philadelphia, Pa.

John E. Loughner, PharmD, BCOP
Supervisor, Oncology Pharmacy
Strong Memorial Hospital
Rochester, N.Y.

Ellyn E. Matthews, RN, PhD, AOCN, CRNI
Assistant Professor
University of Colorado at Denver and Health
Sciences Center
Denver, Colo.

Mary Jane McDevitt, RN, BS
Case Manager
Home Care
Delaware County Memorial Hospital
Drexel Hill, PA

MaryJo Moran, RPh, BCOP
Clinical Pharmacist
Park Ridge Hospital
Rochester, N.Y.

Jose R. Murillo, Jr., BS, PharmD
Clinical Specialist II—Hematology/Oncology
The Methodist Hospital
Houston, Tex.

Cindy L. O'Bryant, PharmD, BCOP
Assistant Professor
University of Colorado at Denver and Health
Sciences Center
School of Pharmacy
Denver, Colo.

Christopher L. Olek, RPh, BCOP
Oncology Pharmacist
Strong Memorial Hospital
Rochester, N.Y.

**Joanna Maudlin Pangilinan, PharmD,
BCOP**
Pharmacist
University of Michigan Health System
and
Cascade Hemophilia Consortium
Ann Arbor, Mich.

Vivian Park, PharmD, BCOP
Clinical Coordinator
Division of Pharmacy Services
Memorial Sloan-Kettering Cancer Center
New York, N.Y.

Martha Polovich, RN, MN, AOCN
Oncology Clinical Nurse Specialist
Southern Regional Medical Center
Riverdale, Ga.

Martha Purrier, RN, MN, AOCN
Oncology Clinical Nurse Specialist
Manager Inpatient Oncology Unit
Virginia Mason Medical Center
Seattle, Wash.

Michele Riccardi, PharmD
Pharmacy Clinical Coordinator
Midstate Medical Center
Meriden, Conn.

Mujahid A. Rizvi, MD, MPH
Fellow, Division of Hematology/Oncology
Northwestern University
Chicago, Ill.

Cynthia Saver, RN, MS
President
CLS Development, Inc.
Columbia, Md.

Nancy Thompson, RN, MS, AOCNS
Clinical Nurse Specialist
Swedish Cancer Institute
Seattle, Wash.

John P. Timoney, PharmD, BCOP
Clinical Pharmacy Specialist
Memorial Sloan-Kettering Cancer Center
New York, N.Y.

Gene A. Wetzstein, PharmD, BCOP
Clinical Specialist, Hematology
H. Lee Moffitt Cancer Center and Research
    Institute
Tampa, Fla.

Robert C. Wolf, PharmD, BCPS, BCOP
Pharmacotherapy Coordinator—
    Hematology/Oncology
Assistant Professor
    Mayo Clinic College of Medicine
Mayo Clinic
Rochester, Minn.

Daisy Yang, PharmD, BCOP
Clinical Pharmacy Specialist
MD Anderson Cancer Center
University of Texas
Houston, Tex.

Preface and user's guide

OVER THE LAST 30 YEARS, we have witnessed substantial progress against cancer. Advances in biomedical knowledge continue to unravel the mysteries of cancer, enhancing our understanding of its causes and mechanisms. For some types of cancer, scientific advances have led to earlier detection and diagnosis and more effective treatments. For instance, using molecular progression models, researchers have identified many cancer markers, such as alpha fetoprotein, lactate hydrogenase, and beta-human chorionic gonadotropin. These markers now are used routinely to guide management decisions for testicular cancer patients.

In addition, newly identified molecular targets are transforming the way oncology drugs are developed. Today, rational drug combinations are used not only to treat cancer but also to cure some cancers that once proved uniformly fatal—such as leukemias, lymphomas, and testicular cancer. Such combinations also have helped to prevent relapse in patients with breast, ovarian, or colorectal cancer and to improve the quality of life in patients with pancreatic and prostate cancer.

In fact, we are beginning to achieve a major goal—a significant drop in the postoperative recurrence rate of common solid tumors. Over the past 5 years, survival rates for patients with breast and colorectal cancers have risen substantially, thanks largely to early diagnosis, new and more effective drugs, and refinements in treatment programs. Use of antiangiogenic and molecularly targeted drugs is likely to yield further postoperative decreases in the relapse rates of advanced breast and colorectal cancers.

Responding to practitioners' needs

As we move closer toward the ultimate goal of curing and eliminating cancer, oncology practitioners face the ever-escalating challenge of keeping up with the rapid pace of developments. Staying abreast of ongoing discoveries and advances is critical for professionals who prescribe or dispense oncology drugs or provide care for cancer patients. To keep your pharmacologic knowledge base up to date, you must have a ready source of current, accurate information.

The Elsevier Guide to Oncology Drugs & Regimens has been developed for just that purpose. Using clear, concise writing and a streamlined design, it provides accurate, comprehensive data on approximately 150 commonly used oncology drugs (including 40 supportive therapy drugs), and more than 180 cancer treatment regimens.

Many of this book's features evolved from research conducted with oncology professionals. Findings from this research revealed the need for an oncology drug resource with better coverage of such topics as new single- and combination-agent regimens, new indications, dosage modifications, off-label uses, administration guidelines, supportive care, management of adverse reactions, and patient education. To help ensure that this book satisfied these demands, a wide range of prominent oncology specialists were recruited. Their counsel informs this book.

How this book is organized

For optimal ease of use, this book is organized in three main sections.

Part 1: Essential general information

Part 1 addresses two subjects of overarching interest to health care professionals who prescribe, dispense, or administer oncology drugs.

• "Chemotherapy principles and practice" provides an overview of cancer chemotherapy It delineates the major oncology drug classifications, describes mechanisms of drug action, and summarizes patient management during cancer treatment.

• "Managing hazardous drugs" details the precautions to take when handling, preparing, or administering hazardous drugs. Based on safety recommendations from major organizations (such as the National Institute for Occupational Safety and Health), this section discusses such vital topics as potential adverse health effects of hazardous drugs; proper labeling, packaging, storage, transport, and disposal of hazardous drugs; personal protective equipment that must be used when handling hazardous drugs; and management of hazardous drug spills and accidental exposure.

Part 2: Drug monographs

Part 2 presents full monographs for the most important and most commonly used chemotherapy and supportive therapy drugs (including analgesics, antiemetics, and hematologic agents). Arranged alphabetically by generic drug name, these monographs present information in a consistent, easily accessible format. Within each monograph, information appears in the order shown below.

Generic name: Generic drug name(s) in the United States, along with salts and other variant names when applicable

Trade name (when applicable): All trade, or brand, names available in the United States

Classification: The drug's pharmacologic class, followed (when applicable) by its therapeutic class

Controlled substance schedule (when applicable): The schedule (I, II, III, IV, or V) assigned to the drug according to the Controlled Substances Act of 1970

Pregnancy risk category: The category (A, B, C, D, X, or NR [not applicable]) assigned to the drug by the Food and Drug Administration (FDA)

Pharmacology: Concise description of the drug's mechanism of action

Pharmacokinetics: Brief summary of the drug's known pharmacokinetic properties, in-

cluding absorption, metabolism, distribution, protein binding, onset of action, time to peak effect, duration of action, half-life, and excretion

How supplied: List of the drug's available forms, along with strengths of each form and, where applicable, details about its release properties (for instance, immediate-, extended-, sustained-, or delayed-release)

Indications and dosages: FDA-approved indications and dosages, followed (when applicable) by selected off-label uses and dosage modifications. Each indication is marked by a red arrow (➡) so you can find it quickly. Only those indications relevant to oncology or supportive care are listed. Where appropriate, adult and pediatric dosages are listed separately.

A special logo (☻) appears next to certain indications to denote orphan designation—a combination of a particular drug and indication that meets the criteria of the Orphan Drug Act. The orphan designation qualifies the product's sponsor for tax credits and marketing exclusivity incentives, as well as direct financial aid to assist in clinical development. (For details on the orphan designation, see http://www.fda.gov/orphan/.)

When applicable, a section on "Off-label uses (selected)" follows FDA-approved indications. Contributors were asked to include the most commonly used off-label uses and dosages prescribed in their practices. In some cases, specific dosages are not included because of variations in patient factors and prescriber preferences. Using drugs for off-label (unlabeled or unapproved) indications is common and acceptable; many off-label uses represent extensively studied, well-documented approaches. Off-label uses are especially common in oncology practice, where freedom in making drug-therapy decisions is critical and drugs approved for treating one type of cancer may subsequently prove to be effective against other cancers. For many off-label indications, a range of dosages and schedules have been used. Before selecting a specific dosage and dosage schedule for a patient, always consult the medical literature.

A note about off-label uses: The FDA does not regulate prescribing practices for legally marketed drugs. The *FDA Drug Bulletin* of April 1982 states that "The Food, Drug, and Cosmetic Act does not limit the manner in which a physician may use an approved drug. Once a product has been approved for marketing, a physician may prescribe it for uses or in treatment regimens or patient populations that are not included in approved labeling. Such 'unapproved' or, more precisely, 'unlabeled' uses may be appropriate and rational in certain circumstances and may, in fact, reflect approaches to drug therapy that have been extensively reported in medical literature." Similarly, the American Society of Health-System Pharmacists views off-label use as "the most appropriate therapy for patients" in many clinical situations—especially since the standards of practice for cancer chemotherapy and certain other drug therapies are dynamic and continually evolving.

The heading "Dosage modifications" appears at the end of the "Indications and dosages" section (where applicable). Here you will find specific instructions on adjusting dosages. Critically important for some patients, dosage modification may be necessitated by such factors as disease severity; patient's age, weight, or general clinical condition; emergence of certain adverse effects; renal, hepatic, or cardiovascular impairment; changes in blood counts in response to initial doses; hematologic, GI, neurologic, and other toxic reactions to preceding doses or other cancer therapies; concomitant drug therapies; or use of the drug in combination regimens or multiple-agent schedules. For easier interpretation, particularly complex dosage modifications are presented in table form.

Warnings (when applicable): "Black box" warnings summarized from the drug label

Contraindications and precautions: Circumstances in which the drug is contraindicated (for example, drug hypersensitivities,

coexisting diseases or disorders, or concomitant drug therapy), followed by a paragraph listing conditions that warrant cautious use of the drug. When a contraindication relates to elderly patients or children, these patient populations appear in bold italic type for quick identification.

Preparation and administration: Succinctly written guidelines to promote safe and effective use of the drug. Common topics include special handling instructions; recommended premedications (such as antiemetics); drug mixing, reconstitution, or preparation methods; appropriate I.V. solutions for dilution; proper infusion rates; appropriate I.M. or subcutaneous injection sites; optimal times of day to administer the drug; whether to give the drug with or without food; and drug storage recommendations.

If the drug poses a risk to health care workers who handle, prepare, or administer it, a warning to this effect appears at the beginning of the "Preparation and administration" section. When the drug is not only hazardous but potentially carcinogenic, a special icon (») accompanies the warning. (For more information on hazardous drugs, see "Managing hazardous drugs" in Part 1.)

Adverse reactions: Common and/or life-threatening adverse reactions to the drug. For quick reference, adverse reactions are organized by body system.

Interactions: Interactions with other drugs (either specific drugs or entire drug classes or categories), diagnostic tests, foods, and herbs. The name of the interacting drug, test, food, or herb appears in italics, followed by the effect of the interaction.

Toxicity and overdose: Clinical effects of overdose or toxicity, followed by appropriate treatment (such as an antidote or supportive therapy)

Special considerations: Key points related to evaluation, monitoring, and follow-up of patients who are receiving the drug (such as specific tests to monitor and expected time of onset of drug toxicities)

Patient education: Important instructions for patients who are receiving the drug, or for family members or other caregivers if the patient is a child or drug administration requires a caregiver's help. These instructions typically relate to the drug's proper use and storage and to measures the patient can take to prevent, minimize, or treat adverse reactions or drug interactions. When applicable, this section includes special instructions or precautions for patients with childbearing potential or for pregnant or breastfeeding patients who are receiving the drug.

Part 3: Chemotherapy regimens and supportive therapy

Part 3 presents a special section on chemotherapy regimens and protocols that covers the most commonly used single- and combination-agent oncology regimens, selected with guidance from oncology practitioners at major cancer centers. Presented alphabetically by cancer-specific disease type, regimens include specific dosages and dosing schedules, along with supporting references. Each regimen is accompanied by detailed information on the supportive therapy that the regimen may necessitate (such as to treat or minimize diarrhea, nausea and vomiting, anemia, or neutropenia).

Appendices and references

• Appendices address carefully chosen topics relevant to oncology practice. They include common oncology abbreviations, formulas for calculating body surface area, a four-page chemotherapy compatibility chart, laboratory test values, patient performance scales, codes used with the Healthcare Common Procedures Coding System, oncology drugs in the pipeline, and online oncology resources. An expanded appendix on supportive therapy describes assessment, treatment, and follow-up care for patients with nausea and vomiting, anemia, febrile neutropenia, diarrhea, and stomatitis.

• References include clinical studies for the off-label uses and dosages, selected regimens, and supportive therapies covered in this book, as well as references for other critical content.

Special features

Inside the front cover, a convenient quick-reference guide titled "Management of chemotherapy-induced nausea and vomiting" explains how to gauge the emetogenic potential of chemotherapy drugs and select the most appropriate treatment. It divides chemotherapy-induced nausea and vomiting (CINV) into the well-established categories of acute-onset, delayed-onset, breakthrough, and anticipatory emesis, and presents specific drugs and dosages for prevention and treatment. This guide is based on recommendations of the National Cancer Institute, National Comprehensive Cancer Network, American Society of Clinical Oncology, and other major organizations.

Despite new antiemetics and other management advances, CINV is perhaps the most dreaded chemotherapy side effect. When prolonged, it can cause dehydration, nutritional deficiencies, anorexia, esophageal tears, wound dehiscence, deterioration of physical and mental status, reduced functional ability, and a poor quality of life. What's worse, patients who experience CINV may refuse subsequent treatment for fear that CINV will recur. Yet for most patients, CINV can be prevented or well controlled—a goal that the author and publisher hope this handy guide will advance.

• The comprehensive index permits you to look up information in five ways—by generic drug name, trade drug name, indication, regimen, and disease type.

• The book's companion website, www.oncologydrugguide.com, features selected full-length drug monographs, regimens, and appendices from this book, plus patient teaching aids that can be downloaded, printed, and given to patients.

Acknowledgments

To all the oncology professionals who have served as advisors and contributors to this book—thank you for your invaluable contributions and guidance. Thanks also to Kevin Hurley, Executive Vice President of Elsevier Health Sciences; and Alan Imhoff, President, International Medical News Group/Elsevier, for their support and encouragement; and to Elizabeth Munn, Executive Director, Medical Practitioner Marketing and Laura Meiskey, Associate Marketing Manager, Medical Practitioner Marketing of Elsevier. Lastly, I would like to give special thanks to Patricia Dwyer Schull, RN, MSN, Director of MedVantage Publishing, and her staff for the countless hours they have spent steering this project from concept through development.

Elsevier Oncology is dedicated to advancing cancer care by providing up-to-date information and educational resources to health care professionals and patients in the fight against cancer. My hope is that *The Elsevier Guide to Oncology Drugs & Regimens* will serve as a valuable tool for practitioners who must make critical and, in some cases, life-or-death decisions regarding cancer treatment.

Anthony Cutrone
President and Publisher, Elsevier Oncology

tions, and pulmonary events. In most cases, symptoms occur during or within 24 hours of administration. Therapy should be interrupted in patients experiencing dyspnea or clinically significant hypotension; patients should be monitored until signs and symptoms resolve completely. Strongly consider drug discontinuation in patients who develop anaphylaxis, angioedema, or adult respiratory distress syndrome.

Contraindications and precautions

No known contraindications exist.

Use cautiously in known hypersensitivity to drug, Chinese hamster ovary cell proteins, or benzyl alcohol; leukopenia; anemia; pregnancy or breastfeeding; and *elderly patients*. Use with extreme caution in patients with cardiac disease. Safety and efficacy in *children* have not been established.

Preparation and administration

- Do not give I.V. push or bolus.
- Do not mix with other drugs or with dextrose solutions.
- Reconstitute each vial with 20 ml bacteriostatic water for injection, 1.1% benzyl alcohol preserved, as supplied, to yield multidose solution containing 21 mg/ml.
- Immediately after reconstitution, label vial in the area marked "Do not use after:" with date that is 28 days from reconstitution date.
- If patient has known hypersensitivity to benzyl alcohol, drug must be reconstituted with sterile water for injection; avoid other reconstitution diluents. Also, reconstituted drug must be used immediately, and any unused portion must be discarded.
- Gently invert bag to mix solution. Do not shake reconstituted drug. After reconstitution, preparation should be a transparent colorless to pale yellow solution.
- Observe patient for fever, chills, and other infusion-associated reactions. If severe reaction occurs, interrupt infusion and provide

supportive therapy, including oxygen, I.V. fluids, beta-agonists, and corticosteroids.
- No incompatibilities exist with polyvinylchloride or polyethylene bags.
- Store at 36° to 46° F (2° to 8° C).

Adverse reactions

CNS: pain, asthenia, headache, insomnia, dizziness, paresthesia, depression
CV: tachycardia, heart failure, cardiomyopathy, ventricular dysfunction
EENT: rhinitis, sinusitis, pharyngitis
GI: abdominal pain, nausea, vomiting, diarrhea, anorexia
GU: urinary tract infection
Hematologic: anemia, leukopenia, pancytopenia
Musculoskeletal: back pain, arthralgia, bone pain
Respiratory: increased cough, dyspnea
Skin: rash
Other: anaphylaxis, angioedema, fever, chills, flulike symptoms, infection, accidental injury, edema, peripheral edema, infusion reaction

Interactions

Drug-herb. *Alpha-lipoic acid, coenzyme Q10, glucosamine, glutamine:* possible decreased chemotherapy efficacy

Toxicity and overdose

- Single doses above 500 mg have not been tested. Anticipated signs and symptoms of toxicity are those of adverse reactions.
- Treatment is supportive and may include diuretics, inotropic agents, ACE inhibitors, beta-adrenergic blockers, isoproterenol, propranolol, and supplemental oxygen, as indicated.

Special considerations

- Severe infusion reaction typically occurs with initial infusion and generally arises during or immediately after infusion. However, onset and clinical course vary, so continue to monitor patient for such reactions throughout therapy.

T

• Beneficial drug effect is limited largely to patients with highest level of HER2 overexpression. Evaluation for HER2 overexpression should be performed by laboratory with demonstrated proficiency in specific technology used.

Patient education
• Caution patient to avoid hazardous tasks; drug may cause dizziness and confusion.
• Instruct patient to report rash and signs or symptoms of infection, including sore throat, fever, diarrhea, and vomiting.
• Advise breastfeeding patient to discontinue breastfeeding during therapy and for 6 months after last dose.

tretinoin, all-*trans* retinoic acid (ATRA)
Vesanoid

Classification: Antineoplastic, retinoid
Pregnancy risk category D

Pharmacology
Tretinoin induces cytodifferentiation and decreases proliferation of acute promyelocytic leukemia (APL) cells in culture and in vivo. In APL, treatment causes initial maturation of primitive promyelocytes derived from leukemic clone, followed by repopulation of bone marrow and peripheral blood by normal, polyclonal hematopoietic cells in patients achieving complete remission. Exact mechanism of action in APL is unknown.

Pharmacokinetics
Drug has good oral bioavailability. It induces its own metabolism in liver, leading to decreased levels with continued administration. (Increasing dosage to correct for this change does not enhance response.) Elimination half-life is approximately 0.5 to 2 hours. Parent compound undergoes no appreciable excretion.

How supplied
Capsules: 10 mg

Indications and dosages

FDA-APPROVED

➡ APL classified M3 by French-American-British system, characterized by presence of t(15:17) translocation and/or PML/RARα gene in patients who are refractory to or have relapsed from anthracycline chemotherapy or for whom anthracycline chemotherapy is contraindicated
Adults and children age 1 and older: 45 mg/m² P.O. daily in two evenly divided doses, discontinued after either 90 days or 30 days after complete remission occurs, whichever comes first

DOSAGE MODIFICATIONS

• Dosage reduction should be considered for children with serious or intolerable toxicity. However, efficacy and safety at dosages below 45 mg/m² daily have not been evaluated in this population.

WARNINGS

• Drug should be given under supervision of physician experienced in managing patients with acute leukemia and in facility with laboratory and supportive services sufficient to monitor drug tolerance and protect and maintain patient compromised by drug toxicity. Drug's possible benefit to patient must outweigh known adverse reactions.
• About 25% of APL patients treated with drug experience retinoic acid-APL (RA-APL) syndrome, marked by fever, dyspnea, weight gain, radiographic evidence of pulmonary infiltrates, and pleural or pericardial effusion.
• High-dose steroids (dexamethasone 10 mg I.V. every 12 hours for 3 days or until symptoms resolve) should be given at first suspi-

cion of RA-APL syndrome to reduce morbidity and mortality. Most patients do not require therapy termination during treatment of syndrome. Chemotherapy may be added to treatment for patients with WBC counts above 5×10^9/L or for rapid WBC increase with leukopenia at start of treatment to reduce risk of RA-APL syndrome. Full-dose chemotherapy (including an anthracycline, unless contraindicated) may be used on day 1 or 2 for patients with WBC counts above 5×10^9/L, or immediately for patients with WBC counts below 5×10^9/L, if WBC count reaches 6×10^9/L or more by day 5, 10×10^9/L or more by day 10, or 15×10^9/L or more by day 28.
• During tretinoin treatment, about 40% of patients develop rapidly evolving leukocytosis, which is associated with higher risk of life-threatening complications.
• Drug use during pregnancy carries high risk of severely deformed infant. If therapy is best available treatment for pregnant woman or woman with childbearing potential, ensure that patient has received full information and warnings of risk to fetus if she were to become pregnant and of risk of possible contraception failure. Also, patient must be instructed to use two reliable contraceptive methods simultaneously during therapy and for 1 month after discontinuation, and must acknowledge her understanding of need to use dual contraception (unless she chooses sexual abstinence).
• Within 1 week before therapy begins, patient should have serum or urine pregnancy test. When possible, therapy should be delayed until negative test result occurs. When delay is not possible, patient should be placed on two reliable contraception methods. Pregnancy testing and contraception counseling should be repeated monthly throughout therapy.

Contraindications and precautions
Contraindicated in hypersensitivity to retinoids and parabens (preservative in gelatin capsule).

Use cautiously in pregnancy and breast-feeding. Safety and efficacy in *children younger than age 1* have not been established.

Preparation and administration
• Follow hazardous drug guidelines for handling, preparation, and administration. (See "Managing hazardous drugs," page 11.)
• Store at 59° to 86° F (15° to 30° C); protect from light.

Adverse reactions
CNS: headache, dizziness, malaise, paresthesia, anxiety, agitation, insomnia, depression, confusion, cerebral hemorrhage, pseudotumor cerebri (benign intracranial hypertension)
CV: heart failure, arrhythmia, hypertension, hypotension, phlebitis
EENT: visual disturbance, ear disorders
GI: nausea, vomiting, diarrhea, constipation, dyspepsia, abdominal distention, anorexia, mucositis, GI hemorrhage
GU: renal insufficiency, dysuria
Hematologic: leukocytosis, hemorrhage, disseminated intravascular coagulation
Hepatic: hepatosplenomegaly
Musculoskeletal: bone pain, flank pain, myalgia
Respiratory: respiratory tract disorders, dyspnea, respiratory insufficiency, pleural effusion, pneumonia, crackles, expiratory wheezing, pulmonary infiltration
Skin: excessive dryness, pallor, flushing, alopecia, blistering, crusting, initial acne flare-up, irritation, photosensitivity, pruritus, rash, cellulitis, temporary hyper- or hypopigmentation
Other: fever, shivering, infection, increased sweating, edema, pain, weight changes, injection site reaction, RA-APL syndrome

Interactions
Drug-drug. *CYP450 inducers (including glucocorticoids, pentobarbital, phenobarbital, and rifampin), CYP450 inhibitors (including cimetidine, cyclosporine, diltiazem, erythromycin, ketoconazole, and verapamil):* possible change in pharmacokinetic properties of tretinoin

Drug-diagnostic tests. *WBCs:* increased
Drug-herb. *Alfalfa, bergamot oil, bishop's weed, St. John's wort:* possible potentiation of photosensitivity

Toxicity and overdose

• No experience with acute overdose has occurred. Maximum tolerated dosage in myelodysplastic syndrome or solid tumor is 195 mg/m² daily. Maximum tolerated dosage in children is 60 mg/m² daily. Overdose with other retinoids has caused transient headache, facial flushing, cheilosis, abdominal pain, dizziness, and ataxia. These symptoms resolve quickly with no apparent residual effects.
• If overdose occurs, provide supportive treatment.

Special considerations

• Drug is used only to induce remission. Optimal consolidation or maintenance regimens have not been determined. Therefore, all patients should receive standard consolidation and maintenance chemotherapy regimen for APL after induction therapy, unless contraindicated.
• Monitor patient for serious adverse reactions, including RA-APL syndrome and leukocytosis.
• Pseudotumor cerebri may occur, particularly in children. Observe for early signs and symptoms (papilledema, headache, nausea, vomiting, and visual disturbances), which may warrant analgesics and lumbar puncture for relief.

Patient education

• Instruct patient to take doses with food.
• Provide full information and warnings to pregnant women and women with childbearing potential on drug's risk to fetus and consequences of contraception failure.
• Advise breastfeeding patient to discontinue breastfeeding before starting drug.

trimethobenzamide hydrochloride

Benzacot, Benzocaine-Trimethobenzamide Adult, Benzocaine-Trimethobenzamide Pediatric, Navogan, Tebamide, Tebamide Pediatric, Tigan, Tigan Adult, Tigan Pediatric

Classifications: Anticholinergic, antiemetic, antivertigo agent
Pregnancy risk category C

Pharmacology

Trimethobenzamide may block dopamine receptors and emetic impulses in chemoreceptor trigger zone of brain, an area in medulla oblongata through which emetic impulses are conveyed to vomiting center.

Pharmacokinetics

Drug is metabolized in liver. With P.O. and P.R. use, onset is approximately 20 to 40 minutes and duration is approximately 3 to 4 hours. With I.M. use, onset is 15 minutes and duration is 2 to 3 hours. It is excreted by kidneys.

How supplied

Capsules: 250 mg, 300 mg
Solution: 100 mg/ml in 2-ml ampules
Suppositories: 100 mg, 200 mg

Indications and dosages

OFF-LABEL USES (SELECTED)

➡ Chemotherapy-induced nausea and vomiting
Adults: Typical dosage is 250 mg P.O. three or four times daily; or 200 mg I.M. or P.R. three or four times daily.
Children weighing 13.6 to 40.8 kg (30 to 90 lb): Typical dosage is 100 to 200 mg P.O. or P.R. three or four times daily.
Children weighing less than 13.6 kg: Typical dosage is 100 mg P.R. three or four times daily.

⊠ WARNINGS

- Use caution when giving drug to child to treat vomiting. Drug is not recommended for treatment of uncomplicated vomiting in children. Its use should be limited to prolonged vomiting of known cause. In children with viral illness (a possible cause of vomiting), drug may contribute to development of Reye's syndrome.
- Drug may cause extrapyramidal symptoms that could be confused with CNS manifestations of undiagnosed primary disease responsible for vomiting, such as Reye's syndrome or other encephalopathy.
- Drug has hepatotoxic potential, which may unfavorably alter course of Reye's syndrome. It should be avoided in children whose signs and symptoms could represent Reye's syndrome. Because salicylates and acetaminophen also are hepatotoxic at large doses, these drugs should be avoided in children whose signs and symptoms could represent Reye's syndrome, unless alternative fever-control methods fail.

Contraindications and precautions

Contraindicated in hypersensitivity to drug or benzocaine (suppositories), premature or newborn infants (suppositories), and *children* (injectable form).

Use cautiously in recent treatment with other CNS-acting agents and in severe emesis.

Preparation and administration

- Although drug may provide some relief from nausea and vomiting associated with chemotherapy, available data indicate that other agents are more effective and are preferred (in absence of well-controlled clinical trials).
- Injectable form is for I.M. use only; it is not recommended for I.V. use.
- I.M. administration may cause pain, stinging, burning, redness, and swelling at injection site. Such effects may be minimized by

deep injection into upper outer quadrant of gluteal region.
- Discontinue drug at first sign of hypersensitivity.
- Store at 59° to 86° F (15° to 30° C).

Adverse reactions

CNS: drowsiness, coma, seizures, opisthotonos, parkinsonian-like symptoms
CV: hypotension (parenteral administration)
Hematologic: blood dyscrasia
Skin: rash, urticaria, flushing
Other: burning at injection site, hypersensitivity reaction

Interactions

Drug-drug. *Other CNS depressants:* additive CNS depression
Drug-diagnostic tests. *Urinary amphetamine:* false positive
Drug-herb. *Aloe, cascara, rhubarb:* possible decreased trimethobenzamide absorption due to reduced GI transit time

Toxicity and overdose

- Signs and symptoms of overdose may include coma, seizures, and opisthotonos.
- If overdose occurs, discontinue drug and provide supportive treatment.

Special considerations

- Do not treat severe emesis with antiemetic drug alone.
- Monitor patient's hydration status. Avoid overhydration, which may lead to cerebral edema (especially in children and in elderly or debilitated patients).
- Drug may render diagnosis more difficult in such conditions as appendicitis, and may mask ototoxic symptoms associated with antibiotics.

Patient education

- Inform patient that drug may cause drowsiness. Caution him not to drive or perform other hazardous activities until response to drug is known.

T

• Explain possible adverse reactions. Stress importance of discontinuing drug and contacting prescriber if these reactions (especially rash) occur.
• Caution patient not to drink alcoholic beverages during therapy.

triptorelin pamoate
Trelstar Depot, Trelstar LA

Classification: Antineoplastic, hormone/hormone modifier, gonadotropin-releasing hormone (GnRH) analogue
Pregnancy risk category X

Pharmacology

Triptorelin is a potent inhibitor of gonadotropin secretion. Initially, it causes transient surge in circulating levels of luteinizing hormone (LH), follicle-stimulating hormone (FSH), testosterone, and estradiol. With chronic and continuous use (usually 2 to 4 weeks), a sustained decrease in LH and FSH secretion occurs, and testicular and ovarian steroidogenesis is markedly reduced. In men, serum testosterone concentration decreases to levels typically seen in surgically castrated men. Tissues and functions that depend on these hormones for maintenance become quiescent. Effects usually reverse after therapy ends.

Pharmacokinetics

Drug has slow onset, peaks in 1 to 3 hours, and has duration of approximately 1 month (depot) or 3 months (long-acting form). Terminal half-life is 3 hours in healthy males. Drug is eliminated by liver and kidneys.

How supplied

Microgranules for injection: 3.75 mg (depot), 11.25 mg (long-acting)

Indications and dosages

➡ Palliative treatment of advanced prostate cancer
Adults: 3.75 mg (depot) I.M. every 4 weeks as single injection; or 11.25 mg (long-acting) I.M. every 12 weeks as single injection

Contraindications and precautions

Contraindicated in hypersensitivity to drug or its components, use of LH-releasing hormone (LHRH) or other LHRH agonists, and women who are pregnant or may become pregnant during therapy.

Use cautiously in increased serum testosterone level, spinal cord compression, renal impairment, and breastfeeding. Safety and efficacy in *children* have not been established.

Preparation and administration

• Follow hazardous drug guidelines for handling, preparation, and administration. (See "Managing hazardous drugs," page 11.)
• Monitor serum levels of testosterone and prostate-specific antigen immediately before and during dosing to determine response to therapy.
• Reconstitute microgranules with sterile water. Do not use other diluents.
• Discard suspension if it is not used immediately after reconstitution.
• Rotate I.M. injection sites.
• Store Trelstar Depot at 77° F (25° C) and Trelstar LA at 68° to 77° F (20° to 25° C); excursions are permitted to 59° to 86° F (15° to 30° C).

Adverse reactions

CNS: headache, dizziness, fatigue, spinal cord compression, insomnia
CV: hypertension
GI: nausea (long-acting form), diarrhea, vomiting
GU: dysuria (long-acting form), erectile dysfunction, urinary retention, urinary infection
Hematologic: altered blood counts

Only common or life-threatening adverse reactions are listed.

Musculoskeletal: skeletal pain, osteoneuralgia
Other: leg edema (long-acting form), hot flashes, injection site pain, hypersensitivity, anaphylaxis

Interactions

Drug-drug. *Hyperprolactinemic drugs (such as dopamine):* possible reduction in number of pituitary GnRH receptors, causing decreased triptorelin efficacy
Drug-diagnostic tests. *Hemoglobin, progesterone, RBCs, testosterone:* decreased
Serum ALP, ALT, AST, BUN, estradiol, FSH, glucose, LH, testosterone (transient effect): increased

Toxicity and overdose

• Overdose is unlikely.
• In suspected overdose, discontinue drug immediately and provide appropriate supportive and symptomatic treatment.

Special considerations

• Transient serum testosterone increase may be associated with temporary worsening of prostate cancer symptoms during first weeks of treatment. Patient may experience worsening symptoms or onset of new symptoms, including bone pain, neuropathy, hematuria, and urethral or bladder outlet obstruction.
• Drug has caused spinal cord compression, which may contribute to paralysis with or without fatal complications. Institute standard treatment and, in extreme cases, consider immediate orchiectomy.
• Patients with renal or hepatic impairment may show two- to fourfold higher exposure than healthy young males. Need for dosage adjustment is unknown, but monitor kidney and liver function tests.

Patient education

• Assure patient that temporary worsening of symptoms does not mean that drug is not effective.
• Instruct patient to immediately report signs and symptoms of hypersensitivity reaction (such as rash and itching) or spinal cord compression (such as weakness or paralysis of lower extremities).
• Emphasize importance of complying with dosage schedule and follow-up visits for medical care.

valrubicin
Valstar

Classification: Antineoplastic, antibiotic (anthracycline)
Pregnancy risk category C

Pharmacology

Valrubicin affects various interrelated biological functions, most of which involve nucleic acid metabolism. It readily penetrates cells, where it inhibits incorporation of nucleosides into nucleic acids, causes extensive chromosomal damage, and arrests cell cycle in G_2 phase. Although drug does not bind strongly to DNA, it interferes with normal DNA breaking-resealing action of DNA topoisomerase II.

Pharmacokinetics

Drug is well absorbed into bladder wall. Negligible systemic absorption occurs during bladder retention (depending on bladder condition). If bladder is perforated, systemic exposure increases. Drug is not metabolized. It is excreted almost completely in urine.

How supplied

Solution for intravesical instillation: 200 mg/5 ml

Indications and dosages

FDA-APPROVED

⊜ Bacillus Calmette-Guérin (BCG)–refractory urinary bladder cancer in patients for whom immediate cystectomy is unacceptable
Adults: 800 mg intravesically every week for 6

V

weeks, starting 14 or more days after fulguration or transurethral resection

Contraindications and precautions
Contraindicated in hypersensitivity to anthracyclines or Cremophor EL, urinary tract infection, and small bladder capacity.

Use cautiously in perforated bladder, compromised bladder mucosa integrity, severe symptoms of irritable bladder, and pregnancy or breastfeeding. Safety and efficacy in *children* have not been established.

Preparation and administration
• Follow hazardous drug guidelines for handling, preparation, and administration. (See "Managing hazardous drugs," page 11.)
• For each instillation, allow four 5-ml vials (200 mg valrubicin/5 ml per vial) to warm slowly to room temperature. Do not heat vials. Dilute 20 ml of drug with 55 ml normal saline solution injection, yielding 75 ml of diluted solution.
• For intravesical instillation, urethral catheter is inserted into bladder under aseptic conditions. Bladder is drained, and diluted 75-ml valrubicin solution is instilled slowly by gravity flow over several minutes. Catheter is then withdrawn. Patient should retain drug for 2 hours.
• Some patients will be unable to retain drug for full 2 hours.
• Ensure that patient maintains adequate hydration after treatment.
• Prepare and store solution in glass, polypropylene, or polyolefin containers and tubing. Use non-DEHP containing administration sets (such as those that are polyethylene-lined).
• Solution is clear and red. Inspect for particulates and discoloration before administration. At temperatures below 39° F (4° C), Cremophor EL may begin to form waxy precipitate. If this happens, warm vial in hand until solution is clear. If particulates remain, do not administer drug.
• When diluted in normal saline solution injection, drug is stable for 12 hours at temperatures up to 77° F (25°C). Do not mix with other drugs.
• Store refrigerated between 36° and 46° F (2° and 8° C) in original carton.

Adverse reactions
CNS: headache, malaise, fever, dizziness
CV: chest pain, vasodilation
GI: nausea, vomiting, diarrhea, abdominal pain
GU: urinary tract infection, urinary retention, hematuria
Hematologic: anemia
Musculoskeletal: myalgia
Skin: rash
Other: asthenia, back pain

Interactions
Drug-herb. *Alpha-lipoic acid, coenzyme Q10, glucosamine, glutamine:* possible decreased chemotherapy efficacy

Toxicity and overdose
• Overdose signs and symptoms resemble those of irritable bladder. Myelosuppression also may occur with inadvertent systemic administration or systemic absorption from intravesical instillation.
• No known antidote exists. Provide supportive treatment.

Special considerations
• Do not clamp catheter in patients with severe irritable bladder symptoms, including spasms.
• Evaluate patient for bladder rupture. If it occurs, monitor for myelosuppression.
• Drug induces complete response in only about 1 of 5 patients with BCG-refractory carcinoma in situ (CIS). Delaying cystectomy could lead to development of metastatic bladder cancer, which is lethal. If patient does not demonstrate complete response to treatment after 3 months or if CIS recurs, reconsider cystectomy.

Only common or life-threatening adverse reactions are listed.

Patient education

• Inform patient that irritable bladder symptoms may occur during drug instillation and retention and for a limited time after voiding. Tell patient that for first 24 hours after administration, urine typically is red-tinged. Instruct him to immediately report prolonged irritable bladder symptoms or prolonged passage of red-tinged urine.

• Advise women with childbearing potential not to become pregnant during therapy. Advise men to refrain from engaging in sexual activities during therapy.

• Urge patient to use effective contraception during therapy.

vinblastine sulfate

Classification: Antineoplastic, vinca alkaloid
Pregnancy risk category D

Pharmacology

Vinblastine may interfere with metabolic amino acid pathways leading from glutamic acid to citric acid cycle and then to urea, producing stathmokinetic effect. It affects cell-energy production required for mitosis, interferes with nucleic acid synthesis, and inhibits microtubule formation in mitotic spindle. These actions cause arrest of dividing cells at metaphase.

Pharmacokinetics

Drug undergoes deacetylation in liver to active metabolite, followed by further metabolism. It is widely distributed; elimination half-life is approximately 20 hours. Excretion is predominantly through bile.

How supplied

Powder for injection: 10-mg vial

Indications and dosages

➡ Palliative treatment of advanced testicular cancer, Hodgkin's disease (Stages III and IV, Ann Arbor modification of Rye staging system), lymphocytic lymphoma, histiocytic lymphoma, mycosis fungoides, histiocytosis, Kaposi's sarcoma, choriocarcinoma resistant to other chemotherapeutic agents, breast carcinoma unresponsive to appropriate endocrine surgery and hormonal therapy
Adults: 0.1 mg/kg or 3.7 mg/m² I.V. weekly or every 2 weeks, not to exceed 0.5 mg/kg or 18.5 mg/m² weekly
Children: Initially 2.5 mg/m² I.V., followed by 3.75 mg/m², 5 mg/m², 6.25 mg/m², and then 7.5 mg/m² I.V. at 7-day intervals

OFF-LABEL USES (SELECTED)

➡ Bladder, cervical, and head and neck cancer
Adults: Typical regimens include vinblastine 3 mg/m² I.V. on days 2, 15, and 22 in combination with methotrexate, doxorubicin, and cisplatin (MVAC), with cycle repeated every 28 days.
➡ Melanoma
Adults: Combination therapy using dacarbazine, cisplatin, vinblastine, interferon, and interleukin-2 is considered alternative treatment of choice.
➡ Non-small-cell lung cancer
Adults: Typical regimens include combination therapy as alternative treatment (vinblastine and cisplatin or vinblastine with cisplatin and mitomycin), with vinblastine dosages of 4 mg/m² I.V. daily from days 1 to 29, then every 2 weeks after day 43 and continuing until last cisplatin administration.
➡ Germ cell tumors
Adults: Typical regimen includes vinblastine 0.11 mg/kg I.V. daily on days 1 and 2 in combination with cisplatin and ifosfamide.

V

DOSAGE MODIFICATIONS

- Hematologic intolerance should guide dosage.
- Dosage reduction of 50% is recommended for patients with direct serum bilirubin level above 3 mg/dl.

⊠ WARNINGS

- Drug should be given only by individuals experienced in administration of chemotherapeutic agents.
- Drug is for I.V. use only and is fatal if given intrathecally. I.V. needle or catheter must be properly positioned before drug is injected. Leakage into surrounding tissue may cause marked irritation. If extravasation occurs, discontinue injection immediately, and introduce remaining portion into another vein. Local hyaluronidase injection and application of moderate heat may help disperse extravasated drug and minimize discomfort and risk of cellulitis.
- Extemporaneously prepared syringes containing product must be packaged in overwrap labeled, "Do not remove covering until moment of injection. Fatal if given intrathecally. For I.V. use only."
- With inadvertent intrathecal administration, immediate neurosurgical intervention is needed to prevent ascending paralysis leading to death. Although life-threatening paralysis and subsequent death may be averted, intrathecal administration generally causes devastating neurologic effects and limited recovery; no published cases of survival after intrathecal administration exist. If drug is mistakenly given by intrathecal route, remove as much cerebrospinal fluid (CSF) as possible through lumbar access. Insert epidural catheter into subarachnoid space through intervertebral space above initial lumbar access, and irrigate CSF with lactated Ringer's solution. Add 25 ml fresh frozen plasma to every liter of lactated Ringer's solution. Intraventricular drain or catheter should be inserted by neurosurgeon

and continuous CSF irrigation should be used, with fluid removed through lumbar access connected to closed drainage system. Lactated Ringer's solution should be given by continuous infusion at 150 ml/hour, or at 75 ml/hour when fresh frozen plasma has been added. Infusion rate should be adjusted to maintain CSF protein level at 150 mg/dl.
- To further reduce neurotoxicity from intrathecal administration, glutamic acid 10 g I.V. over 24 hours may be given, followed by 500 mg P.O. three times daily for 1 month. Folinic acid may be given I.V. as 100-mg bolus and then infused at 25 mg/hour for 24 hours, and then given as bolus doses of 25 mg every 6 hours for 1 week. Pyridoxine may be given as 50 mg I.V. infusion over 30 minutes every 8 hours.

Contraindications and precautions

Contraindicated in significant granulocytopenia and bacterial infection.

Use cautiously in leukopenia, preexisting pulmonary dysfunction, renal impairment, hepatic insufficiency, concurrent radiation therapy, and pregnancy or breastfeeding. *Elderly patients* with cachexia or skin ulceration are more susceptible to leukopenic effects.

Injection contains benzyl alcohol, which may cause allergic reactions in susceptible individuals. Also, large amounts of benzyl alcohol have been associated with potentially fatal toxicity in neonates (gasping syndrome); avoid giving drug to neonates.

Preparation and administration

- Follow hazardous drug guidelines for handling preparation, and administration. (See "Managing hazardous drugs," page 11.)
- Syringe containing specific dose must be labeled, using auxiliary sticker provided, "Fatal if given intrathecally. For I.V. use only."
- Reconstitute powder with 10 ml normal saline solution to concentration of 1 mg/ml.

Inject I.V. dose into tubing of running I.V. line or by direct injection over 1 minute.
- Except in off-label uses, administer no more often than once every 7 days (due to variations in depth of leukopenic response).
- To initiate therapy in adults, administer single I.V. dose of 3.7 mg/m^2 (except in off-label uses). Thereafter, obtain WBC count to determine patient's sensitivity to drug.
- Store refrigerated at 36° to 46° F (2° to 8° C) in original carton.

Adverse reactions

CNS: weakness, malaise, paresthesia, peripheral neuropathy, neuritis, numbness, loss of deep tendon reflexes, seizures
CV: myocardial infarction, hypotension, hypertension, phlebitis
GI: nausea, vomiting, ileus, anorexia, stomatitis, constipation, GI bleeding
Hematologic: anemia, thrombocytopenia, leukopenia, myelosuppression
Hepatic: hepatotoxicity
Musculoskeletal: bone pain, pain in tumor-containing tissue, jaw pain, muscle pain
Respiratory: bronchospasm
Skin: rash, alopecia
Other: weight loss

Interactions

Drug-drug. *Bleomycin:* synergistic effect
CYP450 3A inhibitors (such as erythromycin): increased vinblastine toxicity
Methotrexate: increased methotrexate action
Mitomycin: acute shortness of breath, severe bronchospasm
Phenytoin: decreased phenytoin level
Drug-diagnostic tests. *WBCs:* decreased
Drug-food. *Grapefruit, pomegranate:* possible increased vinblastine levels
Drug-herb. *Alpha-lipoic acid, coenzyme Q10, glucosamine, glutamine:* possible decreased chemotherapy efficacy
Cat's claw, devil's claw, feverfew, garlic, ginkgo, goldenseal, kava, licorice, milk thistle, valerian: possible increased vinblastine levels

Toxicity and overdose

- Excessive doses cause myelosuppression, which may be life-threatening.
- No specific antidote exists. If drug was swallowed, give activated charcoal in water slurry, along with cathartic. Protect airway, and support ventilation and perfusion. Meticulously monitor and maintain vital signs, WBC and differential, platelets, blood gases, and serum electrolytes. No information regarding dialysis or cholestyramine efficacy in treating overdose exists.

Special considerations

- Watch closely for infection in patients with WBC counts below 2,000/mm^3.
- In patients with malignant-cell infiltration of bone marrow, WBC and platelet counts may fall precipitously after moderate doses. Further drug use in such patients is inadvisable.
- If acute respiratory problems occur, do not readminister drug.

Patient education

- Instruct patient to immediately report sore throat, fever, chills, sore mouth, or other serious medical event.
- Advise patient to avoid constipation by increasing dietary bulk, drinking adequate fluids, and exercising.
- Inform patient that drug may cause alopecia, jaw pain, and pain in organs containing tumor tissue. Reassure patient that scalp hair will regrow to pretreatment extent even with continued treatment.
- Advise women with childbearing potential not to become pregnant while taking drug.
- Provide guidance to help breastfeeding patient decide whether to discontinue breastfeeding or stop drug.

V

vincristine sulfate
Oncovin, Vincasar PFS

Classification: Antineoplastic, antimitotic agent, vinca alkaloid
Pregnancy risk category D

Pharmacology
Vincristine inhibits mitotic activity and arrests cell cycle at metaphase. It also inhibits RNA synthesis and blocks cellular use of glutamic acid needed for purine synthesis.

Pharmacokinetics
Drug is metabolized in liver and is distributed quickly and widely throughout body, except cerebrospinal fluid (CSF). Elimination half-life varies but usually exceeds 10 hours. Parent drug and metabolites are excreted primarily in bile and feces.

How supplied
Solution for injection: 1 mg/ml, 2 mg/ml

Indications and dosages

FDA-APPROVED

➤ Hodgkin's disease, non-Hodgkin's lymphoma, acute leukemia, nephroblastoma, rhabdomyosarcoma
Adults: 0.03 to 1.4 mg/m^2 I.V. weekly; maximum dosage is 2 mg.
Children weighing more than 10 kg (22 lb): 1.5 to 2 mg/m^2 I.V. weekly (varies with protocol)
Children weighing 10 kg (22 lb) or less: 0.05 mg/kg I.V. weekly (varies with protocol)

OFF-LABEL USES (SELECTED)

➤ AIDS-related Kaposi's sarcoma, intracranial tumor, hepatic carcinoma, small-cell lung carcinoma, testicular cancer, ovarian cancer, malignant pheochromocytoma
Adults: Usual dosage is 0.03 to 1.4 mg/m^2 I.V. weekly; maximum dosage is 2 mg.

DOSAGE MODIFICATIONS
• Dosage reduction of 50% is recommended for patients with direct serum bilirubin concentrations above 3 mg/dl.
• Dosage limitation depends on patient response and protocol used.

⊠ WARNINGS
• Drug should be given only by individuals experienced in administration of chemotherapeutic agents.
• Drug is for I.V. use only.
• Extemporaneously prepared syringes containing product must be packaged in overwrap labeled, "Do not remove covering until moment of injection. Fatal if given intrathecally. For I.V. use only."
• If intrathecal administration occurs, treatment includes immediate removal of CSF and flushing with lactated Ringer's or other solution. Treatment must begin immediately after intrathecal injection. As much CSF should be removed as can safely be done through lumbar access. Subarachnoid space should be flushed with lactated Ringer's solution infused continuously through catheter in cerebral lateral ventricle at 150 ml/hour. Fluid should be removed through lumbar access. Fresh frozen plasma (25 ml diluted in 1 L lactated Ringer's solution) should be infused through cerebral ventricular catheter at 75 ml/hour, with fluid removed through lumbar access. Infusion rate should be adjusted to maintain CSF protein level of 150 mg/dl. Glutamic acid 10 g should be infused I.V. over 24 hours, followed by 500 mg P.O. three times daily for 1 month or until neurologic dysfunction stabilizes.

Contraindications and precautions
Contraindicated in hypersensitivity to drug and demyelinating form of Charcot-Marie-Tooth syndrome.
    Use cautiously in leukopenia, preexisting pulmonary dysfunction or neuromuscular disease, renal impairment, hepatic insufficiency,

---

Only common or life-threatening adverse reactions are listed.

concurrent radiation therapy, pregnancy or breastfeeding, and frail *elderly patients* at risk for neurotoxicity.

Preparation and administration

>> Follow hazardous drug guidelines for handling, preparation, and administration. (See "Managing hazardous drugs," page 11.)
• Syringe containing specific dose must be labeled, using auxiliary sticker provided, "Fatal if given intrathecally. For I.V. use only."
• Administer dose through intact, free-flowing I.V. needle or catheter within 1 minute.
• Ensure that I.V. needle or catheter is properly positioned before drug injection, to prevent extravasation. If extravasation occurs, discontinue injection immediately and introduce remaining portion of dose into another vein. Local hyaluronidase injection and application of moderate heat helps disperse drug and may minimize discomfort and reduce possibility of cellulitis.
• Store in refrigerator between 36° and 46° F (2° and 8° C).

Adverse reactions

CNS: decreased reflexes, paresthesia, weakness, CNS depression, cranial nerve paralysis, seizures, peripheral neuropathy, coma
CV: hypotension, hypertension, phlebitis
GI: nausea, vomiting, stomatitis, constipation, abdominal pain or cramping, intestinal necrosis
Hematologic: thrombocytopenia, leukopenia, myelosuppression
Hepatic: hepatotoxicity
Metabolic: hyperuricemia
Musculoskeletal: wrist and foot drop
Other: hypersensitivity, syndrome of inappropriate antidiuretic hormone secretion
Respiratory: shortness of breath
Skin: alopecia

Interactions

Drug-drug. *Anticoagulants, methotrexate:* increased actions of these drugs
CYP450 inhibitors (such as erythromycin): in-

creased neurotoxicity (from reduced vincristine clearance)
Digoxin, phenytoin: decreased levels of these drugs
L-asparaginase: decreased vincristine clearance
Mitomycin: acute pulmonary reactions, including bronchospasm
Drug-diagnostic tests. *WBCs:* decreased
Drug-herb. *Alpha-lipoic acid, coenzyme Q10, glucosamine, glutamine:* possible decreased chemotherapy efficacy
Cat's claw, devil's claw, feverfew, garlic, ginkgo, goldenseal, kava, milk thistle, licorice, valerian: possible increased vincristine levels

Toxicity and overdose

• Toxicity effects are dose-related. In children, death has occurred after doses of 10 times the recommended amounts. Expect adults to experience severe symptoms after single doses of 3 mg/m² or more. Toxicity manifests as exaggerated adverse reactions.
• Provide supportive care, including fluid restriction and possibly a diuretic that affects function of Henle's loop and distal tubule, along with anticonvulsants, enemas, or cathartics to prevent ileus (in some instances, GI tract decompression may be necessary), cardiovascular system monitoring, and daily WBC and differential and platelet counts for guidance in transfusion requirements. Also monitor blood gases and serum electrolytes.

Special considerations

• Monitor CBC before each dose.
• Monitor serum uric acid level during first 3 to 4 weeks of therapy.
• If acute respiratory problems occur, do not readminister drug.

Patient education

• Instruct patient to immediately report sore throat, fever, chills, gait changes, numbness in extremities, and bleeding, white spots, or ulcerations in mouth.
• Inform patient that drug may cause alopecia. Reassure patient that scalp hair will re-

grow to pretreatment extent even with continued treatment.

• Advise patient to avoid constipation by increasing dietary bulk, drinking adequate fluids, and exercising.

• Caution women with childbearing potential not to become pregnant while taking drug.

• Provide guidance to help breastfeeding patient decide whether to discontinue breastfeeding or stop drug.

vinorelbine tartrate
Navelbine

Classification: Antineoplastic, antimitotic agent, vinca alkaloid
Pregnancy risk category D

Pharmacology
Vinorelbine has antitumor activity that may stem primarily from mitosis inhibition at metaphase through its interaction with tubulin. Drug also may interfere with amino acid, cyclic AMP, and glutathione metabolism; calmodulin-dependent calcium-transport ATPase activity; cellular respiration; and nucleic acid and lipid biosynthesis.

Pharmacokinetics
Drug has fair oral bioavailability but is available only as I.V. preparation. It is metabolized in liver; elimination half-life is approximately 24 hours. It is excreted predominantly through bile.

How supplied
Solution: 10 mg/ml in 1-ml and 5-ml vials

Indications and dosages

➡ Unresectable, advanced (stage IV) non-small-cell lung cancer
Adults: As single agent, 30 mg/m^2 I.V. given over 6 to 10 minutes every week. Vinorel-

bine 30 mg/m^2 I.V. may be given weekly in combination with cisplatin on days 1 and 29, then every 6 weeks at a dosage of 120 mg/m^2; or vinorelbine 25 mg/m^2 I.V. may be given weekly in combination with cisplatin administered every 4 weeks.

➡ Unresectable, advanced (stage III) non-small-cell lung cancer stage
Adults: As combination therapy, vinorelbine 30 mg/m^2 I.V. may be given weekly in combination with cisplatin on days 1 and 29, then every 6 weeks at a dosage of 120 mg/m^2; or vinorelbine 25 mg/m^2 I.V. weekly in combination with cisplatin given every 4 weeks.

OFF-LABEL USES (SELECTED)

➡ Metastatic breast cancer, recurrent ovarian cancer, cervical cancer
Adults: 30 mg/m^2 I.V. weekly until disease progression or dose-limiting toxicity occurs

DOSAGE MODIFICATIONS

• Dosage should be adjusted according to hematologic toxicity or hepatic insufficiency (hyperbilirubinemia), whichever results in lower dosage for corresponding starting dosage.

• Reduce dosage to 50% of starting dosage if granulocyte count is 1,000 to 1,499/mm^3 on day of treatment. If patient experiences fever or sepsis on initial therapy or if two consecutive doses were withheld because of granulocytopenia, subsequent doses should be 75% of starting dosage for absolute neutrophil count (ANC) of 1,500/mm^3 or more. If ANC is 1,000 to 1,499/mm^3, dosage should be 37.5% of starting dosage.

• In patients with total bilirubin level of 2.1 to 3 mg/dl, use 50% of starting dosage. For total bilirubin level above 3 mg/dl, use 25% of starting dosage. Total bilirubin level of 2 or below does not necessitate dosage modification.

• If Grade 2 or higher neurotoxicity develops during therapy, discontinue drug.

Only common or life-threatening adverse reactions are listed.

☒ WARNINGS

- Product is for I.V. use only. Intrathecal administration may result in death. Syringes containing drug should be labeled, "Warning—for I.V. use only. Fatal if given intrathecally."
- Severe granulocytopenia may occur, causing increased susceptibility to infection. Granulocyte count should be 1,000/mm³ or more before administration. Dosage should be adjusted according to CBC with differential obtained on day of treatment.
- Drug is a vesicant. I.V. needle or catheter must be properly positioned before drug is injected. Drug administration may result in extravasation, causing severe local tissue necrosis, thrombophlebitis, or both.

Contraindications and precautions

Contraindicated in pretreatment granulocyte count below 1,000/mm³.

Use cautiously in myelosuppression, preexisting pulmonary dysfunction, hepatic disease, and pregnancy or breastfeeding. Safety and efficacy in *children* have not been established.

Preparation and administration

- Follow hazardous drug guidelines for handling, preparation, and administration. (See "Managing hazardous drugs," page 11.)
- For I.V. injection, dilute each 10 mg (1 ml) in syringe with at least 2 to 5 ml normal saline for injection or D₅W for desired concentration of 1.5 to 3 mg/ml. Administer diluted drug over 6 to 10 minutes into side port of free-flowing I.V. line closest to I.V. bag; then flush with at least 75 to 125 ml of recommended solution.
- For intermittent I.V. infusion, dilute each 10 mg (1 ml) with 4 to 19 ml normal saline for injection, D₅W, half-normal saline solution, D₅W in half-normal saline solution, Ringer's solution, or lactated Ringer's solution for desired concentration of 0.5 to 2 mg/ml. Administer diluted drug over 6 to 20 minutes into

side port of free-flowing I.V. line, or give directly into large central vein and then flush with at least 75 to 125 ml of recommended solution.
- Diluted drug may be used for up to 24 hours under normal room lighting when stored in polypropylene syringe or polyvinylchloride bag at 41° to 86° F (5° to 30° C).

Adverse reactions

CNS: paresthesia, peripheral neuropathy, depression, headache, seizures, weakness, jaw pain
CV: chest pain
GI: nausea, vomiting, ileus, anorexia, stomatitis, severe constipation, abdominal pain, diarrhea
Hematologic: anemia, thrombocytopenia, granulocytopenia
Musculoskeletal: myalgia
Respiratory: shortness of breath, interstitial pulmonary changes, adult respiratory distress syndrome (ARDS)
Skin: rash, alopecia, photosensitivity
Other: hypersensitivity, syndrome of inappropriate antidiuretic hormone secretion

Interactions

Drug-drug. *CYP450 inhibitors (such as erythromycin):* increased adverse reactions to vinorelbine
Mitomycin: acute pulmonary reaction
Drug-diagnostic tests. *AST, bilirubin:* increased
WBCs: decreased
Drug-food. *Grapefruit, pomegranate:* possible increased vinorelbine levels
Drug-herb. *Alpha-lipoic acid, coenzyme Q10, glucosamine, glutamine:* possible decreased chemotherapy efficacy
Cat's claw, devil's claw, feverfew, garlic, ginkgo, goldenseal, kava, milk thistle, licorice, valerian: possible increased vinorelbine levels

Toxicity and overdose

- Toxicities include paralytic ileus, stomatitis, esophagitis, bone marrow aplasia, sepsis, and

V

paresis. Deaths have occurred after overdose.
• No known antidote exists. If overdose occurs, monitor WBC and differential and platelet counts. Provide general supportive measures, appropriate blood transfusions, growth factors, and antibiotics.

Special considerations
• Monitor patient frequently for myelosuppression during and after therapy.
• Acute dyspnea and severe bronchospasm may occur (most commonly when drug is used in combination with mitomycin). Treat with supplemental oxygen, bronchodilators, and corticosteroids, particularly if patient had preexisting pulmonary dysfunction.
• Potentially fatal interstitial pulmonary changes and ARDS may occur in patients treated with single-agent therapy. Mean time-to-onset of these symptoms is 1 week after therapy begins. Promptly evaluate patients with alterations in baseline pulmonary symptoms or with new onset of dyspnea, cough, hypoxia, or other symptoms.
• Drug may cause severe constipation, paralytic ileus, intestinal obstruction, necrosis, or perforation.
• If patient has history of or preexisting neuropathy (regardless of cause), monitor closely for new or worsening signs and symptoms of neuropathy during therapy.
• "Radiation recall" may occur if drug is given to patient who has received radiation therapy.

Patient education
• Inform patient that major side effects relate to bone marrow toxicity and include granulocytopenia with increased susceptibility to infection.
• Instruct patient to report fever or chills immediately.
• Tell patient to contact prescriber for cough, increased shortness of breath, or other new pulmonary symptoms or if abdominal pain or constipation occurs.

• Advise women with childbearing potential to avoid becoming pregnant during therapy.
• Provide guidance to help breastfeeding patient decide whether to discontinue breastfeeding or stop drug.

Only common or life-threatening adverse reactions are listed.

Part 3

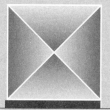

Chemotherapy Regimens and Supportive Therapy

Chemotherapy regimens and supportive therapy

FOR MANY NEOPLASTIC DISEASES, chemotherapy is the primary treatment method. For others, it is used as an adjunct to surgery, radiation, or both. Generally, combination chemotherapy is more effective (although more toxic) than single-agent chemotherapy, even though some combinations may produce antagonistic effects.

The goal of administering combination chemotherapy in cycles or specific sequences is to produce additive or synergistic therapeutic effects while delaying emergence of drug resistance and minimizing overwhelming toxicities. Each drug used in a combination regimen should not only be effective alone against the specific cancer but should potentiate the effects of other drugs in the combination. High-dose intermittent chemotherapy usually is more effective and less toxic than low-dose continuous chemotherapy because most normal tissues have a greater repair capacity than neoplastic tissues and may recover during drug-free periods.

For most cancers, optimum treatment schedules have not been established. However, sequence and timing of drug administration are crucial because the goal is to affect the largest numbers of cells during their susceptible phase.

Another major factor influencing the success of therapy is the use of supportive therapies that allow patients to better tolerate toxic effects of chemotherapeutic agents and experience improved quality of life during treatment.

Selected regimens

Hundreds of combination chemotherapy regimens exist. The regimens listed here are the most commonly used. They were chosen with guidance from oncology practitioners at major cancer centers throughout the United States. This selection is not meant to be all-inclusive or to direct a practitioner's specific choice of therapy, nor do the authors or publisher endorse or recommend any specific regimen.

Determining which regimen is best for a particular patient is based on professional judgment, experience, and the patient's diagnosis and clinical status; one must carefully weigh the regimen's anticipated benefits against potential risks. Typically, oncologists choose drugs, dosages, and administration routes based on efficacy, toxicity, the patient's condition, and previous treatment.

Organization

This section is arranged alphabetically by neoplastic disease. Within each disease entry, chemotherapy regimens are listed alphabetically by drug names. (Regimens for children are not included because, for most children, treatment is based on a national group protocol.) One or more shortened references follow each regimen; some pertain to the original study, others to follow-up investigations or trials. (For the complete reference, see *References*.)

For each regimen, you will find a detailed description of supportive therapy for complications that the regimen is likely to cause (for example, nausea and vomiting, diarrhea, anemia, or neutropenia). (See the front endpaper for specific antiemetic therapies.) These practical guidelines were developed in consultation with the same oncology experts who guided regimen selection. Keep in mind that some patients may require additional supportive care or may experience adverse effects not addressed here. For more detail on these supportive therapies, see Appendix F.

Acute myeloid leukemia

AIDA (all-*trans* retinoic acid, idarubicin) for promyelocytic leukemia

All-trans retinoic acid (ATRA) 45 mg/m² P.O. daily until complete remission or maximum of 90 days and *idarubicin* 12 mg/m² I.V. on days 2, 4, 6, and 8
Followed by three monthly consolidation cycles—
First cycle: *idarubicin* 5 mg/m² I.V. daily on days 1 through 4
Second cycle: *mitoxantrone* 10 mg/m² I.V. daily on days 1 through 5
Third cycle: *idarubicin* 12 mg/m² I.V. on day 1 only
Follow consolidation cycles with maintenance therapy until polymerase chain reaction is negative—
ATRA 45 mg/m² P.O. for 15 days every 3 months with or without methotrexate 15 mg/m² P.O. weekly and 6-mercaptopurine (6-MP) 90 mg/m² P.O. daily
Continue maintenance therapy for 2 years.
Reference: Sanz MA, et al. *Blood.* 1999;94:3015-3021; Avvisati G, et al. *Blood.* 1996;88:1390-1398.

Supportive therapy

For nausea and vomiting
On ATRA-only days, follow acute-onset antiemetic regimen for level 1 risk.
On days 2, 4, 6, and 8, follow acute-onset antiemetic regimen for level 3 risk. Anticipatory, breakthrough, and delayed-onset regimens are recommended as needed.
On ATRA plus 6-MP days, follow acute-onset antiemetic regimen for level 2 risk. Anticipatory, breakthrough, and delayed-onset regimens are recommended as needed.
On ATRA plus 6-MP plus methotrexate days, follow acute-onset antiemetic regimen for level 3 risk. Anticipatory, breakthrough, and delayed-onset regimens are recommended as needed.

For idarubicin and mitoxantrone consolidation courses, follow acute-onset antiemetic regimen for level 3 risk. Anticipatory, breakthrough, and delayed-onset regimens are recommended as needed. For maintenance therapy, follow acute-onset antiemetic regimen for level 1 risk.
For neutropenia (high risk)
To prevent neutropenia, start *one* of the following colony-stimulating factors 1 to 3 days after completion of chemotherapy and continue through postnadir recovery:
• Filgrastim 5 mcg/kg daily or
• Pegfilgrastim 6 mg once for each treatment cycle.

Cytarabine, daunorubicin (7+3)

Cytarabine 100 mg/m² I.V. daily for 7 days
Daunorubicin 45 mg/m² I.V. daily on days 1 through 3
After 14 days, if more than 5% of remaining nucleated cells are leukemic, give:
Cytarabine 100 mg/m² I.V. daily for 5 days
Daunorubicin 45 mg/m² I.V. daily on days 1 and 2
Reference: Volger WR. *J Clin Oncol.* 1992;10:1103-1111; Mayer RJ. *N Engl J Med.* 1994;331:896-903.

Supportive therapy

For nausea and vomiting
On days 1 through 3, follow acute-onset antiemetic regimen for level 4 risk. Anticipatory, breakthrough, and delayed-onset regimens are recommended as needed.
On days 4 through 7, follow acute-onset antiemetic regimen for level 2 risk. Anticipatory, breakthrough, and delayed-onset regimens are recommended as needed.
For neutropenia (high risk)
To prevent neutropenia, start *one* of the following colony-stimulating factors 1 to 3 days after completion of chemotherapy and continue through postnadir recovery:

- Filgrastim 5 mcg/kg daily or
- Pegfilgrastim 6 mg once for each treatment cycle.

For diarrhea (likely)
Prescribe antidiarrheal as indicated.

Gemtuzumab

Gemtuzumab 6 to 9 mg/m² I.V. over 2 hours on days 1 and 15. Third dose may be given if bone marrow polymerase chain reaction is negative.
Reference: Lo Coco F, et al. *Blood.* 2004;104:1995-1999; Larson RA, et al. *Leukemia.* 2002;16:1627-1636.

Supportive therapy
For nausea and vomiting
Follow acute-onset antiemetic regimen for level 1 risk.

For neutropenia (high risk)
To prevent neutropenia, start *one* of the following colony-stimulating factors 1 to 3 days after completion of chemotherapy and continue through postnadir recovery:
- Filgrastim 5 mcg/kg daily or
- Pegfilgrastim 6 mg once for each treatment cycle.

For infusion reactions
Consider premedication with acetaminophen and diphenhydramine to prevent infusion reactions.

HDAC, HiDAC (high-dose cytarabine)

Cytarabine 3 g/m² I.V. over 3 hours every 12 hours on days 1, 3, and 5
Give for four cycles.
Reference: Cassileth PA, et al. *N Engl J Med.* 1998;339:1649-1656.

Supportive therapy
For nausea and vomiting
Follow acute-onset antiemetic regimen for level 4 risk. Anticipatory, breakthrough, and delayed-onset regimens are recommended as needed.

For neutropenia (high risk)
To prevent neutropenia, start *one* of the following colony-stimulating factors 1 to 3 days after completion of chemotherapy and continue through postnadir recovery:
- Filgrastim 5 mcg/kg daily or
- Pegfilgrastim 6 mg once for each treatment cycle.

Diarrhea (likely)
Prescribe antidiarrheal as indicated.

For conjunctivitis
To prevent conjunctivitis associated with cytarabine syndrome, administer saline or steroid eyedrops to both eyes daily until 24 hours after completion of therapy.

Idarubicin, cytarabine (5+2)

Idarubicin 12 mg/m² I.V. daily for 2 days
Cytarabine Initial dose, 25 mg/m² I.V., then 100 mg/m² I.V. for 5 days
Reference: Cassileth PA, et al. *N Engl J Med.* 1998;339:1649-1656; Wiernik PH, et al. *Blood.* 1992;79:313-319.

Supportive therapy
For nausea and vomiting
On days 1 and 2, follow acute-onset antiemetic regimen for level 4 risk. Anticipatory, breakthrough, and delayed-onset regimens are recommended as needed.

On days 3 through 5, follow acute-onset antiemetic regimen for level 2 risk. Anticipatory, breakthrough, and delayed-onset regimens are recommended as needed.

For neutropenia (high risk)
To prevent neutropenia, start *one* of the following colony-stimulating factors 1 to 3 days after completion of chemotherapy and continue through postnadir recovery:
- Filgrastim 5 mcg/kg daily or
- Pegfilgrastim 6 mg once for each treatment cycle.

For diarrhea (likely)
Prescribe antidiarrheal as indicated.

Idarubicin, cytarabine (7+3)

Idarubicin 12 mg/m² I.V. daily for 3 days
Cytarabine 100 mg/m² I.V. for 7 days
May give second cycle after bone marrow evaluation on day 14.
Reference: Cassileth PA, et al. *N Engl J Med.* 1998;339:1649-1656; Wiernik PH, et al. *Blood.* 1992;79:313-319.

Supportive therapy
For nausea and vomiting
On days 1 through 3, follow acute-onset antiemetic regimen for level 4 risk. Anticipatory, breakthrough, and delayed-onset regimens are recommended as needed.

On days 4 through 7, follow acute-onset antiemetic regimen for level 2 risk. Anticipatory, breakthrough, and delayed-onset regimens are recommended as needed.
For neutropenia (high risk)
To prevent neutropenia, start *one* of the following colony-stimulating factors 1 to 3 days after completion of chemotherapy and continue through postnadir recovery:
• Filgrastim 5 mcg/kg daily or
• Pegfilgrastim 6 mg once for each treatment cycle.
For diarrhea (likely)
Prescribe antidiarrheal as indicated.

Bladder cancer

Cisplatin, docetaxel

Cisplatin 75 mg/m² I.V. on day 1
Docetaxel 75 mg/m² I.V. on day 1
Repeat cycle every 21 days.
Reference: Dimopoulos MA, et al. *Ann Oncol.* 1999;10:1385-1388; Sengelov L, et al. *J Clin Oncol.* 1998;3392-3397.

Supportive therapy
For nausea and vomiting
On day 1, follow acute-onset antiemetic regimen for level 5 risk. Anticipatory, breakthrough, and delayed-onset regimens are recommended.
For anemia (likely)
If hemoglobin level is less than 10 g/dl, *one* of the following is recommended:
• Epoetin alfa 150 units/kg subcutaneously three times weekly. If unsatisfactory response, may increase to 300 units/kg three times weekly.
• Epoetin alfa 40,000 units subcutaneously weekly; may increase to 60,000 units if unsatisfactory response.
• Darbepoetin alfa 3 mcg/kg subcutaneously every 2 weeks; may increase to 5 mcg/kg if unsatisfactory response.
• Darbepoetin alfa 200 mcg subcutaneously every 2 weeks; may increase to 300 mcg if unsatisfactory response.
For neutropenia (high risk)
To prevent neutropenia, start *one* of the following colony-stimulating factors 1 to 3 days after completion of chemotherapy and continue through postnadir recovery:
• Filgrastim 5 mcg/kg daily or
• Pegfilgrastim 6 mg once for each treatment cycle.
For hypersensitivity reactions
To prevent hypersensitivity reactions, administer dexamethasone 8 mg P.O. twice daily for 3 days starting 1 day before administration of docetaxel.
For cisplatin-induced nephrotoxicity
Maintain urine output of at least 75 ml/hour for several hours before and after each cisplatin dose. Consider amifostine for prevention of cisplatin-induced nephrotoxicity.

CMV (cisplatin, methotrexate, vinblastine)

Methotrexate 30 to 40 mg/m² I.V. on days 1 and 8
Vinblastine 4 mg/m² I.V. on days 1 and 8
Cisplatin 100 mg/m² I.V. over 4 hours on day 2
Repeat cycle every 21 days.

Reference: Harker WG, et al. *J Clin Oncol.*
1985;3:1463-1470; Wie CH, et al. *J Urol.*
1996;155:118-125.

Supportive therapy

For nausea and vomiting
On days 1 and 8, follow acute-onset antiemetic regimen for level 1 risk.
    On day 2, follow acute-onset antiemetic regimen for level 5 risk. Anticipatory, breakthrough, and delayed-onset regimens are recommended.

For anemia (likely)
If hemoglobin level is less than 10 g/dl, *one* of the following is recommended:
* Epoetin alfa 150 units/kg subcutaneously three times weekly. If unsatisfactory response, may increase to 300 units/kg three times weekly.
* Epoetin alfa 40,000 units subcutaneously weekly; may increase to 60,000 units if unsatisfactory response.
* Darbepoetin alfa 3 mcg/kg subcutaneously every 2 weeks; may increase to 5 mcg/kg if unsatisfactory response.
* Darbepoetin alfa 200 mcg subcutaneously every 2 weeks; may increase to 300 mcg if unsatisfactory response.

For neutropenia (high risk)
To prevent neutropenia, start *one* of the following colony-stimulating factors 1 to 3 days after completion of chemotherapy and continue through postnadir recovery:
* Filgrastim 5 mcg/kg daily or
* Pegfilgrastim 6 mg once for each treatment cycle.

For diarrhea (likely)
Prescribe antidiarrheal as indicated.

For cisplatin-induced nephrotoxicity
Maintain urine output of at least 75 ml/hour for several hours before and after each cisplatin dose. Consider amifostine for prevention of cisplatin-induced nephrotoxicity.

Gemcitabine

Gemcitabine 1,200 mg/m^2 I.V on, days 1, 8, and 15
Repeat every 28 days for maximum of six cycles.
Reference: von der Maase H. *Crit Rev Oncol Hematol.* 2000;34(3):175-183.

Supportive therapy

For nausea and vomiting
Follow acute-onset antiemetic regimen for level 2 risk. Anticipatory, breakthrough, and delayed-onset regimens are recommended as needed.

For anemia (likely)
If hemoglobin level is less than 10 g/dl, *one* of the following is recommended:
* Epoetin alfa 150 units/kg subcutaneously three times weekly. If unsatisfactory response, may increase to 300 units/kg three times weekly.
* Epoetin alfa 40,000 units subcutaneously weekly; may increase to 60,000 units if unsatisfactory response.
* Darbepoetin alfa 3 mcg/kg subcutaneously every 2 weeks; may increase to 5 mcg/kg if unsatisfactory response.
* Darbepoetin alfa 200 mcg subcutaneously every 2 weeks; may increase to 300 mcg if unsatisfactory response.

Gemcitabine, cisplatin

Gemcitabine 1,000 mg/m^2 I.V. on days 1, 8, and 15
Cisplatin 70 mg/m^2 I.V. on day 2
Repeat cycle every 28 days for maximum of six cycles.
Reference: von der Masse H, et al. *J Clin Oncol.* 2000;17:3068-3077.

Supportive therapy

For nausea and vomiting
On days 1, 8, and 15, follow acute-onset antiemetic regimen for level 2 risk. Anticipa-

tory, breakthrough, and delayed-onset regimens are recommended as needed.

On day 2, follow acute-onset antiemetic regimen for level 5 risk. Anticipatory, breakthrough, and delayed-onset regimens are recommended.

For anemia (likely)
If hemoglobin level is less than 10 g/dl, *one* of the following is recommended:
• Epoetin alfa 150 units/kg subcutaneously three times weekly. If unsatisfactory response, may increase to 300 units/kg three times weekly.
• Epoetin alfa 40,000 units subcutaneously weekly; may increase to 60,000 units if unsatisfactory response.
• Darbepoetin alfa 3 mcg/kg subcutaneously every 2 weeks; may increase to 5 mcg/kg if unsatisfactory response.
• Darbepoetin alfa 200 mcg subcutaneously every 2 weeks; may increase to 300 mcg if unsatisfactory response.

For neutropenia (high risk)
To prevent neutropenia, start *one* of the following colony-stimulating factors 1 to 3 days after completion of chemotherapy and continue through postnadir recovery:
• Filgrastim 5 mcg/kg daily or
• Pegfilgrastim 6 mg once for each treatment cycle.

For cisplatin-induced nephrotoxicity
Maintain urine output of at least 75 ml/hour for several hours before and after each cisplatin dose. Consider amifostine for prevention of cisplatin-induced nephrotoxicity.

ITP (ifosfamide, paclitaxel [Taxol], cisplatin [Platinol-AQ])

Ifosfamide 1,500 mg/m^2 I.V. on days 1 through 3 with mesna 300 mg/m^2 I.V. for three doses (30 minutes before start of ifosfamide, 4 hours later, and 8 hours later) on days 1 through 3
Paclitaxel 200 mg/m^2 I.V. over 3 hours on day 1
Cisplatin 70 mg/m^2 on day 1
Repeat cycle every 28 days.

Reference: Bajorin DF. *Cancer.* 2000;88:1671-1678.

Supportive therapy
For nausea and vomiting
On day 1, follow acute-onset antiemetic regimen for level 5 risk. Anticipatory, breakthrough, and delayed-onset regimens are recommended.

On days 2 and 3, follow acute-onset antiemetic regimen for level 3 risk. Anticipatory, breakthrough, and delayed-onset regimens are recommended as needed.

For anemia (likely)
If hemoglobin level is less than 10 g/dl, *one* of the following is recommended:
• Epoetin alfa 150 units/kg subcutaneously three times weekly. If unsatisfactory response, may increase to 300 units/kg three times weekly.
• Epoetin alfa 40,000 units subcutaneously weekly; may increase to 60,000 units if unsatisfactory response.
• Darbepoetin alfa 3 mcg/kg subcutaneously every 2 weeks; may increase to 5 mcg/kg if unsatisfactory response.
• Darbepoetin alfa 200 mcg subcutaneously every 2 weeks; may increase to 300 mcg if unsatisfactory response.

For neutropenia (high risk)
To prevent neutropenia, start *one* of the following colony-stimulating factors 1 to 3 days after completion of chemotherapy and continue through postnadir recovery:
• Filgrastim 5 mcg/kg daily or
• Pegfilgrastim 6 mg once for each treatment cycle.

For hypersensitivity reactions
To prevent hypersensitivity reactions, give the following before paclitaxel administration: dexamethasone 20 mg P.O. 12 hours and 6 hours before, diphenhydramine 50 mg I.V. 30 to 60 minutes before, *and* cimetidine 300 mg I.V. or ranitidine 50 mg I.V. 30 to 60 minutes before.

For cisplatin-induced nephrotoxicity
Maintain urine output of at least 75 ml/hour

for several hours before and after each cisplatin dose. Consider amifostine for prevention of cisplatin-induced nephrotoxicity.

MVAC (methotrexate, vinblastine, doxorubicin [Adriamycin], cisplatin)

Methotrexate 30 mg/m^2 I.V. on days 1, 15, and 22
Vinblastine 3 mg/m^2 I.V. on days 2, 15, and 22
Doxorubicin 30 mg/m^2 I.V. on day 2
Cisplatin 70 mg/m^2 I.V. on day 2
Repeat cycle every 28 days.
Reference: von der Masse H, et al. *J Clin Oncol.* 2000;17:3068-3077.

Supportive therapy
For nausea and vomiting
On days 1, 15, and 22, follow acute-onset antiemetic regimen for level 1 risk.

On day 2, follow acute-onset antiemetic regimen for level 5 risk. Anticipatory, breakthrough, and delayed-onset regimens are recommended.
For neutropenia (high risk)
To prevent neutropenia, start *one* of the following colony-stimulating factors 1 to 3 days after completion of chemotherapy and continue through postnadir recovery:
• Filgrastim 5 mcg/kg daily or
• Pegfilgrastim 6 mg once for each treatment cycle.
For cisplatin-induced nephrotoxicity
Maintain urine output of at least 75 ml/hour for several hours before and after each cisplatin dose. Consider amifostine for prevention of cisplatin-induced nephrotoxicity.

Paclitaxel

Paclitaxel 250 mg/m^2 I.V. over 24 hours on day 1
Repeat every 21 days.
Reference: Roth BJ, et al. *J Clin Oncol.* 1994;12:2264-2270.

Supportive therapy
For nausea and vomiting
Follow acute-onset antiemetic regimen for level 2 risk. Anticipatory, breakthrough, and delayed-onset regimens are recommended as needed.
For anemia (likely)
If hemoglobin level is less than 10 g/dl, *one* of the following is recommended:
• Epoetin alfa 150 units/kg subcutaneously three times weekly. If unsatisfactory response, may increase to 300 units/kg three times weekly.
• Epoetin alfa 40,000 units subcutaneously weekly; may increase to 60,000 units if unsatisfactory response.
• Darbepoetin alfa 3 mcg/kg subcutaneously every 2 weeks; may increase to 5 mcg/kg if unsatisfactory response.
• Darbepoetin alfa 200 mcg subcutaneously every 2 weeks; may increase to 300 mcg if unsatisfactory response.
For neutropenia (high risk)
To prevent neutropenia, start *one* of the following colony-stimulating factors 1 to 3 days after completion of chemotherapy and continue through postnadir recovery:
• Filgrastim 5 mcg/kg daily or
• Pegfilgrastim 6 mg once for each treatment cycle.
For hypersensitivity reactions
To prevent hypersensitivity reactions, give the following before paclitaxel administration: dexamethasone 20 mg P.O. 12 hours and 6 hours before, diphenhydramine 50 mg I.V. 30 to 60 minutes before, *and* cimetidine 300 mg I.V. or ranitidine 50 mg I.V. 30 to 60 minutes before.

Paclitaxel, gemcitabine

Paclitaxel 200 mg/m^2 by I.V. infusion over 1 hour on day 1
Gemcitabine 1,000 mg/m^2 I.V. on days 1, 8, and 15
Repeat cycle every 21 days.

Reference: Meluch AA, et al. *J Clin Oncol.* 2001;19:3018-3024.

Supportive therapy
For nausea and vomiting
On day 1, follow acute-onset antiemetic regimen for level 3 risk. Anticipatory, breakthrough, and delayed-onset regimens are recommended as needed.

On days 8 and 15, follow acute-onset antiemetic regimen for level 2 risk. Anticipatory, breakthrough, and delayed-onset regimens are recommended as needed.
For anemia (likely)
If hemoglobin level is less than 10 g/dl, *one* of the following is recommended:
• Epoetin alfa 150 units/kg subcutaneously three times weekly. If unsatisfactory response, may increase to 300 units/kg three times weekly.
• Epoetin alfa 40,000 units subcutaneously weekly; may increase to 60,000 units if unsatisfactory response.
• Darbepoetin alfa 3 mcg/kg subcutaneously every 2 weeks; may increase to 5 mcg/kg if unsatisfactory response.
• Darbepoetin alfa 200 mcg subcutaneously every 2 weeks; may increase to 300 mcg if unsatisfactory response.
For neutropenia (high risk)
To prevent neutropenia, start *one* of the following colony-stimulating factors 1 to 3 days after completion of chemotherapy and continue through postnadir recovery:
• Filgrastim 5 mcg/kg daily or
• Pegfilgrastim 6 mg once for each treatment cycle.
For hypersensitivity reactions
To prevent hypersensitivity reactions, give the following before paclitaxel administration: dexamethasone 20 mg P.O. 12 hours and 6 hours before, diphenhydramine 50 mg I.V. 30 to 60 minutes before, *and* cimetidine 300 mg I.V. or ranitidine 50 mg I.V. 30 to 60 minutes before.

PC (paclitaxel, carboplatin)

Paclitaxel 225 mg/m^2 I.V. over 3 hours on day 1
Carboplatin to AUC of 6 mg/ml/minute I.V. on day 1, given 15 minutes after paclitaxel
Repeat cycle every 21 days.
Reference: Dreicer R. *Cancer.* 2004;100:1639-1645.

Supportive therapy
For nausea and vomiting
Follow acute-onset antiemetic regimen for level 5 risk. Anticipatory, breakthrough, and delayed-onset regimens are recommended.
For neutropenia (high risk)
To prevent neutropenia, start *one* of the following colony-stimulating factors 1 to 3 days after completion of chemotherapy and continue through postnadir recovery:
• Filgrastim 5 mcg/kg daily or
• Pegfilgrastim 6 mg once for each treatment cycle.
For hypersensitivity reactions
To prevent hypersensitivity reactions, give the following before paclitaxel administration: dexamethasone 20 mg P.O. 12 hours and 6 hours before, diphenhydramine 50 mg I.V. 30 to 60 minutes before, *and* cimetidine 300 mg I.V. or ranitidine 50 mg I.V. 30 to 60 minutes before.
For cisplatin-induced nephrotoxicity
Maintain urine output of at least 75 ml/hour for several hours before and after each cisplatin dose. Consider amifostine for prevention of cisplatin-induced nephrotoxicity.

Bone sarcoma

CAV (cyclophosphamide, doxorubicin [Adriamycin], vincristine) alternating with IE (ifosfamide, etoposide)

CAV
Cyclophosphamide 1,200 mg/m^2 I.V. and mes-

na 240 mg/m² I.V. on day 1; repeat mesna every 3 hours for three to four doses
Doxorubicin 75 mg/m² I.V. on day 1 (after 375 mg/m² cumulative dose of doxorubicin, substitute dactinomycin 1.25 mg/m² I.V.)
Vincristine 2 mg I.V. on day 1

IE

Ifosfamide 1,800 mg/m² I.V. with mesna 360 mg/m² I.V. for three doses (given initially with ifosfamide, then 4 hours later, and 8 hours later) on days 1 through 5
Etoposide 100 mg/m² I.V.on days 1 through 5
Alternate CAV with IE regimens every 21 days for total of 17 cycles.

Reference: Holcombe E, et al. *N Engl J Med.* 2003;348:694-671.

Supportive therapy
For nausea and vomiting
On CAV day 1, follow acute-onset antiemetic regimen for level 5 risk. Anticipatory, breakthrough, and delayed-onset regimens are recommended.

On IE days 1 to 5, follow acute-onset antiemetic regimen for level 4 risk. Anticipatory, breakthrough, and delayed-onset regimens are recommended as needed.

For neutropenia (high risk)
To prevent neutropenia, start *one* of the following colony-stimulating factors 1 to 3 days after completion of chemotherapy and continue through postnadir recovery:
• Filgrastim 5 mcg/kg daily or
• Pegfilgrastim 6 mg once for each treatment cycle.

Methotrexate, leucovorin

Methotrexate 800 to 1,200 mg/m² I.V. on days 1, 8, 29, and 36 before resection
Leucovorin 10 to 15 mg P.O. every 6 hours for 10 doses, starting 20 hours after each methotrexate dose and discontinued when serum methotrexate level is less than 100 nmol/L
Reference: Pazdur R (ed), et al. *Cancer Management: A Multidisciplinary Approach.* 9th ed. CMP Healthcare Media; 2005.

Supportive therapy
For nausea and vomiting
Follow acute-onset antiemetic regimen for level 4 emetic risk. Anticipatory, breakthrough, and delayed-onset regimens are recommended as needed.

For anemia (likely)
If hemoglobin level is less than 10 g/dl, *one* of the following is recommended:
• Epoetin alfa 150 units/kg subcutaneously three times weekly. If unsatisfactory response, may increase to 300 units/kg three times weekly.
• Epoetin alfa 40,000 units subcutaneously weekly; may increase to 60,000 units if unsatisfactory response.
• Darbepoetin alfa 3 mcg/kg subcutaneously every 2 weeks; may increase to 5 mcg/kg if unsatisfactory response.
• Darbepoetin alfa 200 mcg subcutaneously every 2 weeks; may increase to 300 mcg if unsatisfactory response.

For neutropenia (high risk)
To prevent neutropenia, start *one* of the following colony-stimulating factors 1 to 3 days after completion of chemotherapy and continue through postnadir recovery:
• Filgrastim 5 mcg/kg daily or
• Pegfilgrastim 6 mg once for each treatment cycle.

For diarrhea (likely)
Prescribe antidiarrheal as indicated.

Breast cancer

AC (doxorubicin [Adriamycin], cyclophosphamide)

Doxorubicin 60 mg/m² I.V. on day 1
Cyclophosphamide 600 mg/m² I.V. on day 1
Repeat cycle every 21 days.

Reference: Fisher B, et al. *J Clin Oncol.* 1990;8:2150-2156; Fisher B, et al. *J Clin Oncol.* 1997;15:1858-1869.

Supportive therapy
For nausea and vomiting
Follow acute-onset antiemetic regimen for level 5 risk. Anticipatory, breakthrough, and delayed-onset regimens are recommended.
For neutropenia (high risk)
To prevent neutropenia, start *one* of the following colony-stimulating factors 1 to 3 days after completion of chemotherapy and continue through postnadir recovery:
- Filgrastim 5 mcg/kg daily or
- Pegfilgrastim 6 mg once for each treatment cycle.

Bevacizumab, paclitaxel

Bevacizumab 10 mg/kg I.V. over 90 minutes on days 1 and 15; if tolerated, may decrease rate of infusion to 30 to 60 minutes
Paclitaxel 90 mg/m^2 I.V. on days 1, 8, and 15
Repeat cycle every 28 days.
Reference: Sledge GW. *Breast Cancer Update* [Online]. 2005; Shulman LN, et al. *Medscape.* 2005; Miller KD, et al. Presentation at ASCO Meeting; 2005.

Supportive therapy
For nausea and vomiting
Follow acute-onset antiemetic regimen for level 2 risk. Anticipatory, breakthrough, and delayed-onset regimens are recommended as needed.
For hypersensitivity reactions
To prevent hypersensitivity reactions, give the following before paclitaxel administration: dexamethasone 20 mg P.O. 12 hours and 6 hours before, diphenhydramine 50 mg I.V. 30 to 60 minutes before, *and* cimetidine 300 mg I.V. or ranitidine 50 mg I.V. 30 to 60 minutes before.

Capecitabine

Capecitabine 1,250 mg/m^2 P.O. twice daily on days 1 through 14
Repeat every 21 days.

Reference: Fumoleau P, et al. *Eur J Cancer.* 2004;40:536-542.

Supportive therapy
For nausea and vomiting
Follow acute-onset antiemetic regimen for level 2 risk. Anticipatory, breakthrough, and delayed-onset regimens are recommended as needed.
For anemia (likely)
If hemoglobin level is less than 10 g/dl, *one* of the following is recommended:
- Epoetin alfa 150 units/kg subcutaneously three times weekly. If unsatisfactory response, may increase to 300 units/kg three times weekly.
- Epoetin alfa 40,000 units subcutaneously weekly; may increase to 60,000 units if unsatisfactory response.
- Darbepoetin alfa 3 mcg/kg subcutaneously every 2 weeks; may increase to 5 mcg/kg if unsatisfactory response.
- Darbepoetin alfa 200 mcg subcutaneously every 2 weeks; may increase to 300 mcg if unsatisfactory response.
For neutropenia (intermediate risk)
To prevent neutropenia, consider starting *one* of the following colony-stimulating factors 1 to 3 days after completion of chemotherapy and continuing through postnadir recovery:
- Filgrastim 5 mcg/kg daily or
- Pegfilgrastim 6 mg once for each treatment cycle.
For diarrhea (likely)
Prescribe antidiarrheal as indicated.

CMF (cyclophosphamide, methotrexate, 5-fluorouracil)

Patients younger than age 60:
Cyclophosphamide 100 mg/m^2 P.O. on days 1 through 14
Methotrexate 40 mg/m^2 I.V. on days 1 and 8
5-Fluorouracil (5-FU) 600 mg/m^2 I.V. on days 1 and 8
Repeat cycle every 28 days.

Patients older than age 60:
Cyclophosphamide 100 mg/m² P.O. on days 1 through 14
Methotrexate 30 mg/m² I.V. on days 1 and 8
5-FU 400 mg/m² I.V. on days 1 and 8
Repeat cycle every 28 days.
Reference: Bonadonna G, et al. *N Engl J Med.* 1976;294:405-410; Bonadonna G, et al. *N Engl J Med.* 1995;332:901-906; Amadori D, et al. *J Clin Oncol.* 2000;18:3125-3134.

Supportive therapy
For nausea and vomiting
On days 1 and 8, follow acute-onset antiemetic regimen level 4 risk. Anticipatory, breakthrough, and delayed-onset regimens are recommended as needed.

On days 2 through 7 and 9 through 14, follow acute-onset antiemetic regimen for level 3 risk. Anticipatory, breakthrough, and delayed-onset regimens are recommended as needed.
For anemia (likely)
If hemoglobin level is less than 10 g/dl, *one* of the following is recommended:
• Epoetin alfa 150 units/kg subcutaneously three times weekly. If unsatisfactory response, may increase to 300 units/kg three times weekly.
• Epoetin alfa 40,000 units subcutaneously weekly; may increase to 60,000 units if unsatisfactory response.
• Darbepoetin alfa 3 mcg/kg subcutaneously every 2 weeks; may increase to 5 mcg/kg if unsatisfactory response.
• Darbepoetin alfa 200 mcg subcutaneously every 2 weeks; may increase to 300 mcg if unsatisfactory response.
For neutropenia (high risk)
To prevent neutropenia, start *one* of the following colony-stimulating factors 1 to 3 days after completion of chemotherapy and continue through postnadir recovery:
• Filgrastim 5 mcg/kg daily or
• Pegfilgrastim 6 mg once for each treatment cycle.

Docetaxel

Docetaxel 60 to 100 mg/m² I.V. over 1 hour on day 1
Repeat every 21 days.
Reference: Nabholtz J-M, et al. *J Clin Oncol.* 1999;17:1413-1424; docetaxel prescribing information.

Supportive therapy
For nausea and vomiting
Follow acute-onset antiemetic regimen for level 2 risk. Anticipatory, breakthrough, and delayed-onset regimens are recommended as needed.
For anemia (likely)
If hemoglobin level is less than 10 g/dl, *one* of the following is recommended:
• Epoetin alfa 150 units/kg subcutaneously three times weekly. If unsatisfactory response, may increase to 300 units/kg three times weekly.
• Epoetin alfa 40,000 units subcutaneously weekly; may increase to 60,000 units if unsatisfactory response.
• Darbepoetin alfa 3 mcg/kg subcutaneously every 2 weeks; may increase to 5 mcg/kg if unsatisfactory response.
• Darbepoetin alfa 200 mcg subcutaneously every 2 weeks; may increase to 300 mcg if unsatisfactory response.
For neutropenia (high risk)
To prevent neutropenia, start *one* of the following colony-stimulating factors 1 to 3 days after completion of chemotherapy and continue through postnadir recovery:
• Filgrastim 5 mcg/kg daily or
• Pegfilgrastim 6 mg once for each treatment cycle.
For diarrhea (likely)
Prescribe antidiarrheal as indicated.
For hypersensitivity reactions
To prevent hypersensitivity reactions, administer dexamethasone 8 mg P.O. twice daily for 3 days starting 1 day before administration of docetaxel.

Doxorubicin

Doxorubicin 60 to 75 mg/m^2 I.V. on day 1
Repeat every 21 days.
Or
Doxorubicin 20 mg/m^2 I.V. on day 1
Repeat every 7 days.
Reference: Breast cancer. NCCN Practice
Guidelines in Oncology, 2005.

Supportive therapy
For nausea and vomiting
With doxorubicin 60 to 75 mg/m^2, follow
acute-onset antiemetic regimen for level 4
risk. Anticipatory, breakthrough, and delayed-
onset regimens are recommended as needed.
   With doxorubicin 20 mg/m^2, follow acute-
onset antiemetic regimen for level 3 risk. Anticipatory, breakthrough, and delayed-onset
regimens are recommended as needed.
For neutropenia (intermediate risk)
To prevent neutropenia, consider starting *one*
of the following colony-stimulating factors 1
to 3 days after completion of chemotherapy
and continuing through postnadir recovery:
• Filgrastim 5 mcg/kg daily or
• Pegfilgrastim 6 mg once for each treatment
cycle.

Epirubicin

Epirubicin 60 to 90 mg/m^2 I.V. on day 1
Repeat every 21 days.
Reference: Breast cancer. NCCN Practice
Guidelines in Oncology, 2005.

Supportive therapy
For nausea and vomiting
Follow acute-onset antiemetic regimen for level 3 risk. Anticipatory, breakthrough, and delayed-onset regimens are recommended as
needed.
For neutropenia (intermediate risk)
To prevent neutropenia, consider starting *one*
of the following colony-stimulating factors 1
to 3 days after completion of chemotherapy
and continuing through postnadir recovery:

• Filgrastim 5 mcg/kg daily or
• Pegfilgrastim 6 mg once for each treatment
cycle.

FAC (or CAF) (5-fluorouracil, doxoru-bicin [Adriamycin], cyclophospha-mide)

5-Fluorouracil (5-FU) 500 mg/m^2 I.V. on day 1
Doxorubicin 50 mg/m^2 I.V. on day 1
Cyclophosphamide 500 mg/m^2 I.V. on day 1
Repeat cycle every 21 days.
Or
Cyclophosphamide 600 mg/m^2 I.V. on day 1
Doxorubicin 60 mg/m^2 I.V. on day 1
5-FU 600 mg/m^2 I.V. on days 1 and 8
Repeat cycle every 28 days.
Reference: Stewart DJ, et al. *J Clin Oncol.*
1997;15:1897-1905; Budman DR, et al. *J Natl
Cancer Inst.* 1998;90:1205-1211.

Supportive therapy
For nausea and vomiting
On day 1, follow acute-onset antiemetic regimen for level 5 risk. Anticipatory, breakthrough, and delayed-onset regimens are recommended.
   On day 8, follow acute-onset antiemetic
regimen for level 2 risk. Anticipatory, breakthrough, and delayed-onset regimens are recommended as needed.
For anemia (likely)
If hemoglobin level is less than 10 g/dl, *one* of
the following is recommended:
• Epoetin alfa 150 units/kg subcutaneously
three times weekly. If unsatisfactory response,
may increase to 300 units/kg three times
weekly.
• Epoetin alfa 40,000 units subcutaneously
weekly; may increase to 60,000 units if unsatisfactory response.
• Darbepoetin alfa 3 mcg/kg subcutaneously
every 2 weeks; may increase to 5 mcg/kg if
unsatisfactory response.
• Darbepoetin alfa 200 mcg subcutaneously
every 2 weeks; may increase to 300 mcg if unsatisfactory response.

For neutropenia (high risk)
To prevent neutropenia, start **one** of the following colony-stimulating factors 1 to 3 days after completion of chemotherapy and continue through postnadir recovery:
- Filgrastim 5 mcg/kg daily or
- Pegfilgrastim 6 mg once for each treatment cycle.

For diarrhea (likely)
Prescribe antidiarrheal as indicated.

For constipation (likely)
Order stool softener or laxative as indicated.

FEC-100 (5-fluorouracil, epirubicin, cyclophosphamide)

5-Fluorouracil 500 mg/m^2 I.V. on day 1
Epirubicin 100 mg/m^2 I.V. on day 1
Cyclophosphamide 500 mg/m^2 I.V. on day 1
Repeat cycle every 21 days.
Reference: French Epirubicin Study Group. *J Clin Oncol.* 200;18:3115-3124.

Supportive therapy

For nausea and vomiting
Follow acute-onset antiemetic regimen for level 5 risk. Anticipatory, breakthrough, and delayed-onset regimens are recommended.

For anemia (likely)
If hemoglobin level is less than 10 g/dl, **one** of the following is recommended:
- Epoetin alfa 150 units/kg subcutaneously three times weekly. If unsatisfactory response, may increase to 300 units/kg three times weekly.
- Epoetin alfa 40,000 units subcutaneously weekly; may increase to 60,000 units if unsatisfactory response.
- Darbepoetin alfa 3 mcg/kg subcutaneously every 2 weeks; may increase to 5 mcg/kg if unsatisfactory response.
- Darbepoetin alfa 200 mcg subcutaneously every 2 weeks; may increase to 300 mcg if unsatisfactory response.

For neutropenia (high risk)
To prevent neutropenia, start **one** of the following colony-stimulating factors 1 to 3 days

after completion of chemotherapy and continue through postnadir recovery:
- Filgrastim 5 mcg/kg daily or
- Pegfilgrastim 6 mg once for each treatment cycle.

For diarrhea (likely)
Prescribe antidiarrheal as indicated.

GT (gemcitabine, paclitaxel [Taxol])

Paclitaxel 175 mg/m^2 I.V. over 3 hours on day 1 only before gemcitabine
Gemcitabine 1,250 mg/m^2 I.V. over 30 minutes on days 1 and 8
Repeat cycle every 21 days.
Reference: Albain K, et al. *ASCO.* 2004;23: Abstract #510.

Supportive therapy

For nausea and vomiting
Follow acute-onset antiemetic regimen for level 3 risk. Anticipatory, breakthrough, and delayed-onset regimens are recommended as needed.

For anemia (likely)
If hemoglobin level is less than 10 g/dl, **one** of the following is recommended:
- Epoetin alfa 150 units/kg subcutaneously three times weekly. If unsatisfactory response, may increase to 300 units/kg three times weekly.
- Epoetin alfa 40,000 units subcutaneously weekly; may increase to 60,000 units if unsatisfactory response.
- Darbepoetin alfa 3 mcg/kg subcutaneously every 2 weeks; may increase to 5 mcg/kg if unsatisfactory response.
- Darbepoetin alfa 200 mcg subcutaneously every 2 weeks; may increase to 300 mcg if unsatisfactory response.

For neutropenia (high risk)
To prevent neutropenia, start **one** of the following colony-stimulating factors 1 to 3 days after completion of chemotherapy and continue through postnadir recovery:
- Filgrastim 5 mcg/kg daily or

• Pegfilgrastim 6 mg once for each treatment cycle.

For hypersensitivity reactions

To prevent hypersensitivity reactions, give the following before paclitaxel administration: dexamethasone 20 mg P.O. 12 hours and 6 hours before, diphenhydramine 50 mg I.V. 30 to 60 minutes before, *and* cimetidine 300 mg I.V. or ranitidine 50 mg I.V. 30 to 60 minutes before.

Paclitaxel

Paclitaxel 175 or 250 mg/m² I.V. over 3 hours on day 1

Repeat every 21 days.

Or

Paclitaxel 80 mg/m² I.V. over 1 hour on day 1

Repeat every 7 days.

Reference: Seidman AD, et al. *J Clin Oncol.* 1995;13:2575-2581; Smith RE, et al. *J Clin Oncol.* 1999;17:3403-3411; *Breast cancer.* NCCN Practice Guidelines in Oncology, 2005.

Supportive therapy

For nausea and vomiting

Follow acute-onset antiemetic regimen for level 2 risk. Anticipatory, breakthrough, and delayed-onset regimens are recommended as needed.

For anemia (likely)

If hemoglobin level is less than 10 g/dl, *one* of the following is recommended:

• Epoetin alfa 150 units/kg subcutaneously three times weekly. If unsatisfactory response, may increase to 300 units/kg three times weekly.

• Epoetin alfa 40,000 units subcutaneously weekly; may increase to 60,000 units if unsatisfactory response.

• Darbepoetin alfa 3 mcg/kg subcutaneously every 2 weeks; may increase to 5 mcg/kg if unsatisfactory response.

• Darbepoetin alfa 200 mcg subcutaneously every 2 weeks; may increase to 300 mcg if unsatisfactory response.

For neutropenia (high risk)

To prevent neutropenia, start *one* of the following colony-stimulating factors 1 to 3 days after completion of chemotherapy and continue through postnadir recovery:

• Filgrastim 5 mcg/kg daily or

• Pegfilgrastim 6 mg once for each treatment cycle.

For diarrhea (likely)

Prescribe antidiarrheal as indicated.

For hypersensitivity reactions

To prevent hypersensitivity reactions, give the following before paclitaxel administration: dexamethasone 20 mg P.O. 12 hours and 6 hours before, diphenhydramine 50 mg I.V. 30 to 60 minutes before, *and* cimetidine 300 mg I.V. or ranitidine 50 mg I.V. 30 to 60 minutes before.

Pegylated liposomal doxorubicin

Pegylated liposomal doxorubicin 45 mg/m² I.V. over 1 hour on day 1

Repeat every 21 days.

Reference: Ransom MR, et al. *J Clin Oncol.* 1997;15:3185-3191.

Supportive therapy

For nausea and vomiting

Follow acute-onset antiemetic regimen for level 2 risk. Anticipatory, breakthrough, and delayed-onset regimens are recommended as needed.

For neutropenia (intermediate risk)

To prevent neutropenia, consider starting *one* of the following colony-stimulating factors 1 to 3 days after completion of chemotherapy and continuing through postnadir recovery:

• Filgrastim 5 mcg/kg daily or

• Pegfilgrastim 6 mg once for each treatment cycle.

Trastuzumab, vinorelbine

Trastuzumab 4 mg/kg I.V. over 90 minutes on day 1 of first cycle. Give 2 mg/kg I.V. over 30 minutes in subsequent cycles.

Vinorelbine 25 mg/m² I.V. over 6 to 10 minutes (given after trastuzumab). Follow with 125 ml of saline I.V.
Repeat cycle every 7 days.
Reference: Burstein HJ, et al. *J Clin Oncol.* 2001;19:2722-2730; Burstein HJ, et al. *J Clin Oncol.* 2003;21:2889-2895.

Supportive therapy
For nausea and vomiting
Follow acute-onset antiemetic regimen for level 1 risk.
For anemia (likely)
If hemoglobin level is less than 10 g/dl, *one* of the following is recommended:
• Epoetin alfa 150 units/kg subcutaneously three times weekly. If unsatisfactory response, may increase to 300 units/kg three times weekly.
• Epoetin alfa 40,000 units subcutaneously weekly; may increase to 60,000 units if unsatisfactory response.
• Darbepoetin alfa 3 mcg/kg subcutaneously every 2 weeks; may increase to 5 mcg/kg if unsatisfactory response.
• Darbepoetin alfa 200 mcg subcutaneously every 2 weeks; may increase to 300 mcg if unsatisfactory response.
For neutropenia (intermediate risk)
To prevent neutropenia, consider starting *one* of the following colony-stimulating factors 1 to 3 days after completion of chemotherapy and continuing through postnadir recovery:
• Filgrastim 5 mcg/kg daily or
• Pegfilgrastim 6 mg once for each treatment cycle.
For diarrhea (likely)
Prescribe antidiarrheal as indicated.

Cervical cancer
Carboplatin

Carboplatin 300 mg/m² I.V. over 30 minutes on day 1 with concurrent pelvic radiation therapy
Repeat every 21 days.
Reference: Dubay RA, et al. *Gynecol Oncol.* 2004;94(1):121-124

Supportive therapy
For nausea and vomiting
Follow acute-onset antiemetic regimen for level 4 risk. Anticipatory, breakthrough, and delayed-onset regimens are recommended as needed.
For anemia (likely)
If hemoglobin level is less than 10 g/dl, *one* of the following is recommended:
• Epoetin alfa 150 units/kg subcutaneously three times weekly. If unsatisfactory response, may increase to 300 units/kg three times weekly.
• Epoetin alfa 40,000 units subcutaneously weekly; may increase to 60,000 units if unsatisfactory response.
• Darbepoetin alfa 3 mcg/kg subcutaneously every 2 weeks; may increase to 5 mcg/kg if unsatisfactory response.
• Darbepoetin alfa 200 mcg subcutaneously every 2 weeks; may increase to 300 mcg if unsatisfactory response.
For neutropenia (high risk)
To prevent neutropenia, start *one* of the following colony-stimulating factors 1 to 3 days after completion of chemotherapy and continue through postnadir recovery:
• Filgrastim 5 mcg/kg daily or
• Pegfilgrastim 6 mg once for each treatment cycle.
For diarrhea (likely)
Prescribe antidiarrheal as indicated.
For constipation (likely)
Order stool softener or laxative as indicated.

Cisplatin

Cisplatin 50 to 100 mg/m² I.V. on day 1
Repeat every 21 days.
Reference: Bonomi P, et al. *J Clin Oncol.*
1985;3(8):1079-1085.

Supportive therapy

For nausea and vomiting
Follow acute-onset antiemetic regimen for level 4 risk. Anticipatory, breakthrough, and delayed-onset regimens are recommended as needed.

For anemia (likely)
If hemoglobin level is less than 10 g/dl, *one* of the following is recommended:
• Epoetin alfa 150 units/kg subcutaneously three times weekly. If unsatisfactory response, may increase to 300 units/kg three times weekly.
• Epoetin alfa 40,000 units subcutaneously weekly; may increase to 60,000 units if unsatisfactory response.
• Darbepoetin alfa 3 mcg/kg subcutaneously every 2 weeks; may increase to 5 mcg/kg if unsatisfactory response.
• Darbepoetin alfa 200 mcg subcutaneously every 2 weeks; may increase to 300 mcg if unsatisfactory response.

For neutropenia (intermediate risk)
To prevent neutropenia, consider starting *one* of the following colony-stimulating factors 1 to 3 days after completion of chemotherapy and continuing through postnadir recovery:
• Filgrastim 5 mcg/kg daily or
• Pegfilgrastim 6 mg once for each treatment cycle.

For diarrhea (likely)
Prescribe antidiarrheal as indicated.

For cisplatin-induced nephrotoxicity
Maintain urine output of at least 75 ml/hour for several hours before and after each cisplatin dose. Consider amifostine for prevention of cisplatin-induced nephrotoxicity.

Cisplatin, paclitaxel

Paclitaxel 135 mg/m² I.V. over 24 hours on day 1
Cisplatin 50 mg/m² I.V. on day 2
Repeat cycle every 21 days.
Reference: Moore DH, et al. *J Clin Oncol.*
2004;22:3113-3119.

Supportive therapy

For nausea and vomiting
On day 1, follow acute-onset antiemetic regimen for level 2 risk. Anticipatory, breakthrough, and delayed-onset regimens are recommended as needed.

On day 2, follow acute-onset antiemetic regimen for level 5 risk. Anticipatory, breakthrough, and delayed-onset regimens are recommended.

For anemia (likely)
If hemoglobin level is less than 10 g/dl, *one* of the following is recommended:
• Epoetin alfa 150 units/kg subcutaneously three times weekly. If unsatisfactory response, may increase to 300 units/kg three times weekly.
• Epoetin alfa 40,000 units subcutaneously weekly; may increase to 60,000 units if unsatisfactory response.
• Darbepoetin alfa 3 mcg/kg subcutaneously every 2 weeks; may increase to 5 mcg/kg if unsatisfactory response.
• Darbepoetin alfa 200 mcg subcutaneously every 2 weeks; may increase to 300 mcg if unsatisfactory response.

For neutropenia (high risk)
To prevent neutropenia, start *one* of the following colony-stimulating factors 1 to 3 days after completion of chemotherapy and continue through postnadir recovery:
• Filgrastim 5 mcg/kg daily or
• Pegfilgrastim 6 mg once for each treatment cycle.

For diarrhea (likely)
Prescribe antidiarrheal as indicated.

For hypersensitivity reactions

To prevent hypersensitivity reactions, give the following before paclitaxel administration: dexamethasone 20 mg P.O. 12 hours and 6 hours before, diphenhydramine 50 mg I.V. 30 to 60 minutes before, *and* cimetidine 300 mg I.V. or ranitidine 50 mg I.V. 30 to 60 minutes before.

For cisplatin-induced nephrotoxicity

Maintain urine output of at least 75 ml/hour for several hours before and after each cisplatin dose. Consider amifostine for prevention of cisplatin-induced nephrotoxicity.

Cisplatin, topotecan

Cisplatin 50 mg/m^2 I.V. on day 1
Topotecan 0.75 mg/m^2 I.V. on days 1 through 3

Repeat cycle every 21 days.

Reference: Long HJ, et al. *J Clin Oncol.* 2005;23:4626-4633.

Supportive therapy

For nausea and vomiting
On day 1, follow acute-onset antiemetic regimen for level 5 risk. Anticipatory, breakthrough, and delayed-onset regimens are recommended.

On days 2 and 3, follow acute-onset antiemetic regimen for level 2 risk. Anticipatory, breakthrough, and delayed-onset regimens are recommended as needed.

For anemia (likely)
If hemoglobin level is less than 10 g/dl, *one* of the following is recommended:

• Epoetin alfa 150 units/kg subcutaneously three times weekly. If unsatisfactory response, may increase to 300 units/kg three times weekly.

• Epoetin alfa 40,000 units subcutaneously weekly; may increase to 60,000 units if unsatisfactory response.

• Darbepoetin alfa 3 mcg/kg subcutaneously every 2 weeks; may increase to 5 mcg/kg if unsatisfactory response.

• Darbepoetin alfa 200 mcg subcutaneously every 2 weeks; may increase to 300 mcg if unsatisfactory response.

For neutropenia (high risk)
To prevent neutropenia, start *one* of the following colony-stimulating factors 1 to 3 days after completion of chemotherapy and continue through postnadir recovery:

• Filgrastim 5 mcg/kg daily or
• Pegfilgrastim 6 mg once for each treatment cycle.

For diarrhea (likely)
Prescribe antidiarrheal as indicated.

For cisplatin-induced nephrotoxicity
Maintain urine output of at least 75 ml/hour for several hours before and after each cisplatin dose. Consider amifostine for prevention of cisplatin-induced nephrotoxicity.

Docetaxel

Docetaxel 100 mg/m^2 I.V. over 1 hour on day 1

Repeat every 21 days.

Reference: Vallejo CT, et al. *Am J Clin Oncol.* 2003;26:477-482.

Supportive therapy

For nausea and vomiting
Follow acute-onset antiemetic regimen for level 2 risk. Anticipatory, breakthrough, and delayed-onset regimens are recommended as needed.

For anemia (likely)
If hemoglobin level is less than 10 g/dl, *one* of the following is recommended:

• Epoetin alfa 150 units/kg subcutaneously three times weekly. If unsatisfactory response, may increase to 300 units/kg three times weekly.

• Epoetin alfa 40,000 units subcutaneously weekly; may increase to 60,000 units if unsatisfactory response.

• Darbepoetin alfa 3 mcg/kg subcutaneously every 2 weeks; may increase to 5 mcg/kg if unsatisfactory response.

- Darbepoetin alfa 200 mcg subcutaneously every 2 weeks; may increase to 300 mcg if unsatisfactory response.

For neutropenia (high risk)

To prevent neutropenia, start *one* of the following colony-stimulating factors 1 to 3 days after completion of chemotherapy and continue through postnadir recovery:

- Filgrastim 5 mcg/kg daily or
- Pegfilgrastim 6 mg once for each treatment cycle.

For hypersensitivity reactions

To prevent hypersensitivity reactions, administer dexamethasone 8 mg P.O. twice daily for 3 days starting 1 day before administration of docetaxel.

Gemcitabine, cisplatin

Cisplatin 50 mg/m² I.V. over 30 minutes on day 1

Gemcitabine 1,250 mg/m² I.V. over 30 minutes on days 1 and 8

Repeat cycle every 21 days.

Reference: Burnett AF, et al. *Gynecol Oncol.* 2000;76:63-66.

Supportive therapy

For nausea and vomiting

On day 1, follow acute-onset antiemetic regimen for level 5 risk. Anticipatory, breakthrough, and delayed-onset regimens are recommended.

On day 8, follow acute-onset antiemetic regimen for level 2 risk. Anticipatory, breakthrough, and delayed-onset regimens are recommended as needed.

For anemia (likely)

If hemoglobin level is less than 10 g/dl, *one* of the following is recommended:

- Epoetin alfa 150 units/kg subcutaneously three times weekly. If unsatisfactory response, may increase to 300 units/kg three times weekly.
- Epoetin alfa 40,000 units subcutaneously weekly; may increase to 60,000 units if unsatisfactory response.

- Darbepoetin alfa 3 mcg/kg subcutaneously every 2 weeks; may increase to 5 mcg/kg if unsatisfactory response.
- Darbepoetin alfa 200 mcg subcutaneously every 2 weeks; may increase to 300 mcg if unsatisfactory response.

For neutropenia (high risk)

To prevent neutropenia, start *one* of the following colony-stimulating factors 1 to 3 days after completion of chemotherapy and continue through postnadir recovery:

- Filgrastim 5 mcg/kg daily or
- Pegfilgrastim 6 mg once for each treatment cycle.

For diarrhea (likely)

Prescribe antidiarrheal as indicated.

For cisplatin-induced nephrotoxicity

Maintain urine output of at least 75 ml/hour for several hours before and after each cisplatin dose. Consider amifostine for prevention of cisplatin-induced nephrotoxicity.

ICM (ifosfamide, carboplatin, mesna)

Ifosfamide 5,000 mg/m² by continuous I.V. infusion on day 1 with *mesna* 9,200 mg/m² on day 1 only (infuse over 36 hours)

Carboplatin 300 mg/m² I.V. over 30 minutes on day 1

Repeat cycle every 28 days.

Reference: Kuhnle H, et al. *Cancer Chemother Pharmacol.* 1990;26:S33-S35.

Supportive therapy

For nausea and vomiting

Follow acute-onset antiemetic regimen for level 5 risk. Anticipatory, breakthrough, and delayed-onset regimens are recommended.

For anemia (likely)

If hemoglobin level is less than 10 g/dl, *one* of the following is recommended:

- Epoetin alfa 150 units/kg subcutaneously three times weekly. If unsatisfactory response, may increase to 300 units/kg three times weekly.

See front endpaper for specific antiemetic therapies.

- Epoetin alfa 40,000 units subcutaneously weekly; may increase to 60,000 units if unsatisfactory response.
- Darbepoetin alfa 3 mcg/kg subcutaneously every 2 weeks; may increase to 5 mcg/kg if unsatisfactory response.
- Darbepoetin alfa 200 mcg subcutaneously every 2 weeks; may increase to 300 mcg if unsatisfactory response.

For neutropenia (high risk)
To prevent neutropenia, start *one* of the following colony-stimulating factors 1 to 3 days after completion of chemotherapy and continue through postnadir recovery:

- Filgrastim 5 mcg/kg daily or
- Pegfilgrastim 6 mg once for each treatment cycle.

For diarrhea (likely)
Prescribe antidiarrheal as indicated.

For constipation (likely)
Order stool softener or laxative as indicated.

Paclitaxel

Paclitaxel 170 mg/m^2 I.V. over 24 hours on day 1
Repeat every 21 days.
Reference: Curtin JP, et al. *J Clin Oncol.* 2001;19:1275-1278.

Supportive therapy

For nausea and vomiting
Follow acute-onset antiemetic regimen for level 2 risk. Anticipatory, breakthrough, and delayed-onset regimens are recommended as needed.

For anemia (likely)
If hemoglobin level is less than 10 g/dl, *one* of the following is recommended:

- Epoetin alfa 150 units/kg subcutaneously three times weekly. If unsatisfactory response, may increase to 300 units/kg three times weekly.
- Epoetin alfa 40,000 units subcutaneously weekly; may increase to 60,000 units if unsatisfactory response.

- Darbepoetin alfa 3 mcg/kg subcutaneously every 2 weeks; may increase to 5 mcg/kg if unsatisfactory response.
- Darbepoetin alfa 200 mcg subcutaneously every 2 weeks; may increase to 300 mcg if unsatisfactory response.

For neutropenia (intermediate risk)
To prevent neutropenia, consider starting *one* of the following colony-stimulating factors 1 to 3 days after completion of chemotherapy and continuing through postnadir recovery:

- Filgrastim 5 mcg/kg daily or
- Pegfilgrastim 6 mg once for each treatment cycle.

For hypersensitivity reactions
To prevent hypersensitivity reactions, give the following before paclitaxel administration: dexamethasone 20 mg P.O. 12 hours and 6 hours before, diphenhydramine 50 mg I.V. 30 to 60 minutes before, *and* cimetidine 300 mg I.V. or ranitidine 50 mg I.V. 30 to 60 minutes before.

Chronic myelogenous leukemia

Imatinib mesylate

Imatinib 400 mg/day P.O. (chronic phase) daily
Or
Imatinib 600 mg/day P.O. (accelerated phase blast crisis) daily
Continue treatment until disease progresses.
Reference: O'Brien SG, et al. *N Engl J Med.* 2003;348:994-1004; Talpaz M, et. al. *Blood.* 2002;99:1928-1937.

Supportive therapy

For nausea and vomiting
Follow acute-onset antiemetic regimen for level 1 risk.

For diarrhea (likely)
Prescribe antidiarrheal as indicated.

Interferon alfa-2b, cytarabine

Interferon alfa-2b increased as tolerated to target dosage of 5 million units/m^2 subcutaneously daily
Cytarabine 20 mg/m^2 subcutaneously daily for 10 days (maximum daily dosage, 40 mg).
Start cytarabine once tolerated dosage of interferon is achieved.
Repeat cytarabine cycle monthly.

Reference: O'Brien SG, et al. *N Engl J Med.* 2003;348:994-1004.

Supportive therapy
For nausea and vomiting
On days 1 through 10, follow acute-onset antiemetic regimen for level 2 risk. Anticipatory, breakthrough, and delayed-onset regimens are recommended as needed.
For neutropenia (intermediate risk)
To prevent neutropenia, consider starting *one* of the following colony-stimulating factors 1 to 3 days after completion of chemotherapy and continuing through postnadir recovery:
• Filgrastim 5 mcg/kg daily or
• Pegfilgrastim 6 mg once for each treatment cycle.
For diarrhea (likely)
Prescribe antidiarrheal as indicated.

CNS tumors

Carmustine

Carmustine 200 mg/m^2 I.V. as single dose
Repeat every 6 to 8 weeks.

Reference: Selker RG, et al. *Neurosurgery.* 2002;51:343-355.

Supportive therapy
For nausea and vomiting
Follow acute-onset antiemetic regimen for level 4 risk. Anticipatory, breakthrough, and delayed-onset regimens are recommended as needed.

For anemia (likely)
If hemoglobin level is less than 10 g/dl, *one* of the following is recommended:
• Epoetin alfa 150 units/kg subcutaneously three times weekly. If unsatisfactory response, may increase to 300 units/kg three times weekly.
• Epoetin alfa 40,000 units subcutaneously weekly; may increase to 60,000 units if unsatisfactory response.
• Darbepoetin alfa 3 mcg/kg subcutaneously every 2 weeks; may increase to 5 mcg/kg if unsatisfactory response.
• Darbepoetin alfa 200 mcg subcutaneously every 2 weeks; may increase to 300 mcg if unsatisfactory response.
For neutropenia (high risk 4 to 6 weeks after chemotherapy)
To prevent neutropenia, give filgrastim 5 mcg/kg daily or pegfilgrastim, one dose of 6 mg per cycle of treatment subcutaneously; continue through postnadir recovery.

PCV (procarbazine, lomustine [CeeNu], vincristine)

Lomustine 110 mg/m^2 P.O. on day 1
Procarbazine 60 mg/m^2 P.O. on days 8 through 21
Vincristine 1.4 mg/m^2 I.V. on days 8 and 29
Repeat cycle every 6 to 8 weeks.

Reference: Levin VA, et al. *Clin Cancer Res.* 2000;6:3878-3884.

Supportive therapy
For nausea and vomiting
On day 1, follow acute-onset antiemetic regimen for level 3 risk. Anticipatory, breakthrough, and delayed-onset regimens are recommended as needed.

On days 8 through 21, follow acute-onset antiemetic regimen for level 4 risk. Anticipatory, breakthrough, and delayed-onset regimens are recommended as needed.

On day 29, follow acute-onset antiemetic regimen for level 1 risk.

For anemia (likely)
If hemoglobin level is less than 10 g/dl, *one* of the following is recommended:

- Epoetin alfa 150 units/kg subcutaneously three times weekly. If unsatisfactory response, may increase to 300 units/kg three times weekly.
- Epoetin alfa 40,000 units subcutaneously weekly; may increase to 60,000 units if unsatisfactory response.
- Darbepoetin alfa 3 mcg/kg subcutaneously every 2 weeks; may increase to 5 mcg/kg if unsatisfactory response.
- Darbepoetin alfa 200 mcg subcutaneously every 2 weeks; may increase to 300 mcg if unsatisfactory response.

For neutropenia (high risk)
To prevent neutropenia, start *one* of the following colony-stimulating factors 1 to 3 days after completion of chemotherapy and continue through postnadir recovery:

- Filgrastim 5 mcg/kg daily or
- Pegfilgrastim 6 mg once for each treatment cycle.

For constipation (likely)
Order stool softener or laxative as indicated.

Temozolomide

Temozolomide 200 mg/m^2 P.O. daily (chemotherapy naive) *or* 150 mg/m^2 P.O. daily (prior chemotherapy) on days 1 through 5
Repeat every 28 days.
Reference: Yung WK. *J Clin Oncol.* 1999;17:2762-2771.

Supportive therapy

For nausea and vomiting
Follow acute-onset antiemetic regimen for level 2 risk. Anticipatory, breakthrough, and delayed-onset regimens are recommended as needed.

For neutropenia (intermediate risk)
To prevent neutropenia, consider starting *one* of the following colony-stimulating factors 1 to 3 days after completion of chemotherapy and continuing through postnadir recovery:

- Filgrastim 5 mcg/kg daily or
- Pegfilgrastim 6 mg once for each treatment cycle.

Colon, rectal, and anal cancers

Bolus or infusional 5-fluorouracil, leucovorin

Mayo
5-Fluorouracil (5-FU) 425 mg/m^2 daily by I.V. bolus 1 hour after start of leucovorin on days 1 through 5
Leucovorin 20 mg/m^2 daily by I.V. bolus on days 1 through 5
Repeat cycle in 4 weeks and 8 weeks, then every 5 weeks.
Reference: Poon MA, et al. *J Clin Oncol.* 1991;11:1967.

Roswell Park
5-FU 600 mg/m^2 by I.V. bolus 1 hour after start of leucovorin on days 1, 8, 15, 22, 29, 36
Leucovorin 500 mg/m^2 I.V. over 2 hours on days 1, 8, 15, 22, 29, 36
Repeat cycle every 8 weeks.
Reference: Petrelli N, et al. *J Clin Oncol.* 1987;5:1559-1565.

de Gramont
5-FU Initial dose, 400 mg/m^2 by I.V. bolus, then 600 mg/m^2 by continuous I.V. infusion over 22 hours on days 1 and 2 every 2 weeks
Leucovorin 200 mg/m^2 daily I.V. over 2 hours on days 1 and 2 every 2 weeks (before 5-FU)
References: de Gramont A, et al. *J Clin Oncol.* 1997;15:808-815; de Gramont A, et al. *J Clin Oncol.* 2000;18:2938-2947.

Supportive therapy

For nausea and vomiting
Follow acute-onset antiemetic regimen for level 2 risk. Anticipatory, breakthrough, and delayed-onset regimens are recommended as needed.

For anemia (likely)
If hemoglobin level is less than 10 g/dl, *one* of the following is recommended:

• Epoetin alfa 150 units/kg subcutaneously three times weekly. If unsatisfactory response, may increase to 300 units/kg three times weekly.

• Epoetin alfa 40,000 units subcutaneously weekly; may increase to 60,000 units if unsatisfactory response.

• Darbepoetin alfa 3 mcg/kg subcutaneously every 2 weeks; may increase to 5 mcg/kg if unsatisfactory response.

• Darbepoetin alfa 200 mcg subcutaneously every 2 weeks; may increase to 300 mcg if unsatisfactory response.

For diarrhea (very likely)
An antidiarrheal is recommended.

Capecitabine

Capecitabine 2,500 mg/m^2 P.O. daily in two divided doses on days 1 through 14
Repeat every 21 days.

Reference: Scherthauer W, et al. *Annals Oncol.* 2003;14:1735-1743.

Supportive therapy
For nausea and vomiting
Follow acute-onset antiemetic regimen for level 2 risk. Anticipatory, breakthrough, and delayed-onset regimens are recommended as needed.

For anemia (likely)
If hemoglobin level is less than 10 g/dl, *one* of the following is recommended:

• Epoetin alfa 150 units/kg subcutaneously three times weekly. If unsatisfactory response, may increase to 300 units/kg three times weekly.

• Epoetin alfa 40,000 units subcutaneously weekly; may increase to 60,000 units if unsatisfactory response.

• Darbepoetin alfa 3 mcg/kg subcutaneously every 2 weeks; may increase to 5 mcg/kg if unsatisfactory response.

• Darbepoetin alfa 200 mcg subcutaneously

every 2 weeks; may increase to 300 mcg if unsatisfactory response.
For diarrhea (likely)
Prescribe antidiarrheal as indicated.

Cetuximab

For irinotecan-intolerant patient:
Cetuximab Initial dose, 400 mg/m^2 I.V. over 120 minutes, then 250 mg/m^2 I.V. over 60 minutes
Repeat every 7 days.

Reference: Cunningham D, et al. *N Engl J Med.* 2004;351:337-345.

Supportive therapy
For nausea and vomiting
Follow acute-onset antiemetic regimen for level 2 risk. Anticipatory, breakthrough, and delayed-onset regimens are recommended as needed.

For hypersensitivity reactions
To prevent hypersensitivity reactions, administer an antihistamine such as diphenhydramine 50 mg I.V. before chemotherapy.

Cetuximab, irinotecan

Cetuximab Initial dose, 400 mg/ m^2 I.V. over 120 minutes, then 250 mg/m^2 I.V. over 60 minutes weekly
Irinotecan 350 mg/m^2 I.V. over 90 minutes
Repeat cycle every 21 days.
Or
Cetuximab Initial dose, 400 mg/ m^2 I.V. over 120 minutes, then 250 mg/m^2 I.V. over 60 minutes weekly
Irinotecan 180 mg/m^2 I.V. over 90 minutes
Repeat cycle every 14 days.

Reference: Cunningham D, et al. *N Engl J Med.* 2004;351:337-345.

Supportive therapy
For nausea and vomiting
On irinotecan and cetuximab days, follow acute-onset antiemetic regimen for level 3

risk. Anticipatory, breakthrough, and delayed-onset regimens are recommended as needed.

On cetuximab only days, follow acute-onset antiemetic regimen for level 1 risk.

For anemia (likely)
If hemoglobin level is less than 10 g/dl, *one* of the following is recommended:
• Epoetin alfa 150 units/kg subcutaneously three times weekly. If unsatisfactory response, may increase to 300 units/kg three times weekly.
• Epoetin alfa 40,000 units subcutaneously weekly; may increase to 60,000 units if unsatisfactory response.
• Darbepoetin alfa 3 mcg/kg subcutaneously every 2 weeks; may increase to 5 mcg/kg if unsatisfactory response.
• Darbepoetin alfa 200 mcg subcutaneously every 2 weeks; may increase to 300 mcg if unsatisfactory response.

For neutropenia (high risk)
To prevent neutropenia, start *one* of the following colony-stimulating factors 1 to 3 days after completion of chemotherapy and continue through postnadir recovery:
• Filgrastim 5 mcg/kg daily or
• Pegfilgrastim 6 mg once for each treatment cycle.

For diarrhea (likely)
Prescribe antidiarrheal as indicated.

For hypersensitivity reactions
To prevent hypersensitivity reactions, administer an antihistamine such as diphenhydramine 50 mg I.V. before chemotherapy.

5-Fluorouracil

5-Fluorouracil 1,000 mg/m^2 by continuous I.V. infusion daily on days 1 through 5
Repeat every 28 days.

References: Kemeny N, et al. J Clin Oncol. 1990;8:313-318; Schmoll HJ. Eur J Cancer. 1996;32A(suppl):S18-S22.

Supportive therapy
For nausea and vomiting
Follow acute-onset antiemetic regimen for lev-el 2 risk. Anticipatory, breakthrough, and delayed-onset regimens are recommended as needed.

For anemia (likely)
If hemoglobin level is less than 10 g/dl, *one* of the following is recommended:
• Epoetin alfa 150 units/kg subcutaneously three times weekly. If unsatisfactory response, may increase to 300 units/kg three times weekly.
• Epoetin alfa 40,000 units subcutaneously weekly; may increase to 60,000 units if unsatisfactory response.
• Darbepoetin alfa 3 mcg/kg subcutaneously every 2 weeks; may increase to 5 mcg/kg if unsatisfactory response.
• Darbepoetin alfa 200 mcg subcutaneously every 2 weeks; may increase to 300 mcg if unsatisfactory response.

For diarrhea (likely)
Prescribe antidiarrheal as indicated.

5-Fluorouracil, leucovorin, oxaliplatin combinations

FOLFOX4
Oxaliplatin 85 mg/m^2 I.V. over 2 hours on day 1
Leucovorin 200 mg/m^2 I.V. over 2 hours (on days 1 and 2); then
5-Fluorouracil (5-FU) 400 mg/m^2 by I.V. bolus, followed by 600 mg/m^2 by continuous I.V. infusion over 22 hours on days 1 and 2
Repeat cycle every 14 days.

FOLFOX6
Oxaliplatin 100 mg/m^2 I.V. over 2 hours on day 1
Leucovorin 400 mg/m^2 I.V. over 2 hours (on days 1 and 2); then
5-FU 400 mg/m^2 by I.V. bolus, followed by 2,400 mg/m^2 by continuous I.V. infusion over 46 hours
Repeat cycle every 14 days. If no toxicity greater than grade 1 occurs after first two cycles, increase 5-FU dosage to 3,000 mg/m^2.

mFOLFOX6

Oxaliplatin 85 mg/m² I.V. over 2 hours on day 1
Leucovorin 400 mg/m² I.V. over 2 hours on days 1 and 2; then
5-FU 400 mg/m² by I.V. bolus, followed by 2,400 mg/m² by continuous I.V. infusion over 46 hours
Repeat cycle every 14 days. If no toxicity greater than grade 1 occurs after first two cycles, increase 5-FU dosage to 3,000 mg/m².

FOLFOX7

Oxaliplatin 130 mg/m² I.V. over 2 hours on day 1
Leucovorin 400 mg/m² I.V. over 2 hours on days 1 and 2; then
5-FU 400 mg/m² by I.V. bolus, followed by 2,400 mg/m² by continuous I.V. infusion over 46 to 48 hours
Repeat cycle every 14 days. If no toxicity greater than grade 1 occurs after first two cycles, increase 5-FU to 3,000 mg/m².

References: Colucci G, et al. *J Clin Oncol.* 2005;23:4866-4875; Tournigand C, et al. *J Clin Oncol.* 2004;22:229-237; Cheeseman SL, et al. *Br J Cancer.* 2002;87:393-399; Maindrault-Goebel F, et al. *Euro J Cancer.* 2002;37:1000-1005.

Supportive therapy

For nausea and vomiting
On day 1, follow acute-onset antiemetic regimen for level 4 risk. Anticipatory, breakthrough, and delayed-onset regimens are recommended as needed.

On 5-FU days only, follow acute-onset antiemetic regimen for level 2 risk. Anticipatory, breakthrough, and delayed-onset regimens are recommended as needed.

For anemia (likely)
If hemoglobin level is less than 10 g/dl, *one* of the following is recommended:
• Epoetin alfa 150 units/kg subcutaneously three times weekly. If unsatisfactory response, may increase to 300 units/kg three times weekly.

• Epoetin alfa 40,000 units subcutaneously weekly; may increase to 60,000 units if unsatisfactory response.
• Darbepoetin alfa 3 mcg/kg subcutaneously every 2 weeks; may increase to 5 mcg/kg if unsatisfactory response.
• Darbepoetin alfa 200 mcg subcutaneously every 2 weeks; may increase to 300 mcg if unsatisfactory response.

For neutropenia (intermediate risk)
To prevent neutropenia, consider starting *one* of the following colony-stimulating factors 1 to 3 days after completion of chemotherapy and continuing through postnadir recovery:
• Filgrastim 5 mcg/kg daily or
• Pegfilgrastim 6 mg once for each treatment cycle.

For diarrhea (very likely)
An antidiarrheal is recommended.

IFL/BV (irinotecan, 5-fluorouracil, leucovorin, bevacizumab)

Irinotecan 125 mg/m² I.V. over 90 minutes on days 1, 8, 15, and 22
Leucovorin 20 mg/m² daily by I.V. bolus on days 1, 8, 15, 22
5-Fluorouracil 500 mg/m² daily by I.V. bolus on days 1, 8, 15, and 22
Bevacizumab 5 mg/kg I.V. over 90 minutes, then decrease to 30 to 60 minutes, if tolerated, every 14 days
Repeat cycle every 6 weeks.

Reference: Hurwitz H, et al. *N Engl J Med.* 2004;350:2335-2342.

Supportive therapy

For nausea and vomiting
On days 1, 8, 15, and 22, follow acute-onset antiemetic regimen for level 4 risk. Anticipatory, breakthrough, and delayed-onset regimens are recommended as needed.

For anemia (likely)
If hemoglobin level is less than 10 g/dl, *one* of the following is recommended:
• Epoetin alfa 150 units/kg subcutaneously three times weekly. If unsatisfactory response,

---

may increase to 300 units/kg three times weekly.
- Epoetin alfa 40,000 units subcutaneously weekly; may increase to 60,000 units if unsatisfactory response.
- Darbepoetin alfa 3 mcg/kg subcutaneously every 2 weeks; may increase to 5 mcg/kg if unsatisfactory response.
- Darbepoetin alfa 200 mcg subcutaneously every 2 weeks; may increase to 300 mcg if unsatisfactory response.

For neutropenia (intermediate risk)
To prevent neutropenia, consider starting *one* of the following colony-stimulating factors 1 to 3 days after completion of chemotherapy and continuing through postnadir recovery:
- Filgrastim 5 mcg/kg daily or
- Pegfilgrastim 6 mg once for each treatment cycle.

For diarrhea (very likely)
An antidiarrheal is recommended.

Irinotecan

Irinotecan 125 mg/m^2 I.V. over 90 minutes on days 1, 8, 15, and 22
Repeat every 6 weeks.
Or
Irinotecan 350 mg/m^2 I.V. over 90 minutes on day 1
Repeat every 21 days.
Reference: Rougier P, et al. *J Clin Oncol.* 1997;15:251-260; Conti JA, et al. *J Clin Oncol.* 1996;14:709-715; Cunningham D, et al. *Lancet.* 1998;352:1413-1418.

Supportive therapy
For nausea and vomiting
Follow acute-onset antiemetic regimen for level 3 risk. Anticipatory, breakthrough, and delayed-onset regimens are recommended as needed.
For anemia (likely)
If hemoglobin level is less than 10 g/dl, *one* of the following is recommended:
- Epoetin alfa 150 units/kg subcutaneously three times weekly. If unsatisfactory response,

may increase to 300 units/kg three times weekly.
- Epoetin alfa 40,000 units subcutaneously weekly; may increase to 60,000 units if unsatisfactory response.
- Darbepoetin alfa 3 mcg/kg subcutaneously every 2 weeks; may increase to 5 mcg/kg if unsatisfactory response.
- Darbepoetin alfa 200 mcg subcutaneously every 2 weeks; may increase to 300 mcg if unsatisfactory response.

For diarrhea (likely)
Prescribe antidiarrheal as indicated.

Irinotecan, leucovorin, 5-fluorouracil combinations

Douillard
Irinotecan 180 mg/m^2 I.V. over 2 hours on day 1
Leucovorin 200 mg/m^2 I.V. over 2 hours on days 1 and 2
5-Fluorouracil (5-FU) Initial dose, 400 mg/m^2 by I.V. bolus, then 600 mg/m^2 by continuous I.V. infusion over next 22 hours on days 1 and 2. Start 5-FU after leucovorin.
Repeat cycle every 14 days.
FOLFIRI
Irinotecan 180 mg/m^2 I.V. over 90 minutes on day 1
Leucovorin 400 mg/m^2 I.V. over 2 hours during irinotecan infusion
5-FU Initial dose, 400 mg/m^2 by I.V. bolus, then 2,400 mg/m^2 by continuous I.V. infusion over next 46 hours. Start 5-FU after leucovorin.
Repeat cycle every 14 days.
IFL (Saltz)
Irinotecan 125 mg/m^2 I.V. over 90 minutes on days 1, 8, 15, and 22
Leucovorin 20 mg/m^2 by I.V. bolus on days 1, 8, 15, and 22
5-FU 500 mg/m^2 I.V. bolus on days 1, 8, 15, and 22
Repeat cycle every 6 weeks.
Reference: Douillard JY, et al. *Lancet.* 2000;355:1041-1047; Tournigand C, et al.

J Clin Oncol. 2004;22:229-237; Saltz LB, et al. *N Engl J Med.* 2000;343:905-914.

Supportive therapy

For nausea and vomiting

On irinotecan and 5-FU days, follow acute-onset antiemetic regimen for level 4 risk. Anticipatory, breakthrough, and delayed-onset regimens are recommended as needed.

On 5-FU days only, follow acute-onset antiemetic regimen for level 2 risk. Anticipatory, breakthrough, and delayed-onset regimens are recommended as needed.

For anemia (likely)

If hemoglobin level is less than 10 g/dl, *one* of the following is recommended:
- Epoetin alfa 150 units/kg subcutaneously three times weekly. If unsatisfactory response, may increase to 300 units/kg three times weekly.
- Epoetin alfa 40,000 units subcutaneously weekly; may increase to 60,000 units if unsatisfactory response.
- Darbepoetin alfa 3 mcg/kg subcutaneously every 2 weeks; may increase to 5 mcg/kg if unsatisfactory response.
- Darbepoetin alfa 200 mcg subcutaneously every 2 weeks; may increase to 300 mcg if unsatisfactory response.

For neutropenia (intermediate risk)

To prevent neutropenia, consider starting *one* of the following colony-stimulating factors 1 to 3 days after completion of chemotherapy and continuing through postnadir recovery:
- Filgrastim 5 mcg/kg daily or
- Pegfilgrastim 6 mg once for each treatment cycle.

For diarrhea (very likely)

Prescribe antidiarrheal as indicated.

XELOX (capecitabine [Xeloda], oxaliplatin)

Oxaliplatin 130 mg/m^2 I.V. over 2 hours on day 1

Capecitabine 1,000 mg/m^2 P.O. twice daily from evening of day 1 to morning of day 15

Repeat cycle every 21 days.

Reference: Makatsoris T, et al. *Int J Gastro Cancer.* 2005;35:103-109; Cassidy J, et al. *J Clin Oncol.* 2004;22:2084-2091.

Supportive therapy

For nausea and vomiting

On day 1, follow acute-onset antiemetic regimen for level 4 risk. Anticipatory, breakthrough, and delayed-onset regimens are recommended as needed.

On days 2 through 15, follow acute-onset antiemetic regimen for level 2 risk. Anticipatory, breakthrough, and delayed-onset regimens are recommended as needed.

For anemia (likely)

If hemoglobin level is less than 10 g/dl, *one* of the following is recommended:
- Epoetin alfa 150 units/kg subcutaneously three times weekly. If unsatisfactory response, may increase to 300 units/kg three times weekly.
- Epoetin alfa 40,000 units subcutaneously weekly; may increase to 60,000 units if unsatisfactory response.
- Darbepoetin alfa 3 mcg/kg subcutaneously every 2 weeks; may increase to 5 mcg/kg if unsatisfactory response.
- Darbepoetin alfa 200 mcg subcutaneously every 2 weeks; may increase to 300 mcg if unsatisfactory response.

For neutropenia (high risk)

To prevent neutropenia, start *one* of the following colony-stimulating factors 1 to 3 days after completion of chemotherapy and continue through postnadir recovery:
- Filgrastim 5 mcg/kg daily or
- Pegfilgrastim 6 mg once for each treatment cycle.

For diarrhea (likely)

Prescribe antidiarrheal as indicated.

Esophageal cancer

Cisplatin, 5-fluorouracil

Cisplatin 75 mg/m² I.V. on day 1 of weeks 1, 5, 8, and 11
5-Fluorouracil (5-FU) 1,000 mg/m² daily by continuous I.V. infusion on days 1 through 4 of weeks 1, 5, 8, and 11
Radiation therapy 50 Gy in 25 fractions over 5 weeks

Reference: Cooper JS, et al. *JAMA.* 1999;281:1623-1627.

Or

Cisplatin 75 mg/m² by I.V. bolus over 30 minutes on day 1
5-FU 1,000 mg/m² by continuous I.V. infusion on days 1 through 4
Radiation therapy 1.8 Gy/day, 5 days a week of weeks 1 through 5 or weeks 1 through 7
Repeat cycle after 4-week rest from radiation (week 9).

Reference: Minsky BD, et al. *J Clin Oncol.* 2002;20:1167-1174.

Or

5-FU 15 mg/kg I.V. over 16 hours on days 1 through 5
Cisplatin 75 mg/m² I.V. over 8 hours on day 7 of weeks 1 and 6
Radiation therapy 40 Gy in 15 fractions over 3 weeks, beginning concurrently with first course of chemotherapy
Repeat cycle in 6 weeks.

Reference: Walsh TN, et al. *N Engl J Med.* 1996;335:462-467.

Or

Cisplatin 80 mg/m² I.V. over 4 hours on day 1
5-FU 1,000 mg/m² by continuous I.V. infusion daily for 4 days, followed by surgical resection after 2 cycles
Repeat cycle every 21 days.

Reference: Medical Research Council Oesophageal Cancer Working Group. *Lancet.* 2002;359:1727-1733.

Supportive therapy

For nausea and vomiting
On cisplatin days, follow acute-onset antiemetic regimen for level 5 risk. Anticipatory, breakthrough, and delayed-onset regimens are recommended.

On 5-FU days only, follow acute-onset antiemetic regimen for level 2 risk. Anticipatory, breakthrough, and delayed-onset regimens are recommended as needed.

For anemia (likely)
If hemoglobin level is less than 10 g/dl, *one* of the following is recommended:

- Epoetin alfa 150 units/kg subcutaneously three times weekly. If unsatisfactory response, may increase to 300 units/kg three times weekly.
- Epoetin alfa 40,000 units subcutaneously weekly; may increase to 60,000 units if unsatisfactory response.
- Darbepoetin alfa 3 mcg/kg subcutaneously every 2 weeks; may increase to 5 mcg/kg if unsatisfactory response.
- Darbepoetin alfa 200 mcg subcutaneously every 2 weeks; may increase to 300 mcg if unsatisfactory response.

For neutropenia (high risk)
To prevent neutropenia, start *one* of the following colony-stimulating factors 1 to 3 days after completion of chemotherapy and continue through postnadir recovery:

- Filgrastim 5 mcg/kg daily or
- Pegfilgrastim 6 mg once for each treatment cycle.

For diarrhea (very likely)
An antidiarrheal is recommended.

For cisplatin-induced nephrotoxicity
Maintain urine output of at least 75 ml/hour for several hours before and after each cisplatin dose. Consider amifostine for prevention of cisplatin-induced nephrotoxicity.

Cisplatin, paclitaxel

Cisplatin 75 mg/m² I.V. over 2 hours on day 1
Paclitaxel 60 mg/m² I.V. over 3 hours on days 1, 8, 15, and 22

Radiation therapy 1.5 Gy twice daily on days 1 to 5, 8 to 12, and 15 through 19

Reference: Urba SG, et al. *Cancer.* 2003;98:2177-2183.

Supportive therapy

For nausea and vomiting
On day 1, follow acute-onset antiemetic regimen for level 5 risk. Anticipatory, breakthrough, and delayed-onset regimens are recommended.

On days 8, 15, and 22, follow acute-onset antiemetic regimen for level 2 risk. Anticipatory, breakthrough, and delayed-onset regimens are recommended as needed.

For anemia (likely)
If hemoglobin level is less than 10 g/dl, *one* of the following is recommended:
• Epoetin alfa 150 units/kg subcutaneously three times weekly. If unsatisfactory response, may increase to 300 units/kg three times weekly.
• Epoetin alfa 40,000 units subcutaneously weekly; may increase to 60,000 units if unsatisfactory response.
• Darbepoetin alfa 3 mcg/kg subcutaneously every 2 weeks; may increase to 5 mcg/kg if unsatisfactory response.
• Darbepoetin alfa 200 mcg subcutaneously every 2 weeks; may increase to 300 mcg if unsatisfactory response.

For neutropenia (high risk)
To prevent neutropenia, start *one* of the following colony-stimulating factors 1 to 3 days after completion of chemotherapy and continue through postnadir recovery:
• Filgrastim 5 mcg/kg daily or
• Pegfilgrastim 6 mg once for each treatment cycle.

For hypersensitivity reactions
To prevent hypersensitivity reactions, give the following before paclitaxel administration: dexamethasone 20 mg P.O. 12 hours and 6 hours before, diphenhydramine 50 mg I.V. 30 to 60 minutes before, *and* cimetidine 300 mg I.V. or ranitidine 50 mg I.V. 30 to 60 minutes before.

For cisplatin-induced nephrotoxicity
Maintain urine output of at least 75 ml/hour for several hours before and after each cisplatin dose. Consider amifostine for prevention of cisplatin-induced nephrotoxicity.

Cisplatin, vinorelbine

Cisplatin 80 mg/m^2 I.V. over 30 minutes on day 1
Vinorelbine 25 mg/m^2 by I.V. bolus on days 1 and 8 (20 mg/m^2 for patients with documented cirrhosis)
Repeat cycle every 21 days.

Reference: Conroy T, et al. *Ann Oncol.* 2002;13:721-729.

Supportive therapy

For nausea and vomiting
On day 1, follow acute-onset antiemetic regimen for level 5 risk. Anticipatory, breakthrough, and delayed-onset regimens are recommended.

On day 8, follow acute-onset antiemetic regimen for level 1 risk.

For anemia (likely)
If hemoglobin level is less than 10 g/dl, *one* of the following is recommended:
• Epoetin alfa 150 units/kg subcutaneously three times weekly. If unsatisfactory response, may increase to 300 units/kg three times weekly.
• Epoetin alfa 40,000 units subcutaneously weekly; may increase to 60,000 units if unsatisfactory response.
• Darbepoetin alfa 3 mcg/kg subcutaneously every 2 weeks; may increase to 5 mcg/kg if unsatisfactory response.
• Darbepoetin alfa 200 mcg subcutaneously every 2 weeks; may increase to 300 mcg if unsatisfactory response.

For neutropenia (high risk)
To prevent neutropenia, start *one* of the following colony-stimulating factors 1 to 3 days after completion of chemotherapy and continue through postnadir recovery:
• Filgrastim 5 mcg/kg daily or

- Pegfilgrastim 6 mg once for each treatment cycle.

For constipation (likely)
Order stool softener or laxative as indicated.

For cisplatin-induced nephrotoxicity
Maintain urine output of at least 75 ml/hour for several hours before and after each cisplatin dose. Consider amifostine for prevention of cisplatin-induced nephrotoxicity.

CPT-11 + CDDP (irinotecan + cisplatin)

Irinotecan 65 mg/m^2 I.V. over 90 minutes on days 1, 8, 15, and 22
Cisplatin 30 mg/m^2 I.V. over 2 hours on days 1, 8, 15, and 22
After 2-week rest, repeat cycle every 6 weeks.
Or
Irinotecan 65 mg/m^2 I.V. over 90 minutes on days 1 and 8
Cisplatin 30 mg/m^2 I.V. over 2 hours on days 1 and 8
After 1-week rest, repeat cycle every 21 days.
Reference: Ilson DH, et al. *J Clin Oncol.* 1999;17:3270-3275; Ilson DH. *Oncology.* 2004;18(14):22-25.

Supportive therapy
For nausea and vomiting
On days 1 and 8, follow acute-onset antiemetic regimen for level 5 risk. Anticipatory, breakthrough, and delayed-onset regimens are recommended.

For neutropenia (high risk)
To prevent neutropenia, start *one* of the following colony-stimulating factors 1 to 3 days after completion of chemotherapy and continue through postnadir recovery:
- Filgrastim 5 mcg/kg daily or
- Pegfilgrastim 6 mg once for each treatment cycle.

For diarrhea (very likely)
Give atropine 0.5 to 1 mg I.V. for diarrhea or abdominal cramping during or within 1 hour

after irinotecan administration; Prescribe antidiarrheal as indicated.

For cisplatin-induced nephrotoxicity
Maintain urine output of at least 75 ml/hour for several hours before and after each cisplatin dose. Consider amifostine for prevention of cisplatin-induced nephrotoxicity.

ECF (epirubicin, cisplatin, 5-fluorouracil)

Epirubicin 50 mg/m^2 I.V. on day 1
Cisplatin 60 mg/m^2 I.V. on day 1
Repeat above cycle every 21 days with:
5-Fluorouracil (5-FU) 200 mg/m^2 daily by continuous I.V. infusion (for up to 6 months)
Reference: Waters JS, et al. *Br J Cancer.* 1999;80:269-272; Ross P, et al. *J Clin Oncol.* 2002;20:1996-2004.

Supportive therapy
For nausea and vomiting
On day 1, follow acute-onset antiemetic regimen for level 5 risk. Anticipatory, breakthrough, and delayed-onset regimens are recommended.

On 5-FU days only, follow acute-onset antiemetic regimen for level 2 risk. Anticipatory, breakthrough, and delayed-onset regimens are recommended as needed.

For anemia (likely)
If hemoglobin level is less than 10 g/dl, *one* of the following is recommended:
- Epoetin alfa 150 units/kg subcutaneously three times weekly. If unsatisfactory response, may increase to 300 units/kg three times weekly.
- Epoetin alfa 40,000 units subcutaneously weekly; may increase to 60,000 units if unsatisfactory response.
- Darbepoetin alfa 3 mcg/kg subcutaneously every 2 weeks; may increase to 5 mcg/kg if unsatisfactory response.
- Darbepoetin alfa 200 mcg subcutaneously every 2 weeks; may increase to 300 mcg if unsatisfactory response.

For neutropenia (high risk)
To prevent neutropenia, start *one* of the following colony-stimulating factors 1 to 3 days after completion of chemotherapy and continue through postnadir recovery:

• Filgrastim 5 mcg/kg daily or
• Pegfilgrastim 6 mg once for each treatment cycle.

For diarrhea (very likely)
An antidiarrheal is recommended.

For cisplatin-induced nephrotoxicity
Maintain urine output of at least 75 ml/hour for several hours before and after each cisplatin dose. Consider amifostine for prevention of cisplatin-induced nephrotoxicity.

HLFP (hydroxyurea, leucovorin, 5-fluorouracil, cisplatin [Platinol-AQ])

Hydroxyurea 1,000 mg/m² P.O. on days 0, 1, and 2
Leucovorin 200 mg/m² I.V. over 2 hours on days 1 and 2
5-Fluorouracil 400 mg/m² by I.V. bolus on days 1 and 2, then 600 mg/m² I.V. over 22 hours on days 1 and 2
Repeat above cycle every 14 days.
Cisplatin 80 mg/m² I.V. is given every two cycles on day 3

Reference: Taïeb J, et al. *Eur J Cancer.* 2002;38:661-666.

Supportive therapy

For nausea and vomiting
On day 0, follow acute-onset antiemetic regimen for level 1 risk.

On days 1 and 2, follow acute-onset antiemetic regimen for level 2 risk. Anticipatory, breakthrough, and delayed-onset regimens are recommended as needed.

On day 3, follow acute-onset antiemetic regimen for level 5 risk. Anticipatory, breakthrough, and delayed-onset regimens are recommended.

For anemia (likely)
If hemoglobin level is less than 10 g/dl, *one* of the following is recommended:

• Epoetin alfa 150 units/kg subcutaneously three times weekly. If unsatisfactory response, may increase to 300 units/kg three times weekly.
• Epoetin alfa 40,000 units subcutaneously weekly; may increase to 60,000 units if unsatisfactory response.
• Darbepoetin alfa 3 mcg/kg subcutaneously every 2 weeks; may increase to 5 mcg/kg if unsatisfactory response.
• Darbepoetin alfa 200 mcg subcutaneously every 2 weeks; may increase to 300 mcg if unsatisfactory response.

For neutropenia (high risk)
To prevent neutropenia, start *one* of the following colony-stimulating factors 1 to 3 days after completion of chemotherapy and continue through postnadir recovery:

• Filgrastim 5 mcg/kg daily or
• Pegfilgrastim 6 mg once for each treatment cycle.

For diarrhea (very likely)
An antidiarrheal is recommended.

For cisplatin-induced nephrotoxicity
Maintain urine output of at least 75 ml/hour for several hours before and after each cisplatin dose. Consider amifostine for prevention of cisplatin-induced nephrotoxicity.

MCF (mitomycin, cisplatin, 5-fluorouracil)

Mitomycin 7 mg/m² I.V. every 6 weeks for four cycles
Cisplatin 60 mg/m² by I.V. infusion every 3 weeks to maximum of eight cycles
5-Fluorouracil 300 mg/m² daily by continuous I.V. infusion (for up to 6 months)

Reference: Ross P, et al. *J Clin Oncol.* 2002;20:1996-2004.

Supportive therapy

For nausea and vomiting
Follow acute-onset antiemetic regimen for level 5 risk. Anticipatory, breakthrough, and delayed-onset regimens are recommended.

See front endpaper for specific antiemetic therapies.

For anemia (likely)
If hemoglobin level is less than 10 g/dl, *one* of the following is recommended:
• Epoetin alfa 150 units/kg subcutaneously three times weekly. If unsatisfactory response, may increase to 300 units/kg three times weekly.
• Epoetin alfa 40,000 units subcutaneously weekly; may increase to 60,000 units if unsatisfactory response.
• Darbepoetin alfa 3 mcg/kg subcutaneously every 2 weeks; may increase to 5 mcg/kg if unsatisfactory response.
• Darbepoetin alfa 200 mcg subcutaneously every 2 weeks; may increase to 300 mcg if unsatisfactory response.
For neutropenia (high risk)
To prevent neutropenia, start *one* of the following colony-stimulating factors 1 to 3 days after completion of chemotherapy and continue through postnadir recovery:
• Filgrastim 5 mcg/kg daily or
• Pegfilgrastim 6 mg once for each treatment cycle.
For diarrhea (very likely)
An antidiarrheal is recommended.
For cisplatin-induced nephrotoxicity
Maintain urine output of at least 75 ml/hour for several hours before and after each cisplatin dose. Consider amifostine for prevention of cisplatin-induced nephrotoxicity.

Paclitaxel

Paclitaxel 250 mg/m² by I.V. infusion over 24 hours on day 1 only
Repeat every 21 days.
Reference: Ajani JA, et al. *J Natl Cancer Inst.* 1994;86:1086-1091; Ajani JA, et al. *Semin Oncol.* 1996;(5, Suppl 12):S55-S58.

Supportive therapy
For nausea and vomiting
Follow acute-onset antiemetic regimen for level 2 risk. Anticipatory, breakthrough, and delayed-onset regimens are recommended as needed.

For anemia (likely)
If hemoglobin level is less than 10 g/dl, *one* of the following is recommended:
• Epoetin alfa 150 units/kg subcutaneously three times weekly. If unsatisfactory response, may increase to 300 units/kg three times weekly.
• Epoetin alfa 40,000 units subcutaneously weekly; may increase to 60,000 units if unsatisfactory response.
• Darbepoetin alfa 3 mcg/kg subcutaneously every 2 weeks; may increase to 5 mcg/kg if unsatisfactory response.
• Darbepoetin alfa 200 mcg subcutaneously every 2 weeks; may increase to 300 mcg if unsatisfactory response.
For neutropenia (high risk)
To prevent neutropenia, start *one* of the following colony-stimulating factors 1 to 3 days after completion of chemotherapy and continue through postnadir recovery:
• Filgrastim 5 mcg/kg daily or
• Pegfilgrastim 6 mg once for each treatment cycle.
For hypersensitivity reactions
To prevent hypersensitivity reactions, give the following before paclitaxel administration: dexamethasone 20 mg P.O. 12 hours and 6 hours before, diphenhydramine 50 mg I.V. 30 to 60 minutes before, *and* cimetidine 300 mg I.V. or ranitidine 50 mg I.V. 30 to 60 minutes before.

Paclitaxel, cisplatin, 5-fluorouracil

Paclitaxel 175 mg/m² by I.V. infusion over 3 hours on day 1
Cisplatin 20 mg/m² I.V. daily on days 1 through 5 for first three cycles; 15 mg/m² I.V. daily on days 1 through 5 from cycle 4 on
5-Fluorouracil 750 mg/m² by continuous I.V. infusion on days 1 through 5
Repeat cycle every 28 days.
Reference: Ilson DH, et al. *J Clin Oncol.* 1998;16:1826-1834.

Supportive therapy

For nausea and vomiting
On days 1 through 5, follow acute-onset antiemetic regimen for level 5 risk. Anticipatory, breakthrough, and delayed-onset regimens are recommended.

For anemia (likely)
If hemoglobin level is less than 10 g/dl, *one* of the following is recommended:
- Epoetin alfa 150 units/kg subcutaneously three times weekly. If unsatisfactory response, may increase to 300 units/kg three times weekly.
- Epoetin alfa 40,000 units subcutaneously weekly; may increase to 60,000 units if unsatisfactory response.
- Darbepoetin alfa 3 mcg/kg subcutaneously every 2 weeks; may increase to 5 mcg/kg if unsatisfactory response.
- Darbepoetin alfa 200 mcg subcutaneously every 2 weeks; may increase to 300 mcg if unsatisfactory response.

For neutropenia (high risk)
To prevent neutropenia, start *one* of the following colony-stimulating factors 1 to 3 days after completion of chemotherapy and continue through postnadir recovery:
- Filgrastim 5 mcg/kg daily or
- Pegfilgrastim 6 mg once for each treatment cycle.

For hypersensitivity reactions
To prevent hypersensitivity reactions, give the following before paclitaxel administration: dexamethasone 20 mg P.O. 12 hours and 6 hours before, diphenhydramine 50 mg I.V. 30 to 60 minutes before, *and* cimetidine 300 mg I.V. or ranitidine 50 mg I.V. 30 to 60 minutes before.

For diarrhea (very likely)
An antidiarrheal is recommended.

For cisplatin-induced nephrotoxicity
Maintain urine output of at least 75 ml/hour for several hours before and after each cisplatin dose. Consider amifostine for prevention of cisplatin-induced nephrotoxicity.

Gastric cancer

DCF (or TCF) (docetaxel [Taxotere], cisplatin, 5-fluorouracil)

Docetaxel 85 mg/m² I.V. on day 1
Cisplatin 75 mg/m² I.V. on day 1
5-Fluorouracil 300 mg/m² by continuous I.V. infusion on days 1 through 14
Repeat cycle every 21 days for maximum of eight cycles.

Reference: Roth D, et al. *J Clin Oncol.* 2004;22(14S):4020.

Supportive therapy

For nausea and vomiting
On day 1, follow acute-onset antiemetic regimen for level 5 risk. Anticipatory, breakthrough, and delayed-onset regimens are recommended.

On days 2 through 14, follow acute-onset antiemetic regimen for level 2 risk. Anticipatory, breakthrough, and delayed-onset regimens are recommended as needed.

For anemia (likely)
If hemoglobin level is less than 10 g/dl, *one* of the following is recommended:
- Epoetin alfa 150 units/kg subcutaneously three times weekly. If unsatisfactory response, may increase to 300 units/kg three times weekly.
- Epoetin alfa 40,000 units subcutaneously weekly; may increase to 60,000 units if unsatisfactory response.
- Darbepoetin alfa 3 mcg/kg subcutaneously every 2 weeks; may increase to 5 mcg/kg if unsatisfactory response.
- Darbepoetin alfa 200 mcg subcutaneously every 2 weeks; may increase to 300 mcg if unsatisfactory response.

For neutropenia (high risk)
To prevent neutropenia, start *one* of the following colony-stimulating factors 1 to 3 days after completion of chemotherapy and continue through postnadir recovery:
- Filgrastim 5 mcg/kg daily or

• Pegfilgrastim 6 mg once for each treatment cycle.
For diarrhea (very likely)
An antidiarrheal is recommended.
For hypersensitivity reactions
To prevent hypersensitivity reactions, give dexamethasone 8 mg P.O. twice daily for 3 days, starting 1 day before administration of docetaxel.
For cisplatin-induced nephrotoxicity
Maintain urine output of at least 75 ml/hour for several hours before and after each cisplatin dose. Consider amifostine for prevention of cisplatin-induced nephrotoxicity.

DXP (docetaxel, capecitabine [Xeloda], cisplatin [Platinol-AQ])

Capecitabine 1,875 mg/m^2 P.O. daily in two equally divided doses on days 1 through 14
Docetaxel 60 mg/m^2 I.V. on day 1
Cisplatin 60 mg/m^2 I.V. on day 1
Repeat cycle every 21 days.
Reference: Kang YK, et al. *J Clin Oncol.* 2004;22(14S):4066.

Supportive therapy
For nausea and vomiting
On day 1, follow acute-onset antiemetic regimen for level 5 risk. Anticipatory, breakthrough, and delayed-onset regimens are recommended.
On days 2 through 14, follow acute-onset antiemetic regimen for level 2 risk. Anticipatory, breakthrough, and delayed-onset regimens are recommended as needed.
For anemia (likely)
If hemoglobin level is less than 10 g/dl, *one* of the following is recommended:
• Epoetin alfa 150 units/kg subcutaneously three times weekly. If unsatisfactory response, may increase to 300 units/kg three times weekly.
• Epoetin alfa 40,000 units subcutaneously weekly; may increase to 60,000 units if unsatisfactory response.

• Darbepoetin alfa 3 mcg/kg subcutaneously every 2 weeks; may increase to 5 mcg/kg if unsatisfactory response.
• Darbepoetin alfa 200 mcg subcutaneously every 2 weeks; may increase to 300 mcg if unsatisfactory response.
For neutropenia (high risk)
To prevent neutropenia, start *one* of the following colony-stimulating factors 1 to 3 days after completion of chemotherapy and continue through postnadir recovery:
• Filgrastim 5 mcg/kg daily or
• Pegfilgrastim 6 mg once for each treatment cycle.
For diarrhea (likely)
Prescribe antidiarrheal as indicated.
For hypersensitivity reactions
To prevent hypersensitivity reactions, give dexamethasone 8 mg P.O. twice daily for 3 days, starting 1 day before administration of docetaxel.
For cisplatin-induced nephrotoxicity
Maintain urine output of at least 75 ml/hour for several hours before and after each cisplatin dose. Consider amifostine for prevention of cisplatin-induced nephrotoxicity.

ECF (epirubicin, cisplatin, 5-fluorouracil)

Epirubicin 50 mg/m^2 by I.V. bolus on day 1,
Cisplatin 60 mg/m^2 I.V. over 2 hours on day 1
5-Fluorouracil 200 mg/m^2 daily by continuous I.V. infusion on days 1 through 21
Repeat cycle every 21 to 28 days.
Reference: Waters JS, et al. *Br J Cancer.* 1999;80:269-272; Webb A, et al. *J Clin Oncol.* 1997;15:261-267; Findlay M, et al. *Ann Oncol.* 1994;5:609-616.

Supportive therapy
For nausea and vomiting
On day 1, follow acute-onset antiemetic regimen for level 5 risk. Anticipatory, breakthrough, and delayed-onset regimens are recommended.

On days 2 through 21, follow acute-onset antiemetic regimen for level 2 risk. Anticipatory, breakthrough, and delayed-onset regimens are recommended as needed.

For anemia (likely)

If hemoglobin level is less than 10 g/dl, *one* of the following is recommended:

• Epoetin alfa 150 units/kg subcutaneously three times weekly. If unsatisfactory response, may increase to 300 units/kg three times weekly.

• Epoetin alfa 40,000 units subcutaneously weekly; may increase to 60,000 units if unsatisfactory response.

• Darbepoetin alfa 3 mcg/kg subcutaneously every 2 weeks; may increase to 5 mcg/kg if unsatisfactory response.

• Darbepoetin alfa 200 mcg subcutaneously every 2 weeks; may increase to 300 mcg if unsatisfactory response.

For neutropenia (high risk, day 2)

To prevent neutropenia, give filgrastim 5 mcg/kg daily *or* pegfilgrastim, one dose of 6 mg per cycle of treatment subcutaneously. Start colony-stimulating factors 1 to 3 days after completion of chemotherapy; continue through postnadir recovery.

For diarrhea (very likely)

An antidiarrheal is recommended.

For cisplatin-induced nephrotoxicity

Maintain urine output of at least 75 ml/hour for several hours before and after each cisplatin dose. Consider amifostine for prevention of cisplatin-induced nephrotoxicity.

ELF (etoposide, leucovorin, 5-fluorouracil)

Leucovorin 150 mg/m² I.V. daily over 10 minutes on days 1 through 3, then
Etoposide 120 mg/m² I.V. daily over 30 minutes on days 1 through 3, then
5-Fluorouracil (5-FU) 500 mg/m² I.V. daily over 10 minutes on days 1 through 3
Repeat cycle every 21 days.

Or

Leucovorin 300 mg/m² I.V. daily over 10 minutes on days 1 through 3, then
Etoposide 120 mg/m² I.V. daily over 50 minutes on days 1 through 3, then
5-FU 500 mg/m² daily by I.V. bolus over 10 minutes on days 1 through 3
Repeat cycle every 21 days.

Reference: di Bartolomeo M, et al. *Oncology.* 1995;52:41-44; Vanhoefer U, et al. *J Clin Oncol.* 2000;18:2648-2657; Moehler M, et al. *Br J Cancer.* 2005;92:2122-2128; Wilke H. *Cancer Treat Res.* 1991;55:363-373.

Supportive therapy

For nausea and vomiting

On days 1 through 3, follow acute-onset antiemetic regimen for level 3 risk. Anticipatory, breakthrough, and delayed-onset regimens are recommended as needed.

For anemia (likely)

If hemoglobin level is less than 10 g/dl, *one* of the following is recommended:

• Epoetin alfa 150 units/kg subcutaneously three times weekly. If unsatisfactory response, may increase to 300 units/kg three times weekly.

• Epoetin alfa 40,000 units subcutaneously weekly; may increase to 60,000 units if unsatisfactory response.

• Darbepoetin alfa 3 mcg/kg subcutaneously every 2 weeks; may increase to 5 mcg/kg if unsatisfactory response.

• Darbepoetin alfa 200 mcg subcutaneously every 2 weeks; may increase to 300 mcg if unsatisfactory response.

For neutropenia (high risk)

To prevent neutropenia, start *one* of the following colony-stimulating factors 1 to 3 days after completion of chemotherapy and continue through postnadir recovery:

• Filgrastim 5 mcg/kg daily or

• Pegfilgrastim 6 mg once for each treatment cycle.

For diarrhea (very likely)

An antidiarrheal is recommended.

FAMTX (5-fluorouracil, doxorubicin [Adriamycin], methotrexate)

Methotrexate 1,500 mg/m² I.V. on day 1
5-Fluorouracil 1,500 mg/m² I.V. on day 1 given 1 hour after methotrexate dose
Leucovorin 15 mg/m² P.O. given 24 hours after methotrexate dose and every 6 hours for 48 hours
Doxorubicin 30 mg/m² I.V., day 15
Repeat cycle every 28 days.

Reference: Wills J, et al. *J Clin Oncol.* 1986;4:1799-1803; Vanhoefer U, et al. *J Clin Oncol.* 2000;18:2648-2657.

Supportive therapy

For nausea and vomiting
On day 1, follow acute-onset antiemetic regimen for level 4 risk. Anticipatory, breakthrough, and delayed-onset regimens are recommended as needed.

On day 15, follow acute-onset antiemetic regimen for level 3 risk. Anticipatory, breakthrough, and delayed-onset regimens are recommended as needed.

For anemia (likely)
If hemoglobin level is less than 10 g/dl, *one* of the following is recommended:
• Epoetin alfa 150 units/kg subcutaneously three times weekly. If unsatisfactory response, may increase to 300 units/kg three times weekly.
• Epoetin alfa 40,000 units subcutaneously weekly; may increase to 60,000 units if unsatisfactory response.
• Darbepoetin alfa 3 mcg/kg subcutaneously every 2 weeks; may increase to 5 mcg/kg if unsatisfactory response.
• Darbepoetin alfa 200 mcg subcutaneously every 2 weeks; may increase to 300 mcg if unsatisfactory response.

For neutropenia (high risk)
To prevent neutropenia, start *one* of the following colony-stimulating factors 1 to 3 days after completion of chemotherapy and continue through postnadir recovery:

• Filgrastim 5 mcg/kg daily or
• Pegfilgrastim 6 mg once for each treatment cycle.

For diarrhea (very likely)
An antidiarrheal is recommended.

For methotrexate-induced nephrotoxicity
Maintain urine output of at least 75 ml/hour for several hours before and after each methotrexate dose. Consider amifostine for prevention of methotrexate-induced nephrotoxicity.

FOLFOX6 (oxaliplatin, leucovorin, 5-fluorouracil)

Oxaliplatin 100 mg/m² I.V. on day 1
Leucovorin 400 mg/m² I.V. over 2 hours on day 1, followed by
5-Fluorouracil (5-FU) Initial dose, 400 mg/m² I.V. on day 1, then 3,000 mg/m² by continuous I.V. infusion over next 46 hours
Repeat cycle every 14 days.

Reference: Louvet C, et al. *J Clin Oncol.* 2002;20:4543-4548.

Supportive therapy

For nausea and vomiting
On day 1, follow acute-onset antiemetic regimen for level 4 risk. Anticipatory, breakthrough, and delayed-onset regimens are recommended as needed.

On 5-FU days only, follow acute-onset antiemetic regimen for level 2 risk. Anticipatory, breakthrough, and delayed-onset regimens are recommended as needed.

For anemia (likely)
If hemoglobin level is less than 10 g/dl, *one* of the following is recommended:
• Epoetin alfa 150 units/kg subcutaneously three times weekly. If unsatisfactory response, may increase to 300 units/kg three times weekly.
• Epoetin alfa 40,000 units subcutaneously weekly; may increase to 60,000 units if unsatisfactory response.

- Darbepoetin alfa 3 mcg/kg subcutaneously every 2 weeks; may increase to 5 mcg/kg if unsatisfactory response.
- Darbepoetin alfa 200 mcg subcutaneously every 2 weeks; may increase to 300 mcg if unsatisfactory response.

For neutropenia (high risk)

To prevent neutropenia, start *one* of the following colony-stimulating factors 1 to 3 days after completion of chemotherapy and continue through postnadir recovery:

- Filgrastim 5 mcg/kg daily or
- Pegfilgrastim 6 mg once for each treatment cycle.

For diarrhea (very likely)

An antidiarrheal is recommended.

FUP (5-fluorouracil, cisplatin [Platinol-AQ])

5-Fluorouracil 1,000 mg/m² by continuous I.V. infusion on days 1 through 5
Cisplatin 100 mg/m² I.V. over 1 hour on day 2
Repeat cycle every 28 days.

Reference: Vanhoefer U, et al. *J Clin Oncol.* 2000;18:2648-2657.

Supportive therapy

For nausea and vomiting

On days 1, 3, 4, 5, follow acute-onset antiemetic regimen for level 2 risk. Anticipatory, breakthrough, and delayed-onset regimens are recommended as needed.

On day 2, follow acute-onset antiemetic regimen for level 5 risk. Anticipatory, breakthrough, and delayed-onset regimens are recommended.

For anemia (likely)

If hemoglobin level is less than 10 g/dl, *one* of the following is recommended:

- Epoetin alfa 150 units/kg subcutaneously three times weekly. If unsatisfactory response, may increase to 300 units/kg three times weekly.
- Epoetin alfa 40,000 units subcutaneously weekly; may increase to 60,000 units if unsatisfactory response.

- Darbepoetin alfa 3 mcg/kg subcutaneously every 2 weeks; may increase to 5 mcg/kg if unsatisfactory response.
- Darbepoetin alfa 200 mcg subcutaneously every 2 weeks; may increase to 300 mcg if unsatisfactory response.

For neutropenia (high risk)

To prevent neutropenia, start *one* of the following colony-stimulating factors 1 to 3 days after completion of chemotherapy and continue through postnadir recovery:

- Filgrastim 5 mcg/kg daily or
- Pegfilgrastim 6 mg once for each treatment cycle.

For diarrhea (very likely)

An antidiarrheal is recommended.

For cisplatin-induced nephrotoxicity

Maintain urine output of at least 75 ml/hour for several hours before and after each cisplatin dose. Consider amifostine for prevention of cisplatin-induced nephrotoxicity.

Irinotecan, 5-fluorouracil, leucovorin

Irinotecan 180 mg/m² by I.V. infusion over 2 hours on day 1
Leucovorin 200 mg/m² by I.V. infusion over 2 hours on days 1 and 2
5-Fluorouracil Initial dose, 400 mg/m² by I.V. bolus on days 1 and 2, then 600 mg/m² by continuous I.V. infusion over 22 hours on days 1 and 2
Repeat cycle every 14 days.

Reference: Bouche O, et al. *J Clin Oncol.* 2004;22:4319-4328.

Supportive therapy

For nausea and vomiting

On day 1, follow acute-onset antiemetic regimen for level 4 risk. Anticipatory, breakthrough, and delayed-onset regimens are recommended as needed.

On day 2, follow acute-onset antiemetic regimen for level 2 risk. Anticipatory, breakthrough, and delayed-onset regimens are recommended as needed.

See front endpaper for specific antiemetic therapies.

For anemia (likely)
If hemoglobin level is less than 10 g/dl, **one** of the following is recommended:
• Epoetin alfa 150 units/kg subcutaneously three times weekly. If unsatisfactory response, may increase to 300 units/kg three times weekly.
• Epoetin alfa 40,000 units subcutaneously weekly; may increase to 60,000 units if unsatisfactory response.
• Darbepoetin alfa 3 mcg/kg subcutaneously every 2 weeks; may increase to 5 mcg/kg if unsatisfactory response.
• Darbepoetin alfa 200 mcg subcutaneously every 2 weeks; may increase to 300 mcg if unsatisfactory response.

For neutropenia (high risk)
To prevent neutropenia, start **one** of the following colony-stimulating factors 1 to 3 days after completion of chemotherapy and continue through postnadir recovery:
• Filgrastim 5 mcg/kg daily or
• Pegfilgrastim 6 mg once for each treatment cycle.

For diarrhea (very likely)
An antidiarrheal is recommended.

Paclitaxel, cisplatin, 5-fluorouracil, leucovorin

Paclitaxel 175 mg/m² I.V. over 3 hours on days 1 and 22
Cisplatin 50 mg/m² I.V. over 1 hour on days 8 and 29
Leucovorin 500 mg/m² I.V. over 2 hours on days 1, 8, 15, 22, 29, and 36, followed by
5-Fluorouracil 2,000 mg/m² by continuous I.V. infusion over 24 hours on days 1, 8, 15, 22, 29, and 36
Repeat cycle every 6 weeks, with 2 weeks of rest between cycles.

Reference: Kollmannsberger C, et al. *Br J Cancer.* 2000;83:458-462.

Supportive therapy
For nausea and vomiting
On days 1 and 22, follow acute-onset antiemetic regimen for level 3 risk. Anticipatory, breakthrough, and delayed-onset regimens are recommended as needed.
On days 8 and 29, follow acute-onset antiemetic regimen for level 5 risk. Anticipatory, breakthrough, and delayed-onset regimens are recommended.
On days 15 and 36, follow acute-onset antiemetic regimen for level 2 risk. Anticipatory, breakthrough, and delayed-onset regimens are recommended as needed.

For anemia (likely)
If hemoglobin level is less than 10 g/dl, **one** of the following is recommended:
• Epoetin alfa 150 units/kg subcutaneously three times weekly. If unsatisfactory response, may increase to 300 units/kg three times weekly.
• Epoetin alfa 40,000 units subcutaneously weekly; may increase to 60,000 units if unsatisfactory response.
• Darbepoetin alfa 3 mcg/kg subcutaneously every 2 weeks; may increase to 5 mcg/kg if unsatisfactory response.
• Darbepoetin alfa 200 mcg subcutaneously every 2 weeks; may increase to 300 mcg if unsatisfactory response.

For neutropenia (high risk)
To prevent neutropenia, start **one** of the following colony-stimulating factors 1 to 3 days after completion of chemotherapy and continue through postnadir recovery:
• Filgrastim 5 mcg/kg daily or
• Pegfilgrastim 6 mg once for each treatment cycle.

For diarrhea (very likely)
An antidiarrheal is recommended.

For hypersensitivity reactions
To prevent hypersensitivity reactions, give the following before paclitaxel administration: Dexamethasone 20 mg P.O. 12 hours and 6 hours before, diphenhydramine 50 mg I.V. 30 to 60 minutes before, *and* cimetidine 300 mg I.V. *or* ranitidine 50 mg I.V. 30 to 60 minutes before.

For cisplatin-induced nephrotoxicity
Maintain urine output of at least 75 ml/hour

for several hours before and after each cisplatin dose. Consider amifostine for prevention of cisplatin-induced nephrotoxicity.

TC (docetaxel [Taxotere], cisplatin)

Docetaxel 85 mg/m^2 I.V. over 1 hour on day 1 followed by
Cisplatin 75 mg/m^2 I.V. over 1 hour on day 1
Repeat cycle every 21 days for maximum of eight cycles.

Reference: Roth AD, et al. *Ann Oncol.* 2000;11:301-306.

Supportive therapy

For nausea and vomiting
On day 1, follow acute-onset antiemetic regimen for level 5 risk. Anticipatory, breakthrough, and delayed-onset regimens are recommended.

For anemia (likely)
If hemoglobin level is less than 10 g/dl, *one* of the following is recommended:
• Epoetin alfa 150 units/kg subcutaneously three times weekly. If unsatisfactory response, may increase to 300 units/kg three times weekly.
• Epoetin alfa 40,000 units subcutaneously weekly; may increase to 60,000 units if unsatisfactory response.
• Darbepoetin alfa 3 mcg/kg subcutaneously every 2 weeks; may increase to 5 mcg/kg if unsatisfactory response.
• Darbepoetin alfa 200 mcg subcutaneously every 2 weeks; may increase to 300 mcg if unsatisfactory response.

For neutropenia (high risk)
To prevent neutropenia, start *one* of the following colony-stimulating factors 1 to 3 days after completion of chemotherapy and continue through postnadir recovery:
• Filgrastim 5 mcg/kg daily or
• Pegfilgrastim 6 mg once for each treatment cycle. .

For hypersensitivity reactions
To prevent hypersensitivity reactions, give dexamethasone 8 mg P.O. twice daily for 3

days, starting 1 day before administration of docetaxel and continuing for 4 days.
For cisplatin-induced nephrotoxicity
Maintain urine output of at least 75 ml/hour for several hours before and after each cisplatin dose. Consider amifostine for prevention of cisplatin-induced nephrotoxicity.

Head and neck cancers

Cisplatin

Cisplatin 100 mg/m^2 I.V. on days 1, 22, and 43 of radiation therapy regimen
Reference: Bernier J, et al. *N Engl J Med.* 2004;350:1945-1952.

Supportive therapy

For nausea and vomiting
On days 1, 22, and 43, follow acute-onset antiemetic regimen for level 5 risk. Anticipatory, breakthrough, and delayed-onset regimens are recommended.

For anemia (likely)
If hemoglobin level is less than 10 g/dl, *one* of the following is recommended:
• Epoetin alfa 150 units/kg subcutaneously three times weekly. If unsatisfactory response, may increase to 300 units/kg three times weekly.
• Epoetin alfa 40,000 units subcutaneously weekly; may increase to 60,000 units if unsatisfactory response.
• Darbepoetin alfa 3 mcg/kg subcutaneously every 2 weeks; may increase to 5 mcg/kg if unsatisfactory response.
• Darbepoetin alfa 200 mcg subcutaneously every 2 weeks; may increase to 300 mcg if unsatisfactory response.

For neutropenia (high risk)
To prevent neutropenia, start *one* of the following colony-stimulating factors 1 to 3 days after completion of chemotherapy and continue through postnadir recovery:
• Filgrastim 5 mcg/kg daily or

- Pegfilgrastim 6 mg once for each treatment cycle.

For cisplatin-induced nephrotoxicity
Maintain urine output of at least 75 ml/hour for several hours before and after each cisplatin dose. Consider amifostine for prevention of cisplatin-induced nephrotoxicity.

Cisplatin, 5-fluorouracil

Cisplatin 100 mg/m² by continuous I.V. infusion over 24 hours on day 1
5-Fluorouracil (5-FU) 5,000 mg/m² by continuous I.V. infusion over 120 hours on days 1 through 5
Repeat cycle every 21 days.
Reference: DeAndres L, et al. *J Clin Oncol.* 1995;13:1493-1500.
Or
Cisplatin 100 mg/m² I.V. over 1 hour on days 1 and 29
5-FU 1,000 mg/m² on days 1 through 4 and 29 through 32. Both drugs given in combination with radiation.
Give for one cycle.
Reference: Poole ME, et al. *Arch Otolaryngol Head Neck Surg.* 2001;127:1446-1450.
Or
Cisplatin 100 mg/m² by I.V. infusion on day 1
5-FU 1,000 mg/m² I.V. over 120 hours. Both drugs given in combination with radiation.
Give for three cycles.
Reference: Lewin F, et al. *Radiother Oncol.* 1997;43:23-28.

Supportive therapy
For nausea and vomiting
On cisplatin days, follow acute-onset antiemetic regimen for level 5 risk. Anticipatory, breakthrough, and delayed-onset regimens are recommended.

On 5-FU days, follow acute-onset antiemetic regimen for level 2 risk. Anticipatory, breakthrough, and delayed-onset regimens are recommended as needed.

For anemia (likely)
If hemoglobin level is less than 10 g/dl, *one* of the following is recommended:
- Epoetin alfa 150 units/kg subcutaneously three times weekly. If unsatisfactory response, may increase to 300 units/kg three times weekly.
- Epoetin alfa 40,000 units subcutaneously weekly; may increase to 60,000 units if unsatisfactory response.
- Darbepoetin alfa 3 mcg/kg subcutaneously every 2 weeks; may increase to 5 mcg/kg if unsatisfactory response.
- Darbepoetin alfa 200 mcg subcutaneously every 2 weeks; may increase to 300 mcg if unsatisfactory response.

For neutropenia (high risk)
To prevent neutropenia, start *one* of the following colony-stimulating factors 1 to 3 days after completion of chemotherapy and continue through postnadir recovery:
- Filgrastim 5 mcg/kg daily or
- Pegfilgrastim 6 mg once for each treatment cycle.

For diarrhea (very likely)
An antidiarrheal is recommended.

For cisplatin-induced nephrotoxicity
Maintain urine output of at least 75 ml/hour for several hours before and after each cisplatin dose. Consider amifostine for prevention of cisplatin-induced nephrotoxicity.

Hepatobiliary cancer

5-Fluorouracil

5-Fluorouracil 200 mg/m² by continuous I.V. infusion daily, starting on day 1 of radiation and continuing through course of radiation (may last 5 to 7 weeks)
Reference: Whittington R, et al. *J Clin Oncol.* 1995;13:227-232.

Supportive therapy
For nausea and vomiting
Follow acute-onset antiemetic regimen for lev-

el 2 risk. Anticipatory, breakthrough, and delayed-onset regimens are recommended as needed.

For anemia (likely)

If hemoglobin level is less than 10 g/dl, *one* of the following is recommended:

• Epoetin alfa 150 units/kg subcutaneously three times weekly. If unsatisfactory response, may increase to 300 units/kg three times weekly.

• Epoetin alfa 40,000 units subcutaneously weekly; may increase to 60,000 units if unsatisfactory response.

• Darbepoetin alfa 3 mcg/kg subcutaneously every 2 weeks; may increase to 5 mcg/kg if unsatisfactory response.

• Darbepoetin alfa 200 mcg subcutaneously every 2 weeks; may increase to 300 mcg if unsatisfactory response.

For neutropenia (high risk)

To prevent neutropenia, start *one* of the following colony-stimulating factors 1 to 3 days after completion of chemotherapy and continue through postnadir recovery:

• Filgrastim 5 mcg/kg daily or
• Pegfilgrastim 6 mg once for each treatment cycle.

For diarrhea (very likely)

An antidiarrheal is recommended.

5-Fluorouracil, leucovorin

Leucovorin 25 mg/m² daily by I.V. infusion over 2 hours on days 1 through 5
5-Fluorouracil 375 mg/m² daily by I.V. infusion on days 1 through 5
Repeat cycle every 21 to 28 days.

Reference: Choi CW. *Am J Clin Oncol.* 2000;23:425-428.

Supportive therapy

For nausea and vomiting

Follow acute-onset antiemetic regimen for level 2 risk. Anticipatory, breakthrough, and delayed-onset regimens are recommended as needed.

For anemia (likely)

If hemoglobin level is less than 10 g/dl, *one* of the following is recommended:

• Epoetin alfa 150 units/kg subcutaneously three times weekly. If unsatisfactory response, may increase to 300 units/kg three times weekly.

• Epoetin alfa 40,000 units subcutaneously weekly; may increase to 60,000 units if unsatisfactory response.

• Darbepoetin alfa 3 mcg/kg subcutaneously every 2 weeks; may increase to 5 mcg/kg if unsatisfactory response.

• Darbepoetin alfa 200 mcg subcutaneously every 2 weeks; may increase to 300 mcg if unsatisfactory response.

For diarrhea (very likely)

An antidiarrheal is recommended.

Gemcitabine

Gemcitabine 1,000 mg/m² I.V. over 30 minutes for 3 weeks
Repeat every 28 days.

Reference: Kubicka S, et al. *Hepatogastroenterology.* 2001;48:783-789.

Supportive therapy

For nausea and vomiting

Follow acute-onset antiemetic regimen for level 2 risk. Anticipatory, breakthrough, and delayed-onset regimens are recommended as needed.

For anemia (likely)

If hemoglobin level is less than 10 g/dl, *one* of the following is recommended:

• Epoetin alfa 150 units/kg subcutaneously three times weekly. If unsatisfactory response, may increase to 300 units/kg three times weekly.

• Epoetin alfa 40,000 units subcutaneously weekly; may increase to 60,000 units if unsatisfactory response.

• Darbepoetin alfa 3 mcg/kg subcutaneously every 2 weeks; may increase to 5 mcg/kg if unsatisfactory response.

- Darbepoetin alfa 200 mcg subcutaneously every 2 weeks; may increase to 300 mcg if unsatisfactory response.

Hodgkin's disease

ABVD (doxorubicin [Adriamycin], bleomycin, vinblastine, dacarbazine)

Doxorubicin 25 mg/m^2 I.V. on days 1 and 15
Bleomycin 10 units/m^2 I.V. on days 1 and 15
Vinblastine 6 mg/m^2 I.V. on days 1 and 15
Dacarbazine (DTIC) 375 mg/m^2 I.V. on days 1 and 15
Repeat cycle every 28 days.
Reference: Bonadonna G, et al. *Am Soc Clin Oncol.* 2004;22:2835-2841.

Supportive therapy
For nausea and vomiting
On days 1 and 15, follow acute-onset antiemetic regimen for level 5 risk. Anticipatory, breakthrough, and delayed-onset regimens are recommended.
For anemia (likely)
If hemoglobin level is less than 10 g/dl, *one* of the following is recommended:
- Epoetin alfa 150 units/kg subcutaneously three times weekly. If unsatisfactory response, may increase to 300 units/kg three times weekly.
- Epoetin alfa 40,000 units subcutaneously weekly; may increase to 60,000 units if unsatisfactory response.
- Darbepoetin alfa 3 mcg/kg subcutaneously every 2 weeks; may increase to 5 mcg/kg if unsatisfactory response.
- Darbepoetin alfa 200 mcg subcutaneously every 2 weeks; may increase to 300 mcg if unsatisfactory response.
For neutropenia (high risk)
To prevent neutropenia, start *one* of the following colony-stimulating factors 1 to 3 days after completion of chemotherapy and continue through postnadir recovery:

- Filgrastim 5 mcg/kg daily or
- Pegfilgrastim 6 mg once for each treatment cycle.
For diarrhea (likely)
Prescribe antidiarrheal as indicated.

BEACOPP (bleomycin, etoposide, doxorubicin [Adriamycin], cyclophosphamide, vincristine [Oncovin], procarbazine, prednisone)

Bleomycin 10 mg/m^2 I.V. on day 8
Etoposide 100 mg/m^2 I.V. on days 1 through 3
Doxorubicin 25 mg/m^2 I.V. on day 1
Cyclophosphamide 650 mg/m^2 I.V. on day 1
Vincristine 1.4 mg/m^2 I.V. on day 1 or day 8
Procarbazine 100 mg/m^2 P.O. on days 1 through 7
Prednisone 40 mg/m^2 P.O. on days 1 through 14
Repeat cycle every 21 days.
Reference: Tesch H, et al. Blood. 1998;92:4560-4567; Pazdur R, et al., eds. *Cancer Management: A Multidisciplinary Approach.* 9th ed. Lawrence, KS: CMP Media; 2005.

Supportive therapy
For nausea and vomiting
On days 1 through 3, follow acute-onset antiemetic regimen for level 5 risk. Anticipatory, breakthrough, and delayed-onset regimens are recommended.

On days 4 through 8, follow acute-onset antiemetic regimen for level 4 risk. Anticipatory, breakthrough, and delayed-onset regimens are recommended as needed.
For anemia (likely)
If hemoglobin level is less than 10 g/dl, *one* of the following is recommended:
- Epoetin alfa 150 units/kg subcutaneously three times weekly. If unsatisfactory response, may increase to 300 units/kg three times weekly.
- Epoetin alfa 40,000 units subcutaneously weekly; may increase to 60,000 units if unsatisfactory response.

- Darbepoetin alfa 3 mcg/kg subcutaneously every 2 weeks; may increase to 5 mcg/kg if unsatisfactory response.
- Darbepoetin alfa 200 mcg subcutaneously every 2 weeks; may increase to 300 mcg if unsatisfactory response.

For neutropenia (high risk)

To prevent neutropenia, start *one* of the following colony-stimulating factors 1 to 3 days after completion of chemotherapy and continue through postnadir recovery:

- Filgrastim 5 mcg/kg daily or
- Pegfilgrastim 6 mg once for each treatment cycle.

For diarrhea (likely)

Prescribe antidiarrheal as indicated.

For constipation (likely)

Order stool softener or laxative as indicated.

Stanford V (doxorubicin, vinblastine, mechlorethamine, vincristine, bleomycin, etoposide, prednisone)

Doxorubicin 25 mg/m^2 I.V. on days 1 and 15
Vinblastine 6 mg/m^2 I.V. on days 1 and 15
Mechlorethamine 6 mg/m^2 I.V. on day 1
Vincristine 1.4 mg/m^2 I.V. on days 8 and 22
Bleomycin 5 units/m^2 I.V. on days 8 and 22
Etoposide 60 mg/m^2 I.V. on days 15 and 16
Prednisone 40 mg/m^2 P.O. every other day for 10 weeks; then taper dosage downward by 10 mg every other day.

Repeat chemotherapy agents every 28 days for three cycles. Give prednisone continuously for 10 weeks, then taper as noted above.

Reference: Horning SJ, et al. *J Clin Oncol.* 2002;20:630-637; Pazdur R, et al., eds. *Cancer Management. A Multidisciplinary Approach.* 9th ed. Lawrence, KS: CMP Media; 2005.

Supportive therapy

For nausea and vomiting

On day 1, follow acute-onset antiemetic regimen for level 5 risk. Anticipatory, break-through, and delayed-onset regimens are recommended.

On days 8 and 22, follow acute-onset antiemetic regimen for level 1 risk.

On day 15, follow acute-onset antiemetic regimen for level 4 risk. Anticipatory, break-through, and delayed-onset regimens are recommended as needed.

On day 16, follow acute-onset antiemetic regimen for level 2 risk. Anticipatory, break-through, and delayed-onset regimens are recommended as needed.

For anemia (likely)

If hemoglobin level is less than 10 g/dl, *one* of the following is recommended:

- Epoetin alfa 150 units/kg subcutaneously three times weekly. If unsatisfactory response, may increase to 300 units/kg three times weekly.
- Epoetin alfa 40,000 units subcutaneously weekly; may increase to 60,000 units if unsatisfactory response.
- Darbepoetin alfa 3 mcg/kg subcutaneously every 2 weeks; may increase to 5 mcg/kg if unsatisfactory response.
- Darbepoetin alfa 200 mcg subcutaneously every 2 weeks; may increase to 300 mcg if unsatisfactory response.

For neutropenia (high risk)

To prevent neutropenia, start *one* of the following colony-stimulating factors 1 to 3 days after completion of chemotherapy and continue through postnadir recovery:

- Filgrastim 5 mcg/kg daily or
- Pegfilgrastim 6 mg once for each treatment cycle.

For diarrhea (likely)

Prescribe antidiarrheal as indicated.

For constipation (likely)

Order stool softener or laxative as indicated.

See front endpaper for specific antiemetic therapies.

Kidney cancer

Interferon alfa-2a, interleukin-2

Interleukin-2 (IL-2) 18 million units/m^2 daily by continuous I.V. infusion on days 1 through 5; repeat after 6 days of rest (induction), followed 3 weeks later by 18 million units/m^2 daily by continuous I.V. infusion on days 1 through 5 (maintenance).

Repeat maintenance cycle for four cycles, with 3 weeks' rest after each cycle.

Interferon alfa-2a 6 million units subcutaneously three times per week during each IL-2 cycle (induction and maintenance)

Reference: Negrier S, et al. *N Engl J Med.* 1998;338:1273-1278; Dutcher JP, et al. *Cancer J Sci Am.* 1997;3:157-162.

Supportive therapy

For nausea and vomiting
Follow acute-onset antiemetic regimen for level 3 risk. Anticipatory, breakthrough, and delayed-onset regimens are recommended as needed.

For diarrhea (likely)
Prescribe antidiarrheal as indicated.

For flulike symptoms
To avoid flulike symptoms, give indomethacin, acetaminophen, and ranitidine, starting night before first dose of IL-2 and continuing until 24 hours after IL-2 therapy stops.

For infection
To prevent infection, consider prophylactic antibiotic in patients with central lines.

Interleukin-2

High dose:
Interleukin-2 (IL-2) 600,000 to 720,000 units/kg I.V. over 15 minutes every 8 hours until toxicity occurs or 14 doses have been given over 5 days, followed by 7 to 10 days of rest.
Repeat cycle twice.

Low dose:
IL-2 Give 72,000 units/kg I.V. over 15 minutes every 8 hours until toxicity occurs or 14 doses have been given over 5 days; follow by 7 to 10 days of rest.
Repeat cycle up to three times.
Or
IL-2 Give 3 million units/m^2 daily by continuous I.V. infusion on days 1 through 5 and 12 through 17
Repeat second cycle every 28 days for four cycles.

Reference: Fyfe G, et al. *J Clin Oncol.* 1995;13:688-696; Pazdur R (ed), et al. *Cancer Management: A Multidisciplinary Approach.* 8th ed. CMP Healthcare Media; 2005; Yang JC, et al. *J Clin Oncol.* 2003;21:3127-3132.

Supportive therapy

For nausea and vomiting
Follow acute-onset antiemetic regimen for level 3 risk. Anticipatory, breakthrough, and delayed-onset regimens are recommended as needed.

For diarrhea (likely)
Prescribe antidiarrheal as indicated.

For flulike symptoms
To avoid flulike symptoms, give indomethacin, acetaminophen, and ranitidine, starting night before first dose of IL-2 and continuing until 24 hours after IL-2 therapy stops.

For infection
To prevent infection, consider prophylactic antibiotic in patients with central lines.

Vinblastine, interferon alfa-2a

Vinblastine 0.1 mg/kg I.V. every 3 weeks
Interferon alfa-2a 3 million units subcutaneously three times per week for first week, then 18 million units three times per week for subsequent weeks (9 million units for those unable to tolerate higher doses)

Reference: Pyrhonen S, et al. *J Clin Oncol.* 1999;17:2859-2867.

Supportive therapy

For nausea and vomiting
Follow acute-onset antiemetic regimen for level 1 risk.

For anemia (likely)
If hemoglobin level is less than 10 g/dl, *one* of the following is recommended:
- Epoetin alfa 150 units/kg subcutaneously three times weekly. If unsatisfactory response, may increase to 300 units/kg three times weekly.
- Epoetin alfa 40,000 units subcutaneously weekly; may increase to 60,000 units if unsatisfactory response.
- Darbepoetin alfa 3 mcg/kg subcutaneously every 2 weeks; may increase to 5 mcg/kg if unsatisfactory response.
- Darbepoetin alfa 200 mcg subcutaneously every 2 weeks; may increase to 300 mcg if unsatisfactory response.

For constipation (likely)
Order stool softener or laxative as indicated.

Lung cancer (non-small-cell)

Carboplatin, paclitaxel

Carboplatin to AUC of 5 or 6 I.V. on day 1
Paclitaxel 175 to 225 mg/m² I.V. over 3 hours on day 1
Repeat cycle every 21 days.
Reference: Strauss GM. *J Clin Oncol.* 2004;22(14S):7019.

Supportive therapy

For nausea and vomiting
On day 1, follow acute-onset antiemetic regimen for level 5 risk. Anticipatory, breakthrough, and delayed-onset regimens are recommended.

For anemia (likely)
If hemoglobin level is less than 10 g/dl, *one* of the following is recommended:
- Epoetin alfa 150 units/kg subcutaneously three times weekly. If unsatisfactory response, may increase to 300 units/kg three times weekly.
- Epoetin alfa 40,000 units subcutaneously weekly; may increase to 60,000 units if unsatisfactory response.
- Darbepoetin alfa 3 mcg/kg subcutaneously every 2 weeks; may increase to 5 mcg/kg if unsatisfactory response.
- Darbepoetin alfa 200 mcg subcutaneously every 2 weeks; may increase to 300 mcg if unsatisfactory response.

For neutropenia (high risk)
To prevent neutropenia, start *one* of the following colony-stimulating factors 1 to 3 days after completion of chemotherapy and continue through postnadir recovery:
- Filgrastim 5 mcg/kg daily or
- Pegfilgrastim 6 mg once for each treatment cycle.

For diarrhea (likely)
Prescribe antidiarrheal as indicated.

For constipation (likely)
Order stool softener or laxative as indicated.

For hypersensitivity reactions
To prevent hypersensitivity reactions, give the following before paclitaxel administration: dexamethasone 20 mg P.O. 12 hours and 6 hours before, diphenhydramine 50 mg I.V. 30 to 60 minutes before, *and* cimetidine 300 mg I.V. *or* ranitidine 50 mg I.V. 30 to 60 minutes before.

Cisplatin, docetaxel

Cisplatin 75 mg/m² I.V. on day 1
Docetaxel 75 mg/m² I.V. on day 1
Repeat cycle every 21 days.
Reference: Fossella F, et al. *Am Soc Clin Oncol.* 2003;21:3016-3024.

Supportive therapy

For nausea and vomiting
On day 1, follow acute-onset antiemetic regimen for level 5 risk. Anticipatory, breakthrough, and delayed-onset regimens are recommended.

For anemia (likely)
If hemoglobin level is less than 10 g/dl, *one* of the following is recommended:
• Epoetin alfa 150 units/kg subcutaneously three times weekly. If unsatisfactory response, may increase to 300 units/kg three times weekly.
• Epoetin alfa 40,000 units subcutaneously weekly; may increase to 60,000 units if unsatisfactory response.
• Darbepoetin alfa 3 mcg/kg subcutaneously every 2 weeks; may increase to 5 mcg/kg if unsatisfactory response.
• Darbepoetin alfa 200 mcg subcutaneously every 2 weeks; may increase to 300 mcg if unsatisfactory response.
For neutropenia (high risk)
To prevent neutropenia, start *one* of the following colony-stimulating factors 1 to 3 days after completion of chemotherapy and continue through postnadir recovery:
• Filgrastim 5 mcg/kg daily or
• Pegfilgrastim 6 mg once for each treatment cycle.
For diarrhea (likely)
Prescribe antidiarrheal as indicated.
For hypersensitivity reactions
To prevent hypersensitivity reactions, give dexamethasone 8 mg P.O. twice daily for 3 days, starting 1 day before administration of docetaxel.
For cisplatin-induced nephrotoxicity
Maintain urine output of at least 75 ml/hour for several hours before and after each cisplatin dose. Consider amifostine for prevention of cisplatin-induced nephrotoxicity.

Cisplatin, gemcitabine

Cisplatin 100 mg/m^2 I.V. on day 1
Gemcitabine 1,200 mg/m^2 I.V. on days 1 and 8
Repeat cycle every 21 days.
Reference: Gridelli C, et al. *Am Soc Clin Oncol.* 2003;21:3025-3034.
Or
Gemcitabine 1,000 mg/m^2 I.V. on days 1, 8, and 15

Cisplatin 100 mg/m^2 I.V. on day 2
Repeat cycle every 28 days.
Reference: Crino L, et al. *J Clin Oncol.* 1999;17:3522-3530.

Supportive therapy
For nausea and vomiting
For cisplatin days and days on which cisplatin and gemcitabine are given on same day, follow acute-onset antiemetic regimen for level 5 risk. Anticipatory, breakthrough, and delayed-onset regimens are recommended.
For gemcitabine days only, follow acute-onset antiemetic regimen for level 2 risk. Anticipatory, breakthrough, and delayed-onset regimens are recommended as needed.
For anemia (likely)
If hemoglobin level is less than 10 g/dl, *one* of the following is recommended:
• Epoetin alfa 150 units/kg subcutaneously three times weekly. If unsatisfactory response, may increase to 300 units/kg three times weekly.
• Epoetin alfa 40,000 units subcutaneously weekly; may increase to 60,000 units if unsatisfactory response.
• Darbepoetin alfa 3 mcg/kg subcutaneously every 2 weeks; may increase to 5 mcg/kg if unsatisfactory response.
• Darbepoetin alfa 200 mcg subcutaneously every 2 weeks; may increase to 300 mcg if unsatisfactory response.
For neutropenia (high risk)
To prevent neutropenia, start *one* of the following colony-stimulating factors 1 to 3 days after completion of chemotherapy and continue through postnadir recovery:
• Filgrastim 5 mcg/kg daily or
• Pegfilgrastim 6 mg once for each treatment cycle.
For diarrhea (likely)
Prescribe antidiarrheal as indicated.
For constipation (likely)
Order stool softener or laxative as indicated.
For cisplatin-induced nephrotoxicity
Maintain urine output of at least 75 ml/hour for several hours before and after each cis-

platin dose. Consider amifostine for prevention of cisplatin-induced nephrotoxicity.

Cisplatin, paclitaxel

Cisplatin 80 mg/m^2 I.V. over 30 minutes on day 1
Paclitaxel 175 mg/m^2 I.V. over 3 hours on day 1
Repeat cycle every 21 days.

Reference: Gatzemeier U. *J Clin Oncol.* 2000;18:3390-3399.

Supportive therapy
For nausea and vomiting
On day 1, follow acute-onset antiemetic regimen for level 5 risk. Anticipatory, breakthrough, and delayed-onset regimens are recommended.

For anemia (likely)
If hemoglobin level is less than 10 g/dl, *one* of the following is recommended:
• Epoetin alfa 150 units/kg subcutaneously three times weekly. If unsatisfactory response, may increase to 300 units/kg three times weekly.
• Epoetin alfa 40,000 units subcutaneously weekly; may increase to 60,000 units if unsatisfactory response.
• Darbepoetin alfa 3 mcg/kg subcutaneously every 2 weeks; may increase to 5 mcg/kg if unsatisfactory response.
• Darbepoetin alfa 200 mcg subcutaneously every 2 weeks; may increase to 300 mcg if unsatisfactory response.

For neutropenia (high risk)
To prevent neutropenia, start *one* of the following colony-stimulating factors 1 to 3 days after completion of chemotherapy and continue through postnadir recovery:
• Filgrastim 5 mcg/kg daily or
• Pegfilgrastim 6 mg once for each treatment cycle.

For diarrhea (likely)
Prescribe antidiarrheal as indicated.

For hypersensitivity reactions
To prevent hypersensitivity reactions, give the

following before paclitaxel administration: dexamethasone 20 mg P.O. 12 hours and 6 hours before, diphenhydramine 50 mg I.V. 30 to 60 minutes before, and cimetidine 300 mg I.V. or ranitidine 50 mg I.V. 30 to 60 minutes before.

For cisplatin-induced nephrotoxicity
Maintain urine output of at least 75 ml/hour for several hours before and after each cisplatin dose. Consider amifostine for prevention of cisplatin-induced nephrotoxicity.

Docetaxel

Docetaxel 100 mg/m^2 I.V. over 1 hour on day 1
Or
Docetaxel 75 mg/m^2 I.V. over 1 hour on day 1
Repeat every 21 days.

Reference: Gandara DR, et al. *J Clin Oncol.* 2000;18:131-135; Fossella FV, et al. *J Clin Oncol.* 2000;18:2354-2362.

Supportive therapy
For nausea and vomiting
Follow acute-onset antiemetic regimen for level 2 risk. Anticipatory, breakthrough, and delayed-onset regimens are recommended as needed.

For anemia (likely)
If hemoglobin level is less than 10 g/dl, *one* of the following is recommended:
• Epoetin alfa 150 units/kg subcutaneously three times weekly. If unsatisfactory response, may increase to 300 units/kg three times weekly.
• Epoetin alfa 40,000 units subcutaneously weekly; may increase to 60,000 units if unsatisfactory response.
• Darbepoetin alfa 3 mcg/kg subcutaneously every 2 weeks; may increase to 5 mcg/kg if unsatisfactory response.
• Darbepoetin alfa 200 mcg subcutaneously every 2 weeks; may increase to 300 mcg if unsatisfactory response.

For neutropenia (high risk)
To prevent neutropenia, start *one* of the fol-

lowing colony-stimulating factors 1 to 3 days after completion of chemotherapy and continue through postnadir recovery:

- Filgrastim 5 mcg/kg daily or
- Pegfilgrastim 6 mg once for each treatment cycle.

For hypersensitivity reactions

To prevent hypersensitivity reactions, give dexamethasone 8 mg P.O. twice daily for 3 days, starting 1 day before administration of docetaxel.

Erlotinib

Erlotinib 150 mg P.O. daily 2 hours after ingestion of food. Continue treatment until disease progresses or unacceptable toxicity occurs.

Reference: Pérez-Soler R. *J Clin Oncol.* 2004;22:3238-3247.

Supportive therapy

For nausea and vomiting

Follow acute-onset antiemetic regimen for level 1 risk.

For diarrhea (likely)

Prescribe antidiarrheal as indicated.

Gemcitabine

Gemcitabine 1,000 mg/m^2 I.V. on days 1, 8, and 15

Repeat every 28 days.

Reference: Baka S. *J Clin Oncol.* 2005;23:2136-2144.

Supportive therapy

For nausea and vomiting

Follow acute-onset antiemetic regimen for level 2 risk. Anticipatory, breakthrough, and delayed-onset regimens are recommended as needed.

For anemia (likely)

If hemoglobin level is less than 10 g/dl, *one* of the following is recommended:

- Epoetin alfa 150 units/kg subcutaneously three times weekly. If unsatisfactory response,

may increase to 300 units/kg three times weekly.

- Epoetin alfa 40,000 units subcutaneously weekly; may increase to 60,000 units if unsatisfactory response.
- Darbepoetin alfa 3 mcg/kg subcutaneously every 2 weeks; may increase to 5 mcg/kg if unsatisfactory response.
- Darbepoetin alfa 200 mcg subcutaneously every 2 weeks; may increase to 300 mcg if unsatisfactory response.

For neutropenia (high risk)

To prevent neutropenia, start *one* of the following colony-stimulating factors 1 to 3 days after completion of chemotherapy and continue through postnadir recovery:

- Filgrastim 5 mcg/kg daily or
- Pegfilgrastim 6 mg once for each treatment cycle.

For diarrhea (likely)

Prescribe antidiarrheal as indicated.

For constipation (likely)

Order stool softener or laxative as indicated.

Gemcitabine, docetaxel

Gemcitabine 1,000 mg/m^2 I.V. on days 1 and 8
Docetaxel 100 mg/m^2 I.V. on day 8
Repeat cycle every 21 days.

Reference: Georgoulias V, et al. *J Clin Oncol.* 2005;23:2937-2945.

Supportive therapy

For nausea and vomiting

Follow acute-onset antiemetic regimen for level 3 risk. Anticipatory, breakthrough, and delayed-onset regimens are recommended as needed.

For anemia (likely)

If hemoglobin level is less than 10 g/dl, *one* of the following is recommended:

- Epoetin alfa 150 units/kg subcutaneously three times weekly. If unsatisfactory response, may increase to 300 units/kg three times weekly.
- Epoetin alfa 40,000 units subcutaneously

weekly; may increase to 60,000 units if unsatisfactory response.

- Darbepoetin alfa 3 mcg/kg subcutaneously every 2 weeks; may increase to 5 mcg/kg if unsatisfactory response.
- Darbepoetin alfa 200 mcg subcutaneously every 2 weeks; may increase to 300 mcg if unsatisfactory response.

For neutropenia (high risk)
To prevent neutropenia, give filgrastim 150 mcg/m^2 subcutaneously on days 9 through 15.

For diarrhea (likely)
Prescribe antidiarrheal as indicated.

For constipation (likely)
Order stool softener or laxative as indicated.

For hypersensitivity reactions
To prevent hypersensitivity reactions, give dexamethasone 8 mg P.O. twice daily for 3 days, starting 1 day before administration of docetaxel.

Gemcitabine, paclitaxel

Gemcitabine 1,000 mg/m^2 I.V. on days 1 and 8
Paclitaxel 200 mg/m^2 I.V. over 3 hours on day 1
Repeat cycle every 21 days.
Reference: Kosmidis P, et al. *J Clin Oncol.* 2002;20:3578-3585.

Supportive therapy
For nausea and vomiting
Follow acute-onset antiemetic regimen for level 3 risk. Anticipatory, breakthrough, and delayed-onset regimens are recommended as needed.

For anemia (likely)
If hemoglobin level is less than 10 g/dl, *one* of the following is recommended:

- Epoetin alfa 150 units/kg subcutaneously three times weekly. If unsatisfactory response, may increase to 300 units/kg three times weekly.
- Epoetin alfa 40,000 units subcutaneously weekly; may increase to 60,000 units if unsatisfactory response.

- Darbepoetin alfa 3 mcg/kg subcutaneously every 2 weeks; may increase to 5 mcg/kg if unsatisfactory response.
- Darbepoetin alfa 200 mcg subcutaneously every 2 weeks; may increase to 300 mcg if unsatisfactory response.

For neutropenia (high risk)
To prevent neutropenia, start *one* of the following colony-stimulating factors 1 to 3 days after completion of chemotherapy and continue through postnadir recovery:

- Filgrastim 5 mcg/kg daily or
- Pegfilgrastim 6 mg once for each treatment cycle.

For diarrhea (likely)
Prescribe antidiarrheal as indicated.

For constipation (likely)
Order stool softener or laxative as indicated.

For hypersensitivity reactions
To prevent hypersensitivity reactions, give the following before paclitaxel administration: dexamethasone 20 mg P.O. 12 hours and 6 hours before, diphenhydramine 50 mg I.V. 30 to 60 minutes before, *and* cimetidine 300 mg I.V. *or* ranitidine 50 mg I.V. 30 to 60 minutes before.

Gemcitabine, vinorelbine

Gemcitabine 1,200 mg/m^2 I.V. on days 1 and 8
Vinorelbine 30 mg/m^2 I.V. on days 1 and 8
Repeat cycle every 21 days.
Or
Gemcitabine 800 to 1,000 mg/m^2 I.V. on days 1, 8, and 15
Vinorelbine 20 mg/m^2 I.V. on days 1, 8, and 15
Repeat cycle every 28 days.
Reference: Frasci G, et al. *J Clin Oncol.* 2000;18:2529-2536; Chen YM, et al. *Chest.* 2000;117:1583-1589; Hainsworth JD, et al. *Cancer.* 2000;88:1353-1358.

Supportive therapy
For nausea and vomiting
Follow acute-onset antiemetic regimen for level 2 risk. Anticipatory, breakthrough, and

See front endpaper for specific antiemetic therapies.

delayed-onset regimens are recommended as needed.

For anemia (likely)

If hemoglobin level is less than 10 g/dl, *one* of the following is recommended:

- Epoetin alfa 150 units/kg subcutaneously three times weekly. If unsatisfactory response, may increase to 300 units/kg three times weekly.
- Epoetin alfa 40,000 units subcutaneously weekly; may increase to 60,000 units if unsatisfactory response.
- Darbepoetin alfa 3 mcg/kg subcutaneously every 2 weeks; may increase to 5 mcg/kg if unsatisfactory response.
- Darbepoetin alfa 200 mcg subcutaneously every 2 weeks; may increase to 300 mcg if unsatisfactory response.

For neutropenia (high risk)

To prevent neutropenia, start *one* of the following colony-stimulating factors 1 to 3 days after completion of chemotherapy and continue through postnadir recovery:

- Filgrastim 5 mcg/kg daily or
- Pegfilgrastim 6 mg once for each treatment cycle.

For diarrhea (likely)

Prescribe antidiarrheal as indicated.

For constipation (likely)

Order stool softener or laxative as indicated.

Vinorelbine

Vinorelbine 25 to 30 mg/m² I.V. weekly
Repeat every 7 days.

Reference: Vokes EE, et al. *J Clin Oncol.* 2002;20:4191-4198.

Supportive therapy

For nausea and vomiting

Follow acute-onset antiemetic regimen for level 1 risk.

For anemia (likely)

If hemoglobin level is less than 10 g/dl, *one* of the following is recommended:

- Epoetin alfa 150 units/kg subcutaneously three times weekly. If unsatisfactory response,

may increase to 300 units/kg three times weekly.

- Epoetin alfa 40,000 units subcutaneously weekly; may increase to 60,000 units if unsatisfactory response.
- Darbepoetin alfa 3 mcg/kg subcutaneously every 2 weeks; may increase to 5 mcg/kg if unsatisfactory response.
- Darbepoetin alfa 200 mcg subcutaneously every 2 weeks; may increase to 300 mcg if unsatisfactory response.

For neutropenia (high risk)

To prevent neutropenia, start *one* of the following colony-stimulating factors 1 to 3 days after completion of chemotherapy and continue through postnadir recovery:

- Filgrastim 5 mcg/kg daily or
- Pegfilgrastim 6 mg once for each treatment cycle.

For constipation (likely)

Order stool softener or laxative as indicated.

Lung cancer (small-cell)

CAE (or ACE) (cyclophosphamide, doxorubicin [Adriamycin], etoposide)

Cyclophosphamide 1,000 mg/m² I.V. on day 1
Doxorubicin 45 mg/m² I.V. on day 1
Etoposide 100 mg/m² I.V. on days 1 through 3
Repeat cycle every 21 days.

Reference: Ardizzoni A, et al. *J Clin Oncol.* 2002;20:3947-3955.

Supportive therapy

For nausea and vomiting

On day 1, follow acute-onset antiemetic regimen for level 5 risk. Anticipatory, breakthrough, and delayed-onset regimens are recommended.

On days 2 and 3, follow acute-onset antiemetic regimen for level 2 risk. Anticipatory, breakthrough, and delayed-onset regimens are recommended as needed.

For anemia (likely)
If hemoglobin level is less than 10 g/dl, *one* of the following is recommended:
• Epoetin alfa 150 units/kg subcutaneously three times weekly. If unsatisfactory response, may increase to 300 units/kg three times weekly.
• Epoetin alfa 40,000 units subcutaneously weekly; may increase to 60,000 units if unsatisfactory response.
• Darbepoetin alfa 3 mcg/kg subcutaneously every 2 weeks; may increase to 5 mcg/kg if unsatisfactory response.
• Darbepoetin alfa 200 mcg subcutaneously every 2 weeks; may increase to 300 mcg if unsatisfactory response.

For neutropenia (high risk)
To prevent neutropenia, start *one* of the following colony-stimulating factors 1 to 3 days after completion of chemotherapy and continue through postnadir recovery:
• Filgrastim 5 mcg/kg daily or
• Pegfilgrastim 6 mg once for each treatment cycle.

For diarrhea (likely)
Prescribe antidiarrheal as indicated.

Carboplatin, etoposide

Carboplatin to AUC of 5 or 6 I.V. on day 1
Etoposide 100 mg/m^2 I.V. on days 1 through 3
Repeat cycle every 21 to 28 days.

Reference: Pazdur R, et al., eds. *Cancer Management. A Multidisciplinary Approach.* 9th ed. Lawrence, KS: CMP Media; 2005; Skarlos DV, et al. *Ann Oncol.* 2001;12:1231-1238.

Supportive therapy
For nausea and vomiting
On day 1, follow acute-onset antiemetic regimen for level 5 risk. Anticipatory, breakthrough, and delayed-onset regimens are recommended.

On days 2 and 3, follow acute-onset antiemetic regimen for level 2 risk. Anticipatory, breakthrough, and delayed-onset regimens are recommended as needed.

For anemia (likely)
If hemoglobin level is less than 10 g/dl, *one* of the following is recommended:
• Epoetin alfa 150 units/kg subcutaneously three times weekly. If unsatisfactory response, may increase to 300 units/kg three times weekly.
• Epoetin alfa 40,000 units subcutaneously weekly; may increase to 60,000 units if unsatisfactory response.
• Darbepoetin alfa 3 mcg/kg subcutaneously every 2 weeks; may increase to 5 mcg/kg if unsatisfactory response.
• Darbepoetin alfa 200 mcg subcutaneously every 2 weeks; may increase to 300 mcg if unsatisfactory response.

For neutropenia (high risk)
To prevent neutropenia, start *one* of the following colony-stimulating factors 1 to 3 days after completion of chemotherapy and continue through postnadir recovery:
• Filgrastim 5 mcg/kg daily or
• Pegfilgrastim 6 mg once for each treatment cycle.

For diarrhea (likely)
Prescribe antidiarrheal as indicated.

For constipation (likely)
Order stool softener or laxative as indicated.

Carboplatin, paclitaxel, etoposide

Carboplatin to AUC of 5 or 6 I.V. on day 1
Paclitaxel 135 to 200 mg/m^2 I.V. over 1 hour on day 1
Etoposide 50 mg P.O. alternating with 100 mg P.O. on days 1 through 10
Repeat cycle every 21 days.

Reference: Hainsworth JD, et al. *J Clin Oncol.* 1997;15:3464-3470.

Supportive therapy
For nausea and vomiting
On day 1, follow acute-onset antiemetic regimen for level 5 risk. Anticipatory, breakthrough, and delayed-onset regimens are recommended.

See front endpaper for specific antiemetic therapies.

On days 2 through 10, follow acute-onset antiemetic regimen for level 2 risk. Anticipatory, breakthrough, and delayed-onset regimens are recommended as needed.

For anemia (likely)
If hemoglobin level is less than 10 g/dl, *one* of the following is recommended:

• Epoetin alfa 150 units/kg subcutaneously three times weekly. If unsatisfactory response, may increase to 300 units/kg three times weekly.

• Epoetin alfa 40,000 units subcutaneously weekly; may increase to 60,000 units if unsatisfactory response.

• Darbepoetin alfa 3 mcg/kg subcutaneously every 2 weeks; may increase to 5 mcg/kg if unsatisfactory response.

• Darbepoetin alfa 200 mcg subcutaneously every 2 weeks; may increase to 300 mcg if unsatisfactory response.

For neutropenia (high risk)
To prevent neutropenia, start *one* of the following colony-stimulating factors 1 to 3 days after completion of chemotherapy and continue through postnadir recovery:

• Filgrastim 5 mcg/kg daily or
• Pegfilgrastim 6 mg once for each treatment cycle.

For hypersensitivity reactions
To prevent hypersensitivity reactions, give the following before paclitaxel administration: dexamethasone 20 mg P.O. 12 hours and 6 hours before, diphenhydramine 50 mg I.V. 30 to 60 minutes before, *and* cimetidine 300 mg I.V. *or* ranitidine 50 mg I.V. 30 to 60 minutes before.

CAV (cyclophosphamide, doxorubicin [Adriamycin], vincristine)

Cyclophosphamide 800 to 1,000 mg/m² I.V. on day 1
Doxorubicin 40 to 50 mg/m² I.V. on day 1
Vincristine 1 to 1.4 mg/m² I.V. on day 1
Repeat cycle every 21 to 28 days.

Reference: Fukuda M, et al. *J Natl Cancer Inst.* 1991;83:855-861; *Facts and Comparisons.* St. Louis, MO: Wolters Kluwer Business; 2005.

Supportive therapy
For nausea and vomiting
On day 1, follow acute-onset antiemetic regimen for level 5 risk. Anticipatory, breakthrough, and delayed-onset regimens are recommended.

For anemia (likely)
If hemoglobin level is less than 10 g/dl, *one* of the following is recommended:

• Epoetin alfa 150 units/kg subcutaneously three times weekly. If unsatisfactory response, may increase to 300 units/kg three times weekly.

• Epoetin alfa 40,000 units subcutaneously weekly; may increase to 60,000 units if unsatisfactory response.

• Darbepoetin alfa 3 mcg/kg subcutaneously every 2 weeks; may increase to 5 mcg/kg if unsatisfactory response.

• Darbepoetin alfa 200 mcg subcutaneously every 2 weeks; may increase to 300 mcg if unsatisfactory response.

For neutropenia (high risk)
To prevent neutropenia, start *one* of the following colony-stimulating factors 1 to 3 days after completion of chemotherapy and continue through postnadir recovery:

• Filgrastim 5 mcg/kg daily or
• Pegfilgrastim 6 mg once for each treatment cycle.

For diarrhea (likely)
Prescribe antidiarrheal as indicated.

For constipation (likely)
Order stool softener or laxative as indicated.

CAV (cyclophosphamide, doxorubicin [Adriamycin], vincristine) alternating with EP (etoposide, cisplatin [Platinol-AQ])

CAV
Cyclophosphamide 1,000 mg/m² I.V. on day 1
Doxorubicin 50 mg/m² I.V. on day 1

Vincristine 1.2 mg/m² I.V. on day 1
EP
Etoposide 100 mg/m² I.V. on days 1 through 3
Cisplatin 25 mg/m² I.V. on days 1 through 3
Alternate CAV and EP regimens every 21 days.
Reference: Murray N, et al. *J Clin Oncol.* 1999;17:2300-2308.

Supportive therapy
For nausea and vomiting
On day 1 (CAV), follow acute-onset antiemetic regimen for level 5 risk. Anticipatory, breakthrough, and delayed-onset regimens are recommended.

On days 1 to 3 (EP), follow acute-onset antiemetic regimen for level 5 risk. Anticipatory, breakthrough, and delayed-onset regimens are recommended.

For anemia (likely)
If hemoglobin level is less than 10 g/dl, *one* of the following is recommended:
• Epoetin alfa 150 units/kg subcutaneously three times weekly. If unsatisfactory response, may increase to 300 units/kg three times weekly.
• Epoetin alfa 40,000 units subcutaneously weekly; may increase to 60,000 units if unsatisfactory response.
• Darbepoetin alfa 3 mcg/kg subcutaneously every 2 weeks; may increase to 5 mcg/kg if unsatisfactory response.
• Darbepoetin alfa 200 mcg subcutaneously every 2 weeks; may increase to 300 mcg if unsatisfactory response.
For neutropenia (high risk)
To prevent neutropenia, start *one* of the following colony-stimulating factors 1 to 3 days after completion of chemotherapy and continue through postnadir recovery:
• Filgrastim 5 mcg/kg daily or
• Pegfilgrastim 6 mg once for each treatment cycle.
For diarrhea (likely)
Prescribe antidiarrheal as indicated.
For constipation (likely)
Order stool softener or laxative as indicated.

For cisplatin-induced nephrotoxicity
Maintain urine output of at least 75 ml/hour for several hours before and after each cisplatin dose. Consider amifostine for prevention of cisplatin-induced nephrotoxicity.

Cisplatin, etoposide

Cisplatin 60 to 80 mg/m² I.V. on day 1
Etoposide 80 to 120 mg/m² I.V. on days 1 through 3
Repeat cycle every 21 to 28 days.
Or
Cisplatin 25 mg/m² I.V. on days 1 through 3
Etoposide 100 mg/m² I.V. on days 1 through 3
Repeat cycle every 21 days.
Reference: Pazdur R, et al., eds. *Cancer Management. A Multidisciplinary Approach.* 9th ed. Lawrence, KS: CMP Media; 2005; Turrisi AT 3rd, et al. *N Engl J Med.* 1999;340:265-271; Sundstrom S, et al. *J Clin Oncol.* 2002;20:4665-4672.

Supportive therapy
For nausea and vomiting
On days when cisplatin and etoposide are given on same day, follow acute-onset antiemetic regimen for level 5 risk. Anticipatory, breakthrough, and delayed-onset regimens are recommended.

On etoposide-only days, follow acute-onset antiemetic regimen for level 2 risk. Anticipatory, breakthrough, and delayed-onset regimens are recommended as needed.
For anemia (likely)
If hemoglobin level is less than 10 g/dl, *one* of the following is recommended:
• Epoetin alfa 150 units/kg subcutaneously three times weekly. If unsatisfactory response, may increase to 300 units/kg three times weekly.
• Epoetin alfa 40,000 units subcutaneously weekly; may increase to 60,000 units if unsatisfactory response.
• Darbepoetin alfa 3 mcg/kg subcutaneously every 2 weeks; may increase to 5 mcg/kg if unsatisfactory response.

See front endpaper for specific antiemetic therapies.

• Darbepoetin alfa 200 mcg subcutaneously every 2 weeks; may increase to 300 mcg if unsatisfactory response.

For neutropenia (high risk)
To prevent neutropenia, start *one* of the following colony-stimulating factors 1 to 3 days after completion of chemotherapy and continue through postnadir recovery:
• Filgrastim 5 mcg/kg daily or
• Pegfilgrastim 6 mg once for each treatment cycle.

For diarrhea (likely)
Prescribe antidiarrheal as indicated.

For cisplatin-induced nephrotoxicity
Maintain urine output of at least 75 ml/hour for several hours before and after each cisplatin dose. Consider amifostine for prevention of cisplatin-induced nephrotoxicity.

Irinotecan, cisplatin

Cisplatin 60 mg/m² I.V. on day 1
Irinotecan 60 mg/m² I.V. on days 1, 8, and 15
Repeat cycle every 28 days.

Reference: Noda K, et al. *N Engl J Med.* 2002;346:85-91; Pazdur R, et al., eds. *Cancer Management. A Multidisciplinary Approach.* 9th ed. Lawrence, KS: CMP Media; 2005.

Supportive therapy
For nausea and vomiting
On day 1, follow acute-onset antiemetic regimen for level 5 risk. Anticipatory, breakthrough, and delayed-onset regimens are recommended.

On days 8 and 15, follow antiemetic regimen for level 3 risk.

For anemia (likely)
If hemoglobin level is less than 10 g/dl, *one* of the following is recommended:
• Epoetin alfa 150 units/kg subcutaneously three times weekly. If unsatisfactory response, may increase to 300 units/kg three times weekly.
• Epoetin alfa 40,000 units subcutaneously weekly; may increase to 60,000 units if unsatisfactory response.

• Darbepoetin alfa 3 mcg/kg subcutaneously every 2 weeks; may increase to 5 mcg/kg if unsatisfactory response.
• Darbepoetin alfa 200 mcg subcutaneously every 2 weeks; may increase to 300 mcg if unsatisfactory response.

For neutropenia (high risk)
To prevent neutropenia, start *one* of the following colony-stimulating factors 1 to 3 days after completion of chemotherapy and continue through postnadir recovery:
• Filgrastim 5 mcg/kg daily or
• Pegfilgrastim 6 mg once for each treatment cycle.

For diarrhea (very likely)
An antidiarrheal is recommended.

For cisplatin-induced nephrotoxicity
Maintain urine output of at least 75 ml/hour for several hours before and after each cisplatin dose. Consider amifostine for prevention of cisplatin-induced nephrotoxicity.

Topotecan

Topotecan 1.5 mg/m² I.V. daily over 30 minutes on days 1 through 5
Repeat every 21 days.

Reference: Schiller JH. *J Clin Oncol.* 2001;19:2114-2122.

Supportive therapy
For nausea and vomiting
Follow acute-onset antiemetic regimen for level 2 risk. Anticipatory, breakthrough, and delayed-onset regimens are recommended as needed.

For anemia (likely)
If hemoglobin level is less than 10 g/dl, *one* of the following is recommended:
• Epoetin alfa 150 units/kg subcutaneously three times weekly. If unsatisfactory response, may increase to 300 units/kg three times weekly.
• Epoetin alfa 40,000 units subcutaneously weekly; may increase to 60,000 units if unsatisfactory response.

- Darbepoetin alfa 3 mcg/kg subcutaneously every 2 weeks; may increase to 5 mcg/kg if unsatisfactory response.
- Darbepoetin alfa 200 mcg subcutaneously every 2 weeks; may increase to 300 mcg if unsatisfactory response.

For neutropenia (high risk)

To prevent neutropenia, start *one* of the following colony-stimulating factors 1 to 3 days after completion of chemotherapy and continue through postnadir recovery:

- Filgrastim 5 mcg/kg daily or
- Pegfilgrastim 6 mg once for each treatment cycle.

For diarrhea (likely)

Prescribe antidiarrheal as indicated.

For constipation (likely)

Order laxative or stool softener as indicated.

Multiple myeloma

Bortezomib

Bortezomib 1.3 mg/m^2 I.V. on days 1, 4, 8, and 11

Repeat every 21 days.

Reference: Richardson PG, et al. *N Engl J Med.* 2003;348:2609-2617.

Supportive therapy

For nausea and vomiting

Follow acute-onset antiemetic regimen for level 1 risk.

For anemia (likely)

If hemoglobin level is less than 10 g/dl, *one* of the following is recommended:

- Epoetin alfa 150 units/kg subcutaneously three times weekly. If unsatisfactory response, may increase to 300 units/kg three times weekly.
- Epoetin alfa 40,000 units subcutaneously weekly; may increase to 60,000 units if unsatisfactory response.

- Darbepoetin alfa 3 mcg/kg subcutaneously every 2 weeks; may increase to 5 mcg/kg if unsatisfactory response.
- Darbepoetin alfa 200 mcg subcutaneously every 2 weeks; may increase to 300 mcg if unsatisfactory response.

For diarrhea (likely)

Prescribe antidiarrheal as indicated.

DVd (pegylated liposomal doxorubicin, vincristine, dexamethasone)

Pegylated liposomal doxorubicin 40 mg/m^2 I.V. on day 1

Vincristine 2 mg I.V. on day 1

Dexamethasone 40 mg P.O. or I.V. on days 1 through 4

Repeat cycle every 28 days for minimum of six cycles and for two cycles after maximum response.

Reference: Hussein MA, et al. *Cancer.* 2002;95:2160-2168.

Supportive therapy

For nausea and vomiting

On day 1, follow acute-onset antiemetic regimen for level 3 risk. Anticipatory, breakthrough, and delayed-onset regimens are recommended as needed.

On days 2 through 4, no routine prophylaxis is needed.

For anemia (likely)

If hemoglobin level is less than 10 g/dl, *one* of the following is recommended:

- Epoetin alfa 150 units/kg subcutaneously three times weekly. If unsatisfactory response, may increase to 300 units/kg three times weekly.
- Epoetin alfa 40,000 units subcutaneously weekly; may increase to 60,000 units if unsatisfactory response.
- Darbepoetin alfa 3 mcg/kg subcutaneously every 2 weeks; may increase to 5 mcg/kg if unsatisfactory response.
- Darbepoetin alfa 200 mcg subcutaneously every 2 weeks; may increase to 300 mcg if unsatisfactory response.

For constipation (likely)
Order stool softener or laxative as indicated.

DVd-T (pegylated liposomal doxorubicin, vincristine, dexamethasone, thalidomide)

Pegylated liposomal doxorubicin 40 mg/m^2 I.V. over 2 to 3 hours on day 1
Vincristine 2 mg I.V. on day 1
Dexamethasone 40 mg P.O. or I.V. on days 1 through 4
Thalidomide 50 mg P.O. daily, increased by 50 mg daily every week until maximum dose of 400 mg daily is reached
Repeat cycle every 28 days for minimum of six cycles and for two cycles after maximum response.
Maintenance therapy
Prednisone 50 mg P.O. every other day
Thalidomide Maximum tolerated dose P.O. daily. Continue maintenance therapy until disease progresses or toxicity occurs.
Reference: Hussein MA. *Oncologist.* 2003;8(suppl 3):39-45.

Supportive therapy
For nausea and vomiting
On day 1, follow acute-onset antiemetic regimen for level 3 risk. Anticipatory, breakthrough, and delayed-onset regimens are recommended as needed.

On dexamethasone and thalidomide days, follow acute-onset antiemetic regimen for level 1 risk.
For anemia (likely)
If hemoglobin level is less than 10 g/dl, *one* of the following is recommended:
• Epoetin alfa 150 units/kg subcutaneously three times weekly. If unsatisfactory response, may increase to 300 units/kg three times weekly.
• Epoetin alfa 40,000 units subcutaneously weekly; may increase to 60,000 units if unsatisfactory response.
• Darbepoetin alfa 3 mcg/kg subcutaneously

every 2 weeks; may increase to 5 mcg/kg if unsatisfactory response.
• Darbepoetin alfa 200 mcg subcutaneously every 2 weeks; may increase to 300 mcg if unsatisfactory response.
For neutropenia (high risk)
To prevent neutropenia, start *one* of the following colony-stimulating factors 1 to 3 days after completion of chemotherapy and continue through postnadir recovery:
• Filgrastim 5 mcg/kg daily or
• Pegfilgrastim 6 mg once for each treatment cycle.
For constipation (likely)
Order stool softener or laxative as indicated.
For deep vein thrombosis
Consider anticoagulants for patients at high risk for deep vein thrombosis who are receiving thalidomide.
For infection
Consider acyclovir for patients with previous exposure to herpes simplex virus, and fluoroquinolone for bacterial prophylaxis.

MP (melphalan, prednisone)

Melphalan 8 to 10 mg/m^2 P.O. on days 1 through 4
Prednisone 60 mg/m^2 P.O. on days 1 through 4
Repeat cycle every 6 weeks.
Reference: Oken MM, et al. *Arch Int Med.* 1975;135:147-152; Oken MM, et al. *Cancer.* 1997;79:1561-1567.

Supportive therapy
For nausea and vomiting
Follow acute-onset antiemetic regimen for level 1 risk.
For anemia (likely)
If hemoglobin level is less than 10 g/dl, *one* of the following is recommended:
• Epoetin alfa 150 units/kg subcutaneously three times weekly. If unsatisfactory response, may increase to 300 units/kg three times weekly.
• Epoetin alfa 40,000 units subcutaneously

weekly; may increase to 60,000 units if unsatisfactory response.

- Darbepoetin alfa 3 mcg/kg subcutaneously every 2 weeks; may increase to 5 mcg/kg if unsatisfactory response.
- Darbepoetin alfa 200 mcg subcutaneously every 2 weeks; may increase to 300 mcg if unsatisfactory response.

For neutropenia (intermediate risk)
To prevent neutropenia, consider starting *one* of the following colony-stimulating factors 1 to 3 days after completion of chemotherapy and continuing through postnadir recovery:

- Filgrastim 5 mcg/kg daily or
- Pegfilgrastim 6 mg once for each treatment cycle.

Thalidomide

Thalidomide 200 to 800 mg P.O. daily at bedtime

Reference: Shingal S, et al. *N Engl J Med.* 1999;341:1565-1571.

Supportive therapy
For nausea and vomiting
Follow acute-onset antiemetic regimen for level 1 risk.

For anemia (likely)
If hemoglobin level is less than 10 g/dl, *one* of the following is recommended:

- Epoetin alfa 150 units/kg subcutaneously three times weekly. If unsatisfactory response, may increase to 300 units/kg three times weekly.
- Epoetin alfa 40,000 units subcutaneously weekly; may increase to 60,000 units if unsatisfactory response.
- Darbepoetin alfa 3 mcg/kg subcutaneously every 2 weeks; may increase to 5 mcg/kg if unsatisfactory response.
- Darbepoetin alfa 200 mcg subcutaneously every 2 weeks; may increase to 300 mcg if unsatisfactory response.

For constipation (likely)
Order stool softener or laxative as indicated.

For deep vein thrombosis
Consider anticoagulants for patients at high risk for deep vein thrombosis who are receiving thalidomide.

Thalidomide, dexamethasone

Thalidomide 200 mg P.O. daily at bedtime for 2 weeks, then increase by 200 mg daily every 2 weeks to maximum of 800 mg daily, as tolerated

Dexamethasone 40 mg P.O. on days 1 through 4, 9 through 12, and 17 through 20 of odd cycles and 40 mg P.O. on days 1 through 4 only during even cycles

Repeat cycle every 28 days.

Reference: Rajkumar SV, et al. *J Clin Oncol.* 2002;20:4319-4323.

Supportive therapy
For nausea and vomiting
Follow acute-onset antiemetic regimen for level 1 risk.

For anemia (likely)
If hemoglobin level is less than 10 g/dl, *one* of the following is recommended:

- Epoetin alfa 150 units/kg subcutaneously three times weekly. If unsatisfactory response, may increase to 300 units/kg three times weekly.
- Epoetin alfa 40,000 units subcutaneously weekly; may increase to 60,000 units if unsatisfactory response.
- Darbepoetin alfa 3 mcg/kg subcutaneously every 2 weeks; may increase to 5 mcg/kg if unsatisfactory response.
- Darbepoetin alfa 200 mcg subcutaneously every 2 weeks; may increase to 300 mcg if unsatisfactory response.

For deep vein thrombosis
Consider anticoagulants for patients at high risk for deep vein thrombosis who are receiving thalidomide.

VAD (vincristine, doxorubicin [Adria-mycin], dexamethasone)

Vincristine 0.4 mg daily by continuous I.V. infusion on days 1 through 4
Doxorubicin 9 mg/m^2 daily by continuous I.V. infusion on days 1 through 4
Dexamethasone 40 mg P.O.on days 1 through 4, 9 through 12, and 17 through 20
Repeat cycle every 28 days.
Reference: Barlogie B, et al. *N Engl J Med.* 1984;310:1353-1356; Alexian R. *Am J Hematol.* 1990;33:86-89.

Supportive therapy
For nausea and vomiting
On days 1 through 4, follow acute-onset antiemetic regimen for level 4 risk. Anticipatory, breakthrough, and delayed-onset regimens are recommended as needed.
   On dexamethasone days, no routine prophylaxis is recommended.
For anemia (likely)
If hemoglobin level is less than 10 g/dl, *one* of the following is recommended:
• Epoetin alfa 150 units/kg subcutaneously three times weekly. If unsatisfactory response, may increase to 300 units/kg three times weekly.
• Epoetin alfa 40,000 units subcutaneously weekly; may increase to 60,000 units if unsatisfactory response.
• Darbepoetin alfa 3 mcg/kg subcutaneously every 2 weeks; may increase to 5 mcg/kg if unsatisfactory response.
• Darbepoetin alfa 200 mcg subcutaneously every 2 weeks; may increase to 300 mcg if unsatisfactory response.
For neutropenia (high risk)
To prevent neutropenia, start *one* of the following colony-stimulating factors 1 to 3 days after completion of chemotherapy and continue through postnadir recovery:
• Filgrastim 5 mcg/kg daily *or*
• Pegfilgrastim 6 mg once for each treatment cycle.

For constipation (likely)
Order stool softener or laxative as indicated.

Myelodysplastic syndrome (MDS)

Azacitidine

Azacitidine 75 mg/m^2 subcutaneously daily for 7 days
Repeat every 28 days.
Reference: Silverman LR, et al. *J Clin Oncol.* 2002;20:2429-2440.

Supportive therapy
For nausea and vomiting
Follow acute-onset antiemetic regimen for level 4 risk. Anticipatory, breakthrough, and delayed-onset regimens are recommended as needed.
For anemia (likely)
Give epoetin alfa 40,000 to 60,000 units subcutaneously two to three times per week for 2 to 3 months.
For neutropenia
To prevent neutropenia, give filgrastim *or* pegfilgrastim, 1 to 2 mg/kg subcutaneously two to three times per week.

Decitabine

Decitabine 15 mg/m^2 I.V. over 4 hours every 8 hours for 3 days (for total of 45 mg/m^2 daily for 3 days)
Repeat every 6 weeks.
Reference: Wijermans P, et al. *J Clin Oncol.* 2000;18:956-962.

Supportive therapy
For nausea and vomiting
Follow acute-onset antiemetic regimen for level 1 risk.
For anemia (likely)
Give epoetin alfa 40,000 to 60,000 units

subcutaneously two to three times per week for 2 to 3 months.

For neutropenia

To prevent neutropenia, give filgrastim *or* peg-filgrastim, 1 to 2 mg/kg subcutaneously two to three times per week.

Neuroendocrine tumors

Doxorubicin, streptozocin

Streptozocin 500 mg/m² I.V. on days 1 through 5

Doxorubicin 50 mg/m² I.V. on days 1 and 22

Repeat cycle every 6 weeks.

Reference: Moertel CG, et al. *N Engl J Med.* 1992;326:519.

Supportive therapy

For nausea and vomiting

On days 1 through 5, follow acute-onset antiemetic regimen for level 5 risk. Anticipatory, breakthrough, and delayed-onset regimens are recommended.

On day 22, follow acute-onset antiemetic regimen for level 3 risk. Anticipatory, breakthrough, and delayed-onset regimens are recommended as needed.

For anemia (likely)

If hemoglobin level is less than 10 g/dl, *one* of the following is recommended:
- Epoetin alfa 150 units/kg subcutaneously three times weekly. If unsatisfactory response, may increase to 300 units/kg three times weekly.
- Epoetin alfa 40,000 units subcutaneously weekly; may increase to 60,000 units if unsatisfactory response.
- Darbepoetin alfa 3 mcg/kg subcutaneously every 2 weeks; may increase to 5 mcg/kg if unsatisfactory response.
- Darbepoetin alfa 200 mcg subcutaneously every 2 weeks; may increase to 300 mcg if unsatisfactory response.

For neutropenia (intermediate risk)

To prevent neutropenia, consider starting *one* of the following colony-stimulating factors 1 to 3 days after completion of chemotherapy and continuing through postnadir recovery:
- Filgrastim 5 mcg/kg daily or
- Pegfilgrastim 6 mg once for each treatment cycle.

5-Fluorouracil, dacarbazine, epirubicin

5-Fluorouracil 500 mg/m² by I.V. bolus on days 1 through 3

Dacarbazine 200 mg/m² I.V. over 30 minutes on days 1 through 3

Epirubicin 30 mg/m² by I.V. bolus on days 1 through 3

Repeat cycle every 21 days.

Reference: Bajetta E, et al. *Cancer.* 1998;83:372-378.

Supportive therapy

For nausea and vomiting

On days 1 through 3, follow acute-onset antiemetic regimen for level 5 risk. Anticipatory, breakthrough, and delayed-onset regimens are recommended

For anemia (likely)

If hemoglobin level is less than 10 g/dl, *one* of the following is recommended:
- Epoetin alfa 150 units/kg subcutaneously three times weekly. If unsatisfactory response, may increase to 300 units/kg three times weekly.
- Epoetin alfa 40,000 units subcutaneously weekly; may increase to 60,000 units if unsatisfactory response.
- Darbepoetin alfa 3 mcg/kg subcutaneously every 2 weeks; may increase to 5 mcg/kg if unsatisfactory response.
- Darbepoetin alfa 200 mcg subcutaneously every 2 weeks; may increase to 300 mcg if unsatisfactory response.

For neutropenia (high risk)

To prevent neutropenia, start *one* of the following colony-stimulating factors 1 to 3 days

after completion of chemotherapy and continue through postnadir recovery:
- Filgrastim 5 mcg/kg daily or
- Pegfilgrastim 6 mg once for each treatment cycle.

For diarrhea (likely)
Prescribe antidiarrheal drug as indicated.

Non-Hodgkin's lymphoma

Chlorambucil

Chlorambucil 40 mg/m^2 P.O. on day 1
Repeat every 28 days.

Reference: Rai KR, et al. *N Engl J Med.* 2000;343:1750-1757.

Supportive therapy
For nausea and vomiting
Follow acute-onset antiemetic regimen for level 1 risk.

For anemia (likely)
If hemoglobin level is less than 10 g/dl, *one* of the following is recommended:
- Epoetin alfa 150 units/kg subcutaneously three times weekly. If unsatisfactory response, may increase to 300 units/kg three times weekly.
- Epoetin alfa 40,000 units subcutaneously weekly; may increase to 60,000 units if unsatisfactory response.
- Darbepoetin alfa 3 mcg/kg subcutaneously every 2 weeks; may increase to 5 mcg/kg if unsatisfactory response.
- Darbepoetin alfa 200 mcg subcutaneously every 2 weeks; may increase to 300 mcg if unsatisfactory response.

For neutropenia (intermediate risk)
To prevent neutropenia, consider starting *one* of the following colony-stimulating factors 1 to 3 days after completion of chemotherapy and continuing through postnadir recovery:
- Filgrastim 5 mcg/kg daily or
- Pegfilgrastim 6 mg once for each treatment cycle.

For diarrhea (likely)
Prescribe antidiarrheal as indicated.

CHOP (cyclophosphamide, doxorubicin, vincristine [Oncovin], prednisone)

Cyclophosphamide 750 mg/m^2 I.V. on day 1
Doxorubicin 50 mg/m^2 I.V. on day 1
Vincristine 1.4 mg/m^2 I.V. on day 1
Prednisone 100 mg P.O. on days 1 through 5
Repeat cycle every 21 days.

Reference: Doorduijin JK, et al. *J Clin Oncol.* 2003;21:3041-3050.

Supportive therapy
For nausea and vomiting
On day 1, follow acute-onset antiemetic regimen for level 4 risk. Anticipatory, breakthrough, and delayed-onset regimens are recommended as needed.

For anemia (likely)
If hemoglobin level is less than 10 g/dl, *one* of the following is recommended:
- Epoetin alfa 150 units/kg subcutaneously three times weekly. If unsatisfactory response, may increase to 300 units/kg three times weekly.
- Epoetin alfa 40,000 units subcutaneously weekly; may increase to 60,000 units if unsatisfactory response.
- Darbepoetin alfa 3 mcg/kg subcutaneously every 2 weeks; may increase to 5 mcg/kg if unsatisfactory response.
- Darbepoetin alfa 200 mcg subcutaneously every 2 weeks; may increase to 300 mcg if unsatisfactory response.

For neutropenia (high risk)
To prevent neutropenia, start *one* of the following colony-stimulating factors 1 to 3 days after completion of chemotherapy and continue through postnadir recovery:
- Filgrastim 5 mcg/kg daily or
- Pegfilgrastim 6 mg once for each treatment cycle.

For diarrhea (likely)
Prescribe antidiarrheal as indicated.

For constipation (likely)
Order stool softener or laxative as indicated.

CODOX-M (cyclophosphamide, vincristine [Oncovin], doxorubicin, high-dose methotrexate) alternating with IVAC (ifosfamide, etoposide, high-dose cytarabine)

CODOX-M

Cyclophosphamide 800 mg/m^2 I.V. on day 1 and 200 mg/m^2 I.V. on days 2 through 5
Vincristine 1.5 mg/m^2 I.V. on days 1 and 8 in cycle 1 and days 1, 8, and 15 in cycle 3
Doxorubicin 40 mg/m^2 I.V. on day 1
Cytarabine 70 mg intrathecally on days 1 and 3
Methotrexate 1,200 mg/m^2 I.V. over 1 hour on day 1 followed by 240 mg/m^2 every hour for 23 hours on day 10
Leucovorin 192 mg/m^2 I.V. begun 12 hours after completion of methotrexate for one dose, followed by 12 mg/m^2 I.V. every 6 hours until methotrexate level is below 5×10^{-8} mol/L
Methotrexate 12 mg intrathecally on day 15

Patients presenting with CNS disease receive additional intrathecal therapy with cytarabine on day 5 and methotrexate on day 17.

IVAC

Etoposide 60 mg/m^2 I.V. over 1 hour on days 1 through 5
Ifosfamide 1,500 mg/m^2 I.V. over 1 hour on days 1 through 5 with mesna 360 mg/m^2 I.V., followed by 360 mg/m^2 I.V. every 3 hours over 15 minutes on days 1 through 5
Cytarabine 2,000 mg/m^2 I.V. over 3 hours every 12 hours on days 1 and 2 (four doses total)
Methotrexate 12 mg intrathecally on day 5
Leucovorin 15 mg P.O. 24 hours after intrathecal methotrexate

Patients presenting with CNS disease receive additional intrathecal therapy with cytarabine 70 mg on days 7 and 9 of first IVAC regimen.

Alternate CODOX-M and IVAC regimens for total of four cycles (two of each).
Reference: Magrath I, et al. *J Clin Oncol.* 1996;14:925-934; Mead GM, et al. *Annals Oncol.* 2002;13:1264-1274.

Supportive therapy
For nausea and vomiting
CODOX-M
On day 1, follow acute-onset antiemetic regimen for level 5 risk. Anticipatory, breakthrough, and delayed-onset regimens are recommended.

On days 2 through 5, follow acute-onset antiemetic regimen for level 3 risk. Anticipatory, breakthrough, and delayed-onset regimens are recommended as needed.

On days 8, 15, and 17, follow acute-onset antiemetic regimen for level 1 risk.
IVAC
On days 1 and 2, follow acute-onset antiemetic regimen for level 5 risk. Anticipatory, breakthrough, and delayed-onset regimens are recommended.

On days 3 through 5, follow acute-onset antiemetic regimen for level 4 risk. Anticipatory, breakthrough, and delayed-onset regimens are recommended as needed.

On days 7 and 9, follow acute-onset antiemetic regimen for level 1 risk.
For anemia (likely)
If hemoglobin level is less than 10 g/dl, *one* of the following is recommended:
• Epoetin alfa 150 units/kg subcutaneously three times weekly. If unsatisfactory response, may increase to 300 units/kg three times weekly.
• Epoetin alfa 40,000 units subcutaneously weekly; may increase to 60,000 units if unsatisfactory response.
• Darbepoetin alfa 3 mcg/kg subcutaneously every 2 weeks; may increase to 5 mcg/kg if unsatisfactory response.
• Darbepoetin alfa 200 mcg subcutaneously every 2 weeks; may increase to 300 mcg if unsatisfactory response.
For neutropenia (high risk with CODOX-M)

See front endpaper for specific antiemetic therapies.

To prevent neutropenia, give filgrastim 5 mcg/kg daily *or* pegfilgrastim, one dose of 6 mg per cycle of treatment subcutaneously. Start colony-stimulating factors 3 days after completion of chemotherapy; continue through postnadir recovery.

Fludarabine, rituximab

Fludarabine 25 mg/m^2 I.V. on days 1 through 5

Rituximab 375 mg/m^2 I.V. on days 1, 8, 15, and 22

Repeat cycle every 21 to 28 days.

Reference: Czuczman MS, et al. *J Clin Oncol.* 2005;23:694-704.

Supportive therapy

For nausea and vomiting

Follow acute-onset antiemetic regimen for level 1 risk.

For anemia (likely)

If hemoglobin level is less than 10 g/dl, *one* of the following is recommended:

• Epoetin alfa 150 units/kg subcutaneously three times weekly. If unsatisfactory response, may increase to 300 units/kg three times weekly.

• Epoetin alfa 40,000 units subcutaneously weekly; may increase to 60,000 units if unsatisfactory response.

• Darbepoetin alfa 3 mcg/kg subcutaneously every 2 weeks; may increase to 5 mcg/kg if unsatisfactory response.

• Darbepoetin alfa 200 mcg subcutaneously every 2 weeks; may increase to 300 mcg if unsatisfactory response.

For constipation (likely)

Order stool softener or laxative as indicated.

Hyper CVAD (cyclophosphamide, vincristine, doxorubicin [Adriamycin], dexamethasone) alternating with methotrexate, cytarabine

Hyper CVAD

Cyclophosphamide 300 mg/m^2 I.V. over 3 hours every 12 hours (for six doses) on days 1 through 3 and mesna at same total dose of cyclophosphamide by continuous I.V. infusion, starting with the first cyclophosphamide dose and ending 6 hours after last dose

Vincristine 2 mg I.V. on days 4 and 11

Dexamethasone 40 mg daily I.V. or P.O. on days 1 through 4 and days 11 through 14

Doxorubicin 50 mg/m^2 I.V. on day 4

Methotrexate, cytarabine

Methotrexate 200 mg/^{2} I.V. over 2 hours on day 1, then 800 mg/m^2 I.V. over 24 hours

Cytarabine 3,000 mg/m^2 I.V. over 2 hours every 12 hours for four doses on days 2 and 3

Methylprednisolone 50 mg I.V. twice daily (for six doses) on days 1 through 3

Leucovorin 15 mg I.V. or P.O. every 6 hours until methotrexate level is below 5×10^{-8} mol/L starting 24 hours after methotrexate

Alternate both regimens for total of eight cycles (four of each).

Reference: Kantarjian HM, et al. *J Clin Oncol.* 2000;18:547-561.

Supportive therapy

For nausea and vomiting

Hyper CVAD

On days 1 through 4, follow acute-onset antiemetic regimen for level 3 risk. Anticipatory, breakthrough, and delayed-onset regimens are recommended as needed.

On days 11 through 14, follow acute-onset antiemetic regimen for level 1 risk.

Methotrexate/cytarabine

On day 1, follow acute-onset antiemetic regimen for level 3 risk. Anticipatory, breakthrough, and delayed-onset regimens are recommended as needed.

On days 2 and 3, follow acute-onset antiemetic regimen for level 4 risk. Anticipatory, breakthrough, and delayed-onset regimens are recommended as needed.

For anemia (likely)

If hemoglobin level is less than 10 g/dl, *one* of the following is recommended:

• Epoetin alfa 150 units/kg subcutaneously three times weekly. If unsatisfactory response, may increase to 300 units/kg three times weekly.

- Epoetin alfa 40,000 units subcutaneously weekly; may increase to 60,000 units if unsatisfactory response.
- Darbepoetin alfa 3 mcg/kg subcutaneously every 2 weeks; may increase to 5 mcg/kg if unsatisfactory response.
- Darbepoetin alfa 200 mcg subcutaneously every 2 weeks; may increase to 300 mcg if unsatisfactory response.

For neutropenia (high risk)

To prevent neutropenia, start *one* of the following colony-stimulating factors 1 to 3 days after completion of chemotherapy and continue through postnadir recovery:

- Filgrastim 5 mcg/kg daily or
- Pegfilgrastim 6 mg once for each treatment cycle.

For diarrhea (likely)

Prescribe antidiarrheal as indicated.

For CNS disease

To prevent CNS disease during both cycles, give 12 mg methotrexate intrathecally on day 2 and 100 mg cytarabine intrathecally on day 8 for 16 treatments (high-risk patients), four treatments (low-risk patients), or eight treatments (unknown-risk patients).

For hyperuricemia

Allopurinol is recommended during the Hyper CVAD cycle.

For conjunctivitis

Use corticosteroid eyedrops to prevent conjunctivitis.

For infection

Give empiric antibiotic prophylaxis during dose-intensive phase: ciprofloxacin 500 mg P.O. twice daily or levofloxacin 500 mg P.O. daily, fluconazole 200 mg P.O. daily, and acyclovir 200 mg P.O. twice daily or valacyclovir 500 mg P.O. daily.

For methotrexate-induced nephrotoxicity

Maintain urine output of at least 75 ml/hour for several hours before and 24 hours after each methotrexate dose. Maintain urine pH above 7.

Rituximab

Rituximab 375 mg/m^2 by slow I.V. infusion once weekly for four or eight doses

Reference: Witzig TE, et al. *J Clin Oncol.* 2005;23:1103-1108.

Supportive therapy

For nausea and vomiting

Follow acute-onset antiemetic regimen for level 1 risk.

For anemia (likely)

If hemoglobin level is less than 10 g/dl, *one* of the following is recommended:

- Epoetin alfa 150 units/kg subcutaneously three times weekly. If unsatisfactory response, may increase to 300 units/kg three times weekly.
- Epoetin alfa 40,000 units subcutaneously weekly; may increase to 60,000 units if unsatisfactory response.
- Darbepoetin alfa 3 mcg/kg subcutaneously every 2 weeks; may increase to 5 mcg/kg if unsatisfactory response.
- Darbepoetin alfa 200 mcg subcutaneously every 2 weeks; may increase to 300 mcg if unsatisfactory response.

For infusion reactions

Consider premedication with acetaminophen and diphenhydramine to prevent infusion reactions.

Rituximab/CHOP (cyclophosphamide, doxorubicin, vincristine [Oncovin], prednisone)

Rituximab 375 mg/m^2 I.V. on day 1
Cyclophosphamide 750 mg/m^2 I.V. on day 1
Doxorubicin 50 mg/m^2 I.V. on day 1
Vincristine 1.4 mg/m^2 I.V. on day 1
Prednisone 100 mg P.O. on days 1 through 5
Repeat cycle every 21 days.

Reference: Zinzani PL, et al. *J Clin Oncol.* 2004;22:2654-2661.

Supportive therapy

For nausea and vomiting

On day 1, follow acute-onset antiemetic regimen for level 4 risk. Anticipatory, breakthrough, and delayed-onset regimens are recommended as needed.

On days 2 through 5, follow acute-onset antiemetic regimen for level 1 risk.

For anemia (likely)

If hemoglobin level is less than 10 g/dl, *one* of the following is recommended:

• Epoetin alfa 150 units/kg subcutaneously three times weekly. If unsatisfactory response, may increase to 300 units/kg three times weekly.

• Epoetin alfa 40,000 units subcutaneously weekly; may increase to 60,000 units if unsatisfactory response.

• Darbepoetin alfa 3 mcg/kg subcutaneously every 2 weeks; may increase to 5 mcg/kg if unsatisfactory response.

• Darbepoetin alfa 200 mcg subcutaneously every 2 weeks; may increase to 300 mcg if unsatisfactory response.

For neutropenia (high risk)

To prevent neutropenia, start *one* of the following colony-stimulating factors 1 to 3 days after completion of chemotherapy and continue through postnadir recovery:

• Filgrastim 5 mcg/kg daily or

• Pegfilgrastim 6 mg once for each treatment cycle.

For diarrhea (likely)

Prescribe antidiarrheal as indicated.

For constipation (likely)

Order stool softener or laxative as indicated.

For infusion reactions

Consider premedication with acetaminophen and diphenhydramine to prevent infusion reactions.

Rituximab/EPOCH (etoposide, prednisone, vincristine [Oncovin], doxorubicin, cyclophosphamide)

Rituximab 375 mg/m² I.V. on day 1
Etoposide 50 mg/m² daily (by continuous I.V. infusion over 96 hours) on days 1 through 4
Vincristine 0.4 mg/m² daily (by continuous I.V. infusion over 96 hours) on days 1 through 4
Doxorubicin 10 mg/m² by daily (continuous I.V. infusion over 96 hours) on days 1 through 4
Prednisone 60 mg/m² P.O. on days 1 through 5
Cyclophosphamide 750 mg/m² I.V. on day 5
Repeat cycle every 21 days.

Reference: Gutierrez M, et al. *J Clin Oncol.* 2000;18:3633-3642; Pazdur R, et al., eds. *Cancer Management. A Multidisciplinary Approach.* 9th ed. Lawrence, KS: CMP Media; 2005.

Supportive therapy

For nausea and vomiting

On days 1 through 4, follow acute-onset antiemetic regimen for level 4 risk. Anticipatory, breakthrough, and delayed-onset regimens are recommended as needed.

On day 5, follow acute-onset antiemetic regimen for level 3 risk. Anticipatory, breakthrough, and delayed-onset regimens are recommended as needed.

For anemia (likely)

If hemoglobin level is less than 10 g/dl, *one* of the following is recommended:

• Epoetin alfa 150 units/kg subcutaneously three times weekly. If unsatisfactory response, may increase to 300 units/kg three times weekly.

• Epoetin alfa 40,000 units subcutaneously weekly; may increase to 60,000 units if unsatisfactory response.

• Darbepoetin alfa 3 mcg/kg subcutaneously every 2 weeks; may increase to 5 mcg/kg if unsatisfactory response.

• Darbepoetin alfa 200 mcg subcutaneously every 2 weeks; may increase to 300 mcg if unsatisfactory response.

For neutropenia (high risk)

To prevent neutropenia, start *one* of the following colony-stimulating factors 1 to 3 days after completion of chemotherapy and continue through postnadir recovery:

• Filgrastim 5 mcg/kg daily or

• Pegfilgrastim 6 mg once for each treatment cycle.

For diarrhea (likely)
Prescribe antidiarrheal as indicated.

For constipation (likely)
Order stool softener or laxative as indicated.

For infusion reactions
Consider premedication with acetaminophen and diphenhydramine to prevent infusion reactions.

Rituximab/hyper CVAD (cyclophosphamide, vincristine, doxorubicin [Adriamycin], dexamethasone) alternating with methotrexate, cytarabine

Rituximab/hyper CVAD

Rituximab 375 mg/m^2 I.V. on day 1
Cyclophosphamide 300 mg/m^2 I.V. every 12 hours on days 2 through 4 infused over 3 hours for total of six doses
Doxorubicin 16.7 mg/m^2 I.V. daily over 24 hours on days 5 through 7
Vincristine 1.4 mg/m^2 I.V. on days 5 and 12
Dexamethasone 40 mg I.V. or P.O. daily on days 2 through 5 and days 12 through 15

Methotrexate, cytarabine

Rituximab 375 mg/m^2 I.V. on day 1
Methotrexate 200 mg/m^2 I.V. over 2 hours, then 800 mg/m^2 by continuous I.V. infusion over 22 hours on day 2
Cytarabine 3,000 mg/m^2 I.V. (over 2 hours) every 12 hours for four doses on days 3 through 4
Leucovorin 15 mg P.O. or I.V. every 6 hours until methotrexate level is below 5×10^{-8} mol/L, starting after methotrexate

Alternate regimens every 21 days for total of six to eight cycles.

Reference: Romaguera JE. *J Clin Oncol.* 2005;23:7013-7023.

Supportive therapy

For nausea and vomiting
Rituximab/hyper CVAD
On days 1 through 4, follow acute-onset antiemetic regimen for level 3 risk. Anticipatory, breakthrough, and delayed-onset regimens are recommended as needed.

On days 11 through 14, follow acute-onset antiemetic regimen for level 1 risk.

Methotrexate, cytarabine
On day 1, follow acute-onset antiemetic regimen for level 3 risk. Anticipatory, breakthrough, and delayed-onset regimens are recommended as needed.

On days 2 and 3, follow acute-onset antiemetic regimen for level 4 risk. Anticipatory, breakthrough, and delayed-onset regimens are recommended as needed.

For anemia (likely)
If hemoglobin level is less than 10 g/dl, *one* of the following is recommended:
• Epoetin alfa 150 units/kg subcutaneously three times weekly. If unsatisfactory response, may increase to 300 units/kg three times weekly.
• Epoetin alfa 40,000 units subcutaneously weekly; may increase to 60,000 units if unsatisfactory response.
• Darbepoetin alfa 3 mcg/kg subcutaneously every 2 weeks; may increase to 5 mcg/kg if unsatisfactory response.
• Darbepoetin alfa 200 mcg subcutaneously every 2 weeks; may increase to 300 mcg if unsatisfactory response.

For neutropenia (high risk)
To prevent neutropenia, start *one* of the following colony-stimulating factors 1 to 3 days after completion of chemotherapy and continue through postnadir recovery:
• Filgrastim 5 mcg/kg daily or
• Pegfilgrastim 6 mg once for each treatment cycle.

For diarrhea (likely)
Prescribe antidiarrheal as indicated.

For infusion reactions
Consider premedication with acetaminophen and diphenhydramine to prevent infusion reactions.

Ovarian cancer

Carboplatin, cyclophosphamide

Carboplatin 300 mg/m² I.V. on day 1
Cyclophosphamide 600 mg/m² I.V. on day 1
Repeat cycle every 28 days for six cycles.
Reference: Alberts DS, et al. *J Clin Oncol.*
1992;10:706-717; Swenerton K, et al. *J Clin Oncol.* 1992;10:718-726.

Supportive therapy
For nausea and vomiting
Follow acute-onset antiemetic regimen for level 5 risk. Anticipatory, breakthrough, and delayed-onset regimens are recommended.
For anemia (likely)
If hemoglobin level is less than 10 g/dl, *one* of the following is recommended:
• Epoetin alfa 150 units/kg subcutaneously three times weekly. If unsatisfactory response, may increase to 300 units/kg three times weekly.
• Epoetin alfa 40,000 units subcutaneously weekly; may increase to 60,000 units if unsatisfactory response.
• Darbepoetin alfa 3 mcg/kg subcutaneously every 2 weeks; may increase to 5 mcg/kg if unsatisfactory response.
• Darbepoetin alfa 200 mcg subcutaneously every 2 weeks; may increase to 300 mcg if unsatisfactory response.
For neutropenia (high risk)
To prevent neutropenia, start *one* of the following colony-stimulating factors 1 to 3 days after completion of chemotherapy and continue through postnadir recovery:
• Filgrastim 5 mcg/kg daily or
• Pegfilgrastim 6 mg once for each treatment cycle.
For diarrhea (likely)
Prescribe antidiarrheal as indicated.
For constipation (likely)
Order stool softener or laxative as indicated.

Cisplatin, etoposide

Cisplatin 50 to 70 mg/m² I.V. weekly for 6 weeks
Etoposide 50 mg P.O. once daily for 6 weeks
Reference: van der Burg ME, et al. *Br J Cancer.* 2002;86:19-25.

Supportive therapy
For nausea and vomiting
On cisplatin days, follow acute-onset antiemetic regimen for level 5 risk. Anticipatory, breakthrough, and delayed-onset regimens are recommended.

On etoposide days, follow acute-onset antiemetic regimen for level 2 risk. Anticipatory, breakthrough, and delayed-onset regimens are recommended as needed.
For anemia (likely)
If hemoglobin level is less than 10 g/dl, *one* of the following is recommended:
• Epoetin alfa 150 units/kg subcutaneously three times weekly. If unsatisfactory response, may increase to 300 units/kg three times weekly.
• Epoetin alfa 40,000 units subcutaneously weekly; may increase to 60,000 units if unsatisfactory response.
• Darbepoetin alfa 3 mcg/kg subcutaneously every 2 weeks; may increase to 5 mcg/kg if unsatisfactory response.
• Darbepoetin alfa 200 mcg subcutaneously every 2 weeks; may increase to 300 mcg if unsatisfactory response.
For neutropenia (high risk)
To prevent neutropenia, start *one* of the following colony-stimulating factors 1 to 3 days after completion of chemotherapy and continue through postnadir recovery:
• Filgrastim 5 mcg/kg daily or
• Pegfilgrastim 6 mg once for each treatment cycle.
For diarrhea (likely)
Prescribe antidiarrheal as indicated.
For cisplatin-induced nephrotoxicity
Maintain urine output of at least 75 ml/hour

for several hours before and after each cisplatin dose. Consider amifostine for prevention of cisplatin-induced nephrotoxicity.

Docetaxel

Docetaxel 75 or 100 mg/m² I.V. over 1 hour on day 1
Repeat every 21 days.
Reference: Vershraegen CF, et al. *J Clin Oncol.* 2000;18:2733-2739.

Supportive therapy
For nausea and vomiting
Follow acute-onset antiemetic regimen for level 2 risk. Anticipatory, breakthrough, and delayed-onset regimens are recommended as needed.
For anemia (likely)
If hemoglobin level is less than 10 g/dl, *one* of the following is recommended:
• Epoetin alfa 150 units/kg subcutaneously three times weekly. If unsatisfactory response, may increase to 300 units/kg three times weekly.
• Epoetin alfa 40,000 units subcutaneously weekly; may increase to 60,000 units if unsatisfactory response.
• Darbepoetin alfa 3 mcg/kg subcutaneously every 2 weeks; may increase to 5 mcg/kg if unsatisfactory response.
• Darbepoetin alfa 200 mcg subcutaneously every 2 weeks; may increase to 300 mcg if unsatisfactory response.
For neutropenia (high risk)
To prevent neutropenia, start *one* of the following colony-stimulating factors 1 to 3 days after completion of chemotherapy and continue through postnadir recovery:
• Filgrastim 5 mcg/kg daily or
• Pegfilgrastim 6 mg once for each treatment cycle.
For hypersensitivity reactions
To prevent hypersensitivity reactions, give dexamethasone 8 mg P.O. twice daily for 3 days starting 1 day before docetaxel administration.

Docetaxel, carboplatin

Docetaxel 60 mg/m² I.V. on day 1, followed by *Carboplatin* to AUC of 6 I.V.
Repeat cycle every 21 days.
Reference: Markman M, et al. *J Clin Oncol.* 2001;19:1901-1905.

Supportive therapy
For nausea and vomiting
Follow acute-onset antiemetic regimen for level 5 risk. Anticipatory, breakthrough, and delayed-onset regimens are recommended.
For anemia (likely)
If hemoglobin level is less than 10 g/dl, *one* of the following is recommended:
• Epoetin alfa 150 units/kg subcutaneously three times weekly. If unsatisfactory response, may increase to 300 units/kg three times weekly.
• Epoetin alfa 40,000 units subcutaneously weekly; may increase to 60,000 units if unsatisfactory response.
• Darbepoetin alfa 3 mcg/kg subcutaneously every 2 weeks; may increase to 5 mcg/kg if unsatisfactory response.
• Darbepoetin alfa 200 mcg subcutaneously every 2 weeks; may increase to 300 mcg if unsatisfactory response.
For neutropenia (high risk)
To prevent neutropenia, start *one* of the following colony-stimulating factors 1 to 3 days after completion of chemotherapy and continue through postnadir recovery:
• Filgrastim 5 mcg/kg daily or
• Pegfilgrastim 6 mg once for each treatment cycle.
For diarrhea (likely)
Prescribe antidiarrheal as indicated.
For constipation (likely)
Order stool softener or laxative as indicated.
For hypersensitivity reactions
To prevent hypersensitivity reactions, give dexamethasone 8 mg P.O. twice daily for 3 days starting 1 day before docetaxel administration.

Paclitaxel

Paclitaxel 175 mg/m² I.V. over 3 hours on day 1

Repeat every 21 days.

Reference: Eisenhauer EA, et al. *J Clin Oncol.* 1994;12:2654-2666; Markman M, et al. *J Clin Oncol.* 2003;21:2460-2465.

Supportive therapy

For nausea and vomiting

Follow acute-onset antiemetic regimen for level 2 risk. Anticipatory, breakthrough, and delayed-onset regimens are recommended as needed.

For anemia (likely)

If hemoglobin level is less than 10 g/dl, *one* of the following is recommended:

• Epoetin alfa 150 units/kg subcutaneously three times weekly. If unsatisfactory response, may increase to 300 units/kg three times weekly.

• Epoetin alfa 40,000 units subcutaneously weekly; may increase to 60,000 units if unsatisfactory response.

• Darbepoetin alfa 3 mcg/kg subcutaneously every 2 weeks; may increase to 5 mcg/kg if unsatisfactory response.

• Darbepoetin alfa 200 mcg subcutaneously every 2 weeks; may increase to 300 mcg if unsatisfactory response.

For neutropenia (high risk)

To prevent neutropenia, start *one* of the following colony-stimulating factors 1 to 3 days after completion of chemotherapy and continue through postnadir recovery:

• Filgrastim 5 mcg/kg daily or

• Pegfilgrastim 6 mg once for each treatment cycle.

For hypersensitivity reactions

To prevent hypersensitivity reactions, give the following before paclitaxel administration: dexamethasone 20 mg P.O. 12 hours and 6 hours before, diphenhydramine 50 mg I.V. 30 to 60 minutes before, *and* cimetidine 300 mg I.V. *or* ranitidine 50 mg I.V. 30 to 60 minutes before.

Paclitaxel, carboplatin

Paclitaxel 175 mg/m² I.V. over 3 hours on day 1, followed by

Carboplatin to AUC of 5 to 7.5 I.V. over 1 hour on day 1

Repeat cycle every 21 days.

Reference: Vasey PA, et al. *J Natl Cancer Inst.* 2004;96:1682-1691; Coleman RL, et al. *Cancer J Sci Am.* 1997;3:246-253.

Supportive therapy

For nausea and vomiting

Follow acute-onset antiemetic regimen for level 5 risk. Anticipatory, breakthrough, and delayed-onset regimens are recommended.

For anemia (likely)

If hemoglobin level is less than 10 g/dl, *one* of the following is recommended:

• Epoetin alfa 150 units/kg subcutaneously three times weekly. If unsatisfactory response, may increase to 300 units/kg three times weekly.

• Epoetin alfa 40,000 units subcutaneously weekly; may increase to 60,000 units if unsatisfactory response.

• Darbepoetin alfa 3 mcg/kg subcutaneously every 2 weeks; may increase to 5 mcg/kg if unsatisfactory response.

• Darbepoetin alfa 200 mcg subcutaneously every 2 weeks; may increase to 300 mcg if unsatisfactory response.

For neutropenia (high risk)

To prevent neutropenia, start *one* of the following colony-stimulating factors 1 to 3 days after completion of chemotherapy and continue through postnadir recovery:

• Filgrastim 5 mcg/kg daily or

• Pegfilgrastim 6 mg once for each treatment cycle.

For diarrhea (likely)

Prescribe antidiarrheal as indicated.

For constipation (likely)

Order stool softener or laxative as indicated.

For hypersensitivity reactions

To prevent hypersensitivity reactions, give the

following before paclitaxel administration: dexamethasone 20 mg P.O. 12 hours and 6 hours before, diphenhydramine 50 mg I.V. 30 to 60 minutes before, *and* cimetidine 300 mg I.V. *or* ranitidine 50 mg I.V. 30 to 60 minutes before.

Paclitaxel, cisplatin

Paclitaxel 135 mg/m^2 I.V. over 3 hours on day 1, followed by
Cisplatin 75 mg/m^2 I.V. over 1 hour on day 1
Repeat cycle every 21 days.

Reference: McGuire WP, et al. *N Engl J Med.* 1996;334:1-6; Neijt JP, et al. *J Clin Oncol.* 2000;18:3084-3092; Ozols RF, et al. *J Clin Oncol.* 2003;21:3194-3200.

Supportive therapy

For nausea and vomiting
Follow acute-onset antiemetic regimen for level 5 risk. Anticipatory, breakthrough, and delayed-onset regimens are recommended.

For anemia (likely)
If hemoglobin level is less than 10 g/dl, *one* of the following is recommended:
• Epoetin alfa 150 units/kg subcutaneously three times weekly. If unsatisfactory response, may increase to 300 units/kg three times weekly.
• Epoetin alfa 40,000 units subcutaneously weekly; may increase to 60,000 units if unsatisfactory response.
• Darbepoetin alfa 3 mcg/kg subcutaneously every 2 weeks; may increase to 5 mcg/kg if unsatisfactory response.
• Darbepoetin alfa 200 mcg subcutaneously every 2 weeks; may increase to 300 mcg if unsatisfactory response.

For neutropenia (high risk)
To prevent neutropenia, start *one* of the following colony-stimulating factors 1 to 3 days after completion of chemotherapy and continue through postnadir recovery:
• Filgrastim 5 mcg/kg daily or
• Pegfilgrastim 6 mg once for each treatment cycle.

For diarrhea (likely)
Prescribe antidiarrheal as indicated.

For hypersensitivity reactions
To prevent hypersensitivity reactions, give the following before paclitaxel administration: dexamethasone 20 mg P.O. 12 hours and 6 hours before, diphenhydramine 50 mg I.V. 30 to 60 minutes before, *and* cimetidine 300 mg I.V. *or* ranitidine 50 mg I.V. 30 to 60 minutes before.

For cisplatin-induced nephrotoxicity
Maintain urine output of at least 75 ml/hour for several hours before and after each cisplatin dose. Consider amifostine for prevention of cisplatin-induced nephrotoxicity.

Pancreatic cancer

Capecitabine

Capecitabine 1,250 mg/m^2 P.O. twice daily on days 1 through 14
Repeat every 21 days.

Reference: Cartwright TH, et al. *J Clin Oncol.* 2002;20:160-164.

Supportive therapy

For nausea and vomiting
Follow acute-onset antiemetic regimen for level 2 risk. Anticipatory, breakthrough, and delayed-onset regimens are recommended as needed.

For anemia (likely)
If hemoglobin level is less than 10 g/dl, *one* of the following is recommended:
• Epoetin alfa 150 units/kg subcutaneously three times weekly. If unsatisfactory response, may increase to 300 units/kg three times weekly.
• Epoetin alfa 40,000 units subcutaneously weekly; may increase to 60,000 units if unsatisfactory response.
• Darbepoetin alfa 3 mcg/kg subcutaneously every 2 weeks; may increase to 5 mcg/kg if unsatisfactory response.

See front endpaper for specific antiemetic therapies.

- Darbepoetin alfa 200 mcg subcutaneously every 2 weeks; may increase to 300 mcg if unsatisfactory response.

For diarrhea (likely)
Prescribe antidiarrheal as indicated.

Gemcitabine

Gemcitabine 1,000 mg/m² I.V. every week for 7 weeks, followed by 1 week of rest
Repeat subsequent cycles 3 weeks out of every 4.
Reference: Costanzo FD, et al. *Br J Cancer.* 2005;93:185-189.

Supportive therapy

For nausea and vomiting
Follow acute-onset antiemetic regimen for level 2 risk. Anticipatory, breakthrough, and delayed-onset regimens are recommended as needed.

For anemia (likely)
If hemoglobin level is less than 10 g/dl, *one* of the following is recommended:
- Epoetin alfa 150 units/kg subcutaneously three times weekly. If unsatisfactory response, may increase to 300 units/kg three times weekly.
- Epoetin alfa 40,000 units subcutaneously weekly; may increase to 60,000 units if unsatisfactory response.
- Darbepoetin alfa 3 mcg/kg subcutaneously every 2 weeks; may increase to 5 mcg/kg if unsatisfactory response.
- Darbepoetin alfa 200 mcg subcutaneously every 2 weeks; may increase to 300 mcg if unsatisfactory response.

For neutropenia (intermediate risk)
To prevent neutropenia, consider starting *one* of the following colony-stimulating factors 1 to 3 days after completion of chemotherapy and continuing through postnadir recovery:
- Filgrastim 5 mcg/kg daily or
- Pegfilgrastim 6 mg once for each treatment cycle.

Gemcitabine, cisplatin

Gemcitabine 1,000 mg/m² I.V. over 30 minutes on days 1, 8, and 15, followed by
Cisplatin 50 mg/m² I.V. on days 1 and 15
Repeat cycle every 28 days.
Reference: Philip PA, et al. *Cancer.* 2001;92:569-577.

Supportive therapy

For nausea and vomiting.
On days 1 and 15, follow acute-onset antiemetic regimen for level 5 risk. Anticipatory, breakthrough, and delayed-onset regimens are recommended.

On day 8, follow acute-onset antiemetic regimen for level 2 risk. Anticipatory, breakthrough, and delayed-onset regimens are recommended as needed.

For anemia (likely)
If hemoglobin level is less than 10 g/dl, *one* of the following is recommended:
- Epoetin alfa 150 units/kg subcutaneously three times weekly. If unsatisfactory response, may increase to 300 units/kg three times weekly.
- Epoetin alfa 40,000 units subcutaneously weekly; may increase to 60,000 units if unsatisfactory response.
- Darbepoetin alfa 3 mcg/kg subcutaneously every 2 weeks; may increase to 5 mcg/kg if unsatisfactory response.
- Darbepoetin alfa 200 mcg subcutaneously every 2 weeks; may increase to 300 mcg if unsatisfactory response.

For neutropenia (high risk)
To prevent neutropenia, start *one* of the following colony-stimulating factors 1 to 3 days after completion of chemotherapy and continue through postnadir recovery:
- Filgrastim 5 mcg/kg daily or
- Pegfilgrastim 6 mg once for each treatment cycle.

For diarrhea (likely)
Prescribe antidiarrheal as indicated.

For cisplatin-induced nephrotoxicity
Maintain urine output of at least 75 ml/hour

for several hours before and after each cis-platin dose. Consider amifostine for prevention of cisplatin-induced nephrotoxicity.

Gemcitabine, oxaliplatin

Gemcitabine 1,000 mg/m² I.V. over 100 minutes (10 mg/m²/minute) on day 1
Oxaliplatin 100 mg/m² I.V. over 2 hours on day 2
Repeat cycle every 14 days.
Reference: Louvet C, et al. *J Clin Oncol.* 2002;20:1512-1518.

Supportive therapy
For nausea and vomiting
On day 1, follow acute-onset antiemetic regimen for level 2 risk. Anticipatory, breakthrough, and delayed-onset regimens are recommended as needed.

On day 2, follow acute-onset antiemetic regimen for level 3 risk. Anticipatory, breakthrough, and delayed-onset regimens are recommended as needed.
For anemia (likely)
If hemoglobin level is less than 10 g/dl, *one* of the following is recommended:
• Epoetin alfa 150 units/kg subcutaneously three times weekly. If unsatisfactory response, may increase to 300 units/kg three times weekly.
• Epoetin alfa 40,000 units subcutaneously weekly; may increase to 60,000 units if unsatisfactory response.
• Darbepoetin alfa 3 mcg/kg subcutaneously every 2 weeks; may increase to 5 mcg/kg if unsatisfactory response.
• Darbepoetin alfa 200 mcg subcutaneously every 2 weeks; may increase to 300 mcg if unsatisfactory response.

Infusional 5-fluorouracil

Infusional 5-fluorouracil 200 to 250 mg/m² I.V. daily on days 1 through 5
Repeat every 28 days.

Reference: Rich TA, et al. *Am Soc Clin Oncol.* 2004;22:2214-2232.

Supportive therapy
For nausea and vomiting
Follow acute-onset antiemetic regimen for level 2 risk. Anticipatory, breakthrough, and delayed-onset regimens are recommended as needed.
For anemia (likely)
If hemoglobin level is less than 10 g/dl, *one* of the following is recommended:
• Epoetin alfa 150 units/kg subcutaneously three times weekly. If unsatisfactory response, may increase to 300 units/kg three times weekly.
• Epoetin alfa 40,000 units subcutaneously weekly; may increase to 60,000 units if unsatisfactory response.
• Darbepoetin alfa 3 mcg/kg subcutaneously every 2 weeks; may increase to 5 mcg/kg if unsatisfactory response.
• Darbepoetin alfa 200 mcg subcutaneously every 2 weeks; may increase to 300 mcg if unsatisfactory response.
For diarrhea (very likely)
Prescribe antidiarrheal as indicated.

Prostate cancer

Docetaxel, estramustine

Estramustine 280 mg P.O. three times daily on days 1 through 5
Docetaxel 60 mg/m² I.V. on day 2
Repeat cycle every 21 days for maximum of six cycles.

Reference: Walczak JR, et al. *Urology.* 2003;62(suppl 1):141-146.

Supportive therapy
For nausea and vomiting
On days 1, 3, 4, and 5, follow acute-onset antiemetic regimen for level 1 risk.

On day 2, follow acute-onset antiemetic regimen for level 2 risk. Anticipatory, breakthrough, and delayed-onset regimens are recommended as needed.

For neutropenia (high risk)

To prevent neutropenia, start *one* of the following colony-stimulating factors 1 to 3 days after completion of chemotherapy and continue through postnadir recovery:

• Filgrastim 5 mcg/kg daily or
• Pegfilgrastim 6 mg once for each treatment cycle.

For hypersensitivity reactions

To prevent hypersensitivity reactions, give dexamethasone 8 mg P.O. twice daily for 3 days starting 1 day before docetaxel administration.

Docetaxel, prednisone

Docetaxel 75 mg/m^2 I.V. over 1 hour on day 1
Prednisone 5 mg P.O. twice daily on days 1 through 21
Repeat cycle every 21 days.

Reference: Tannock IF, et al. *N Engl J Med.* 2004;351:1502-1512.

Supportive therapy

For nausea and vomiting

On day 1, follow acute-onset antiemetic regimen for level 2 risk. Anticipatory, breakthrough, and delayed-onset regimens are recommended as needed.

On days 2 through 21, follow acute-onset antiemetic regimen for level 1 risk.

For neutropenia (high risk)

To prevent neutropenia, start *one* of the following colony-stimulating factors 1 to 3 days after completion of chemotherapy and continue through postnadir recovery:

• Filgrastim 5 mcg/kg daily or
• Pegfilgrastim 6 mg once for each treatment cycle.

For hypersensitivity reactions

To prevent hypersensitivity reactions, give dexamethasone 8 mg P.O. twice daily for 3 days starting 1 day before docetaxel administration.

Estramustine

Estramustine 14 mg/kg P.O. daily in three or four divided doses

Reference: Emcyt [package insert]. New York, NY: Pfizer; 2003.

Supportive therapy

For nausea and vomiting

Follow acute-onset antiemetic regimen for level 1 risk.

Estramustine, vinblastine

Estramustine 600 mg/m^2 P.O. in divided doses daily on days 1 through 42
Vinblastine 4 mg/m^2 I.V. weekly for 6 weeks, beginning on day 1
Repeat cycle every 8 weeks.

Reference: Hudes G, et al. *J Clin Oncol.* 1999;17:3160-3166.

Supportive therapy

For nausea and vomiting

Follow acute-onset antiemetic regimen for level 1 risk.

For anemia (likely)

If hemoglobin level is less than 10 g/dl, *one* of the following is recommended:

• Epoetin alfa 150 units/kg subcutaneously three times weekly. If unsatisfactory response, may increase to 300 units/kg three times weekly.
• Epoetin alfa 40,000 units subcutaneously weekly; may increase to 60,000 units if unsatisfactory response.
• Darbepoetin alfa 3 mcg/kg subcutaneously every 2 weeks; may increase to 5 mcg/kg if unsatisfactory response.
• Darbepoetin alfa 200 mcg subcutaneously every 2 weeks; may increase to 300 mcg if unsatisfactory response.

For constipation (likely)

Order stool softener or laxative as indicated.

Hormone therapy

Bicalutamide and leuprolide or goserelin
Bicalutamide 50 mg daily P.O.
Leuprolide depot 7.5 mg I.M. every 28 days
Or
Goserelin implant 3.6 mg subcutaneously every
28 days
Reference: Schellhammer P, et al. Urology.
1995;45:745-752.

FL (flutamide and leuprolide)
Flutamide 250 mg P.O. three times daily
Leuprolide 1 mg daily subcutaneously
Or
Leuprolide depot 7.5 mg I.M. every 28 days
Reference: Sarosdy MF, et al. Urology.
2000;55:391-396.

FZ (flutamide and goserelin [Zoladex])
Flutamide 250 mg P.O. three times daily
Goserelin implant 3.6 mg subcutaneously every
28 days, beginning 8 weeks before radiation
therapy for four cycles; or 10.8 mg subcutaneously 4 weeks before radiotherapy
Reference: Jurincic CD, et al. Semin Oncol.
1991;18(suppl 6):21-25.

Goserelin, leuprolide, or triptorelin
Goserelin implant 3.6 mg subcutaneously every
28 days; or 10.8 mg subcutaneously every 12
weeks
Reference: Pilepich MV, et al. Urology.
1995;45:616-623.
Or
Leuprolide depot 7.5 mg I.M. every 28 days or
22.5 mg I.M. every 3 months; or 30 mg I.M.
every 4 months
Reference: Lupron Depot 7.5 mg, Lupron Depot 22.5 mg, Lupron Depot 30 mg [package
inserts]. Lake Forest, IL: TAP Pharmaceuticals;
2004.
Or
Triptorelin 3.75 mg I.M. every 28 days; or triptorelin LA 11.25 mg I.M. every 84 days
Reference: Kuhn JM, et al. Eur Urol.
1997;32:397-403.

Supportive therapy
For nausea and vomiting
Follow acute-onset antiemetic regimen for level 1 risk.
For osteoporosis
Supplemental calcium and vitamin D are recommended to mitigate bone loss and bisphos-
phonate treatment for men who either meet
diagnostic criteria for osteoporosis or develop
fractures.

Mitoxantrone, prednisone

Mitoxantrone 12 mg/m^2 I.V. on day 1
Prednisone 5 mg P.O. twice daily on days 1
through 21
Repeat cycle every 21 days.
Reference: Tannock IF, et al. J Clin Oncol.
1996;14:1756-1764; Petrylak DP, et al. N Engl
J Med. 2004;351:1513-1520.

Supportive therapy
For nausea and vomiting
On day 1, follow acute-onset antiemetic regimen for level 3 risk. Anticipatory, break-
through, and delayed-onset regimens are rec-
ommended as needed.
  On prednisone days only, follow acute-
onset antiemetic regimen for level 1 risk.
For neutropenia (intermediate risk)
To prevent neutropenia, consider starting *one*
of the following colony-stimulating factors 1
to 3 days after completion of chemotherapy
and continuing through postnadir recovery:
• Filgrastim 5 mcg/kg daily or
• Pegfilgrastim 6 mg once for each treatment
cycle.
For diarrhea (likely)
Prescribe antidiarrheal as indicated.

PE (paclitaxel, estramustine)

Paclitaxel 120 mg/m^2 I.V. daily on days 1
through 4 (continuous infusion over 96 hours)
Estramustine 600 mg/m^2 P.O. daily in two or
three divided doses, starting 24 hours before
paclitaxel

See front endpaper for specific antiemetic therapies.

Repeat cycle every 21 days.

Reference: Hudes GR, et al. *J Clin Oncol.* 1997;15:3156-3163.

Supportive therapy

For nausea and vomiting
On days 1 through 4, follow acute-onset antiemetic regimen for level 2 risk. Anticipatory, breakthrough, and delayed-onset regimens are recommended as needed.

On estramustine days only, follow acute-onset antiemetic regimen for level 1 risk.

For anemia (likely)
If hemoglobin level is less than 10 g/dl, *one* of the following is recommended:
• Epoetin alfa 150 units/kg subcutaneously three times weekly. If unsatisfactory response, may increase to 300 units/kg three times weekly.
• Epoetin alfa 40,000 units subcutaneously weekly; may increase to 60,000 units if unsatisfactory response.
• Darbepoetin alfa 3 mcg/kg subcutaneously every 2 weeks; may increase to 5 mcg/kg if unsatisfactory response.
• Darbepoetin alfa 200 mcg subcutaneously every 2 weeks; may increase to 300 mcg if unsatisfactory response.

For neutropenia (high risk)
To prevent neutropenia, start *one* of the following colony-stimulating factors 1 to 3 days after completion of chemotherapy and continue through postnadir recovery:
• Filgrastim 5 mcg/kg daily or
• Pegfilgrastim 6 mg once for each treatment cycle.

For diarrhea (likely)
Prescribe antidiarrheal as indicated.

For hypersensitivity reactions
To prevent hypersensitivity reactions, give the following before paclitaxel administration: dexamethasone 20 mg P.O. 12 hours and 6 hours before, diphenhydramine 50 mg I.V. 30 to 60 minutes before, *and* cimetidine 300 mg I.V. *or* ranitidine 50 mg I.V. 30 to 60 minutes before.

Skin cancer (melanoma)

Aldesleukin (interleukin-2)

Aldesleukin 600,000 units/kg I.V. over 15 minutes every 8 hours for 5 days for maximum of 14 doses
Repeat after 9 days of rest.

Reference: Atkins MB, et al. *Cancer J Sci Am.* 2000;6(suppl 1):S11–S14.

Supportive therapy

For nausea and vomiting
Follow acute-onset antiemetic regimen for level 3 risk. Anticipatory, breakthrough, and delayed-onset regimens are recommended as needed.

For anemia (likely)
Transfuse packed RBCs to achieve hematocrit of more than 28% during aldesleukin dosing. If hemoglobin level is less than 10 g/dl, *one* of the following is recommended:
• Epoetin alfa 150 units/kg subcutaneously three times weekly. If unsatisfactory response, may increase to 300 units/kg three times weekly.
• Epoetin alfa 40,000 units subcutaneously weekly; may increase to 60,000 units if unsatisfactory response.
• Darbepoetin alfa 3 mcg/kg subcutaneously every 2 weeks; may increase to 5 mcg/kg if unsatisfactory response.
• Darbepoetin alfa 200 mcg subcutaneously every 2 weeks; may increase to 300 mcg if unsatisfactory response.

For diarrhea (likely)
Prescribe antidiarrheal as indicated.

Dacarbazine

Dacarbazine 2 to 4.5 mg/kg I.V. daily on days 1 through 10
Repeat every 21 or 28 days.
Or
Dacarbazine 1,000 mg/m^2 I.V. on day 1
Repeat every 21 days.

Reference: Chapman PB, et al. *J Clin Oncol.*
1999;17:2745-2751; Middleton MR, et al. *J Clin Oncol.* 2000;18:158-166.

Supportive therapy

For nausea and vomiting
On days 1 through 10 or on day 1 only, follow acute-onset antiemetic regimen for level 5 risk. Anticipatory, breakthrough, and delayed-onset regimens are recommended.

For anemia (likely)
If hemoglobin level is less than 10 g/dl, *one* of the following is recommended:
• Epoetin alfa 150 units/kg subcutaneously three times weekly. If unsatisfactory response, may increase to 300 units/kg three times weekly.
• Epoetin alfa 40,000 units subcutaneously weekly; may increase to 60,000 units if unsatisfactory response.
• Darbepoetin alfa 3 mcg/kg subcutaneously every 2 weeks; may increase to 5 mcg/kg if unsatisfactory response.
• Darbepoetin alfa 200 mcg subcutaneously every 2 weeks; may increase to 300 mcg if unsatisfactory response.

For neutropenia (high risk)
To prevent neutropenia, start *one* of the following colony-stimulating factors 1 to 3 days after completion of chemotherapy and continue through postnadir recovery:
• Filgrastim 5 mcg/kg daily or
• Pegfilgrastim 6 mg once for each treatment cycle.

IFN (interferon alfa-2b)

Interferon alfa-2b 20 million units/m² I.V. weekly on days 1 through 5 for 4 weeks, then 10 million units/m² subcutaneously three times weekly for 48 weeks

Reference: Kirkwood JM, et al. *J Clin Oncol.* 1996;14:7-17.

Supportive therapy

For nausea and vomiting
Follow acute-onset antiemetic regimen for

level 1 risk.

For neutropenia (high risk)
To prevent neutropenia, start *one* of the following colony-stimulating factors 1 to 3 days after completion of chemotherapy and continue through postnadir recovery:
• Filgrastim 5 mcg/kg daily or
• Pegfilgrastim 6 mg once for each treatment cycle.

For flulike symptoms
To avoid flulike symptoms, give indomethacin, acetaminophen, and ranitidine, starting night before first dose of IFN and continuing until 24 hours after IFN therapy stops.

Temozolomide

Temozolomide 200 mg/m² P.O. on days 1 through 5
Repeat every 28 days.

Reference: Middleton MR, et al. *Am Soc Clin Oncol.* 2000;18:158-166.

Supportive therapy

For nausea and vomiting
Follow acute-onset antiemetic regimen for level 2 risk. Anticipatory, breakthrough, and delayed-onset regimens are recommended as needed.

For neutropenia (high risk)
To prevent neutropenia, start *one* of the following colony-stimulating factors 1 to 3 days after completion of chemotherapy and continue through postnadir recovery:
• Filgrastim 5 mcg/kg daily or
• Pegfilgrastim 6 mg once for each treatment cycle.

For constipation (likely)
Order stool softener or laxative as indicated.

Skin cancer (Merkel cell)

Carboplatin, etoposide

Carboplatin to AUC of 4.5 I.V. on day 1 of weeks 1, 4, 7, and 10
Etoposide 80 mg/m² I.V. daily on days 1 through 3 of weeks 1, 4, 7, and 10

Reference: Poulsen M, et al. *J Clin Oncol.* 2003;21:4371-4376.

Supportive therapy

For nausea and vomiting
On day 1, follow acute-onset antiemetic regimen for level 5 risk. Anticipatory, breakthrough, and delayed-onset regimens are recommended.

On days 2 and 3, follow acute-onset antiemetic regimen for level 2 risk. Anticipatory, breakthrough, and delayed-onset regimens are recommended as needed.

For anemia (likely)
If hemoglobin level is less than 10 g/dl, *one* of the following is recommended:
• Epoetin alfa 150 units/kg subcutaneously three times weekly. If unsatisfactory response, may increase to 300 units/kg three times weekly.
• Epoetin alfa 40,000 units subcutaneously weekly; may increase to 60,000 units if unsatisfactory response.
• Darbepoetin alfa 3 mcg/kg subcutaneously every 2 weeks; may increase to 5 mcg/kg if unsatisfactory response.
• Darbepoetin alfa 200 mcg subcutaneously every 2 weeks; may increase to 300 mcg if unsatisfactory response.

For neutropenia (high risk)
To prevent neutropenia, start *one* of the following colony-stimulating factors 1 to 3 days after completion of chemotherapy and continue through postnadir recovery:
• Filgrastim 5 mcg/kg daily or
• Pegfilgrastim 6 mg once for each treatment cycle.

For diarrhea (likely)
Prescribe antidiarrheal as indicated.
For constipation (likely)
Order stool softener or laxative as indicated.

Cisplatin, etoposide

Cisplatin 60 mg/m² I.V. on day 1
Etoposide 120 mg/m² I.V. on days 1 through 3
Repeat cycle every 21 days.

Reference: Turrisi AT III, et al. *N Engl J Med.* 1999;340:265-271.

Supportive therapy

For nausea and vomiting
On day 1, follow acute-onset antiemetic regimen for level 5 risk. Anticipatory, breakthrough, and delayed-onset regimens are recommended.

On days 2 and 3, follow acute-onset antiemetic regimen for level 2 risk. Anticipatory, breakthrough, and delayed-onset regimens are recommended as needed.

For anemia (likely)
If hemoglobin level is less than 10 g/dl, *one* of the following is recommended:
• Epoetin alfa 150 units/kg subcutaneously three times weekly. If unsatisfactory response, may increase to 300 units/kg three times weekly.
• Epoetin alfa 40,000 units subcutaneously weekly; may increase to 60,000 units if unsatisfactory response.
• Darbepoetin alfa 3 mcg/kg subcutaneously every 2 weeks; may increase to 5 mcg/kg if unsatisfactory response.
• Darbepoetin alfa 200 mcg subcutaneously every 2 weeks; may increase to 300 mcg if unsatisfactory response.

For neutropenia (high risk)
To prevent neutropenia, start *one* of the following colony-stimulating factors 1 to 3 days after completion of chemotherapy and continue through postnadir recovery:
• Filgrastim 5 mcg/kg daily or
• Pegfilgrastim 6 mg once for each treatment cycle.

For diarrhea (likely)
Prescribe antidiarrheal as indicated.

Topotecan

Topotecan 1.5 mg/m^2 I.V. over 30 minutes on days 1 through 5
Repeat every 21 days.

Reference: NCCN Practice Guidelines in Oncology. Merkel Cell Carcinoma v.2.2005. Available in: Hycamtin prescribing information. Research Triangle Park, NC: GlaxoSmithKline; July 2003.

Supportive therapy

For nausea and vomiting
Follow acute-onset antiemetic regimen for level 2 risk. Anticipatory, breakthrough, and delayed-onset regimens are recommended as needed.

For anemia (likely)
If hemoglobin level is less than 10 g/dl, *one* of the following is recommended:
• Epoetin alfa 150 units/kg subcutaneously three times weekly. If unsatisfactory response, may increase to 300 units/kg three times weekly.
• Epoetin alfa 40,000 units subcutaneously weekly; may increase to 60,000 units if unsatisfactory response.
• Darbepoetin alfa 3 mcg/kg subcutaneously every 2 weeks; may increase to 5 mcg/kg if unsatisfactory response.
• Darbepoetin alfa 200 mcg subcutaneously every 2 weeks; may increase to 300 mcg if unsatisfactory response.

For neutropenia (high risk)
To prevent neutropenia, start *one* of the following colony-stimulating factors 1 to 3 days after completion of chemotherapy and continue through postnadir recovery:
• Filgrastim 5 mcg/kg daily or
• Pegfilgrastim 6 mg once for each treatment cycle.

For diarrhea (likely)
Prescribe antidiarrheal as indicated.

For constipation (likely)
Order stool softener or laxative as indicated.

Soft-tissue sarcoma

AD (doxorubicin [Adriamycin], dacarbazine)

Doxorubicin 15 mg/m^2 daily by continuous I.V. infusion on days 1 through 4
Dacarbazine 250 mg/m^2 daily by continuous I.V. infusion on days 1 through 4
Repeat cycle every 21 days.

Reference: Antman K, et al. *J Clin Oncol.* 1993;11:1276-1285.

Supportive therapy

For nausea and vomiting
On days 1 through 4, follow acute-onset antiemetic regimen for level 5 risk. Anticipatory, breakthrough, and delayed-onset regimens are recommended.

For anemia (likely)
If hemoglobin level is less than 10 g/dl, *one* of the following is recommended:
• Epoetin alfa 150 units/kg subcutaneously three times weekly. If unsatisfactory response, may increase to 300 units/kg three times weekly.
• Epoetin alfa 40,000 units subcutaneously weekly; may increase to 60,000 units if unsatisfactory response.
• Darbepoetin alfa 3 mcg/kg subcutaneously every 2 weeks; may increase to 5 mcg/kg if unsatisfactory response.
• Darbepoetin alfa 200 mcg subcutaneously every 2 weeks; may increase to 300 mcg if unsatisfactory response.

For neutropenia (high risk)
To prevent neutropenia, start *one* of the following colony-stimulating factors 1 to 3 days after completion of chemotherapy and continue through postnadir recovery:
• Filgrastim 5 mcg/kg daily or
• Pegfilgrastim 6 mg once for each treatment cycle.

See front endpaper for specific antiemetic therapies.

AIM (doxorubicin [Adriamycin], ifosfamide, mesna)

Doxorubicin 50 mg/m² by I.V. bolus on day 1
Ifosfamide 5,000 mg/m² by continuous I.V. infusion on day 1
Mesna 600 mg/m² by I.V. bolus before ifosfamide, 2,500 mg/m² by continuous I.V. infusion with ifosfamide, and 1,250 mg/m² I.V. over 12 hours following ifosfamide
Repeat cycle every 21 days.

Reference: Santoro A, et al. *J Clin Oncol.* 1995;13:1537-1545.

Supportive therapy

For nausea and vomiting
On day 1, follow acute-onset antiemetic regimen for level 4 risk. Anticipatory, breakthrough, and delayed-onset regimens are recommended as needed.

For anemia (likely)
If hemoglobin level is less than 10 g/dl, *one* of the following is recommended:

• Epoetin alfa 150 units/kg subcutaneously three times weekly. If unsatisfactory response, may increase to 300 units/kg three times weekly.

• Epoetin alfa 40,000 units subcutaneously weekly; may increase to 60,000 units if unsatisfactory response.

• Darbepoetin alfa 3 mcg/kg subcutaneously every 2 weeks; may increase to 5 mcg/kg if unsatisfactory response.

• Darbepoetin alfa 200 mcg subcutaneously every 2 weeks; may increase to 300 mcg if unsatisfactory response.

For neutropenia (high risk)
To prevent neutropenia, start *one* of the following colony-stimulating factors 1 to 3 days after completion of chemotherapy and continue through postnadir recovery:

• Filgrastim 5 mcg/kg daily or

• Pegfilgrastim 6 mg once for each treatment cycle.

Doxorubicin

Doxorubicin 75 mg/m² I.V. on day 1
Repeat every 21 days.

Reference: Edmonson JH, et al. *J Clin Oncol.* 1993;11:1269-1275; Nielsen OS, et al. *Br J Cancer.* 1998;78:1634-1639; Santoro A, et al. *J Clin Oncol.* 1995;13:1537-1545.

Supportive therapy

For nausea and vomiting
Follow acute-onset antiemetic regimen for level 4 risk. Anticipatory, breakthrough, and delayed-onset regimens are recommended as needed.

For anemia (likely)
If hemoglobin level is less than 10 g/dl, *one* of the following is recommended:

• Epoetin alfa 150 units/kg subcutaneously three times weekly. If unsatisfactory response, may increase to 300 units/kg three times weekly.

• Epoetin alfa 40,000 units subcutaneously weekly; may increase to 60,000 units if unsatisfactory response.

• Darbepoetin alfa 3 mcg/kg subcutaneously every 2 weeks; may increase to 5 mcg/kg if unsatisfactory response.

• Darbepoetin alfa 200 mcg subcutaneously every 2 weeks; may increase to 300 mcg if unsatisfactory response.

For neutropenia (high risk)
To prevent neutropenia, start *one* of the following colony-stimulating factors 1 to 3 days after completion of chemotherapy and continue through postnadir recovery:

• Filgrastim 5 mcg/kg daily or

• Pegfilgrastim 6 mg once for each treatment cycle.

Gemcitabine, docetaxel

For patients who have previously received radiation:
Gemcitabine 675 mg/m² I.V. over 90 minutes on days 1 and 8

Docetaxel 100 mg/m² I.V. over 60 minutes on day 8

Repeat cycle every 21 days.

Or

For patients who have not previously received radiation:

Gemcitabine 900 mg/m² I.V. over 90 minutes on days 1 and 8

Docetaxel 100 mg/m² I.V. over 60 minutes on day 8

Repeat cycle every 21 days.

Reference: Leu KM, et al. *J Clin Oncol.* 2004;22:1706-1712; Hensley ML. *J Clin Oncol.* 2002;20:2824-2831.

Supportive therapy

For nausea and vomiting

On day 1, follow acute-onset antiemetic regimen for level 2 risk. Anticipatory, breakthrough, and delayed-onset regimens are recommended as needed.

On day 8, follow acute-onset antiemetic regimen for level 3 risk. Anticipatory, breakthrough, and delayed-onset regimens are recommended as needed.

For anemia (likely)

If hemoglobin level is less than 10 g/dl, **one** of the following is recommended:

• Epoetin alfa 150 units/kg subcutaneously three times weekly. If unsatisfactory response, may increase to 300 units/kg three times weekly.

• Epoetin alfa 40,000 units subcutaneously weekly; may increase to 60,000 units if unsatisfactory response.

• Darbepoetin alfa 3 mcg/kg subcutaneously every 2 weeks; may increase to 5 mcg/kg if unsatisfactory response.

• Darbepoetin alfa 200 mcg subcutaneously every 2 weeks; may increase to 300 mcg if unsatisfactory response.

For neutropenia (high risk)

To prevent neutropenia, give granulocyte-colony stimulating factor (G-CSF) 150 mcg/m² (dose rounded to 300 or 480 mcg) subcutaneously, days 9 through 15; may stop G-CSF before day 15 if absolute neutrophil count is above 1,200/mm³ on two separate occasions.

For diarrhea (likely)

Prescribe antidiarrheal as indicated.

For hypersensitivity reactions

To prevent hypersensitivity reactions, give dexamethasone 8 mg P.O. twice daily for 3 days starting 1 day before docetaxel administration.

Imatinib mesylate

Imatinib mesylate 400 to 800 mg P.O. daily for 8 weeks or more as tolerated

Reference: Demetri GD, et al. *N Engl J Med.* 2002;347:472-480; Verweij J, et al. *Lancet.* 2004;364:1127-1134.

Supportive therapy

For nausea and vomiting

Follow acute-onset antiemetic regimen for level 1 risk.

For anemia (likely)

If hemoglobin level is less than 10 g/dl, **one** of the following is recommended:

• Epoetin alfa 150 units/kg subcutaneously three times weekly. If unsatisfactory response, may increase to 300 units/kg three times weekly.

• Epoetin alfa 40,000 units subcutaneously weekly; may increase to 60,000 units if unsatisfactory response.

• Darbepoetin alfa 3 mcg/kg subcutaneously every 2 weeks; may increase to 5 mcg/kg if unsatisfactory response.

• Darbepoetin alfa 200 mcg subcutaneously every 2 weeks; may increase to 300 mcg if unsatisfactory response.

For neutropenia (high risk)

To prevent neutropenia, start **one** of the following colony-stimulating factors 1 to 3 days after completion of chemotherapy and continue through postnadir recovery:

• Filgrastim 5 mcg/kg daily or

• Pegfilgrastim 6 mg once for each treatment cycle.

See front endpaper for specific antiemetic therapies.

Liposomal doxorubicin

Liposomal doxorubicin 50 mg/m² by I.V. infusion over 1 hour
Repeat every 28 days.
Reference: Casper ES, et al. *J Clin Oncol.* 1997;15:2111-2117; Judson I, et al. *Eur J Cancer.* 2001;37:870-877; Skubitz, KM. *Cancer Invest,* 2003;21:167-176.

Supportive therapy

For nausea and vomiting
Follow acute-onset antiemetic regimen for level 3 risk. Anticipatory, breakthrough, and delayed-onset regimens are recommended as needed.

For anemia (likely)
If hemoglobin level is less than 10 g/dl, *one* of the following is recommended:
• Epoetin alfa 150 units/kg subcutaneously three times weekly. If unsatisfactory response, may increase to 300 units/kg three times weekly.
• Epoetin alfa 40,000 units subcutaneously weekly; may increase to 60,000 units if unsatisfactory response.
• Darbepoetin alfa 3 mcg/kg subcutaneously every 2 weeks; may increase to 5 mcg/kg if unsatisfactory response.
• Darbepoetin alfa 200 mcg subcutaneously every 2 weeks; may increase to 300 mcg if unsatisfactory response.

For neutropenia (high risk)
To prevent neutropenia, start *one* of the following colony-stimulating factors 1 to 3 days after completion of chemotherapy and continue through postnadir recovery:
• Filgrastim 5 mcg/kg daily or
• Pegfilgrastim 6 mg once for each treatment cycle.

MAID (mesna, doxorubicin [Adriamycin], ifosfamide, dacarbazine)

Regimen A
Ifosfamide 2,500 mg/m² daily by continuous I.V. infusion on days 1 through 3
Mesna 2,500 mg/m² daily by continuous I.V. infusion on days 1 through 4
Doxorubicin 15 mg/m² daily by continuous I.V. infusion on days 1 through 4
Dacarbazine 250 mg/m² daily by continuous I.V. infusion on days 1 through 4
Repeat cycle every 21 days.
Reference: Antman K, et al. *J Clin Oncol.* 1993;11:1276-1285.
Or

Regimen B
Ifosfamide 2,500 mg/m² daily by continuous I.V. infusion on days 1 through 3
Mesna 2,500 mg/m² daily by continuous I.V. infusion on days 1 through 4
Doxorubicin 20 mg/m² daily by continuous I.V. infusion on days 1 through 3
Dacarbazine 300 mg/m² daily by continuous I.V. infusion on days 1 through 3
Repeat cycle every 21 days.
Reference: Elias A, et al. *Semin Oncol.* 1990;17(suppl 4):41-49.

Supportive therapy

For nausea and vomiting
On days 1 through 4 (regimen A), follow acute-onset antiemetic regimen for level 5 risk. Anticipatory, breakthrough, and delayed-onset regimens are recommended.

On days 1 through 3 (regimen B), follow acute-onset antiemetic regimen for level 5 risk. Anticipatory, breakthrough, and delayed-onset regimens are recommended.

For anemia (likely)
If hemoglobin level is less than 10 g/dl, *one* of the following is recommended:
• Epoetin alfa 150 units/kg subcutaneously three times weekly. If unsatisfactory response, may increase to 300 units/kg three times weekly.
• Epoetin alfa 40,000 units subcutaneously weekly; may increase to 60,000 units if unsatisfactory response.
• Darbepoetin alfa 3 mcg/kg subcutaneously every 2 weeks; may increase to 5 mcg/kg if unsatisfactory response.

- Darbepoetin alfa 200 mcg subcutaneously every 2 weeks; may increase to 300 mcg if unsatisfactory response.

For neutropenia (high risk)

To prevent neutropenia, start *one* of the following colony-stimulating factors 1 to 3 days after completion of chemotherapy and continue through postnadir recovery:

- Filgrastim 5 mcg/kg daily or
- Pegfilgrastim 6 mg once for each treatment cycle.

Testicular cancer

BEP (bleomycin, etoposide, cisplatin [Platinol-AQ])

Etoposide 100 mg/m² I.V. daily over 30 to 60 minutes on days 1 through 5
Cisplatin 20 mg/m² I.V. over 30 to 60 minutes on days 1 through 5
Bleomycin 30 units by I.V. bolus on days 2, 9, and 16
Repeat cycle every 21 days.

Reference: Williams SD, et al. *N Engl J Med.* 1987;316:1435-1440.

Supportive therapy

For nausea and vomiting

On days 1 through 5, follow acute-onset antiemetic regimen for level 5 risk. Anticipatory, breakthrough, and delayed-onset regimens are recommended.

For anemia (likely)

If hemoglobin level is less than 10 g/dl, *one* of the following is recommended:

- Epoetin alfa 150 units/kg subcutaneously three times weekly. If unsatisfactory response, may increase to 300 units/kg three times weekly.
- Epoetin alfa 40,000 units subcutaneously weekly; may increase to 60,000 units if unsatisfactory response.

- Darbepoetin alfa 3 mcg/kg subcutaneously every 2 weeks; may increase to 5 mcg/kg if unsatisfactory response.
- Darbepoetin alfa 200 mcg subcutaneously every 2 weeks; may increase to 300 mcg if unsatisfactory response.

For neutropenia (high risk)

To prevent neutropenia, start *one* of the following colony-stimulating factors 1 to 3 days after completion of chemotherapy and continue through postnadir recovery:

- Filgrastim 5 mcg/kg daily or
- Pegfilgrastim 6 mg once for each treatment cycle.

For cisplatin-induced nephrotoxicity

Maintain urine output of at least 75 ml/hour for several hours before and after each cisplatin dose. Consider amifostine for prevention of cisplatin-induced nephrotoxicity.

EP (etoposide, cisplatin [Platinol-AQ])

Etoposide 100 mg/m² I.V. daily on days 1 through 5
Cisplatin 20 mg/m² I.V. daily on days 1 through 5
Repeat cycle once after 21 days.

Reference: Motzer RJ, et al. *J Clin Oncol.* 1995;13:2700-2704.

Supportive therapy

For nausea and vomiting

On days 1 through 5, follow acute-onset antiemetic regimen for level 5 risk. Anticipatory, breakthrough, and delayed-onset regimens are recommended.

For anemia (likely)

If hemoglobin level is less than 10 g/dl, *one* of the following is recommended:

- Epoetin alfa 150 units/kg subcutaneously three times weekly. If unsatisfactory response, may increase to 300 units/kg three times weekly.
- Epoetin alfa 40,000 units subcutaneously weekly; may increase to 60,000 units if unsatisfactory response.

See front endpaper for specific antiemetic therapies.

- Darbepoetin alfa 3 mcg/kg subcutaneously every 2 weeks; may increase to 5 mcg/kg if unsatisfactory response.
- Darbepoetin alfa 200 mcg subcutaneously every 2 weeks; may increase to 300 mcg if unsatisfactory response.

For neutropenia (high risk)
To prevent neutropenia, start *one* of the following colony-stimulating factors 1 to 3 days after completion of chemotherapy and continue through postnadir recovery:
- Filgrastim 5 mcg/kg daily or
- Pegfilgrastim 6 mg once for each treatment cycle.

For cisplatin-induced nephrotoxicity
Maintain urine output of at least 75 ml/hour for several hours before and after each cisplatin dose. Consider amifostine for prevention of cisplatin-induced nephrotoxicity.

Paclitaxel, ifosfamide, cisplatin, mesna

Paclitaxel 250 mg/m² by continuous I.V. infusion over 24 hours on day 1
Ifosfamide 1,500 mg/m² by I.V. infusion over 60 minutes on days 2 through 5 given with *Mesna* 500 mg/m² I.V. before ifosfamide and 4 and 8 hours after ifosfamide for total daily mesna dose of 1,500 mg/m² to match daily ifosfamide dose on days 2 through 5
Cisplatin 25 mg/m² by I.V. infusion over 30 minutes on days 2 through 5
Repeat cycle every 21 days.

Reference: Kondagunta GV, et al. *J Clin Oncol.* 2005;23:6549-6555; Motzer RJ, et al. *J Clin Oncol.* 2000;18:2413-2418.

Supportive therapy
For nausea and vomiting
On day 1, follow acute-onset antiemetic regimen for level 2 risk. Anticipatory, breakthrough, and delayed-onset regimens are recommended as needed.

On days 2 through 5, follow acute-onset antiemetic regimen for level 5 risk. Anticipatory, breakthrough, and delayed-onset regimens are recommended.

For anemia (likely)
If hemoglobin level is less than 10 g/dl, *one* of the following is recommended:
- Epoetin alfa 150 units/kg subcutaneously three times weekly. If unsatisfactory response, may increase to 300 units/kg three times weekly.
- Epoetin alfa 40,000 units subcutaneously weekly; may increase to 60,000 units if unsatisfactory response.
- Darbepoetin alfa 3 mcg/kg subcutaneously every 2 weeks; may increase to 5 mcg/kg if unsatisfactory response.
- Darbepoetin alfa 200 mcg subcutaneously every 2 weeks; may increase to 300 mcg if unsatisfactory response.

For neutropenia (high risk)
To prevent neutropenia, start *one* of the following colony-stimulating factors 1 to 3 days after completion of chemotherapy and continue through postnadir recovery:
- Filgrastim 5 mcg/kg daily or
- Pegfilgrastim 6 mg once for each treatment cycle.

For diarrhea (likely)
Prescribe antidiarrheal as indicated.

For hypersensitivity reactions
To prevent hypersensitivity reactions, give the following before paclitaxel administration: dexamethasone 20 mg P.O. 12 hours and 6 hours before, diphenhydramine 50 mg I.V. 30 to 60 minutes before, *and* cimetidine 300 mg I.V. *or* ranitidine 50 mg I.V. 30 to 60 minutes before.

For cisplatin-induced nephrotoxicity
Maintain urine output of at least 75 ml/hour for several hours before and after each cisplatin dose. Consider amifostine for prevention of cisplatin-induced nephrotoxicity.

PVB (cisplatin [Platinol-AQ], vinblastine, bleomycin)

Vinblastine 0.15 mg/kg daily by I.V. bolus on days 1 and 2

Cisplatin 20 mg/m² I.V. daily over 15 to 30 minutes on days 1 through 5
Bleomycin 30 units daily by I.V. bolus on days 2, 9, and 16
Repeat cycle every 21 days.
Reference: Williams SD, et al. *N Engl J Med.* 1987;316:1435-1440.

Supportive therapy
For nausea and vomiting
On days 1 through 5, follow acute-onset antiemetic regimen for level 4 risk. Anticipatory, breakthrough, and delayed-onset regimens are recommended as needed. .

On days 9 and 16, follow acute-onset antiemetic regimen for level 1 risk.
For anemia (likely)
If hemoglobin level is less than 10 g/dl, *one* of the following is recommended:
• Epoetin alfa 150 units/kg subcutaneously three times weekly. If unsatisfactory response, may increase to 300 units/kg three times weekly.
• Epoetin alfa 40,000 units subcutaneously weekly; may increase to 60,000 units if unsatisfactory response.
• Darbepoetin alfa 3 mcg/kg subcutaneously every 2 weeks; may increase to 5 mcg/kg if unsatisfactory response.
• Darbepoetin alfa 200 mcg subcutaneously every 2 weeks; may increase to 300 mcg if unsatisfactory response.
For neutropenia (high risk)
To prevent neutropenia, start *one* of the following colony-stimulating factors 1 to 3 days after completion of chemotherapy and continue through postnadir recovery:
• Filgrastim 5 mcg/kg daily or
• Pegfilgrastim 6 mg once for each treatment cycle.
For constipation (likely)
Order stool softener or laxative as indicated.
For cisplatin-induced nephrotoxicity
Maintain urine output of at least 75 ml/hour for several hours before and after each cisplatin dose. Consider amifostine for prevention of cisplatin-induced nephrotoxicity.

VeIP (vinblastine, ifosfamide, mesna, cisplatin [Platinol-AQ])

Vinblastine 0.11 mg/kg I.V. daily on days 1 and 2
Ifosfamide 1,200 mg/m² daily on days 1 through 5 by continuous I.V. infusion with *mesna* 400 mg I.V. daily 15 minutes before ifosfamide, followed by 1,200 mg continuous I.V. infusion daily on days 1 through 5
Cisplatin 20 mg/m² I.V. over 30 to 60 minutes on days 1 through 5
Repeat cycle every 21 days.
Reference: Loehrer PJ, et al. *Ann Intern Med.* 1988;109:540-546.

Supportive therapy
For nausea and vomiting
On days 1 through 5, follow acute-onset antiemetic regimen for level 5 risk. Anticipatory, breakthrough, and delayed-onset regimens are recommended.
For anemia (likely)
If hemoglobin level is less than 10 g/dl, *one* of the following is recommended:
• Epoetin alfa 150 units/kg subcutaneously three times weekly. If unsatisfactory response, may increase to 300 units/kg three times weekly.
• Epoetin alfa 40,000 units subcutaneously weekly; may increase to 60,000 units if unsatisfactory response.
• Darbepoetin alfa 3 mcg/kg subcutaneously every 2 weeks; may increase to 5 mcg/kg if unsatisfactory response.
• Darbepoetin alfa 200 mcg subcutaneously every 2 weeks; may increase to 300 mcg if unsatisfactory response.
For neutropenia (high risk)
To prevent neutropenia, start *one* of the following colony-stimulating factors 1 to 3 days after completion of chemotherapy and continue through postnadir recovery:
• Filgrastim 5 mcg/kg daily or
• Pegfilgrastim 6 mg once for each treatment cycle.

For constipation (likely)
Order stool softener or laxative as indicated.
For cisplatin-induced nephrotoxicity
Maintain urine output of at least 75 ml/hour for several hours before and after each cisplatin dose. Consider amifostine for prevention of cisplatin-induced nephrotoxicity.

VIP (etoposide [VePesid], ifosfamide, mesna, cisplatin [Platinol-AQ])

Etoposide 75 mg/m² I.V. daily on days 1 through 5
Ifosfamide 1,200 mg/m² I.V. daily on days 1 through 5 given with *mesna* 400 mg I.V. 15 minutes before ifosfamide, followed by 1,200 mg daily by continuous I.V. infusion on days 1 through 5
Cisplatin 20 mg/m² I.V. over 30 to 60 minutes on days 1 through 5
Repeat cycle every 21 days.
Reference: Loehrer PJ, et al. *Ann Intern Med.* 1988;109:540-546.

Supportive therapy
For nausea and vomiting
On days 1 through 5, follow acute-onset antiemetic regimen for level 5 risk. Anticipatory, breakthrough, and delayed-onset regimens are recommended.
For anemia (likely)
If hemoglobin level is less than 10 g/dl, *one* of the following is recommended:
• Epoetin alfa 150 units/kg subcutaneously three times weekly. If unsatisfactory response, may increase to 300 units/kg three times weekly.
• Epoetin alfa 40,000 units subcutaneously weekly; may increase to 60,000 units if unsatisfactory response.
• Darbepoetin alfa 3 mcg/kg subcutaneously every 2 weeks; may increase to 5 mcg/kg if unsatisfactory response.
• Darbepoetin alfa 200 mcg subcutaneously every 2 weeks; may increase to 300 mcg if unsatisfactory response.

For neutropenia (high risk)
To prevent neutropenia, start *one* of the following colony-stimulating factors 1 to 3 days after completion of chemotherapy and continue through postnadir recovery:
• Filgrastim 5 mcg/kg daily or
• Pegfilgrastim 6 mg once for each treatment cycle.
For cisplatin-induced nephrotoxicity
Maintain urine output of at least 75 ml/hour for several hours before and after each cisplatin dose. Consider amifostine for prevention of cisplatin-induced nephrotoxicity.

Thyroid cancer

CVD (cyclophosphamide, vincristine, dacarbazine)

Cyclophosphamide 750 mg/m² I.V. on day 1
Vincristine 1.4 mg/m² I.V. on day 1
Dacarbazine 600 mg/m² I.V. on days 1 and 2
Repeat cycle every 21 to 28 days.
Reference: Wu LT, et al. *Cancer.* 1994;73:432-436.

Supportive therapy
For nausea and vomiting
On days 1 and 2, follow acute-onset antiemetic regimen for level 5 risk. Anticipatory, breakthrough, and delayed-onset regimens are recommended.
For anemia (likely)
If hemoglobin level is less than 10 g/dl, *one* of the following is recommended:
• Epoetin alfa 150 units/kg subcutaneously three times weekly. If unsatisfactory response, may increase to 300 units/kg three times weekly.
• Epoetin alfa 40,000 units subcutaneously weekly; may increase to 60,000 units if unsatisfactory response.
• Darbepoetin alfa 3 mcg/kg subcutaneously every 2 weeks; may increase to 5 mcg/kg if unsatisfactory response.

- Darbepoetin alfa 200 mcg subcutaneously every 2 weeks; may increase to 300 mcg if unsatisfactory response.

For neutropenia (high risk)

To prevent neutropenia, start **one** of the following colony-stimulating factors 1 to 3 days after completion of chemotherapy and continue through postnadir recovery:

- Filgrastim 5 mcg/kg daily or
- Pegfilgrastim 6 mg once for each treatment cycle.

For diarrhea (likely)

Prescribe antidiarrheal as indicated.

Dacarbazine, 5-fluorouracil

Dacarbazine 250 mg/m² I.V. over 15 to 30 minutes on days 1 through 5
5-Fluorouracil 450 mg/m² I.V. over 12 hours on days 1 through 5
Repeat cycle every 28 days for maximum of six cycles.

Reference: Orlandi F, et al. *Ann Oncol.* 1994;5:763-765.

Supportive therapy

For nausea and vomiting

On days 1 through 5, follow acute-onset antiemetic regimen for level 5 risk. Anticipatory, breakthrough, and delayed-onset regimens are recommended.

For anemia (likely)

If hemoglobin level is less than 10 g/dl, **one** of the following is recommended:

- Epoetin alfa 150 units/kg subcutaneously three times weekly. If unsatisfactory response, may increase to 300 units/kg three times weekly.
- Epoetin alfa 40,000 units subcutaneously weekly; may increase to 60,000 units if unsatisfactory response.
- Darbepoetin alfa 3 mcg/kg subcutaneously every 2 weeks; may increase to 5 mcg/kg if unsatisfactory response.
- Darbepoetin alfa 200 mcg subcutaneously every 2 weeks; may increase to 300 mcg if unsatisfactory response.

For neutropenia (high risk)

To prevent neutropenia, start **one** of the following colony-stimulating factors 1 to 3 days after completion of chemotherapy and continue through postnadir recovery:

- Filgrastim 5 mcg/kg daily or
- Pegfilgrastim 6 mg once for each treatment cycle.

For diarrhea (very likely)

An antidiarrheal is recommended.

Uterine cancer

CAP (cyclophosphamide, doxorubicin [Adriamycin], cisplatin [Platinol-AQ])

Cisplatin 70 mg/m² I.V. on day 1
Doxorubicin 40 mg/m² I.V. on day 1
Cyclophosphamide 500 mg/m² I.V. on day 1
Repeat cycle every 28 days.

Reference: Watanabe Y, et al. *Gynecol Oncol.* 2004;94:333-339.

Supportive therapy

For nausea and vomiting

Follow acute-onset antiemetic regimen for level 5 risk. Anticipatory, breakthrough, and delayed-onset regimens are recommended.

For anemia (likely)

If hemoglobin level is less than 10 g/dl, **one** of the following is recommended:

- Epoetin alfa 150 units/kg subcutaneously three times weekly. If unsatisfactory response, may increase to 300 units/kg three times weekly.
- Epoetin alfa 40,000 units subcutaneously weekly; may increase to 60,000 units if unsatisfactory response.
- Darbepoetin alfa 3 mcg/kg subcutaneously every 2 weeks; may increase to 5 mcg/kg if unsatisfactory response.
- Darbepoetin alfa 200 mcg subcutaneously every 2 weeks; may increase to 300 mcg if unsatisfactory response.

For neutropenia (high risk)
To prevent neutropenia, start *one* of the following colony-stimulating factors 1 to 3 days after completion of chemotherapy and continue through postnadir recovery:
- Filgrastim 5 mcg/kg daily or
- Pegfilgrastim 6 mg once for each treatment cycle.

For diarrhea (likely)
Prescribe antidiarrheal as indicated.

For cisplatin-induced nephrotoxicity
Maintain urine output of at least 75 ml/hour for several hours before and after each cisplatin dose. Consider amifostine for prevention of cisplatin-induced nephrotoxicity.

Cisplatin, doxorubicin

Cisplatin 100 mg/m^2 I.V. on day 1
Doxorubicin 45 to 60 mg/m^2 I.V. on day 1
Repeat cycle every 21 days.

Reference: Peters WA III, et al. *Gynecol Oncol.* 1989;34:323-327; Randall ME, et al. *J Clin Oncol.* 2003;22:237.

Supportive therapy

For nausea and vomiting
Follow acute-onset antiemetic regimen for level 5 risk. Anticipatory, breakthrough, and delayed-onset regimens are recommended.

For anemia (likely)
If hemoglobin level is less than 10 g/dl, *one* of the following is recommended:
- Epoetin alfa 150 units/kg subcutaneously three times weekly. If unsatisfactory response, may increase to 300 units/kg three times weekly.
- Epoetin alfa 40,000 units subcutaneously weekly; may increase to 60,000 units if unsatisfactory response.
- Darbepoetin alfa 3 mcg/kg subcutaneously every 2 weeks; may increase to 5 mcg/kg if unsatisfactory response.
- Darbepoetin alfa 200 mcg subcutaneously every 2 weeks; may increase to 300 mcg if unsatisfactory response.

For neutropenia (high risk)
To prevent neutropenia, start *one* of the following colony-stimulating factors 1 to 3 days after completion of chemotherapy and continue through postnadir recovery:
- Filgrastim 5 mcg/kg daily or
- Pegfilgrastim 6 mg once for each treatment cycle.

For diarrhea (likely)
Prescribe antidiarrheal as indicated.

For cisplatin-induced nephrotoxicity
Maintain urine output of at least 75 ml/hour for several hours before and after each cisplatin dose. Consider amifostine for prevention of cisplatin-induced nephrotoxicity.

Cisplatin, paclitaxel

Radiation therapy, days 1 and 28: 4,500 cGy in 5 weeks, with daily fractions of 1.8 Gy to pelvis, followed by intracavitary single low dose of 20 Gy to vaginal surface; or three high-dose applications totaling 18 Gy to vaginal surface
Cisplatin 50 mg/m^2 I.V. on days 1 and 28
After radiation therapy is completed:
Cisplatin 50 mg/m^2 I.V. on day 1
Paclitaxel 175 mg/m^2 I.V. over 24 hours on day 1
Repeat cisplatin and paclitaxel every 28 days.

Reference: Greven K, et al. *Int J Radiat Oncol Biol Phys.* 2004;59:168-173.

Supportive therapy

For nausea and vomiting
On days 1 and 28, follow acute-onset antiemetic regimen for level 5 risk. Anticipatory, breakthrough, and delayed-onset regimens are recommended.

For anemia (likely)
If hemoglobin level is less than 10 g/dl, *one* of the following is recommended:
- Epoetin alfa 150 units/kg subcutaneously three times weekly. If unsatisfactory response, may increase to 300 units/kg three times weekly.

- Epoetin alfa 40,000 units subcutaneously weekly; may increase to 60,000 units if unsatisfactory response.
- Darbepoetin alfa 3 mcg/kg subcutaneously every 2 weeks; may increase to 5 mcg/kg if unsatisfactory response.
- Darbepoetin alfa 200 mcg subcutaneously every 2 weeks; may increase to 300 mcg if unsatisfactory response.

For neutropenia (high risk)
To prevent neutropenia, start *one* of the following colony-stimulating factors 1 to 3 days after completion of chemotherapy and continue through postnadir recovery:
- Filgrastim 5 mcg/kg daily or
- Pegfilgrastim 6 mg once for each treatment cycle.

For diarrhea (likely)
Prescribe antidiarrheal as indicated.

For hypersensitivity reactions
To prevent hypersensitivity reactions, give the following before paclitaxel administration: dexamethasone 20 mg P.O. 12 hours and 6 hours before, diphenhydramine 50 mg I.V. 30 to 60 minutes before, *and* cimetidine 300 mg I.V. *or* ranitidine 50 mg I.V. 30 to 60 minutes before.

For cisplatin-induced nephrotoxicity
Maintain urine output of at least 75 ml/hour for several hours before and after each cisplatin dose. Consider amifostine for prevention of cisplatin-induced nephrotoxicity.

Doxorubicin

Doxorubicin 60 mg/m^2 I.V. on day 1
Repeat every 28 days.

Reference: Thigpen JT, et al. *J Clin Oncol.* 2004;22:3902-3908; Aapro MS, et al. *Ann Oncol.* 2003;14:441-448.

Supportive therapy
For nausea and vomiting
Follow acute-onset antiemetic regimen for level 4 risk. Anticipatory, breakthrough, and delayed-onset regimens are recommended as needed.

For neutropenia (intermediate risk)
To prevent neutropenia, consider starting *one* of the following colony-stimulating factors 1 to 3 days after completion of chemotherapy and continuing through postnadir recovery:
- Filgrastim 5 mcg/kg daily or
- Pegfilgrastim 6 mg once for each treatment cycle.

Ifosfamide

Ifosfamide 1,500 mg/m^2 I.V. daily on days 1 through 5 given with mesna 300 mg/m^2 I.V. immediately and 4 and 8 hours after ifosfamide
For patients who have previously received radiation therapy:
Ifosfamide 1,200 mg/m^2 I.V. daily on days through 5 given with mesna 240 mg/m^2 I.V. immediately and 4 and 8 hours after ifosfamide
Repeat every 28 days.

Reference: Sutton GP, et al. *Am J Obstet Gynecol.* 1989;161:309-312.

Supportive therapy
For nausea and vomiting
On days 1 through 5, follow acute-onset antiemetic regimen for level 3 risk. Anticipatory, breakthrough, and delayed-onset regimens are recommended as needed.

For anemia (likely)
If hemoglobin level is less than 10 g/dl, *one* of the following is recommended:
- Epoetin alfa 150 units/kg subcutaneously three times weekly. If unsatisfactory response, may increase to 300 units/kg three times weekly.
- Epoetin alfa 40,000 units subcutaneously weekly; may increase to 60,000 units if unsatisfactory response.
- Darbepoetin alfa 3 mcg/kg subcutaneously every 2 weeks; may increase to 5 mcg/kg if unsatisfactory response.
- Darbepoetin alfa 200 mcg subcutaneously every 2 weeks; may increase to 300 mcg if unsatisfactory response.

For neutropenia (high risk)
To prevent neutropenia, start *one* of the following colony-stimulating factors 1 to 3 days after completion of chemotherapy and continue through postnadir recovery:
• Filgrastim 5 mcg/kg daily or
• Pegfilgrastim 6 mg once for each treatment cycle.

Ifosfamide, cisplatin

Ifosfamide 1,500 mg/m^2 I.V. daily given with mesna 1,500 mg/m^2 daily by continuous I.V. infusion on days 1 through 5
Cisplatin 20 mg/m^2 I.V. daily on days 1 through 5
Repeat cycle every 21 days.

Reference: Sutton G, et al. *Gynecol Oncol.* 2000;79:147-153.

Supportive therapy
For nausea and vomiting
On days 1 through 5, follow acute-onset antiemetic regimen for level 5 risk. Anticipatory, breakthrough, and delayed-onset regimens are recommended.
For anemia (likely)
If hemoglobin level is less than 10 g/dl, *one* of the following is recommended:
• Epoetin alfa 150 units/kg subcutaneously three times weekly. If unsatisfactory response, may increase to 300 units/kg three times weekly.
• Epoetin alfa 40,000 units subcutaneously weekly; may increase to 60,000 units if unsatisfactory response.
• Darbepoetin alfa 3 mcg/kg subcutaneously every 2 weeks; may increase to 5 mcg/kg if unsatisfactory response.
• Darbepoetin alfa 200 mcg subcutaneously every 2 weeks; may increase to 300 mcg if unsatisfactory response.
For neutropenia (high risk)
To prevent neutropenia, start *one* of the following colony-stimulating factors 1 to 3 days after completion of chemotherapy and continue through postnadir recovery:

• Filgrastim 5 mcg/kg daily or
• Pegfilgrastim 6 mg once for each treatment cycle.
For cisplatin-induced nephrotoxicity
Maintain urine output of at least 75 ml/hour for several hours before and after each cisplatin dose. Consider amifostine for prevention of cisplatin-induced nephrotoxicity.

MAID (mesna, doxorubicin [Adriamycin], ifosfamide, dacarbazine)

Ifosfamide 2,500 mg/m^2 daily by continuous I.V. infusion on days 1 through 3
Mesna 2,500 mg/m^2 daily by continuous I.V. infusion on days 1 through 4
Doxorubicin 15 mg/m^2 daily by continuous I.V. infusion on days 1 through 4
Dacarbazine 250 mg/m^2 daily by continuous I.V. infusion on days 1 through 4
Repeat cycle every 21 days.

Reference: Antman K, et al. *J Clin Oncol.* 1993;11:1276-1285.

Supportive therapy
For nausea and vomiting
On days 1 through 4, follow acute-onset antiemetic regimen for level 5 risk. Anticipatory, breakthrough, and delayed-onset regimens are recommended.
For anemia (likely)
If hemoglobin level is less than 10 g/dl, *one* of the following is recommended:
• Epoetin alfa 150 units/kg subcutaneously three times weekly. If unsatisfactory response, may increase to 300 units/kg three times weekly.
• Epoetin alfa 40,000 units subcutaneously weekly; may increase to 60,000 units if unsatisfactory response.
• Darbepoetin alfa 3 mcg/kg subcutaneously every 2 weeks; may increase to 5 mcg/kg if unsatisfactory response.
• Darbepoetin alfa 200 mcg subcutaneously every 2 weeks; may increase to 300 mcg if unsatisfactory response.

For neutropenia (high risk)

To prevent neutropenia, start *one* of the following colony-stimulating factors 1 to 3 days after completion of chemotherapy and continue through postnadir recovery:

- Filgrastim 5 mcg/kg daily or
- Pegfilgrastim 6 mg once for each treatment cycle.

TAP (doxorubicin [Adriamycin], cisplatin [Platinol-AQ], paclitaxel [Taxol], filgrastim)

Doxorubicin 45 mg/m^2 I.V. on day 1, followed immediately by

Cisplatin 50 mg/m^2 I.V. on day 1

Paclitaxel 160 mg/m^2 I.V. over 3 hours on day 2

Filgrastim 5 mcg/kg subcutaneously on days 3 through 12

Repeat cycle every 21 days for maximum of seven cycles.

Reference: Fleming GF, et al. *J Clin Oncol.* 2004;22:2159-2166.

Supportive therapy

For nausea and vomiting

On day 1, follow acute-onset antiemetic regimen for level 5 risk. Anticipatory, breakthrough, and delayed-onset regimens are recommended.

On day 2, follow acute-onset antiemetic regimen for level 2 risk. Anticipatory, breakthrough, and delayed-onset regimens are recommended as needed.

For anemia (likely)

If hemoglobin level is less than 10 g/dl, *one* of the following is recommended:

- Epoetin alfa 150 units/kg subcutaneously three times weekly. If unsatisfactory response, may increase to 300 units/kg three times weekly.
- Epoetin alfa 40,000 units subcutaneously weekly; may increase to 60,000 units if unsatisfactory response.

- Darbepoetin alfa 3 mcg/kg subcutaneously every 2 weeks; may increase to 5 mcg/kg if unsatisfactory response.
- Darbepoetin alfa 200 mcg subcutaneously every 2 weeks; may increase to 300 mcg if unsatisfactory response.

For neutropenia

To prevent neutropenia, give filgrastim 5 mcg/kg daily *or* pegfilgrastim, one dose of 6 mg per cycle of treatment subcutaneously. Start colony-stimulating factors 1 to 3 days after completion of chemotherapy; continue through postnadir recovery.

For diarrhea (likely)

Prescribe antidiarrheal as indicated.

For hypersensitivity reactions

To prevent hypersensitivity reactions, give the following before paclitaxel administration: dexamethasone 20 mg P.O. 12 hours and 6 hours before, diphenhydramine 50 mg I.V. 30 to 60 minutes before, *and* cimetidine 300 mg I.V. *or* ranitidine 50 mg I.V. 30 to 60 minutes before.

For cisplatin-induced nephrotoxicity

Maintain urine output of at least 75 ml/hour for several hours before and after each cisplatin dose. Consider amifostine for prevention of cisplatin-induced nephrotoxicity.

See front endpaper for specific antiemetic therapies.

Appendices

■

References

■

Index

Common oncology abbreviations

The abbreviations below are commonly used in oncology practice and research. However, use abbreviations with caution. When in doubt, spell out the word or term rather than risk misinterpretation of an abbreviation.

AA	anaplastic anemia		CRO	contract research organization
AAIR	age-adjusted incidence rate		CSF	colony-stimulating factor, cerebrospinal fluid
ABMT	autologous bone marrow transplant			
ADE	adverse drug event		CT	computerized tomography
ADR	adverse drug reaction		CTC	common toxicity criteria (research and clinical tool to assess toxicity)
AE	adverse event			
AFP	alpha fetoprotein		CTCL	cutaneous T-cell lymphoma
ALCL	anaplastic large-cell lymphoma		DCIS	ductal carcinoma in situ
ALL	acute lymphoblastic or lymphocytic leukemia		DFI	disease-free interval
			DLBCL	diffuse large B-cell lymphoma
AML	acute myeloid leukemia		DLCL	diffuse large-cell lymphoma
ANA	antinuclear antibodies		DTIC	dacarbazine
ANC	absolute neutrophil count		EBV	Epstein-Barr virus
ANLL	acute nonlymphocytic leukemia		ECOG	Eastern Cooperative Oncology Group
Ara-C	cytarabine			
AUC	area under the curve		EFS	event-free survival
BCL	B-cell leukemia, B-cell lymphoma		EPO	epoetin alfa
BCNU	carmustine		FMEN	familial multiple endocrine neoplasia
bleo	bleomycin		FMTC	familial medullary thyroid carcinoma
BMT	bone marrow transplant		FNA	fine-needle aspiration
BRM	biological response modifier		5-FU	5-fluorouracil
BSA	body surface area		G-CSF	granulocyte colony–stimulating factor
BSE	breast self-examination			
Bx	biopsy		GM-CSF	granulocyte-macrophage colony–stimulating factor
CA	cancer, cancer antigen			
CA 125	cancer antigen 125		GPR	good partial remission
CCNU	lomustine		GVHD	graft versus host disease
CEA	carcinoembryonic antigen		Gy	gray (unit of radiation)
CG	control group		HCL	hairy cell leukemia
CGL	chronic granulocytic leukemia		HD	Hodgkin's disease, high dose
cGy	centigray (unit of radiation)		HDC	high-dose chemotherapy
CIS	carcinoma in situ		HEPA	high-efficiency particulate air
CLL	chronic lymphocytic leukemia		HLA	human leukocyte antigens
CML	chronic myelogenous leukemia		HNPCC	hereditary nonpolyposis colorectal cancer
CR	complete remission, complete response			
			HPV	human papilloma virus
CRA	clinical research associate		HR	high risk
			HRT	hormone replacement therapy

HSCT	hematopoietic stem-cell transplant	PEL	permissible exposure limit
IFN	interferon	PFS	progression-free survival
IL-2	interleukin-2	PPE	personal protective equipment
IMRT	intensity-modulated radiotherapy	PR	partial response, partial remission
IRB	institutional review board	PSA	prostate-specific antigen
IU	international units	QALY	quality-adjusted life year
LCIS	lobular cancer in situ	QoL	quality of life
LVEF	left ventricular ejection fraction	RCT	randomized clinical trial
LVSF	left ventricular shortening fraction	REL	recommended exposure limit
Lx	lumpectomy	RT	radiotherapy
m^3	cubic meter	SAE	serious adverse event
mAb	monoclonal antibody	SCC	squamous-cell carcinoma
MBq	megabecquerel	SCLC	small-cell lung cancer
mcg	microgram	SD	stable disease
mCi	millicurie	SIADH	syndrome of inappropriate antidiuretic hormone secretion
MDR	multidrug resistant		
MDS	myelodysplastic syndrome	SWOG	Southwest Oncology Group
mets	metastases	TBI	total body irradiation
mg	milligram	TCC	transitional-cell carcinoma
mM	millimole	TCP	thrombocytopenia
mm	millimeter	6-TG	6-thioguanine
6-MP	6-mercaptopurine	TNF	tumor necrosis factor
MSDS	material safety data sheet	TNFa	tumor necrosis factor alpha
MTD	maximum tolerated dose	TNM	tumor, nodes, metastasis
MTX	methotrexate	TSG	tumor suppressor gene
MUD	matched unrelated donor	VNB	vinorelbine
Mx	mastectomy	VP16	etoposide
ng	nanogram		
NHL	non-Hodgkin's lymphoma		
NIOSH	National Institute for Occupational Safety and Health		
NK	natural killer cells		
NMSC	non-melanoma skin cancer		
NSCLC	non-small-cell lung cancer		
OEL	occupational exposure limit		
OS	osteogenic sarcoma, overall survival		
OSHA	Occupational Safety and Health Administration		
PBSC	peripheral blood stem cell		
PBSCH	peripheral blood stem-cell harvest		
PBSCR	peripheral blood stem-cell rescue		
PBSCT	peripheral blood stem-cell transplant		
PD	progressive disease		

Calculating body surface area

Determining body surface area (BSA) is crucial to ensuring that patients receive optimal doses of chemotherapeutic drugs. Calculating BSA from a mathematical formula is more accurate than using a nomogram. The most commonly used formula for both adults and children is the Mostellar calculation.

Mosteller calculation

$$BSA\ (m^2) = \sqrt{\frac{height\ (cm) \times weight\ (kg)}{3,600}}$$

Average BSAs

Although BSA hinges largely on height and weight, age and gender also play a role, as the average BSAs below illustrate:

- Adult men: 1.9 m^2
- Adult women: 1.6 m^2
- Children ages 12 to 13: 1.33 m^2
- Children age 10: 1.14 m^2
- Children age 9: 1.07 m^2

Sources: Mosteller RD. Simplified calculation of body surface area. *N Engl J Med.* 1987;317:1098; Lam TK, Leung DT. More on simplified calculation of body surface area. *N Engl J Med.* 1988;318:1130.

Chemotherapy admixture compatibilities

Use this chart to determine the compatibility of each drug combination across three fluids—dextrose 5% in water, normal saline solution, and in direct drug-to-drug admixtures.

KEY TO SYMBOLS
C - Compatible
X - Incompatible
Ø - Conflicting data; may be compatible or incompatible
Blank - No data available

Column headers (left to right): 1 Dextrose 5% in water · 2 Normal saline solution · 3 aldesleukin · 4 amifostine · 5 amino acids solution · 6 bleomycin sulfate · 7 carboplatin · 8 carmustine · 9 ceftazidime · 10 ciprofloxacin · 11 cisplatin · 12 cladribine · 13 cyclophosphamide · 14 cytarabine · 15 dacarbazine · 16 dactinomycin · 17 daunorubicin hydrochloride · 18 docetaxel · 19 doxorubicin hydrochloride · 20 doxorubicin hydrochloride liposome · 21 etoposide · 22 etoposide phosphate · 23 fentanyl citrate

(■ = self/diagonal shaded cell)

Drug	1	2	3	4	5	6	7	8	9	10	11	12	13	14	15	16	17	18	19	20	21	22	23
aldesleukin	C		■																				
amifostine		C		■	C	C	C	C	C	X		C	C	C	C	C	C	C		C			
amino acids solution					■								C										
bleomycin sulfate	Ø	C		C		■			C		C		C						C	C		C	
carboplatin	C	Ø		C			■				C	C								C	C	C	
carmustine	Ø	Ø		C				■	C		C											C	
ceftazidime	C	C		C				C	■		C						C		X			C	
ciprofloxacin	C	C		C					C	■							C		C			C	
cisplatin	Ø	Ø			X	C	C	C			■	C	C	C					Ø	C	C	C	
cladribine						C			C		C	■	C				C		C				
cyclophosphamide	C	C		C	C	C				C	C		■	C					C	C		C	
cytarabine	C	C		C						C	C			■		C				C	C	C	
dacarbazine	C			C		C		C					C		■	C			C	C		C	
dactinomycin	C	C		C											C	■						C	
daunorubicin hydrochloride	C	C		C												C	■				C	C	
docetaxel	Ø	Ø		C					C	C								■	X				
doxorubicin hydrochloride	C	C		C		C					Ø	C	C			C			■		C	C	
doxorubicin hydrochloride liposome					C	C		X	C	C	C		C	C	C		X			■	C		
etoposide	C	Ø		C		C					C	C		C				C		C	■	C	
etoposide phosphate	C	C				C	C	C	C	C	C		C	C	C	C	C		C			■	
fentanyl citrate	C																						■
filgrastim		X								C							C				X		
floxuridine		C		C				C					C								C	C	
fludarabine phosphate		C				C	C	C		C		C	C	C	C	X		C		C	C		
fluorouracil		C		C	C	C	X	C			Ø		C		Ø	C			Ø	C	C	C	Ø
gemcitabine hydrochloride	C	C		C		C	C	C	C	C	C		C	C		C	C	C	C		C	C	
granisetron hydrochloride	C	C		C		C	C	C		C		C		C		C	C	C	Ø	C	C	C	
hydromorphone hydrochloride	C	C		C					C								C		C			C	C
idarubicin hydrochloride	C	C		C				C			C	C	C							X	C		

	filgrastim	floxuridine	fludarabine phosphate	fluorouracil	gemcitabine hydrochloride	granisetron hydrochloride	hydromorphone hydrochloride	idarubicin hydrochloride	ifosfamide	leucovorin calcium	levorphanol tartrate	mechlorethamine hydrochloride	melphalan	meperidine hydrochloride	mesna	methotrexate sodium	metoclopramide hydrochloride	metronidazole hydrochloride	mitomycin	mitoxantrone hydrochloride	morphine sulfate	nafcillin sodium	ondansetron hydrochloride	paclitaxel	palonosetron hydrochloride	pentostatin	sargramostim	streptozocin	teniposide	thiotepa	topotecan hydrochloride	total parenteral nutrition solutions	trimethobenzamide hydrochloride	vancomycin hydrochloride	vinblastine sulfate	vincristine sulfate	vinorelbine tartrate
																C					C		C														
	C	C	C	C	C	C	C	C	C		C		C	C	C	C	C	C	C	C	C		C					C	C	C					C	C	C
			C											C		X																					
			C	C	C				C				C			Ø	C		Ø				C	C		C		C	C						C	C	C
	C	C	X	C	C			C					C		X				C	Ø			C			C		C	C	C	C						
			C	C	C	C							C							C			C	C		C		C	C								
	C		C				X						C	C						C			C	C		Ø		C	C		C		Ø				
			C	C												C	C						C	C		C		C	C	C							
	C	C	Ø	C				C	C				C		X	C	Ø		Ø				C	Ø		C		C	X	C	C				C	C	C
			C	C	C			C					C	C		C	C			C	C		C	C					C							C	
	C	C	C			C		C					C		C	C	C	C			C	C	C	C		C	C	C	C					C	C	C
		C	Ø	C	C		C						C			Ø	C		X	C	C		C	C		C	C	C		C					C	C	
		C	C										C		C	C				C	C		C	C		C	C	C				C			
	C		C	C	C						C			C					C		C	C		C	C					C	
		X		C	C							C						C	C										Ø
			C	C	C			C			C	C		C	C			C	C		C		C					C	
	C	Ø	C	Ø				C			C				C	C	Ø		C	C	C	C		C	C	C	X			C	C
			C			C	C		X	C	C	X	C		X	X		C	X				C	C	C	C
	X	C	C	C	C	C		X	C				C			C			C	C		C	C	C	C			C
	C	C	C	C	C	C	C	C	C			C	C	C	C	C	X	C	C		C	C			C	C	C			C	C	C
			Ø		C								C		C	C			C	C		C	C	C
■		X		C								X	X									C	C	C	C
	■	C	C	C	C			C		C				C	C		C	C	C			C	C
	C	■	C	C	C	C		C			C	C	C	C			C	C		C	C			C	C	C	C
X	C	C	■	C	C	C		C	Ø		C		X	Ø		Ø		X		X	C	C		C	Ø	C	C	X	Ø		C	C	X
C	C	C	C	■	C	C	C	C				C	C	X	C	C	X	C	C		C	C	C		Ø	C	C	C	C		C	C	C	C
C	C	C	C	C	■	C	C			C	C	C	C	C	C	C	C	C	C	C	C			C			C	C	C	C		C	C	C	C
		Ø		C		■						C					C				C	C	C		X			C		Ø	C	C				C
			C	C			■					C	X		X	C				X	C	C	C		X	X		X	Ø

(continued)

Chemotherapy admixture compatibilities (continued)

KEY TO SYMBOLS
C - Compatible
X - Incompatible
Ø - Conflicting data; may be compatible or incompatible
Blank - No data available

	Dextrose 5% in water	Normal saline solution	aldesleukin	amifostine	amino acids solution	bleomycin sulfate	carboplatin	carmustine	ceftazidime	ciprofloxacin	cisplatin	cladribine	cyclophosphamide	cytarabine	dacarbazine	dactinomycin	daunorubicin hydrochloride	docetaxel	doxorubicin hydrochloride	doxorubicin hydrochloride liposome	etoposide	etoposide phosphate	fentanyl citrate
ifosfamide	C	C		C		C					C										C	C	C
leucovorin calcium	C	C		C	C						C	C	C						C	C	C	C	
levorphanol tartrate																							
mechlorethamine hydrochloride				C																			
melphalan					C	C	C	C			C		C	C	C	C			C		C		
meperidine hydrochloride	C	C		C				C			C							C		X		C	
mesna	C	C		C		X					X	C	C					C		C		C	
methotrexate sodium	C	C		C	C	Ø					C		C	Ø	C				C	C		C	
metoclopramide hydrochloride	Ø	C	C	C		C			C		Ø	C	C	C	C				C	C	X	C	C
metronidazole hydrochloride			C	X			C	C											C		C	C	C
mitomycin	Ø	Ø		C	Ø						Ø		C							Ø		X	
mitoxantrone hydrochloride				C									C							X		C	
morphine sulfate	C	C	C	C				C			C							C		X		C	
nafcillin sodium	Ø	C											X										C
ondansetron hydrochloride	C	C	C	C		C	C	C	C		C	C	C	C	C	C	C	C	C	C	C	C	C
paclitaxel	C	C			C	Ø			C		Ø	C	C	C	C				C	X	C	C	
palonosetron hydrochloride	C	C									C							C	C				
pentostatin	C	C																					
sargramostim					C	C	C	Ø			C		C	C	C				C		C		C
streptozocin	C	C		C																		C	
teniposide				C	C	C	C	C	C	C	C	C	C	C	C	C			C		C	C	
thiotepa	C	C		C		C	C	C	C	X		C	C	C	C				C		C	C	
topotecan hydrochloride	C	C				C					C		C						C		C		
total parenteral nutrition solutions							C		C	C	C		C	C					X				C
trimethobenzamide hydrochloride																							
vancomycin hydrochloride	C	C		C					Ø										C		C	C	C
vinblastine sulfate	C	C		C							C		C		C				C	C		C	
vincristine sulfate	C	C		C	C						C	C	C						C	C	C	C	
vinorelbine tartrate	C	C		C							C		C	C	C	C	Ø				C		

	filgrastim	floxuridine	fludarabine phosphate	fluorouracil	gemcitabine hydrochloride	granisetron hydrochloride	hydromorphone hydrochloride	idarubicin hydrochloride	ifosfamide	leucovorin calcium	levorphanol tartrate	mechlorethamine hydrochloride	melphalan	meperidine hydrochloride	mesna	methotrexate sodium	metoclopramide hydrochloride	metronidazole hydrochloride	mitomycin	mitoxantrone hydrochloride	morphine sulfate	nafcillin sodium	ondansetron hydrochloride	paclitaxel	palonosetron hydrochloride	pentostatin	sargramostim	streptozocin	teniposide	thiotepa	topotecan hydrochloride	total parenteral nutrition solutions	trimethobenzamide hydrochloride	vancomycin hydrochloride	vinblastine sulfate	vincristine sulfate	vinorelbine tartrate
ifosfamide			C	C	C				■				C		Ø								C	C	C		C		C	C	C	C					C
leucovorin calcium	C		Ø	C	C					■							C	C			C								C	C				C		C	C
levorphanol tartrate											■																								X		
mechlorethamine hydrochloride		C			C							■	C										C						C		C						C
melphalan	C		C		C	C	C	C		C			■		C	C	C	C	C	C	C	C					C		C	C				C	C	C	C
meperidine hydrochloride	C		C		C	C			X		C		C	■		Ø		C					C	C			C		C		C	C			C		C
mesna	C		C		C	C				Ø			C		■		C						C	C			C		C	C				C	C	C	
methotrexate sodium	C		X	X	C			X		C			C			■		Ø		C			C	C			C		C	C				C		C	C
metoclopramide hydrochloride	C		Ø	C	C		C		C				C	C		Ø	■		C		C		C	C			C		C	C	C	C		C		C	C
metronidazole hydrochloride	X				C	C	C						C	C				■			C						C		C		C	C	C				
mitomycin	X		Ø	X	C				C				C						■				C				X	Ø	C	C	X				C	C	X
mitoxantrone hydrochloride		C	C										C							■			C	C			C		C		C	C		C			Ø
morphine sulfate	C		X	C	C								C	X		C	C				■		C	C	C		C		X		C	C		Ø		C	
nafcillin sodium					Ø								X							Ø		■								C	Ø						
ondansetron hydrochloride	C	C		X	C		C		C				C	C	C	C		C	C	C			■		C		C	X	C	C	C	C	Ø		C	C	C
paclitaxel	C		C	C	C	C		C					C	C	C	C			C	C			C	■			C	C			C	C		C	C	C	
palonosetron hydrochloride			C	C						C															■		C										
pentostatin	C												C										C	C		■	C										
sargramostim	C		C		X	C	X	C		C			C	C	C	C		X	C	X		X					■		C		C			C		Ø	C
streptozocin			Ø	C									C					Ø			C							■	C	C	C						C
teniposide	C	C	C	C	C	C		X	C	C			C	C	C	C	C		C	C	C	C	C						■		C	C		C	C	C	C
thiotepa	C	C	C	C	C	C	C		C	C					C	C	C	C	C	C	C		C	C						■	C	C		C	C	C	C
topotecan hydrochloride		X	C	C					C						C						C				X						■			C			C
total parenteral nutrition solutions		Ø		C		Ø	C	C	C	X					C	C	C	C		C	Ø	C	Ø	C					C			■	C		C		
trimethobenzamide hydrochloride					C																												■				
vancomycin hydrochloride	C		C	C	X								C	C					C		Ø	C	C				Ø		C	C		Ø	C	■		C	C
vinblastine sulfate	C		C	C	C						C		C			C	C		C				C	C			C		C		C	C			■		C
vincristine sulfate	C		C	C	C				X		C		C			C	C		C				C	C			C		C		C	C	C			■	
vinorelbine tartrate	C			X	C	C	Ø	C			C	C	C							X	Ø								C	C	X				C		■

Chemotherapy Admixtures Chart © 2006 King Guide Publications, Inc. Adapted with permission.

Normal laboratory values and calculations

Use the values and equations below as a quick-reference to both routine laboratory tests and oncology-related monitoring parameters. (*Note:* Reference values may differ somewhat among laboratories.)

Standard blood tests

Chemistry
Glucose
70 to 100 mg/dl
BUN
8 to 20 mg/dl
Creatinine
Men: 0.8 to 1.2 mg/dl
Women: 0.6 to 1.1 mg/dl
Sodium
135 to 145 mEq/L
Potassium
3.5 to 5 mEq/L
Anion gap
8 to 16 mEq/L
Chloride
100 to 108 mEq/L
Carbon dioxide
22 to 34 mEq/L
Albumin
3.3 to 4.5 g/dl
Calcium
9 to 10.5 mg/dl
Magnesium
1.5 to 2.5 mEq/L
Phosphorus
2.5 to 4.5 mg/dl
Protein
6 to 8.5 g/dl
Uric acid
Men: 4 to 8.5 mg/dl
Women: 2.5 to 7.5 mg/dl

Coagulation studies
Partial thromboplastin time
20 to 36 seconds
Prothrombin time
10 to 14 seconds

International Normalized Ratio (INR)
2 to 3 in patients receiving warfarin
Fibrinogen
215 to 519 mg/dl

Hematology
White blood cell count
4,100 to 10,900/mm^3
Red blood cell count
Men: 4.5 to 6.2 million/mm^3
Women: 4.2 to 5.4 million/mm^3
Hemoglobin
Men: 14 to 18 g/dl
Women: 12 to 16 g/dl
Hematocrit
Men: 42% to 54%
Women: 38% to 46%
Platelet count
40,000 to 400,000/mm^3
Red blood cell indices
MCH: 26 to 32 pg
MCHC: 32 to 36 g/dl
MCV: 80 to 95 μm^3
White blood cell differential
Basophils: 0.3% to 2%
Eosinophils: 0.3% to 7%
Lymphocytes: 16.2% to 43%
Monocytes: 4% to 10%
Neutrophils: 47.6% to 76.8%

Iron studies
Serum iron
40 to 180 mcg/dl
Ferritin
Men: 18 to 270 ng/ml
Women: 18 to 160 ng/ml

Iron-binding capacity
200 to 450 mcg/dl
Transferrin
88 to 341 mg/dl
Transferrin saturation
12% to 57%

Lipids

Low-density lipoproteins
Optimal: < 100 mg/dl
Near optimal: 100 to 129 mg/dl
High-density lipoproteins
Desirable: ≥ 60 mg/dl
Total cholesterol
Desirable: < 200 mg/dl
Triglycerides
Desirable: < 200 mg/dl

Liver function studies

Alanine aminotransferase
Men: 10 to 35 units/L
Women: 9 to 24 units/L
Alkaline phosphatase
39 to 117 units/L

Aspartate aminotransferase
Men: 8 to 20 units/L
Women: 5 to 40 units/L
Serum bilirubin
Direct: ≤ 0.4 mg/dl
Indirect: ≤ 1.3 mg/dl
Total: ≤ 1.3 mg/dl

Pancreatic enzymes

Amylase
30 to 170 U/L
Lipase
7 to 60 U/L

Thyroid studies

Triiodothyronine (T_3)
60 to 181 mg/dl
Thyroxine (T_4)
4.5 to 12.5 mcg/dl
Thyroid-stimulating hormone
0.5 to 4.5 mIU/L
Parathyroid hormone, intact
Ages 2 to 20: 9 to 52 pg/ml
Older than age 20: 8 to 97 pg/ml

Calculating creatinine clearance

Normal creatinine clearance ranges from 72 to 156 ml/minute/1.73 m². The three equations below are commonly used to calculate creatinine clearance.

Calculation using timed urine collection

Creatinine clearance (ml/minute) = $\frac{\text{urine creatinine (mg/dl)}}{\text{serum creatinine (mg/dl)}} \times \frac{\text{urine volume (ml)}}{\text{time*}}$

(* Duration of urine collection: 1,440 minutes = 24 hours, 720 minutes = 12 hours, 480 minutes = 8 hours. Less than 20% variability with 8-, 12-, and 24-hour collection times.)

Estimating creatinine clearance using age, weight, and serum creatinine

Cockcroft-Gault method

Creatinine clearance$_{men}$ (ml/min) = $\frac{[(140-\text{age}) \times (\text{lean body weight in kg})]}{72 \times \text{serum creatinine (mg/dl)}}$

Creatinine clearance$_{women}$ (ml/min) = 0.85 × creatinine clearance$_{men}$

Jelliffe method

This method assumes the patient has normal muscle mass and is used when urine cannot be collected.

Creatinine clearance (ml/min) = 98−[0.8 × (age − 20)]/serum creatinine (mg/dl)

Calculating absolute neutrophil count

The absolute neutrophil count (ANC) is used to track a patient's response to chemotherapy and treatment for neutropenia. ANC should be above $1,500/mm^3$. Here is a commonly used equation for calculating ANC:

$$ANC = \frac{WBCs \times (polymorphonuclear\ cells + bands)}{100}$$

Example:
WBC = 3,000 cells/mm^3
Polymorphonuclear cells = 60%
Bands = 3%,

$$ANC = \frac{3,000 \times (60 + 3)}{100} = 3,000 \times 63 = 1,890\ cells/mm^3$$

Degrees of neutropenia
Mild: 1,000 to 1,500/mm^3
Moderate: 500 to 1,000/mm^3
Severe: < 500/mm^3

Performance scales

Performance scales aid in monitoring a patient's quality of life. Although such scales do not provide a comprehensive picture of the patient's response to treatment, they are useful adjuncts for selecting a course of therapy and evaluating patient response.

Karnofsky performance index

The Karnofsky performance index is used to measure the patient's ability to perform activities of daily living and evaluate progress after a therapeutic intervention.

Score	Description
100	Normal; no complaints, no signs or symptoms of disease
90	Able to carry on normal activity; minor signs or symptoms of disease
80	Normal activity with effort; some signs or symptoms of disease
70	Cares for self; unable to perform normal activity or active work
60	Requires occasional assistance; able to care for most of his or her needs
50	Requires considerable assistance and frequent medical care
40	Disabled; dependent; requires special care and assistance
30	Severely disabled; hospitalization indicated (although death not imminent)
20	Very sick; hospitalization and active supportive treatment needed (although death not imminent)
10	Moribund; fatal processes progressing quickly
0	Expired

ECOG performance status scale

Daily functional performance commonly varies among patients. Patients may have "good" days and "bad" days that do not reflect their general performance ability. The Eastern Cooperative Oncology Group (ECOG) scale (also called the WHO or Zubrod scale) is used to measure the patient's general performance ability—not a particular day's activity.

Grade	Description
0	Fully active; able to perform all predisease activities without restriction
1	Restricted in physically strenuous activity but ambulatory and able to perform light or sedentary work (such as light housework or office work)
2	Ambulatory and capable of all self-care but unable to perform any work activities. Up and about more than 50% of waking hours
3	Capable of only limited self-care; confined to bed or chair more than 50% of waking hours
4	Completely disabled; cannot perform self-care; totally confined to bed or chair
5	Expired

Sources: Karnofsky DA, Abelmann, WH, Craver LF, et al. The use of the nitrogen mustards in the palliative treatment of carcinoma with particular reference to bronchogenic carcinoma. *Cancer.* 1948;1:634-656. Scale available online at http://en.wikipedia.org/wiki/Zubrod_scale#ECOG.2FWHO.2FZubrod_score

Oken MM, Creech RH, Tormey DC, et al. Toxicity and response criteria of the Eastern Cooperative Oncology Group. *Am J Clin Oncol.* 1982;5:649-655. Scale available online at http://www.ecog.org/general/perf_stat.html

Supportive therapy for cancer patients

This appendix presents guidelines for identifying and managing adverse reactions to chemotherapy or to the disease process, including nausea and vomiting, anemia, neutropenia, diarrhea, and mucositis.

Managing chemotherapy-induced nausea and vomiting

Despite advances in pharmacotherapeutics, chemotherapy-induced nausea and vomiting (CINV) can be difficult to treat and control once it has become established. Therefore, the goal of therapy is to prevent CINV.

Types of CINV

CINV may be acute-onset, delayed-onset, breakthrough, or anticipatory.
• *Acute-onset* CINV occurs within the first 24 hours of chemotherapy administration. It is best managed by assessing the emetic potential of the patient's regimen and ordering appropriate antiemetic agents.
• *Delayed-onset* CINV occurs more than 24 hours after the first chemotherapy administration and may last up to 120 hours. It warrants treatment with an antiemetic from a class other than the one the patient is currently receiving.
• *Breakthrough* CINV occurs during a chemotherapy cycle when the prescribed antiemetic regimen is ineffective. Although as-needed medications can be used to manage breakthrough CINV, the best prevention is an effective initial CINV regimen.
• *Anticipatory* CINV occurs before the start of a new chemotherapy cycle. It has a strong psychological component and a poor response to antiemetic therapy. The most effective approach is to prevent nausea and vomiting during the initial chemotherapy cycle.

Risk factors

Certain patient-specific factors increase the likelihood that CINV will occur. Such factors include:
• female gender
• age younger than 50
• dehydration
• history of motion sickness
• history of morning sickness with past pregnancies
• nausea and vomiting with previous chemotherapy or radiation therapy.
    On the other hand, a history of alcohol abuse decreases the risk of CINV.

Chemotherapy-specific risk levels

Chemotherapeutic agents fall into five levels of emetogenic potential—from level 1 agents, which have the least emetogenic potential, to level 5 agents, which have the greatest potential. The risk level of a patient's chemotherapy regimen guides CINV management. (See chart at right.) *Note:* Emesis frequency refers to the percentage of patients who experience emesis in the absence of effective antiemetic prophylaxis.

Risk level	Chemotherapy agent
Level 5: High emetic risk Emesis frequency: More than 90%	altretamine carmustine > 250 mg/m^2 cisplatin $\geq$ 50 mg/m^2 cyclophosphamide > 1,500 mg/m^2 dacarbazine doxorubicin or epirubicin with cyclophosphamide lomustine > 60 mg/m^2 mechorethamine streptozocin
Level 4: Moderate emetic risk Emesis frequency: 60% to 90%	amifostine > 500 mg/m^2 busulfan > 4 mg daily carboplatin carmustine $\leq$ 250 mg/m^2 cisplatin < 50 mg/m^2 cyclophosphamide > 750 mg/m^2 to $\leq$ 1,500 mg/m^2 cytarabine (except in low doses) dactinomycin doxorubicin $\geq$ 60 mg/m^2 epirubicin > 90 mg/m^2 melphalan > 50 mg/m^2 methotrexate > 1,000 mg/m^2 procarbazine (oral)
Level 3: Moderate emetic risk Emesis frequency: 30% to 60%	aldesleukin amifostine > 300 to $\leq$ 500 mg/m^2 arsenic trioxide cyclophosphamide $\leq$ 750 mg/m^2 cyclophosphamide (oral) daunorubicin doxorubicin 20 to < 60 mg/m^2 doxorubicin liposomal epirubicin $\leq$ 90 mg/m^2 hexamethylmelamine (oral) idarubicin ifosfamide interleukin-2 > 12 to 15 million units/m^2 irinotecan lomustine < 60 mg/m^2 methotrexate 250 to 1,000 mg/m^2 mitoxantrone < 15 mg/m^2 oxaliplatin > 75 mg/m^2
Level 2: Low emetic risk Emesis frequency: 10% to 30%	amifostine $\leq$ 300 mg asparaginase bexarotene bortezomib cytarabine 100 to 200 mg/m^2 capecitabine docetaxel doxorubicin < 20 mg/m^2

(continued)

Risk level	Chemotherapy agent
Level 2: Low emetic risk *(continued)* Emesis frequency: 10% to 30%	etoposide fludarabine fluorouracil gemcitabine mercaptopurine methotrexate > 50 to < 250 mg/m^2 mitomycin paclitaxel pemetrexed temozolomide teniposide thiotepa trimetrexate topotecan
Level 1: Minimal emetic risk Emesis frequency: Less than 10%	alemtuzumab asparaginase azacitidine bevacizumab bleomycin bortezomib busulfan cetuximab chlorambucil (oral) cladribine denileukin diftitox dexrazoxane erlotinib estramustine fludarabine gefitinib gemtuzumab ozogamicin hormones hydroxyurea imatinib mesylate interferon alfa melphalan (oral low dose) methotrexate ≤ 50 mg/m^2 mitotane pegaspargase pentostatin rituximab thioguanine (oral) tositumomab trastuzumab uracil valrubicin vinblastine vincristine vinorelbine

Treatment

For patients receiving combination chemotherapy, determine the emetogenic potential by identifying the most emetogenic agent in the combination and then assessing the relative potential of the other agents. The following rules apply:

- Level 1 drugs do not contribute to the emetogenic potential of a combination.
- A drug from level 2, 3, or 4 increases emetogenic potential by one level greater than the most emetogenic drug in the combination.

General principles of antiemetic therapy

- Determine the emetogenic risk level for each day of chemotherapy.
- Choose the appropriate antiemetic regimen based on the drug's emetogenic risk level and any patient risk factors. Protect patients throughout the full risk period (usually 4 days for most highly or moderately emetogenic chemotherapy regimens).
- To prevent acute- or delayed-onset emesis, use the most active antiemetic regimen appropriate for the chemotherapy the patient is receiving. Order the antiemetic regimen before the initial chemotherapy cycle begins.
- Do not use dexamethasone if the patient's chemotherapy regimen includes a corticosteroid.
- Use aprepitant for multiday chemotherapy regimens that have high emetogenic potential and are associated with a significant risk of delayed-onset nausea and vomiting (such as those containing cisplatin). Also consider prescribing aprepitant for patients receiving carboplatin, cyclophosphamide, doxorubicin, epirubicin, ifosfamide, irinotecan, or methotrexate.
- Prescribe delayed-onset antiemetic regimens for all patients receiving actinomycin D, carmustine, carboplatin, cisplatin, cyclophosphamide, cytarabine, dacarbazine, daunorubicin, doxorubicin, epirubicin, hexamethylmelamine, idarubicin, ifosfamide, lomustine, mechlorethamine, or streptozocin.
- Prescribe antiemetics for breakthrough nausea and vomiting as needed. Use an additional drug from a different antiemetic class for breakthrough nausea and vomiting.
- Prescribe antiemetics for anticipatory nausea and vomiting as needed.
  (For specific drug therapies for each type and level of CINV, see the front endpaper.)

References

Gralla RJ, Osoba D, Kris MG, et al. Recommendations for the use of antiemetics: Evidence-based, clinical practice guidelines. *J Clin Oncol.* 1999;17:2971-2994.

Grunberg SM. Chemotherapy-induced nausea and vomiting: Prevention, detection, and treatment—how are we doing? J Support Oncol. 2004; 2(suppl 1):1-12.

Hesketh PJ, Kris MG, Grunberg SM, et al. Proposal for classifying the acute emetogenicity of cancer chemotherapy. *J Clin Oncol.* 1997;15:116-123.

NCCN Practice Guidelines in Oncology: Antiemesis (v.1.2005). Available online at http://www.nccn.org/professionals/physician_gls/PDF/antiemesis.pdf. Accessed January 12, 2006.

Polovich M, White JM, Kelleher LO, eds. *Chemotherapy and Biotherapy Guidelines and Recommendations for Practice.* 2nd ed. Pittsburgh, Pa: Oncology Nursing Society; 2005:20-44, 111-112.

Managing anemia

Anemia occurs in nearly half of cancer patients even before treatment begins. Once chemotherapy starts, anemia is a near certainty. Anemia and the associated fatigue are more than a quality-of-life issue; they can significantly affect patient outcome as well.

Risk factors
The following factors increase a cancer patient's risk of developing symptomatic anemia:
• blood transfusion within the past 6 months
• previous myelosuppressive therapy
• radiotherapy to more than 20% of the skeleton
• potential for myelosuppression related to current cancer therapy (including duration, schedule, and agents)
• low hemoglobin
• advanced age.

Determining severity
Anemia severity commonly is graded according to the patient's hemoglobin value. In the scales below, developed by the National Cancer Institute (NCI) and World Health Organization (WHO), the hemoglobin value varies slightly.

Grade	Severity	Hemoglobin (g/dl) NCI scale	WHO scale
0	None	Normal	> 11
1	Mild	10	9.5 to 10
2	Moderate	8 to 10	8 to 9.4
3	Severe	6.5 to 7.9	6.5 to 7.9
4	Life-threatening	< 6.5	< 6.5

Treatment
The guidelines below focus on cancer- or treatment-related anemia. Also consider other possible causes of anemia (such as bleeding, hemolysis, nutritional deficiency, hereditary factors, and renal dysfunction), and treat accordingly.

Optimally, hemoglobin should be maintained at 12 g/dl or higher. If it falls below 11 g/dl and immediate correction is needed, transfuse blood products as indicated, based on facility guidelines. If immediate correction is not required, conduct a complete symptom assessment using fatigue and anemia scales, activity level, and performance status. Evaluate risk factors for developing symptomatic anemia (as described above), and intervene appropriately. If the patient is asymptomatic and lacks risk factors, observe the patient and reevaluate periodically.

If the patient is asymptomatic but has risk factors for anemia:
• Observe the patient, and consider erythropoietic therapy.
• If erythropoietic therapy is being considered, obtain iron studies and prescribe iron supplements as indicated. Typically, such supplements are indicated by a ferritin level below 100 mcg/ml or transferrin saturation below 20%. Titrate dosages to maintain an optimal hemoglobin value (12 g/dl).
• Reevaluate symptoms and hemoglobin at each follow-up visit.
• If hemoglobin is 12 g/dl, or more than 2 g/dl lower than the initial level, and symptoms have not improved, consider erythropoietic therapy. If hemoglobin is 12 g/dl, or more than 2 g/dl lower than the initial level, and symptoms have improved, titrate the dosage of the erythropoietic agent or iron preparation to maintain a hemoglobin level of at least 12 g/dl.

If the patient is symptomatic:
• Transfuse appropriate blood products. If hemoglobin is 10 to 11 g/dl, consider erythropoietic therapy; if hemoglobin is below 10 g/dl, strongly consider erythropoietic therapy.
• Obtain iron studies and administer iron supplements as indicated (for ferritin level below 100 mcg/ml or transferrin saturation below 20%). Titrate dosage to maintain optimal hemoglobin (12 g/dl).
• Reevaluate symptoms and hemoglobin at each follow-up visit.
• If hemoglobin is 12 g/dl, or more than 2 g/dl lower than the initial level, and symptoms have improved, titrate the dosage of the erythropoietic agent or iron preparation to maintain a hemoglobin level of at least 12 g/dl.

Erythropoietic therapy
When indicated, prescribe epoetin alfa or darbepoetin alfa to treat anemia. Commonly used regimens include the following:
• Epoetin alfa: 150 units/kg subcutaneously three times weekly. If unsatisfactory response, may increase to 300 units/kg. Or 40,000 units subcutaneously weekly; if unsatisfactory response, may increase to 60,000 units.
• Darbepoetin alfa: 3 mcg/kg subcutaneously every 2 weeks; If unsatisfactory response, may increase to 5 mcg/kg. Or 200 mcg subcutaneously every 2 weeks; if unsatisfactory response, may increase up to 300 mcg.
    If hemoglobin increases by more than 1 g/dl in a 2-week period, reduce the dosage by 25%. If hemoglobin exceeds 12 g/dl, withhold therapy; reinitiate therapy if hemoglobin falls below 12 g/dl at 25% reduction from previous dosage.
    If unsatisfactory response occurs after 4 weeks for epoetin alfa or after 6 weeks for darbepoetin alfa, increase the dosage and add oral or I.V. iron therapy. If the patient responds (as shown by a hemoglobin increase of 1 g/dl at 8 to 12 weeks), titrate the dosage to maintain a hemoglobin level of at least 12 g/dl. If hemoglobin fails to respond, discontinue erythropoietic therapy and administer transfusions as indicated.

Parenteral iron administration
Consider prescribing parenteral iron for patients with iron deficiency who cannot tolerate or do not respond to oral iron therapy and in those with functional iron deficiency. To minimize adverse effects, give diphenhydramine and acetaminophen before iron administration. The table on page 476 shows test doses, dosages, and administration routes for various iron preparations.

Iron preparation	Test dose	Dosage	Administration route
Iron dextran	Required: 25 mg I.M. or by slow I.V. push	100 mg over 5 minutes. Larger doses can be given over several hours.	I.M. (INFeD), I.V. infusion
Ferric gluconate	At physician's discretion: 25 mg slow I.V. push or infusion	125 mg over 10 minutes. Repeated dosing given one to three times weekly.	I.V. injection or infusion
Iron sucrose	At physician's discretion: 25 mg slow I.V. push	100 mg one to three times weekly	I.V. injection or infusion

References

Auerbach M, Ballard H, Trout JR, et al. Intravenous iron optimizes the response to recombinant human erythropoietin in cancer patients with chemotherapy-related anemia: A multicenter, open-label, randomized trial. *J Clin Oncol.* 2004;22:1301-1307.

Earlier initiation of treatment recommended in using erythropoietic agents in chemotherapy-induced anemia. *J Support Oncol.* 2004;2(4):319.

Groopman JL, Itri LM. Chemotherapy-induced anemia in adults: Incidence and treatment. *J Natl Cancer Inst.* 1999;91:1616-1634.

NCCN Practice Guidelines in Oncology. National Comprehensive Cancer Network Practice. 2005;April 21:1-27.

Waltzman RJ, Capo G. Cancer-related anemia, fatigue, and quality of life. *Oncology Special Edition.* 2005;8:51-55.

Managing febrile neutropenia

Neutropenia increases a cancer patient's mortality risk, lengthens hospitalization, and increases medical costs. In many cases, fever is the first—and sometimes only—sign of neutropenia. The following guidelines on neutropenia evaluation and management are based on recommendations from the National Comprehensive Cancer Network and the Infectious Diseases Society of America.

Morbidity risk factors

Treatment decisions must take into account whether the patient is at high or low risk for neutropenia-associated morbidity.

Identifying high-risk neutropenia patients

In patients with neutropenia, the presence of any of the following factors indicates a high risk of morbidity:

- hospitalized at fever onset
- leukemia without remission
- nonleukemic cancer disease progression after more than two chemotherapy courses
- significant comorbidity or clinical instability
- absolute neutrophil count (ANC) below 100 cells/mm^3
- anticipated neutropenia duration longer than 7 days
- serum creatinine level above 2 mg/dl, liver function values more than three times normal
- complex infection, such as pneumonia, at clinical presentation.

High-risk patients should be hospitalized and treated with I.V. antibiotics.

Identifying low-risk neutropenia patients

Low-risk patients have none of the high-risk factors listed above, but do have most of the following:

- outpatient status at fever onset
- lack of neurologic changes, appearance of illness, abdominal pain, infection, or comorbidity (such as shock, hypoxia, vomiting, diarrhea, or pneumonia)
- anticipated neutropenia resolution in less than 10 days
- good performance status.

Low-risk patients can be treated in the hospital, an ambulatory care clinic, or at home if appropriate support is available.

Clinical evaluation

Patients should be further evaluated if they have:

- a single oral temperature of 101° F (38.3° C) or higher, or an oral temperature of 100.4° F (38° C) or higher for 1 hour or longer
- a neutrophil level below 500/mm^3 (or a predicted decrease to that level over the next 48 hours).

Many patients lack signs and symptoms of infection (such as pus, induration, and chest infiltrates); pain at the infection site may be the only clue that an infection is present. Initial evaluation should include a history, physical examination, and diagnostic tests, with the goal of identifying the infection site and causative organism. Infection sites commonly include the GI tract, lungs, eyes, skin (such as bone marrow aspiration sites and vascular catheter access sites), perineum, and anus. (*Note:* An internal rectal examination is contraindicated.)

History

Significant history factors may include history of infections, HIV status, recent travel, pets, tuberculosis exposure, recent antibiotic therapy, major illness, household members with similar symptoms, medications, and time since last chemotherapy administration.

Laboratory and radiologic findings

Obtain CBC with differential and platelet count; BUN, electrolyte, and creatinine levels; and liver function tests. If indicated, also order urinalysis, pulse oximetry, chest X-ray (if the patient has respiratory signs or symptoms), and site-specific imaging studies.

Cultures

Obtain two sets of blood cultures (aerobic and anaerobic; two tubes per set), with at least 10 ml blood per tube. One sample may be obtained from a central line and the other from a peripheral line, or two peripheral samples may be used.

Obtain a urine culture if the patient has symptoms, if urinalysis is abnormal, or if a urinary catheter is present. Site-specific cultures may be warranted, including skin (aspirate or biopsy of skin lesions or wounds) and vascular-access cutaneous sites (if inflamed). Cultures for diarrhea (*Clostridium difficile* assay, enteric pathogen screening) also may be needed.

If indicated, also obtain viral cultures of mucosal or cutaneous vesicular or ulcerated lesions. Obtain throat or nasopharynx cultures if symptoms are present or during seasonal outbreaks of respiratory viral infections.

Treatment

Choose therapy based on risk assessment findings, the patient's condition, clinical evaluation, infection site, and previous antibiotic therapy. Optimally, treatment should start within the first few hours of clinical presentation of signs and symptoms, with follow-up as needed.

Initial therapy

Initial therapy for neutropenia may involve oral combination therapy, I.V. monotherapy, or I.V. dual therapy. Vancomycin therapy is usually avoided due to the emergence of vancomyin-resistant organisms.

Oral combination therapy is used for low-risk adults only. Typically, it involves ciprofloxacin and amoxicillin/clavulanate. In patients with penicillin allergy, substitute clindamycin for amoxicillin/clavulanate.

For *I.V. monotherapy,* choose one of the following:
• carbapenem
• cefepime (check susceptibility for local antibiogram)
• ceftazidime (provides weak gram-positive coverage, is associated with increased breakthrough infections)
• imipenem and cilastatin
• meropenem
• piperacillin and tazobactam (may interfere with galactomannan measurement).

For *I.V. dual therapy,* choose one of these regimens:
• an aminoglycoside and an antipseudomonal penicillin or extended-spectrum cephalosporin (such as cefepime or ceftazidime), with or without a beta-lactamase inhibitor; or an aminoglycoside with an extended-spectrum cephalosporin (such as cefepime or ceftazidime)
• ciprofloxacin and an antipseudomonal penicillin.

Follow-up evaluation and care

Follow-up for neutropenic patients includes a clinical evaluation, review of culture results, and evaluation for drug toxicity. Evaluate the patient's overall response to therapy in 3 to 5 days, and take appropriate actions as indicated.

- Decreasing fever, signs and symptoms of stable or improving infection, and hemodynamic stability indicate the patient is responding to therapy.
- Persistent or intermittent fever, no improvement in infection signs and symptoms, hemodynamic instability, and persistent positive blood cultures indicate the patient is not responding to therapy.

For patients who are responding to therapy, consider the following:

- If an etiologic agent has been identified, adjust therapy as indicated and continue.
- If no etiologic agent has been identified:
  — Discontinue therapy if ANC is 500 cells/mm^3 or higher.
  — If ANC is less than 500 cells/mm^3, continue current regimen if the patient is low risk and has been receiving oral antibiotics. In low-risk patients receiving I.V. antibiotics, switch to oral therapy.

For patients who are not responding to therapy, consider the following:

- If fever continues for 4 days or more after antibiotic therapy begins, consider prescribing an antifungal agent with activity against molds.
- If an etiologic agent has been identified, assess antibiotic appropriateness (susceptibility testing and dosing), and make adjustments as needed. If the patient's condition is expected to worsen, consider administering colony-stimulating factors. Base duration of therapy on ANC, infection site, infecting pathogen, and the patient's underlying illness.
- If no etiologic agent has been identified and the patient is unstable, broaden antibiotic coverage to include anaerobes, resistant gram-negative rods, and resistant gram-positive organisms. Also consider adding colony-stimulating factors. Evaluate for toxoplasmosis as indicated, and consider consulting an infectious disease specialist.

References

Berger A. Selected reviews on the treatment of anemia, neutropenia, and symptom clusters. *J Support Oncol*. 2005;3(6):3-37.

Feld R, Pasemans M, Freifeld AG. Methodology for clinical trials involving patients with cancer who have febrile neutropenia: Updated guidelines of the Immunocompromised Host Society/Multinational Association for Supportive Care in Cancer, with emphasis on outpatient studies. *Clin Infect Dis*. 2002;35:1463-1468.

Hughes WT, Armstrong D, Bodey GP, et al. 2002 guidelines for the use of antimicrobial agents in neutropenic patients with cancer. *Clin Infect Dis*. 2002;34:730-751.

Polovich M, White JM, Kelleher LO, eds. *Chemotherapy and Biotherapy Guidelines and Recommendations for Practice*. 2nd ed. Pittsburgh, Pa: Oncology Nursing Society;2005.

NCCN Practice Guidelines in Oncology. Fever and neutropenia: Treatment guidelines for patients with cancer. v.1.2005 May. 19-31.

NCCN Practice Guidelines in Oncology. National Comprehensive Cancer Network Practice. 2005;April 21:1-27.

Wolff D, Culakova E, Poniewierski S, et al. Predictors of chemotherapy-induced neutropenia and its complications: Results from a prospective nationwide registry. *J Support Oncol*. 2005;3(suppl 4):24-25.

Managing diarrhea

Diarrhea can decrease the patient's quality of life and seriously jeopardize outcome. Based on severity of symptoms, NCI grades diarrhea on a scale from 1 (mild) to 4 (severe or life-threatening).

Assessment

Various factors can contribute to diarrhea in patients receiving chemotherapy:
- dietary habits, such as a high-fiber diet and consumption of milk and dairy products, caffeine, spicy or fatty foods, alcohol, and high-osmolar dietary supplements
- laxative abuse
- endocrine conditions, such as hyperthyroidism and neuroendocrine tumors
- infection, such as *Clostridium difficile, Campylobacter, Escherichia coli, Shigella, Salmonella,* and parasitic infections
- inflammatory conditions, such as Crohn's disease, diverticulitis, irritable bowel syndrome, radiation proctitis, and ulcerative colitis
- malabsorption, such as bowel-wall edema, motility disturbances, partial bowel obstruction, short bowel, and sprue.

Treatment guide

Treatment of diarrhea takes a stepped approach and varies according to NCI grade. For patients with grade 2 diarrhea, withhold cytotoxic chemotherapy until symptoms abate, and consider reducing the dosage of chemotherapy.

Step 1: Immediate management

Immediate management focuses on patient education. Provide the following instructions:
- Stop all lactose-containing products and high-osmolar dietary supplements.
- Drink 8 to 10 glasses of clear liquids (such as Gatorade, broth, or gelatin) daily.
- Eat frequent small meals containing such foods as bananas, rice, peeled apples, toast, and plain pasta.
- Eat foods that are low in residue, roughage, and fat.
- Eat green bananas, which contain an amylase-resistant starch that is digested in the colon and stimulates water and salt absorption.
- Avoid alcohol and caffeine-containing products.
- Drink ginger tea, which has a high pectin level, or eat high-pectin foods (such as bananas, avocados, and asparagus tips).
- Report the number of stools and life-threatening symptoms (such as fever, dizziness, and excessive abdominal cramping).

Step 2: Initial treatment

- Administer loperamide 4 mg P.O. initially, then 2 mg every 4 hours or after every unformed stool. Do not exceed 16 mg daily.
- Discontinue loperamide when the patient has been diarrhea-free for 12 hours.

Step 3: Continued treatment (NCI grade 1 or 2)

- Administer loperamide 2 mg P.O. every 2 hours until the patient has been diarrhea-free for 12 hours. Patients may take 4 mg every 4 hours during the night. (*Note:* This dosage exceeds the manufacturer's recommendation.)

- Administer oral antibiotics.
- If the patient progresses to NCI grade 3 or 4, proceed to step 5.

Step 4: Treatment of persistent diarrhea (NCI grade 1 or 2)

- Evaluate stool specimens, CBC, and electrolytes.
- Examine the abdomen for abnormalities.
- Replace electrolytes as needed.
- Discontinue loperamide and start second-line treatment—octreotide 100 to 150 mcg subcutaneously three times daily, up to 500 mcg three times daily; or tincture of opium 0.6 ml P.O. four times daily.

Step 5: Treatment of severe diarrhea (NCI grade 3 or 4)

- Admit the patient to the hospital.
- Administer octreotide 100 to 150 mcg subcutaneously three times daily. As needed, titrate up to 500 mcg three times daily based on response, or administer 25 to 50 mcg/hour by continuous I.V. infusion.
- Administer I.V. fluids and antibiotics as needed.
- Discontinue cytotoxic chemotherapy until symptoms resolve; then restart at reduced dosage.

References

Benson AB III, Ajani JA, Catalano RB, et al. Recommended guidelines for the treatment of cancer treatment-induced diarrhea. *J Clin Oncol.* 2004;22:2918-2926.

Polovich M, White JM, Kelleher LO, eds. *Chemotherapy and Biotherapy Guidelines and Recommendations for Practice.* 2nd ed. Pittsburgh, Pa: Oncology Nursing Society; 2005:20-44, 118-123.

Viele C, Stern JM, Ippoliti C, et al. Symptom management of chemotherapy-induced diarrhea: A multidisciplinary approach. 27th Annual Congress of Oncology Nursing Society; 2002. Medical Association Communications. Available online at: http://www.cmecorner.com/macmcm/ons/ons2002_05.htm. Accessed January 20, 2006.

Wadler S. Treatment guidelines for chemotherapy-induced diarrhea. *Oncology Special Edition.* 2005;8:105-110.

Managing mucositis

Mucositis occurs in approximately 40% of cancer patients and may involve the oral cavitiy, GI tract, and other mucosal areas. It is a major concern because it can lead to life-threatening conditions, such as sepsis, infection, and malnutrition.

Assessment

Various scales have been developed to grade mucositis. The World Health Organization has developed the scale below.
0 = No symptoms
1 = Soreness with or without erythema; no ulceration
2 = Erythema and ulceration; patient can swallow solid food
3 = Ulcers and extensive erythema; patient cannot swallow solid food
4 = Severe mucositis precluding alimentation.

Treatment guide for oral mucositis

Examine the patient's oral mucosa daily, and teach the patient how to perform this examination at home. Additional recommendations include the following:
• Advise the patient to use bland mouth rinses, such as normal saline solution and sodium bicarbonate.
• If sores crust over, instruct the patient to rinse with equal parts hydrogen peroxide and water or salt water (1 tsp salt in 4 cups water) for no more than 2 days. (A longer period impedes healing).
• Instruct the patient to use a soft, nylon-bristled toothbrush and to avoid dental floss and water-pressure gum cleaners.
• As indicated, prescribe mucosal-coating agents (such as antacid solutions, kaolin solutions, and Amphojel), water-soluble lubricating agents (including artificial saliva for xerostomia), or topical anesthetics (such as 2% viscous lidocaine or benzocaine spray or gel). Instruct the patient to rinse or irrigate the mouth before using these agents, to remove particles and debris.
• Culture mucosal lesions. Candidal lesions appear as whitish plaque.
• Use cryotherapy to cool the oral cavity and help prevent oral mucositis. Cooling causes vasoconstriction, which seems to limit absorption of mucotoxic agents by the oral mucosa.
• For oral bleeding, instruct the patient to rinse the mouth with a mixture of one part 3% hydrogen peroxide to two or three parts saltwater solution (1 tsp salt in 4 cups water) to help clean the wound. Stress the importance of rinsing carefully so as not to disturb clots.
• Instruct the patient to avoid irritating agents, such as commercial mouthwashes containing phenol, astringents, or alcohol, as well as lemon-glycerin swabs and solutions. Also discourage tobacco use and alcohol consumption.

Treatment guide for upper GI mucositis

• In patients who have been receiving the CMF chemotherapy regimen (cyclophosphamide, methotrexate, and 5-fluorouracil) or 5-fluorouracil, prescribe ranitidine or omeprazole to prevent epigastric pain.
• In patients with non-small-cell lung cancer, prescribe amifostine to reduce esophagitis induced by chemotherapy or radiotherapy. Amifostine also has some benefit in preventing mild mucositis in patients receiving radiotherapy for head and neck cancer.

References

Ignatavicius DD. *Clinical Companion for Medical-Surgical Nursing.* 5th ed. St Louis: Elsevier; 2006.

Keefe D, Sonis S. Mucositis following cancer treatment. *Oncology Special Edition.* 2005;8:117-120.

National Cancer Institute. Oral complications of chemotherapy and head/neck radiation (PDQ). Oral mucositis. Available online at http://www.cancer.gov/cancertopics/pdq/supportivecare/oralcomplications/HealthProfessional/page5. Modified November 18, 2005. Accessed January 6, 2006.

Polovich M, White JM, Kelleher LO, eds. *Chemotherapy and Biotherapy Guidelines and Recommendations for Practice.* 2nd ed. Pittsburgh, Pa: Oncology Nursing Society;2005:118-123.

Prevention and treatment of oral mucositis in cancer patients. The Joanna Briggs Institute for Evidence-Based Practice and Midwifery. *South Australia.* 1998;2(2). Available online at http://www.oralcancerfoundation.org/dental/pdf/mucositis.pdf. Accessed January 6, 2006.

Oncology drug codes

This appendix lists Healthcare Common Procedures Coding System (HCPCS) codes for selected antineoplastic agents, drug and fluid administration solutions, and miscellaneous drug administration items. Trade names appear in all capital letters. Although every reasonable effort has been made to ensure coding accuracy, the ultimate responsibility for coding lies with the service provider. For a complete list of HCPCS codes, visit www.oncologydrugguide.com.

Drug name	Quantity	J code	Drug name	Quantity	J code
Adriamycin	10 mg	J9000	Carmustine	100 mg	J9050
ADRUCIL	500 mg	J9190	CERUBIDINE	10 mg	J9150
Aldesleukin	single dose	J9015	Cetuximab	10 mg	J9055
Alemtuzumab	10 mg	J9010	Cisplatin	10 mg	J9060
ALFERON N	250,000 IU	J9215	Cisplatin	50 mg	J9062
ALIMTA	10 mg	J9305	Cladribine	1 mg	J9065
ALKERAN	50 mg	J9245	COSMEGEN	0.5 mg	J9120
ALKERAN, oral	2 mg	J8600	Cyclophosphamide, lyophilized	100 mg	J9093
Arsenic trioxide	1 mg	J9017	Cyclophosphamide, lyophilized	200 mg	J9094
Asparaginase	10,000 U	J9020	Cyclophosphamide, lyophilized	500 mg	J9095
AVASTIN	10 mg	J9035	Cyclophosphamide, lyophilized	1 g	J9096
BCG, intravesical	single dose	J9031	Cyclophosphamide, lyophilized	2 g	J9097
Bevacizumab	10 mg	J9035	Cyclophosphamide, oral	25 mg	J8530
BiCNU	100 mg	J9050	Cyclophosphamide, parenteral	100 mg	J9070
BLENOXANE	15 U	J9040	Cyclophosphamide, parenteral	200 mg	J9080
Bleomycin sulfate	15 U	J9040	Cyclophosphamide, parenteral	500 mg	J9090
Bortezomib	0.1 mg	J9041	Cyclophosphamide, parenteral	1 g	J9091
Busulfan, oral	2 mg	J8510			
CAMPATH	10 mg	J9010			
CAMPTOSAR	20 mg	J9206			
Capecitabine	500 mg	J8521			
Capecitabine	150 mg	J8520			
Carboplatin	50 mg	J9045			

Drug name	Quantity	J code
Cyclophosphamide, parenteral	2 g	J9092
Cytarabine	100 mg	J9100
Cytarabine	500 mg	J9110
Cytarabine, liposomal	10 mg	J9098
CYTOSAR-U	100 mg	J9100
CYTOSAR-U	500 mg	J9110
CYTOXAN, lyophilized	100 mg	J9093
CYTOXAN, lyophilized	200 mg	J9094
CYTOXAN, lyophilized	500 mg	J9095
CYTOXAN, lyophilized	1 g	J9096
CYTOXAN, lyophilized	2 g	J9097
CYTOXAN, oral	25 mg	J8530
Dacarbazine	100 mg	J9130
Dacarbazine	200 mg	J9140
Dactinomycin	0.5 mg	J9120
Daunorubicin	10 mg	J9150
Daunorubicin citrate, liposomal	10 mg	J9151
DAUNOXOME	10 mg	J9151
Denileukin diftitox	300 µg	J9160
DEPOCYT	10 mg	J9098
Docetaxel	20 mg	J9170
DOXIL	10 mg	J9001
Doxorubicin HCl	10 mg	J9000
Doxorubicin HCl, liposomal	10 mg	J9001
DTIC-DOME	100 mg	J9130
DTIC-DOME	200 mg	J9140
ELLENCE	2 mg	J9178
ELLENCE	50 mg	J9180
ELOXATIN	0.5 mg	J9263
ELSPAR	10,000 U	J9020

Drug name	Quantity	J code
Epirubicin HCl	2 mg	J9178
Epirubicin HCl	50 mg	J9180
ERBITUX	10 mg	J9055
Etoposide	10 mg	J9181
Etoposide	100 mg	J9182
Etoposide, oral	50 mg	J8560
FASLODEX	25 mg	J9395
Floxuridine	500 mg	J9200
FLUDARA	50 mg	J9185
Fludarabine phosphate	50 mg	J9185
Fluorouracil	500 mg	J9190
FUDR	500 mg	J9200
Fulvestrant	25 mg	J9395
Gefitinib	250 mg	J8565
Gemcitabine HCl	200 mg	J9201
Gemtuzumab ozogamicin	5 mg	J9300
GEMZAR	200 mg	J9201
HERCEPTIN	10 mg	J9355
HYCAMTIN	4 mg	J9350
IDAMYCIN	5 mg	J9211
Idarubicin HCl	5 mg	J9211
IFEX	1 g	J9208
Ifosfamide	1 g	J9208
Interferon alfa-2a, recombinant	3,000,000 U	J9213
Interferon alfa-2b, recombinant	1,000,000 U	J9214
Interferon alfa-n3, recombinant	250,000 IU	J9215
INTRON A	1,000,000 U	J9214
IRESSA	250 mg	J8565
Irinotecan	20 mg	J9206
Leucovorin calcium	50 mg	J0640

Drug name	Quantity	J code	Drug name	Quantity	J code
Leustatin	1 mg	J9065	Oncovin	5 mg	J9380
Mechlorethamine HCl	10 mg	J9230	Ontak	300 µg	J9160
Melphalan HCl	50 mg	J9245	Oxaliplatin	0.5 mg	J9263
Melphalan, oral	2 mg	J8600	Pacis BCG	single use	J9031
Mesna	200 mg	J9209	Paclitaxel	30 mg	J9265
Mesnex	200 mg	J9209	Paraplatin	50 mg	J9045
Methotrexate, oral	2.5 mg	J8610	Pegaspargase	single dose	J9266
Methotrexate, parenteral	5 mg	J9250	Pemetrexed	10 mg	J9305
Methotrexate, parenteral	50 mg	J9260	Pentostatin	10 mg	J9268
Mexate-AQ	5 mg	J9250	Photofrin	75 mg	J9600
Mexate-AQ	50 mg	J9260	Platinol	10 mg	J9060
Mithracin	2.5 mg	J9270	Platinol	50 mg	J9062
Mitomycin	5 mg	J9280	Plicamycin	2.5 mg	J9270
Mitomycin	20 mg	J9290	Porfimer sodium	75 mg	J9600
Mitomycin	40 mg	J9291	Proleukin	single use	J9015
Mitoxantrone HCl	5 mg	J9293	Rituxan	100 mg	J9310
Mutamycin	5 mg	J9280	Rituximab	100 mg	J9310
Mutamycin	20 mg	J9290	Roferon-A	3,000,000 U	J9213
Mutamycin	40 mg	J9291	Rubex	10 mg	J9000
Myleran	2 mg	J8510	Streptozocin	1 g	J9320
Mylotarg	5 mg	J9300	Taxol	30 mg	J9265
Navelbine	10 mg	J9390	Taxotere	20 mg	J9170
Neosar	100 mg	J9070	Temodar	5 mg	J8700
Neosar	200 mg	J9080	Temozolomide	5 mg	J8700
Neosar	500 mg	J9090	TheraCys	single use	J9031
Neosar	1 g	J9091	Thioplex	15 mg	J9340
Neosar	2 g	J9092	Thiotepa	15 mg	J9340
Nipent	10 mg	J9268	TICE BCG	single use	J9031
Novantrone	5 mg	J9293	Toposar	10 mg	J9181
Oncaspar	single dose	J9266	Toposar	100 mg	J9182
Oncovin	1 mg	J9370	Topotecan	4 mg	J9350
Oncovin	2 mg	J9375	Trastuzumab	10 mg	J9355

Drug name	Quantity	J code
TRELSTAR DEPOT	3.75 mg	J3315
TREXALL	2.5 mg	J8610
Triptorelin pamoate	3.75 mg	J3315
TRISENOX	1 mg	J9017
Valrubicin	200 mg	J9357
VALSTAR	200 mg	J9357
VELBAN	1 mg	J9360
VELCADE	0.1 mg	J9041
VEPESID, oral	50 mg	J8560
VEPESID, parenteral	10 mg	J9181
VEPESID, parenteral	100 mg	J9182
Vinblastine sulfate	1 mg	J9360

Drug name	Quantity	J code
VINCASAR	1 mg	J9370
VINCASAR	2 mg	J9375
VINCASAR	5 mg	J9380
Vincristine sulfate	1 mg	J9370
Vincristine sulfate	2 mg	J9375
Vincristine sulfate	5 mg	J9380
Vinorelbine tartrate	10 mg	J9390
Wellcovorin	50 mg	J0640
XELODA	500 mg	J8521
XELODA	150 mg	J8520
ZANOSAR	1 g	J9320

Solutions for drug and fluid administration

Solution	Quantity	J code
0.9% sodium chloride	2 ml	J2912
25% mannitol	50 ml	J2150
5% dextrose/normal saline	500 ml	J7042
5% dextrose/water (D_5W)	500 ml	J7060
5% dextrose/water (D_5W)	1,000 ml	J7070
Dextran 40	500 ml	J7100
Dextran 75	500 ml	J7110
Hypertonic saline (50/100 mEq)	20 ml	J7130
Normal saline	250 ml	J7050
Normal saline	500 ml	J7040
Normal saline	1,000 ml	J7030
Ringer's lactate	≤ 1,000 ml	J7120
Sterile saline or water	≤ 5 ml	J7051

Source: Oncology Coding Update: HCPCS Level II Codes for Drug Administration. *Community Oncology.* 2005;2(1)Suppl 2. Available online at: http://www.communityoncology.net/journal/0201s2.html. Accessed January 11, 2006.

Miscellaneous Level II drug administration codes

Description	Code
Antineoplastic drug, not otherwise classified	J9999
Chemotherapy administration by both infusion technique and other technique(s) (such as subcutaneous, I.M., push), per visit	Q0085
Chemotherapy administration by infusion technique only, per visit	Q0084
Chemotherapy administration by other than infusion technique only, per visit (such as subcutaneous, I.M., push)	Q0083
Immunosuppressive drug, not otherwise classified	J7599
Prescription drug, oral, chemotherapeutic, not otherwise classified	J8999
Prescription drug, oral, non-chemotherapeutic, not otherwise classified	J8499
Unclassified biologic	J3590
Unclassified drug	J3490

Source: Oncology Coding Update: HCPCS Level II Codes for Drug Administration. *Community Oncology.* 2005;2(1)Suppl 2. Available online at: http://www.communityoncology.net/journal/0201s2.html. Accessed January 11, 2006.

Oncology drugs in the pipeline

This appendix lists selected oncology drugs currently in Phase III development, shown alphabetically by the type of cancer for which they are being investigated. (Many of these drugs are already FDA-approved for other cancer types or indications.) The information appears in this order: generic drug name (product name; manufacturer[s]): comments (where applicable). An asterisk (*) indicates that the product name is not available.

Acute myeloid leukemia

histamine dihydrochloride (Ceplene; Maxim)
oblimersen (Genasense; Genta)
VNP 4010M (Cloretazine; Vion): relapsed

Bladder cancer

BCI immune activator (*; Intracel)
lapatinib (*; GSK)

Breast cancer

atamestane (*; Intarcia)
bevacizumab (Avastin; Genentech, Roche): metastatic
capecitabine (Xeloda; Roche): adjuvant
doxorubicin (Myocet; Elan): metastatic
fulvestrant (Faslodex; AstraZeneca): first line, advanced
Generic name not available (Enhanzyn; Corixa): adjuvant
Generic name not available (Theratope; Biomira)
lapatinib (*; GSK)
lasofoxifene (*; Ligand): prevention
Mab immunotherapeutic CEA vaccine (CEA Vac; Titan)
temsirolimus/CCI-779 (*;Wyeth)
tesmilifene (*; YM Biosciences)
trastuzumab (Herceptin; Roche, Genentech): adjuvant and with hormone therapy
vinorelbine (Navelbine; GSK): advanced

Cervical cancer

HPV recombinant vaccine (Gardasil; Merck): prevention of human papillomavirus (HPV) cervical cancer
recombinant vaccine with MPL adjuvant (Cervarix; GSK, MedImmune, Corixa): prevention of cervical cancer

Chronic lymphocytic leukemia

oblimersen (Genasense; Genta)
rituximab (Rituxan; Biogen, Idec, Genentech): relapsed

CNS tumors

chimeric Mab 14.18 (*; NCI): neuroblastoma
IL 13-PE38QQR (*; Neopharm): glioblastoma, malignant glioma
Interferon beta-1A (Avonex; Biogen)

Colorectal cancer

bevacizumab (Avastin; Genentech, Roche): adjuvant
capecitabine (Xeloda; Roche): adjuvant and metastatic
cetuximab (Erbitux; Bristol-Myers Squibb, ImClone): early stage
edotecarin (*; Pfizer)
Mab immunotherapeutic CEA vaccine (CEA Vac; Titan)
PTK787/ZK 222584 (*; Novartis, Schering): metastatic
tegafur/uracil (UFT; Bristol-Myers Squibb): adjuvant therapy
vaccine (OncoVAX; Intracel): colon cancer
vaccine with combination therapy (Avicine; SuperGen): metastatic

Esophageal cancer

anti-gastrin 17 (Insegia; Aphton)
pegamotecan (*; Enzon): gastroesophageal cancer

Gastric cancer

572016 (*; GSK)
anti-gastrin 17 (Insegia; Aphton): stomach
   cancer
edotecarin (*; Pfizer): stomach cancer
lapatinib (*; GSK)
oxaliplatin (Eloxatin; Sanofi-Aventis)
pegamotecan (*; Enzon)
SU-11248 (*; Pfizer): stomach cancer

Head and neck cancer

gefitinib (Iressa; AstraZeneca)
lapatinib (*; GSK)

Hepatobiliary cancer

nolatrexed (Thymitaq; Eximias): unresectable
   liver cancer
T67 (*; Amgen): hepatocellular cancer
XL119 (*; Exelixis): bile duct tumors

Kidney cancer

AE-941 (Neovastat; Aeterna Zentaris)
bevacizumab (Avastin; Genentech)
HSPPC-96 (Oncophage; Antigenics)
lapatinib (*; GSK)
temsirolimus/CCI-779 (*; Wyeth)

Lung cancer

572016 (*; GSK)
AE-941 (Neovastat; Aeterna Zentaris):
   non-small-cell lung cancer
AG3340 (*; Agouron)
atrasentan (Xinlay; Abbott)
bevacizumab (Avastin; Genentech): non-
   small-cell lung cancer
bexarotene capsules (Targretin; Ligand)
CAI (*; NCI)
cetuximab (Erbitux; Bristol-Myers Squibb,
   ImClone)
exisuline (Aptosyn; NCI)
IMC-BEC2 (*; ImClone): SCLC
lapatinib (*; GSK)
Mab immunotherapeutic CEA vaccine (CEA
   Vac; Titan Pharmaceuticals)
paclitaxel poliglumex/CT-2103 (Xytotax; CTI)
ranpirnase (Onconase; Alfacell)

recombinant interferon beta-1A (*; Serono)
tariquidar (*; QLT)
thalidomide (Thalomid; Celgene)
TLK286 (Telcyta; Telik): non-small-cell lung
   cancer
topotecan (Hycamtin; GSK): small-cell and
   non-small-cell lung cancer
Trp-p8 (*; Dendreon, Genentech)
vinorelbine (Navelbine, GSK)

Melanoma

GMK (*; Progenics)
HSPPC-96 (Oncophage; Anigenics)
Immunotherapy (Canvaxin; CancerVax)
oblimersen (Genasense; Genta)
peginterferon-alfa 2b (PEG-INTRON;
   Schering-Plough)

Multiple myeloma

AMD-3100 (*; AnorMED)
lenalidomide/CC-5013 (Revlimid; Celgene)
oblimersen (Genasense; Genta)
skeletal targeted radiotherapy (STR; NeoRx)

Myelodysplastic syndrome

aldesleukin (Proleukin; Chiron)

Non-Hodgkin's lymphoma

aldesleukin (Proleukin; Chiron)
AMD-3100 (*; AnorMED)
epratuzumab (*; Immunomedics): B-cell
   disease
favid-04 with rituximab (Favld/Rituxan;
   Favrille, Genentech, Biogen Idec): follicular
   disease
Generic name not available (Lymphoscan;
   Immunomedics)
IDEC-In2B8 (*; Idec)
non-Hodgkin's lymphoma vaccine (BIOVI-
   AXID; Accentia)
oblimersen (Genasense; Genta)
pixantrone (*; Cell Therapeutics)
recombinant idiotype conjugated to KLJ
   (MyVax Personalized Immunotherapy;
   Genitope)

rituximab (Rituxan; Biogen Idec, Genentech)

vincristine sulfate liposomes (Marqibo; Inex)

Ovarian cancer

bevacizumab (Avastin; Genentech): first-line treatment

docetaxel (Taxotere; Sanofi-Aventis)

ET-743 (Yondelis; Johnson & Johnson, PharmaMar USA)

gemcitabine (Gemzar; Eli Lilly)

interferon gamma-1b (*; InterMune)

oregovomab (OvaRex; United Therapeutics, Virexx)

pemtumomab/R1549 (*; Roche)

polyglutamate pacitaxel (Xyotax; Cell Therapeutics)

TLK 286 (Telcyta; Telik): advanced disease (with carboplatin)

topotecan (Hycamtin; GSK): first-line treatment

Pancreatic cancer

anti-gastrin 17 (Insegia; Aphton)

bevacizumab (Avastin; Genentech, Roche)

cetuximab (Erbitux; Bristol-Myers Squibb, ImClone)

erlotinib (Tarceva; Genentech, OSI)

Generic name not available (Virulizin; Lorus)

glufosfamide (*; Threshold): second-line treatment

oxaliplatin (Eloxatin; Sanofi-Aventis)

rubitecan (Orathecin; SuperGen)

vaccine (PANVAC-VF; Therion Biologics)

Prostate cancer

adjuvant androgen deprivation therapy (*; NCI)

AG3340 (*; Pfizer)

AMG-162 (*; Amgen): cancer-related bone loss

androgen suppression with radiotherapy (*; NCI)

APC8015 (Provenge; Dendreon)

bevacizumab (Avastin; Genentech)

cancer vaccine (GVAX-Prostate; Northwest Biotherapeutics)

flurbiprofen/MPC-7869 (Flurizan; Myriad Genetics)

ozarelix/SP-153 (*; Spectrum)

PMSA & dendritic cell vaccine (DVAX-Prostate; Northwest Biotherapeutics)

trabectedin (Yondelis; PharmMar)

Online resources for oncology practitioners and patients

The websites listed below offer helpful online resources for oncology practitioners and their patients.

General resources

American Association for Cancer Research (www.aacr.org) provides abstracts and full-text articles of the latest scientific research from five peer-reviewed journals, including *Cancer Research* and *Clinical Cancer Research*. It also features patient resources.

American Cancer Society (www.cancer.org) provides information about cancer treatment, staging, clinical trials, research advances, and research programs and funding.

American College of Radiology (www.acr.org) is an educational portal to a resident education center, webcast theater, and online learning. It also offers Reuters healthcare updates and links to clinical research.

American Joint Committee on Cancer (AJCC) (www.cancerstaging.org/) provides access to the Collaborative Staging System, along with data collection and quality assurance resources.

American Society of Clinical Oncology (ASCO) (www.asco.org) features article reviews, information on ASCO policies, clinical guidelines and abstracts of the latest clinical research, and electronic tools for oncologists.

American Society of Hematology (www.hematology.org) provides abstracts and full-text articles from the journal *Blood*, as well as abstracts from past annual meetings.

American Society for Therapeutic Radiology and Oncology (www.astro.org/) presents information on clinical trials, research highlights, clinical tools, and patient resources.

Ask C/Net (http://www.askcnet.org/dataq/cancer.htm), from C/NET Solutions, provides links to U.S. and international cancer data.

Cancer Information Services (http://cis.nci.nih.gov/), from the National Cancer Institute, provides access to a national information and educational network for healthcare professionals and patients.

Cancernetwork.com (www.cancernetwork.com) features full-text articles from the journal *Oncology*, continuing medical education, a genetics resource center, and patient resources.

CenterWatch (www.centerwatch.com) lists actively recruiting clinical trials and offers access to cancer drug directories, family drug guides, clinical trial results, patient-focused information on clinical trials, and research center profiles.

Coalition of National Cancer Cooperative Groups (http://www.cancertrialshelp.org/medicalCommunity/medicalCommunity.jsp) offers a network of cancer clinical trial specialists and professional support services, as well as Trialcheck, a web-based search engine that locates hundreds of cancer clinical trials.

HemeOncLinx (http://mdlinx.com/HemeOncLinx/), from MDLink, features hematology and oncology news, a drug guide, and links to medical specialty and allied health sites.

International Union Against Cancer (www.uicc.org) spotlights this global association's efforts to act as a catalyst for worldwide dialogue and collective action on cancer by health authorities. It offers a database of international cancer registries, access to cancer prevention publications, and information about global health initiatives.

Journal of Supportive Oncology (www.supportiveoncology.net) provides access to published review articles and original research articles pertaining to palliative and supportive care for patients with cancer.

National Cancer Database (http://www.facs.org/cancer/ncdb/index.html), from the American College of Surgeons, is a clinical surveillance resource that provides physicians with data and resources to compare management of cancer patients.

National Cancer Institute (http://cancer.gov) provides peer-reviewed information, a registry of clinical studies, statistical databases, and updates of NCI highlights.

National Center for Chronic Disease Prevention (www.cdc.gov/nccdphp/), from the Centers for Disease Control and Prevention (CDC), features information on the costs of cancer and other chronic diseases, offers access to data from the CDC's Behavioral Risk Factor Surveillance System, and provides online versions of annual reports on cancer.

National Center for Health Statistics (www.cdc.gov/nchs/datawh.htm), from the CDC, offers access to health statistics from every state.

National Comprehensive Cancer Network (NCCN) (www.nccn.org) features a tool that allows physicians to query NCCN expert faculty and receive a response within 2 days. It also provides NCCN clinical practice guidelines, information about clinical trials, and access to the *NCCN Drugs and Biologic Compendium™*.

North American Association of Central Cancer Registries (NAACCR) (www.naaccr.org) provides statistics and reports, registration standards, cancer incidence data, and information on cancer registry certification.

OncoLink (www.oncolink.com), from the University of Pennsylvania, offers webcasts, cancer news updates, and clinical trial matching. It also features OncoLink Rx, which provides information on the most commonly used chemotherapy drugs.

Oncology Nursing Society (www.ons.org) offers oncology news, FDA updates, drug recall information, full-text articles from *Oncology Nursing Forum* journal, and patient education and clinical information resources.

PubMed (http://pubmed.gov), from the National Library of Medicine and NIH, provides more than 15 million citations from MEDLINE and other life science journals.

Surveillance, Epidemiology, And End Results (SEER) (http://seer.cancer.gov/), from NCI, provides statistical resources pertaining to cancer.

Drug resources

Consumer Drug Info (www.fda.gov/cder/drug/DrugSafety/DrugIndex.htm), from the U.S. Food and Drug Administration (FDA), provides drug information written for patients.

Drug Infonet, Inc. (www.druginfonet.com/) offers drug information (including official package inserts and patient package inserts) and pharmaceutical manufacturer information.

U.S. FDA (www.fda.gov/cder/da/da.htm) provides a list of FDA-approved drugs.

Patient care resources

CancerLinks.com (**www.cancerlinks.com**) provides patient- and family-centered information on cancer, drugs, clinical trials, chemotherapy, and immunotherapy.

CancerSourceMD (**www.cancersourcemd.com**) features drug databases organized for physicians, nurses, and patients as well as cancer updates and articles.

Corporate Angel Network (**www.corpangelnetwork.org**) provides information on free air transportation for cancer patients traveling to and from recognized treatment centers in the United States.

Griefnet.org (**www.griefnet.org**) serves as an Internet community for people dealing with death and loss. It includes a companion site, KidSaid (www.kidsaid.com), where children dealing with grief can participate in online support groups, ask questions, post original writings and art, and find peers.

Lance Armstrong Foundation (**http://laf.org/**) provides cancer information and a search tool for clinical trial matching.

National Hospice and Palliative Care Organization (**www.nhpco.org/**) offers information on end-of-life care, advance directives, and resources.

OncoLink Rx (**www.oncolink.upenn.edu/treatment/section.cfm?c=2&s=10**), from the University of Pennsylvania, features an easy-to-understand guide to the most commonly used chemotherapy agents.

People Living with Cancer (**www.plwc.org/plwc/Home/1,1743,,00.html**) is the patient information website of the American Society of Clinical Oncology. It features information on types of cancer, clinical trials, side effects, and patient support organizations.

References

Aapro MS, van Wijk FH, Bolis G, et al. Doxorubicin versus doxorubicin and cisplatin in endometrial carcinoma: Definitive results of a randomised study (55872) by the EORTC Gynaecological Cancer Group. *Ann Oncol.* 2003;14(3):441-448.

Abeloff MD (ed), Armitage JO, Niederhuber JE, et al. *Clinical Oncology.* 3rd ed. New York, NY: Elsevier Churchill Livingstone; 2004.

Ajani JA, Ilson DH, Daugherty K, et al. Activity of Taxol in patient with squamous cell carcinoma and adenocarcinoma of the esophagus. *J Natl Cancer Inst.* 1994;86:1086-1091.

Ajani JA, Ilson DH, Kelsen DP. Paclitaxel in the treatment of patients with upper gastrointestinal carcinomas. *Semin Oncol.* 1996 Oct;23(suppl 12):55-58.

Albain K, Nag S, Calderillo-Ruiz G, et al. Global phase III study of gemcitabine plus paclitaxel (GT) vs. paclitaxel (T) as frontline therapy for metastatic breast cancer (MBC): First report of overall survival. PASCO 2004;23. Abstract 510.

Alberts DS, et al. Improved therapeutic index of carboplatin plus cyclophosphamide versus cisplatin plus cyclophosphamide: Final report by the Southwest Oncology Group of a phase III randomized trial in stages III and IV ovarian cancer. *J Clin Oncol.* 1992;10:706-717.

Alexian R, Barlogie B, Tucker, S. VAD-based regimens as primary treatment for multiple myeloma. *Am J Hematology.* 1990;33:86-89.

Amadori D, Nanni O, Marangolo M, et al. Disease-free survival advantage of adjuvant cyclophosphamide, methotrexate, and fluorouracil in patients with node-negative, rapidly proliferating breast cancer: A randomized multicenter study. *J Clin Oncol.* 2000;18:3125-3134.

American Society of Clinical Oncology Clinical Practice Guidelines. *J Clin Oncol.* 1999;17:2971-2994.

American Society of Health-System Pharmacists. Available online at: http://www.ashp.org/ahfs/.

American Society of Health-System Pharmacists. ASHP guidelines on handling hazardous drugs. *Am J. Health Syst Pharm.* 2006;63(12):in press.

American Society of Hospital Pharmacists. ASHP statement on the use of medications for unlabeled uses. *Am J Hosp Pharm.* 1992;49:2006-2008.

Antman K, Crowley J, Balcerzak SP, et al. An intergroup phase III randomized study of doxorubicin and dacarbazine with or without ifosfamide and mesna in advanced soft tissue and bone sarcomas. *J Clin Oncol.* 1993;11:1276-1285.

Ardizzoni A, Tjan-Heijnen VC, Postmus PE, et al. Standard versus intensified chemotherapy with granulocyte colony-stimulating factor support in small-cell lung cancer: A prospective European Organization for Research and Treatment of Cancer-Lung Cancer Group phase III trial-08923. *J Clin Oncol.* 2002;20(19):3947-3955.

Association of Community Cancer Centers. Available online at: http://www.naturaldatabase.com.

Atkins MB, Kunkel L. High-dose recombinant interleukin-2 therapy in patients with metastatic melanoma: Long-term survival update. *Cancer J Sci Am.* 2000;6(suppl 1):S11-S14.

Auerbach M, Ballard H, Trout JR, et al. Intravenous iron optimizes the response to recombinant human erythropoietin in cancer patients with chemotherapy-related anemia: A multicenter, open-label, randomized trial. *J Clin Oncol.* 2004;22:1301-1307.

Avvisati G, Lo Coca F, Diverio D, et al. AIDA (all-trans retinoic acid + idarubicin) in newly diagnosed acute promyelocytic leukemia: A Gruppo Italiano Malattie Ematologiche Maligne dell'adulto (GIMEMA) pilot study. *Blood.* 1996;88:1390-1398.

Bajetta E, Rimassa L, Carnaghi C, et al. 5-Fluorouracil, dacarbazine, and epirubicin in the treatment of patients with neuroendocrine tumors. *Cancer.* 1998;83:372-378.

Bajorin DF. Ifosfamide, paclitaxel, and cisplatin for patients with advanced carcinoma of the urithelial tract: final report of a phase II trial evaluating 2 dosing schedules. *Cancer.* 2000;88:1671-1678.

Baka S, Ashcroft L, Anderson H, et al. Phase II study of two gemcitabine schedules for patients with impaired performance status (Karnofsky performance status ≤ 70) and advanced non-small-cell lung cancer. *J Clin Oncol.* 2005;23:2136-2144.

Barlogie B, Smith L, Alexenian R. Effective treatment of advanced multiple myeloma refractory to alkylating agents. *N Engl J Med.* 1984;310:1353-1356.

Baumann TJ, Staddon JE, Horst HM, et al. Minimum urine collection periods for accurate determination of creatinine clearance in critically ill patients. *Clin Pharm.* 1987;6:393-398.

Benjamin RS, Rankin C, Fletcher C, et al. Phase III dose-randomized study of imatinib mesylate (STI571) for GIST: Intergroup S0033 early results. Presented at: 39th Annual Meeting of the American Society of Clinical Oncology; May 31-June 3, 2003; Chicago, Ill. Abstract 3271.

Benson AB III, Ajani JA, Catalano RB, et al. Recommended guidelines for the treatment of cancer treatment-induced diarrhea. *J Clin Oncol.* 2004;22:2918-2926.

Berger A. Selected reviews on the treatment of anemia, neutropenia, and symptom clusters. *J Support Oncol.* 2005;3(6):3-37.

Bernier J, Domenge C, Ozsahin M, et al. Postoperative irradiation with or without concomitant chemotherapy for locally advanced head and neck cancer. European Organization for Research and Treatment of Cancer Trial 22931. *N Engl J Med.* 2004;350(19):1945-1952.

Berruti A, Bitossi R, Gorzegno G, et al. Time to progression in metastatic breast cancer patients treated with epirubicin is not improved by the addition of either cisplatin or lonidamine: Final results of a phase III study with a factorial design. *J Clin Oncol.* 2002;20:4150-4159.

Bonadonna G, Bonfante V, Viviani S, et al. American Society of Clinical Oncology ABVD plus subtotal nodal versus involved-field radiotherapy in early-stage Hodgkin's disease: Long-term results. *J Clin Oncol.* 2004;22(14):2835-2841.

Bonadonna G, Brusamolino E, Vlagussa P, et al. Combination chemotherapy as an adjuvant treatment in operable breast cancer. *N Engl J Med.* 1976;294:405-410.

Bonadonna G, Valagussa P, Moliterni A, et al. Adjuvant cyclophosphamide, methotrexate, and fluorouracil in node-positive breast cancer: The results of 20 years of follow-up. *N Engl J Med.* 1995;332:901-906.

Bonomi P, Blessing JA, Stehman FB, et al. Randomized trial of three cisplatin dose schedules in squamous-cell carcinoma of the cervix: A Gynecologic Oncology Group study. *J Clin Oncol.* 1985;3(8):1079-1085.

Bouche O, Raoul JL, Bonnetain F, et al. Randomized multicenter phase II trial of a biweekly regimen of fluorouracil and leucovorin (LV5FU2), LV5FU2 plus cisplatin, or LV5FU2 plus irinotecan in patients with previously untreated metastatic gastric cancer: A Federation Francophone de Cancerologie Digestive Group study—FFCD 9803. *J Clin Oncol.* 2004;22(21):4319-4328.

Budman DR, Berry DA, Cirrincione CT, et al. Dose and dose intensity as determinants of outcome in the adjuvant treatment of breast cancer. *J Natl Cancer Inst.* 1998;90:1205-1211.

Burnett AF, Roman LD, Garcia AA, et al. A phase II study of gemcitabine and cisplatin in patients with advanced, persistent, or recurrent squamous cell carcinoma of the cervix. *Gynecol Oncol.* 2000;76:63-66.

Burstein HJ, Harris LN, Marcom PK, et al. Trastuzumab and vinorelbine as first-line therapy for HER2-overexpressing metastatic breast cancer: Multicenter phase II trial with clinical outcomes, analysis of serum tumor markers as predictive factors, and cardiac surveillance algorithm. *J Clin Oncol.* 2003;21(15):2889-2895.

Burstein HJ, Kuter I, Campos SM, et al. Clinical activity of trastuzumab and vinorelbine in women with HER2-overexpressing metastatic breast cancer. *J Clin Oncol.* 2001;19:2722-2730.

Burstein HJ (reviewer), Tyagi P, Lee D. Combination of antiangiogenic therapy and chemotherapy prolongs time to progression in metastatic breast cancer. Available online at: http://www.cancerpublications.com/newsletter/breast/OB/v3n8/article.htm. Accessed November 4, 2005.

Cartwright TH, Cohn A, Varkey JA, et al. Phase II study of oral capecitabine in patients with advanced or metastatic pancreatic cancer. *J Clin Oncol.* 2002;20:160-164.

Casper, ES, Schwartz GK, Sugarman A, et al., Phase I trial of dose-intense liposome-encapsulated doxorubicin in patients with advanced sarcoma. *J Clin Oncol.* 1997;15(5):2111-2117.

Cassidy J, Tabernero J, Twelves C, et al. XELOX (capecitabine plus oxaliplatin): Active first-line therapy for patients with metastatic colorectal cancer. *J Clin Oncol.* 2004;22:2084-2091.

Cassileth PA, Harrington DP, Appelbaum FR. Chemotherapy compared with autologous or allogenic bone marrow transplantation in the management of acute myeloid leukemia in first remission. *N Engl J Med.* 1998;339:1649-1656.

Chapman PB, Einhorn LH, Meyers ML, et al. Multicenter randomized trial of the Dartmouth regimen versus dacarbazine in patients with metastatic melanoma. *J Clin Oncol.* 1999;17:2745-2751.

Cheeseman SL, Joel SP, Chester JD, et al. A "modified de Gramont" regimen of fluorouracil, alone and with oxaliplatin, for advanced colorectal cancer. *Br J Cancer.* 2002;87:393-399.

Chen YM, Perng RP, Yang KY, et al. A multicenter phase II trial of vinorelbine plus gemcitabine in previously untreated inoperable (stage IIIB/IV) non-small-cell lung cancer. *Chest.* 2000;117: 1583-1589.

Choi CW, Choi IK, Seo JH, et al. Effects of 5-fluorouracil and leucovorin in the treatment of pancreatic-biliary tract adenocarcinomas. *Am J Clin Oncol.* 2000;23(4):425-428.

Cockcroft DW, Gault MH. Prediction of creatinine clearance from serum creatinine. *Nephron.* 1976;16:31-41.

Coleman RL, Bagnell KG, Townley PM. Carboplatin and short-infusion paclitaxel in high-risk and advanced-stage ovarian carcinoma. *Cancer J Sci Am.* 1997;3:246-253.

Colucci G, Gebbia V, Paoletti G, et al. Phase III randomized trial of FOLFIRI versus FOLFOX4 in the treatment of advanced colorectal cancer: A multicenter study of the Gruppo Oncologico Dell'Italia Meridionale. *J Clin Oncol.* 2005;23(22):4811-4814.

Conroy T, Etienne PL, Adenis A, et al. Vinorelbine and cisplatin in metastatic squamous cell carcinoma of the oesophagus: Response, toxicity, quality of life and survival. *Ann Oncol.* 2002; 13(5):721-729.

Conti JA, Kemeny NE, Saltz LB, et al. Irinotecan is an active agent in untreated patients with metastatic colorectal cancer. *J Clin Oncol.* 1996;14:709-715.

Cooper JS, Guo MD, Herskovic A, et al. Chemoradiotherapy of locally advanced esophageal cancer: Long-term follow-up of a prospective randomized trial (RTOG 85-01). Radiation Therapy Oncology Group. *JAMA.* 1999;281(17):1623-1627.

Costanzo FD, Carlini P, Doni L, et al. Gemcitabine with or without continuous infusion 5-FU in advanced pancreatic cancer: A randomized phase II trial of the Italian Oncology Group for Clinical Research (GOIRC). *Br J Cancer.* 2005;93:185-189.

Cox JV, Pazdur R, Thibault A, et al. A phase III trial of Xeloda (capecitabine) in previously untreated advanced/metastatic colorectal cancer. *Proc Am Soc Clin Oncol.* 1999;18:265a. Abstract 1016a.

Crinò L, Scagliotti GV, Ricci S, et al. Gemcitabine and cisplatin versus mitomycin, ifosfamide, and cisplatin in advanced non-small-cell lung cancer: A randomized phase III study of the Italian Lung Cancer Project. *J Clin Oncol.* 1999;17:3522-3530.

Cunningham D, Humblet Y, Siena S, et al. Cetuximab monotherapy and cetuximab plus irinotecan in irinotecan-refractory metastatic colorectal cancer. *N Engl J Med.* 2004;351:337-345.

Cunningham D, Pyrhonen S, James RD, et al. Randomised trial of irinotecan plus supportive care alone after fluorouracil failure for patients with metastatic colorectal cancer. *Lancet.* 1998;352:1413-1418.

Curtin JP, Blessing JA, Webster, KD, et al. Paclitaxel, an active agent in nonsquamous carcinomas of the uterine cervix: A Gynecologic Oncology Group study. *J Clin Oncol.* 2001;19(5):1275-1278.

Czuczman MS, Koryzna A, Mohr A, et al. Rituximab in combination with fludarabine chemotherapy in low-grade or follicular lymphoma. *J Clin Oncol.* 2005;23(4):694-704.

DeAndres L, Brunt J, Lopez-Pousa A, et al. Randomized trial of neoadjuvant cisplatin and fluorouracil versus carboplatin and fluorouracil in patients with stage IV-M0 head and neck cancer. *J Clin Oncol.* 1995;13:1493-1500.

de Gramont A, Bosset J-F, Milan C, et al. Randomized trial comparing monthly low-dose leucovorin and fluorouracil bolus with bimonthly high-dose leucovorin and fluorouracil bolus plus continuous infusion for advanced colorectal cancer: A French intergroup study. *J Clin Oncol.* 1997;15:808-815.

Demetri GD, von Mehren M, Blanke CD, et al. Efficacy and safety of imatinib mesylate in advanced gastrointestinal stromal tumors. *N Engl J Med.* 2002;347(7):472-480.

di Bartolomeo M, Bajetta E, de Braud F, et al. Phase II study of the etoposide, leucovorin, and fluorouracil combination for patients with advanced gastric cancer unsuitable for aggressive chemotherapy. *Oncology.* 1995;52:41-44.

Dimopoulos MA, Bakoyannis C, Georgoulias V, et al. Docetaxel and cisplatin combination chemotherapy in advanced carcinoma of the urothelium: A multicenter phase II study of the Hellenic Cooperative Oncology Group. *Ann Oncol.* 1999;10(11):1385-1388.

Doorduijn JK, van der Holt B, van Imhoff GW, et al. CHOP compared with CHOP plus granulocyte colony-stimulating factor in elderly patients with aggressive non-Hodgkin's lymphoma. *J Clin Oncol.* 2003;21(16):3041-3050.

Douillard JY, Cunningham D, Roth AD, et al. Irinotecan combined with fluorouracil compared with fluorouracil alone as first-line treatment for metastatic colorectal cancer: A multicentre randomised trial. *Lancet.* 2000;355:1041-1047.

Dreicer R. Phase III trial of methotrexate, vinblastine, doxorubicin, and cisplatin versus carboplatin and paclitaxel in patients with advanced carcinoma of the urothelium. *Cancer.* 2004; 100(8):1639-1645.

Drug Facts and Comparisons. St. Louis, Mo: Wolters Kluwer Health, Inc; 2006. Available online at: http://www.factsandcomparisons.com/.

Dubay RA, Rose PG, O'Malley DM, et al. Evaluation of concurrent and adjuvant carboplatin with radiation therapy for locally advanced cervical cancer. *Gynecol Oncol.* 2004;94(1):121-124.

Dutcher JP, Fisher RI, Weiss G, et al. Outpatient subcutaneous interleukin-2 and interferon-alpha for metastatic renal cell cancer: Five-year follow-up of the Cytokine Working Group Study. *Cancer J Sci Am.* 1997;3(3):157-162.

Earlier initiation of treatment recommended in using erythropoietic agents in chemotherapy-induced anemia. *J Support Oncol.* 2004;2(4):319.

Edmonson JH, Ryan LM, Blum RH, et al. Randomized comparison of doxorubicin alone versus ifosfamide plus doxorubicin or mitomycin, doxorubicin, and cisplatin against advanced soft tissue sarcomas. *J Clin Oncol.* 1993;11(7):1269-1275.

Eisenhauer EA, ten Bokkel Huinink WW, Swenerton KD, et al. European-Canadian randomized trial of paclitaxel in relapsed ovarian cancer: High-dose versus low-dose and long versus short infusion. *J Clin Oncol.* 1994;12:2654-2666.

Elias A, Ryan L, Aisner J, et al. Mesna, doxorubicin, ifosfamide, dacarbazine (MAID) regimen for adults with advanced sarcoma. *Semin Oncol.* 1990;179(suppl 4):41-49.

Environmental Protection Agency. Introduction to containers (40 CFR Parts 264/265, Subpart I; §261.7). Available online at: http://www.epa.gov/epaoswer/hotline/training/cont05.pdf. Accessed March 23, 2006.

Environmental Protection Agency. Introduction to hazardous waste identification (40 CFR Part 261). Available online at: http://www.epa.gov/epaoswer/hotline/training/hwid05.pdf . Accessed March 23, 2006.

Fagioli F, Aglietta M, Tienghi, et al. High-dose chemotherapy in the treatment of relapsed osteosarcoma: An Italian sarcoma group study. *J Clin Oncol.* 2002;20:2150-2156.

FDA Drug Bulletin. 1982;12:4-5.

Feld R, Pasemans M, Freifeld AG. Methodology for clinical trials involving patients with cancer who have febrile neutropenia: Updated guidelines of the Immunocompromised Host Society/Multinational Association for Supportive Care in Cancer, with emphasis on outpatient studies. *Clin Infect Dis.* 2002;35:1463-1468.

Fenaux P, Chastang C, Sanz MA, et al. A randomized comparison of ATRA followed by chemotherapy and ATRA plus chemotherapy, and the role of maintenance therapy in newly diagnosed acute promyelocytic leukemia. *Blood.* 1999;94:1192-1200.

Findlay M, Cunningham D, Norman A, et al. A phase II study in advanced gastric cancer using epirubicin and cisplatin in combination with continuous 5-FU (ECF). *Ann Oncol.* 1994;5:609-616.

Fisher B, Anderson S, Wickerham DL, et al. Increased intensification and total dose of cyclophosphamide in a doxorubicin-cyclophosphamide regimen for the treatment of primary breast cancer: Findings from National Surgical Adjuvant Breast and Bowel Project B-22. *J Clin Oncol.* 1997;15(5):1858-1869.

Fisher B, Brown AM, Dimitrov NV, et al. Two months of doxorubicin-cyclophosphamide with and without interval reinduction therapy compared with 6 months of cyclophosphamide, methotrexate, and fluorouracil in positive-node breast cancer patients with tamoxifen-nonresponsive tumors: Results from the National Surgical Adjuvant Breast and Bowel Project B-15. *J Clin Oncol.* 1990;8(9):1483-1496.

Fleming GF, Brunetto VL, Cella D, et al. Phase III trial of doxorubicin plus cisplatin with or without paclitaxel plus filgrastim in advanced endometrial carcinoma: A Gynecologic Oncology Group study. *J Clin Oncol.* 2004;22:2159-2166.

Food and Drug Administration. List of Orphan Designations and Approvals. Available online at: http://www.naturaldatabase.com.

Food and Drug Administration Center for Drug Evaluation and Research. Available online at: http://www.fda.gov/cder/.

Fossella FV, DeVore R, Kerr RN, et al. Randomized phase III trial of docetaxel versus vinorelbine or ifosfamide in patients with advanced non-small-cell lung cancer previously treated with platinum-containing chemotherapy regimens. The TAX 320 Non-Small-Cell Lung Cancer Study Group. *J Clin Oncol.* 2000;18:2354-2362.

Fossella FV, Pereira JR, von Pawel J, et al. Randomized, multinational, phase III study of docetaxel plus platinum combinations versus vinorelbine plus cisplatin for advanced non-small-cell lung cancer: The TAX 326 Study Group. *J Clin Oncol.* 2003;21(16):3016-3024.

Frasci G, Lorusso V, Panza N, et al. Gemcitabine plus vinorelbine versus vinorelbine alone in elderly patients with advanced non-small-cell lung cancer. *J Clin Oncol.* 2000;18:2529-2536.

French Epirubicin Study Group. Epirubicin-based chemotherapy in metastatic breast cancer patients: Role of dose-intensity and duration of treatment. *J Clin Oncol.* 2000;18(17):3115-3124.

Fukuda M, Furuse K, Saijo N, et al. Randomized trial of cyclophosphamide, doxorubicin, and vincristine versus cisplatin and etoposide versus alternation of these regimens in small-cell lung cancer. *J Natl Cancer Inst.* 1991;83:855-861.

Fumoleau P, Largillier R, Clippe C, et al. Multicentre, phase II study evaluating capecitabine monotherapy in patients with anthracycline- and taxane-pretreated metastatic breast cancer. *Eur J Cancer.* 2004;40:536-542.

Gahart BL, Nazareno AR. *Intravenous Medications: A Handbook for Nurses and Allied Health Professionals.* 21st ed. St. Louis, Mo: Mosby, Inc; 2005.

Gandara DR, Vokes E, Green M, et al. Activity of docetaxel in platinum-treated non-small-cell lung cancer: Results of a phase II multicenter trial. *J Clin Oncol.* 2000;18:131-135.

Gatzemeier U, von Pawel J, Gottfried M, et al. Phase III comparative study of high-dose cisplatin versus a combination of paclitaxel and cisplatin in patients with advanced non-small-cell lung cancer. *J Clin Oncol.* 2000;18(19):3390-3399.

Georgoulias V, Ardavanis A, Tsiafaki X, et al. Vinorelbine plus cisplatin versus docetaxel plus gemcitabine in advanced non-small-cell lung cancer: A phase III randomized trial. *J Clin Oncol.* 2005;23:2937-2945.

Gralla RJ, Osoba D, Kris MG, et al. Recommendations for the use of antiemetics: Evidence-based, clinical practice guidelines. *J Clin Oncol.* 1999;17:2971-2994.

Greven K, Winter K, Underhill K, et al. Preliminary analysis of RTOG 9708: Adjuvant postoperative radiotherapy combined with cisplatin/paclitaxel chemotherapy after surgery for patients with high-risk endometrial cancer. Radiation Therapy Oncology Group. *Int J Radiat Oncol Biol Phys.* 2004;59(1):168-173.

Gridelli C, Ciro Gallo C, Shepherd FA, et al. Gemcitabine plus vinorelbine compared with cisplatin plus vinorelbine or cisplatin plus gemcitabine for advanced non-small-cell lung cancer: A phase III trial of the Italian GEMVIN Investigators and the National Cancer Institute of Canada Clinical Trials Group. *J Clin Oncol.* 2003;21(16):3025-3034.

Grier HE, Krailo MD, Tarbell NJ, et al. Addition of ifosfamide and etoposide to standard chemotherapy for Ewing's sarcoma and primitive neuroectodermal tumor of bone. *N Engl J Med.* 2003; 348:694-671.

Groopman JL, Itri LM. Chemotherapy-induced anemia in adults: Incidence and treatment. *J Natl Cancer Inst.* 1999;91:1616-1634.

Grunberg SM. Chemotherapy-induced nausea and vomiting: Prevention, detection, and treatment—How are we doing? *J Support Oncol.* 2004;2(suppl 1):1-12.

Gutierrez M, Chabner BA, Pearson D, et al. Role of doxorubicin-containing regimen in relapsed and resistant lymphomas: An 8-year follow-up of EPOCH. *J Clin Oncol.* 2000;18:3633-3642.

Hainsworth JD, Burris HA III, Litchy S, et al. Gemcitabine and vinorelbine in the second-line treatment of non-small-cell lung carcinoma patients: A Minnie Pearl Cancer Research Network phase II trial. *Cancer.* 2000;88:1353-1358.

Hainsworth JD, Gray JR, Stroup SL, et al. Paclitaxel, carboplatin, and extended-schedule etoposide in the treatment of small-cell lung cancer: Comparison of sequential phase II trials using different dose intensities. *J Clin Oncol.* 1997;15:3464-3470.

Hansten and Horn Drug Interactions. Available online at: http://www.naturaldatabase.com.

Harker WG, Meyers FJ, Freiha FS, et al. Cisplatin, methotrexate, and vinblastine (CMV): An effective chemotherapy regimen for metastatic transitional cell carcinoma of the urinary tract. *J Clin Oncol.* 1985;3:1463-1470.

Hensley ML, Maki R, Venkatraman E, et al. Gemcitabine and docetaxel in patients with unresectable leiomyosarcoma: Results of a phase II trial. *J Clin Oncol.* 2002;20(12):2824-2831.

Hesketh PJ, Kris MG, Grunberg SM, et al. Proposal for classifying the acute emetogenicity of chemotherapy. *J Clin Oncol.* 1997;15:116-123.

Horning SJ, Hoppe RT, Breslin S, et al. Stanford V and radiotherapy for locally extensive and advanced Hodgkin's disease: Mature results of a prospective clinical trial. *J Clin Oncol.* 2002;20(3):630-637.

Hudes GR, Einhorn L, Ross E, et al. Vinblastine versus vinblastine plus oral estramustine phosphate for patients with hormone-refractory prostate cancer: A Hoosier Oncology Group and Fox Chase Network phase III trial. *J Clin Oncol.* 1999;17:3160-3166.

Hudes GR, Nathan F, Khater C, et al. Phase II trial of 96-hour paclitaxel plus oral estramustine phosphate in metastatic hormone-refractory prostate cancer. *J Clin Oncol.* 1997;15:3156-3163.

Hughes WT, Armstrong D, Bodey GP. 2002 guidelines for the use of antimicrobial agents in neutropenic patients with cancer. *Clin Infect Dis.* 2002;34:730-751.

Hurwitz H, Fehrenbacher L, Novotny W, et al. Bevacizumab plus irinotecan, fluorouracil, and leucovorin for metastatic colorectal cancer. *N Engl J Med.* 2004;350:2335-2342.

Hussein MA. Modifications to therapy for multiple myeloma: Pegylated liposomal doxorubicin in combination with vincristine, reduced-dose dexamethasone, and thalidomide. *Oncologist.* 2003; 8S:39-45.

Hussein MA, Wood L, Hsi E, et al. A phase II trial of pegylated liposomal doxorubicin, vincristine, and reduced-dose dexamethasone combination therapy in newly diagnosed multiple myeloma patients. *Cancer.* 2002;95:2160-2168.

Hycamtin prescribing information. GlaxoSmithKline. Research Triangle Park, NC. July 2003.

Ignatavicius DD. *Clinical Companion for Medical-Surgical Nursing.* 5th ed. St Louis, Mo: Elsevier; 2006.

Ilson DH, Ajani JA, Bhalla K, et al. A phase II trial of paclitaxel, fluorouracil, and cisplatin in patients with advanced carcinoma of the esophagus. *J Clin Oncol.* 1998;16:1826-1834.

Ilson DH, Saltz L, Enzinger P, et al. Phase II trail of weekly irinotecan plus cisplatin in advanced esophageal cancer. *J Clin Oncol.* 1999;17:3270-3275.

Jeliffe RW. Estimation of creatinine clearance when urine cannot be collected. *Lancet.* 1971;1: 975-976.

Judson I, Radford JA, Harris M, et al. Randomised phase II trial of pegylated liposomal doxorubicin (DOXIL/CAELYX) versus doxorubicin in the treatment of advanced or metastatic soft tissue sarcoma: A study by the EORTC Soft Tissue and Bone Sarcoma Group. *Eur J Cancer.* 2001;37(7): 870-877.

Jurincic CD, Horlbeck R, Klippel KF. Combined treatment (goserelin plus flutamide) versus monotherapy (goserelin alone) in advanced prostate cancer: A randomized study. *Semin Oncol.* 1991;18(suppl 6):21-25.

Kang YK, Kim TW, Chang HM, et al. A phase I/II trial of docetaxel, capecitabine, and cisplatin as a first line chemotherapy for advanced gastric cancer. Abstract No: 4066. 2004 ASCO Annual Meeting Proceedings (Post-Meeting Edition). *J Clin Oncol.* 22;14S(July 15 suppl):4066.

Kantarjian HM, O'Brien S, Smith TL, et al. Treatment with hyper-CVAD, a dose-intensive regimen, in adult acute lymphocytic leukemia. *J Clin Oncol.* 2000;18(3):547.

Karnofsky DA, Abelmann WH, Craver LF, et al. The use of the nitrogen mustards in the palliative treatment of carcinoma with particular reference to bronchogenic carcinoma. *Cancer.* 1948;1: 634-656. Scale available online at: http://en.wikipedia.org/wiki/Zubrod_scale#ECOG.2FWHO.2FZubrod_score. Accessed December 17, 2005.

Kasper DL, Braunwald E, Fauci AS, eds. *Harrison's Principles of Internal Medicine.* 16th ed. New York, NY: McGraw Hill Publishing Co; 2005.

Keefe D, Sonis S. Mucositis following cancer treatment. *Oncology Special Edition.* 2005;8:117-120.

Kemeny N, Israel K, Neidzwieki D, et al. Randomized study of continuous-infusion fluorouracil versus fluorouracil plus cisplatin in patients with metastatic colorectal cancer. *J Clin Oncol.* 1990;8:313-318.

Kirkwood JM, Strawderman MH, Ernstoff MS, et al. Interferon alfa-2b adjuvant therapy of high risk resected cutaneous melanoma: The Eastern Cooperative Oncology Group Trial EST 1684. *J Clin Oncol.* 1996;14:7.

Kollmannsberger C, Quietzsch D, Haag C, et al. A phase II study of paclitaxel, weekly, 24-hour continuous-infusion 5-fluorouracil, folinic acid and cisplatin in patients with advanced gastric cancer. *Br J Cancer.* 2000;83(4):458-462.

Kondagunta GV, Bacik J, Donadio A, et al. Combination of paclitaxel, ifosfamide, and cisplatin is an effective second-line therapy for patients with relapsed testicular germ cell tumors. *J Clin Oncol.* 2005;23:6549-6555.

Kosmidis P, Mylonakis N, Nicolaides C, et al. Paclitaxel plus carboplatin versus gemcitabine plus paclitaxel in advanced non-small-cell lung cancer: A phase III randomized trial. *J Clin Oncol.* 2002;20:3578-3585.

Kubicka S, Rudolph KL, Tietze MK, et al. Phase II study of systemic gemcitabine chemotherapy for advanced unresectable hepatobiliary carcinomas. *Hepatogastroenterology.* 2001;48(39):783-789.

Kuhn JM, Abourachid H, Brucher P, et al. A randomized comparison of the clinical and hormonal effects of two GnRH agonists in patients with prostate cancer. *Eur Urol.* 1997;32:397-403.

Kuhnle H, Meerpohl HG, Eiermann W, et al. Phase II study of carboplatin/ifosfamide in untreated advanced cervical cancer. *Cancer Chemother Pharmacol.* 1990;26(suppl):S33-S35.

Lam TK, Leung DT. More on simplified calculation of body-surface area. *N Engl J Med.* 1988;318:1130.

Larson, RA, Boogaerts M, Estey E, et al. Antibody-targeted chemotherapy of older patients with acute myeloid leukemia in first relapse using Mylotarg (gemtuzumab ozogamicin). *Leukemia.* 2002;16(9):1627-1636.

Leu KM, Ostruszka LJ, Shewach D, et al. Laboratory and clinical evidence of synergistic cytotoxicity of sequential treatment with gemcitabine followed by docetaxel in the treatment of sarcoma. *J Clin Oncol.* 2004;22(9):1706-1712.

Levin VA, Uhm JH, Jaeckle KA, et al. Phase III randomized study of postradiotherapy chemotherapy with alpha-difluoromethylornithine-procarbazine, N-(2-chloroethyl)-N'-cyclohexyl-N-nitrosurea, vincristine (DFMO-PCV) versus PCV for glioblastoma multiforme. *Clin Cancer Res.* 2000;6(10):3878-3884.

Lewin F, Damber L, Jonsson H, et al. Neoadjuvant chemotherapy with cisplatin and 5-fluorouracil in advanced squamous cell carcinoma of the head and neck: A randomized phase III study. *Radiother Oncol.* 1997;43(1):23-28.

Lipshultz SE, Rifai N, Dalton VM, et al. The effect of dexrazoxane on myocardial injury in doxorubicin-treated children with acute lymphoblastic leukemia. *N Engl J Med.* 2006;351(2):145-153.

Lo-Coco F, Cimmino G, Breccia M, et al. Gemtuzumab ozogamicin (Mylotarg) as a single agent for molecularly relapsed acute promyelocytic leukemia. *Blood.* 2004;104:1995-1999.

Loehrer PJ, Lauer R, Roth BJ, et al. Salvage therapy in recurrent germ-cell cancer: Ifosfamide and cisplatin plus either vinblastine or etoposide. *Ann Intern Med.* 1988;109:540-546.

Long HJ III, Bundy BN, Grendys EC Jr, et al. Randomized phase III trial of cisplatin with or without topotecan in carcinoma of the uterine cervix: A Gynecologic Oncology Group study. *J Clin Oncol.* 2005;23:4626-4633.

Louvet C, Andre T, Lledo G, et al. Gemcitabine combined with oxaliplatin in advanced pancreatic adenocarcinoma: Final results of a GERCOR multicenter phase II study. *J Clin Oncol.* 2002;20:1512-1518.

Louvet C, André T, Tigaud JM, et al. Phase II study of oxaliplatin, fluorouracil, and folinic acid in locally advanced or metastatic gastric cancer patients. *J Clin Oncol.* 2002;20:4543-4548.

Magrath I, Adde M, Shad A, et al. Adults and children with small non-cleaved-cell lymphoma have a similar excellent outcome when treated with the same chemotherapy regimen. *J Clin Oncol.* 1996;14:925-934.

Maindrault-Goebel F, de Gramont A, Louvet C, et al. High-dose intensity oxaliplatin added to the simplified bimonthly leucovorin and 5-fluorouracil regimen as second-line therapy for metastatic colorectal cancer (FOLFOX 7). Oncology Multidisciplinary Research Group (GERCOR). *Eur J Cancer.* 2001;37(8):1000-1005.

Makatsoris T, Kalofonos HP, Aravantinos G, et al. A phase II study of capecitabine plus oxaliplatin (XELOX): A new first-line option in metastatic colorectal cancer. Hellenic Cooperative Oncology Group. *Int J Gastrointest Cancer.* 2005;35(2):103-109.

Mandelli F, Diverio D, Avvisati G, et al. Molecular remission in PML/RARα-positive acute promyelocytic leukemia by combined all-trans retinoic acid and idarubicin (AIDA) therapy. *Blood.* 1997;90:1014-1021.

Markman M, Kennedy A, Webster K, et al. Combination chemotherapy with carboplatin and docetaxel in the treatment of cancers of the ovary and fallopian tube and primary carcinoma of the peritoneum. *J Clin Oncol.* 2001;19:1901-1905.

Markman M, Liu PY, Wilczynski S, et al. Phase III randomized trial of 12 versus 3 months of maintenance paclitaxel in patients with advanced ovarian cancer after complete response to platinum and paclitaxel-based chemotherapy: A Southwest Oncology Group and Gynecologic Oncology Group trial. *J Clin Oncol.* 2003;21(13):2460-2465.

Martin S. The adverse health effects of occupational exposure to hazardous drugs. Community Oncology. 2005;2(5):397-400.

Mayer RJ, Davis RB, Schiffer CA. Intensive postremission chemotherapy in adults with acute myeloid leukemia. *N Engl J Med.* 1994;331:896-903.

McEvoy GK, Miller J, Litvak K, eds. *AHFS Drug Information 2005.* Bethesda, Md: American Society of Health-System Pharmacists, American Hospital Formulary Service; 2005.

McGuire WP, Hoskins WJ, Brady MF, et al. Cyclophosphamide and cisplatin compared with paclitaxel and cisplatin in patients with stage III and stage IV ovarian cancer. *N Engl J Med.* 1996;334:1-6.

Mead GM, Sydes MR, Walewski J, et al. An international evaluation of CODOX-M and CODOX-M alternating with IVAC in adult Burkitt's lymphoma: Results of United Kingdom Lymphoma Group LV06 study. *Ann Oncol.* 2002;13:1264-1274.

Medical Research Council Oesophageal Cancer Working Group. Surgical resection with or without preoperative chemotherapy in oesophageal cancer: A randomised controlled trial. *Lancet.* 2002;359(9319):1727-1733.

Medical Research Council Renal Cancer Collaborators. Interferon-alpha and survival in metastatic renal carcinoma: Early results of a randomised controlled trial. *Lancet.* 1999;353(9146):14-17.

Meluch AA, Greco FA, Burris HA III, et al. Paclitaxel and gemcitabine chemotherapy for advanced transitional-cell carcinoma of the urothelial tract: A phase II trial of the Minnie Pearl Cancer Research Network. *J Clin Oncol.* 2001;19(12):3018-3024.

Middleton MR, Grob JJ, Aaronson N, et al. Randomized phase III study of temozolomide versus dacarbazine in the treatment of patients with advanced metastatic malignant melanoma. *J Clin Oncol.* 2000;18(1):158.

Miller KD, Wang M, Gralow J, et al. E2100: A randomized phase III trial of paclitaxel versus paclitaxel plus bevacizumab as first-line therapy for locally recurrent or metastatic breast cancer. Paper presented at: 41st Annual Meeting of the American Society of Clinical Oncology; May 13-17, 2005; Orlando, FL. Available online at: http://www.asco.org. Accessed July 20, 2005.

Minsky BD, Pajak TF, Ginsberg RJ, et al. INT 0123 (Radiation Therapy Oncology Group 94-05) phase III trial of combined-modality therapy for esophageal cancer: High-dose versus standard-dose radiation therapy. *J Clin Oncol.* 2002;20(5):1167-1174.

Moehler M, Eimermacher A, Siebler J, et al. Randomised phase II evaluation of irinotecan plus high-dose 5-fluorouracil and leucovorin (ILF) vs 5-fluorouracil, leucovorin, and etoposide (ELF) in untreated metastatic gastric cancer. *Br J Cancer.* 2005;92(12):2122-2128.

Moertel CG, Lefkopoulo M, Lipsitz S, et al. Streptozotocin-doxorubicin, streptozotocin-fluorouracil or chlorozotocin in the treatment of advanced islet cell carcinoma. *N Engl J Med.* 1992;326:519.

Moore DH, Blessing JA, McQuellon RP, et al. Phase III study of cisplatin with or without paclitaxel in stage IVB, recurrent, or persistent squamous cell carcinoma of the cervix: A Gynecologic Oncology Group study. *J Clin Oncol.* 2004;22(15):3113-3119.

Mosby's Drug Consult. St. Louis, Mo: Elsevier Mosby; 2005. Also available online at: http://www.mosbysdrugconsult.com.

Mosby's Drug Consult for Nurses. St. Louis, Mo: Elsevier Mosby; 2005.

Mosby's Medical Drug Reference. St. Louis, Mo: Elsevier Mosby; 2005.

Mosteller RD. Simplified calculation of body-surface area. *N Engl J Med.* 1987;317:1098.

Motzer RJ, Sheinfeld J, Mazumdar M, et al. Etoposide and cisplatin adjuvant therapy for patients with pathologic stage II germ cell tumors. *J Clin Oncol.* 1995;13:2700-2704.

Motzer RJ, Sheinfeld J, Mazumdar M, et al. Paclitaxel, ifosfamide, and cisplatin second-line therapy for patients with relapsed testicular germ cell cancer. *J Clin Oncol.* 2000;18:2413-2418.

Murray N, Livingston RB, Shepherd FA, et al. Randomized study of CODE versus alternating CAV/EP for extensive-stage small-cell lung cancer: An intergroup study of the National Cancer Institute of Canada Clinical Trials Group and the Southwest Oncology Group. *J Clin Oncol.* 1999; 17:2300-2308.

Nabholtz J-M, Senn HJ, Bezwoda WR, et al. Prospective randomized trial of docetaxel versus mitomycin plus vinblastine in patients with metastatic breast cancer progressing despite previous anthracycline-containing chemotherapy. *J Clin Oncol.* 1999;17(5):1413-1424.

National Cancer Institute. Cancer Trends Progress Report, 2005 Update. Available online at: http://progressreport.cancer.gov/introduction.asp.

National Cancer Institute. National Cancer Institute Fact Sheet, Targeted Cancer Therapies: Questions and Answers. Available online at: http://www.cancer.gov/cancertopics/factsheet/ Therapy/targeted.

National Cancer Institute. Oral complications of chemotherapy and head/neck radiation (PDQ). Oral mucositis. Available online at: http://www.cancer.gov/cancertopics/pdq/supportivecare/ oralcomplications/HealthProfessional/page5. Accessed January 6, 2006.

National Comprehensive Cancer Network Practice Guidelines in Oncology. v.1.2005.

National Comprehensive Cancer Network Practice Guidelines in Oncology. Antiemesis. v.1.2006, v.1.2005.

National Comprehensive Cancer Network Practice Guidelines in Oncology. Breast cancer. 2005.

National Comprehensive Cancer Network Practice Guidelines in Oncology. Cancer and treatment-related anemia. v.2.2005.

National Comprehensive Cancer Network Practice Guidelines in Oncology. Fever and neutropenia. v.1.2005.

National Comprehensive Cancer Network Practice Guidelines in Oncology. Merkel cell carcinoma. v.2.2005.

National Institute for Occupational Safety and Health. Preventing occupational exposure to antineoplastic and other hazardous drugs in health care settings. Available online at: http://www.cdc.gov/niosh/docs/2004-165/. Accessed January 8, 2006.

Natural Medicines Comprehensive Database. Available online at: http://www.naturaldatabase.com.

Negrier S, Escudier B, Lasset C, et al. Recombinant human interleukin-2, recombinant human interferon alfa-2a, or both in metastatic renal-cell carcinoma. *N Engl J Med.* 1998;338:1273-1278.

Neijt JP, Engelholm SA, Tuxen MK, et al. Exploratory phase III study of paclitaxel and cisplatin versus paclitaxel and carboplatin in advanced ovarian caner. *J Clin Oncol.* 2000;18:3084-3092.

Nichols CR, Catalano PJ, Crawford ED, et al. Randomized comparison of cisplatin and etoposide and either bleomycin or ifosfamide in treatment of advanced disseminated germ cell tumors: An Eastern Cooperative Oncology Group, Southwest Oncology Group, and Cancer and Leukemia Group B study. *J Clin Oncol.* 1998;16:1287-1293.

Nielsen OS, Dombernowsky P, Mouridsen H, et al. High dose epirubicin is not an alternative to standard dose doxorubicin in the treatment of advanced soft tissue sarcomas: A study of the EORTC soft tissue and bone sarcoma group. *Br J Cancer.* 1998;78:1634-1639.

Noda K, Nishiwaki Y, Kawahara M, et al. Irinotecan plus cisplatin compared with etoposide plus cisplatin for extensive small-cell lung cancer. *N Engl J Med.* 2002;346(2):85-91.

O'Brien SG, Guilhot F, Larson RA, et al. Imatinib compared with interferon and low-dose cytarabine for newly diagnosed chronic-phase chronic myelogenous leukemia. *N Engl J Med.* 2003; 384(11):994-1004.

Occupational Safety and Health Administration. Technical Manual, TED 1-0.15A, Section VI, Chapter 2. Available online at: http://www.osha.gov/dts/osta/otm/otm_vi/otm_vi_2.html. Accessed January 8, 2006.

Oken MM, Creech RH, Tormey DC, et al. Toxicity and response criteria of the Eastern Cooperative Oncology Group. *Am J Clin Oncol.* 1982;5:649-655. Scale available online at: http://www.ecog.org/general/perf_stat.html. Accessed 12/17/05.

Oken MM, et al. Remission maintenance therapy for multiple myeloma. Southwest Oncology Group study. *Arch Intern Med.* 1975;135:147-152.

Oken MM, Harrington DP, Abramson N, et al. Comparison of melphalan and prednisone with vincristine, carmustine, melphalan, cyclophosphamide, and prednisone in the treatment of multiple myeloma: Results of Eastern Cooperative Oncology Group Study E2479. *Cancer.* 1997;79: 1561-1567.

Oncology coding update: HPCPS Level II codes for drug administration. *Community Oncology.* 2005;2(1 suppl 2). Available online at: http://www.communityoncology.net/journal/0201s2.html.

Orlandi F, Caraci P, Berruti A, et al. Chemotherapy with dacarbazine and 5-fluorouracil in advanced medullary thyroid cancer. *Ann Oncol.* 1994;5:763-765.

Ozols RF, Bundy BN, Greer BE, et al. Phase III trial of carboplatin and paclitaxel compared with cisplatin and paclitaxel in patients with optimally resected stage III ovarian cancer: A Gynecologic Oncology Group study. *J Clin Oncol.* 2003;21(17):3194-3200.

Pazdur R, ed. *Cancer Management: A Multidisciplinary Approach.* 9th ed. CMP Healthcare Media: 2005.

PDR. Available online at: http://www.pdr.net/Home/Home.aspx.

Pérez-Soler R, Chachoua A, Hammond LA, et al. Determinants of tumor response and survival with erlotinib in patients with non-small-cell lung cancer. *J Clin Oncol.* 2004;22(16):3238-3247.

Perkins GL, Slater ED, Sanders GK, et al. Serum tumor markers. *Am Fam Physician.* 2003;68: 1075-1082.

Peters WA III, Rivkin SE, Smith MR, et al. Cisplatin and adriamycin combination chemotherapy for uterine stromal sarcomas and mixed mesodermal tumors. *Gynecol Oncol.* 1989;34(3):323-327.

Petrelli N, Herrera L, Rustum Y, et al. A prospective randomized trial of 5-fluorouracil versus 5-fluorouracil and high-dose leucovorin versus 5-fluorouracil and methotrexate in previously untreated patients with advanced colorectal carcinoma. *J Clin Oncol.* 1987;5:1559-1565.

Philip PA, Zalupski MM, Vaitkevicius VK, et al. Phase II study of gemcitabine and cisplatin in the treatment of patients with advanced pancreatic carcinoma. *Cancer.* 2001;92:569-577.

Pilepich MV, Krall JM, Al-Sarraf M, et al. Androgen deprivation with radiation therapy compared with radiation therapy alone for locally advanced prostatic carcinoma: A randomized comparative trial of the Radiation Therapy Oncology Group. *Urology.* 1995;45:616-623.

Polovich M. Developing a hazardous drug safe-handling program. *Community Oncology.* 2005; 2(5):403-405.

Polovich M. Safe handling of hazardous drugs. Available online at: http://www.nursingworld.org/ojin/topic25/tpc25_5.html.

Polovich M, White JM, Kelleher LO, eds. *Chemotherapy and Biotherapy Guidelines and Recommendations for Practice.* 2nd ed. Pittsburgh, Pa: Oncology Nursing Society; 2005:20-44, 111-112, 118-123.

Poole ME, Sailer SL, Roseman JG, et al. Chemoradiation for locally advanced squamous cell carcinoma of the head and neck for organ preservation and palliation. *Arch Otolaryngol Head Neck Surg.* 2001;127:1446-1450.

Poon MA, O'Connell MJ, Wieand HS, et al. Biochemical modulation of 5-fluorouracil with leucovorin: Confirmatory evidence of improved therapeutic efficacy in advanced colorectal cancer. *J Clin. Oncol.* 1991;11:1967.

Poulsen M, Rischin D, Walpole E, et al. High-risk Merkel cell carcinoma of the skin treated with synchronous carboplatin/etoposide and radiation: A trans-tasman radiation. Oncology Group study—TROG 96:07. *J Clin Oncol.* 2003;21:4371-4376.

Prevention and treatment of oral mucosa in cancer patients. The Joanna Briggs Institute for Evidence-Based Practice and Midwifery. *South Australia.* 1998;2(2). Available online at: http://www.oralcancerfoundation.org/dental/pdf/mucositis.pdf. Accessed January 6, 2006.

Pyrhonen S, Salminen E, Ruutu M, et al. Prospective randomized trial of interferon alfa-2a plus vinblastine versus vinblastine alone in patients with advanced renal cell cancer. *J Clin Oncol.* 1999;(9):2859-2867.

Rajkumar SV, Hayman S, Gertz ME, et al. Combination therapy with thalidomide plus dexamethasone for newly diagnosed myeloma. *J Clin Oncol.* 2002;20:4319-4323.

Randall ME, Brunetto G, Muss H, et al. Whole abdominal radiotherapy versus combination doxorubicin-cisplatin chemotherapy in advanced endometrial carcinoma: A randomized phase III trial of the Gynecologic Oncology Group. *Proc Am Soc Clin Oncol.* 2003;22:2. Abstract 3.

Ransom MR, Carmichael J, O'Byrne K, et al. Treatment of advanced breast cancer with sterically stabilized liposomal doxorubicin: Results of a multicenter phase II trial. *J Clin Oncol.* 1997;15: 3185-3191.

Rich TA, Shepard RC, Mosley ST. Four decades of continuing innovation with fluorouracil: Current and future approaches to fluorouracil chemoradiation therapy. *J Clin Oncol.* 2004;22(11): 2214-2232.

Richardson PG, Barlogie B, Berenson J. A phase 2 study of bortezomib in relapsed, refractory myeloma. *N Engl J Med.* 2003;348:2609-2617.

Romaguera JE, Fayad L, Rodriguez MA, et al. High rate of durable remissions after treatment of newly diagnosed aggressive mantle-cell lymphoma with rituximab plus hyper-CVAD alternating with rituximab plus high-dose methotrexate and cytarabine. *J Clin Oncol.* 2005;23(28): 7013-7023.

Ross JS, Schenkein DP, Pietrusko R, et al. Targeted therapies for cancer 2004. *Am J Clin Pathol.* 2004;122(4):598-609.

Ross P, Nicolson M, Cunningham D, et al. Prospective randomized trial comparing mitomycin, cisplatin, and protracted venous-infusion fluorouracil (PVI 5-FU) with epirubicin, cisplatin, and PVI 5-FU in advanced esophagogastric cancer. *J Clin Oncol.* 2002;20(8):1996-2004.

Roth AD, Maibach R, Martinelli G, et al. Docetaxel (Taxotere)-cisplatin (TC): An effective drug combination in gastric carcinoma. *Ann Oncol.* 2000;11:301-306.

Roth BJ, Dreicer R, Einhorn LH, et al. Significant activity of paclitaxel in advanced transitional-cell carcinoma of the urothelium: A phase II trial of the Eastern Cooperative Oncology Group. *J Clin Oncol.* 1994;12:2264-2270.

Roth D, Maibach R, Falk S, et al. Docetaxel-cisplatin-5FU (TCF) versus docetaxel-cisplatin (TC) versus epirubicin-cisplatin-5FU (ECF) as systemic treatment for advanced gastric carcinoma (AGC): A randomized phase II trial of the Swiss Group for Clinical Cancer Research (SAKK). *J Clin Oncol.* 2004(July 15 suppl);22(14S). Abstract 4020.

Rougier P, Bugat R, Douillard JY, et al. Phase II study of irinotecan in the treatment of advanced colorectal cancer in chemotherapy-naïve patients and patients pretreated with fluorouracil-based chemotherapy. *J Clin Oncol.* 1997;15:251-260.

Saltz LB, Cox JV, Blanke C, et al. Irinotecan plus fluorouracil and leucovorin for metastatic colorectal cancer. *N Engl J Med.* 2000;343:905-914.

Santoro A, Tursz T, Mouridsen H, et al. Doxorubicin versus CYVADIC versus doxorubicin plus ifosfamide in first-line treatment of advanced soft tissue sarcoma: A randomized study of the European Organization for Research and Treatment of Cancer Soft Tissue and Bone Sarcoma Group. *J Clin Oncol.* 1995;13:1537-1545.

Sanz MA, Tallman MS. Tricks of the trade for the appropriate management of newly diagnosed acute promyelocytic leukemia. *Blood.* 2005;105(8):3019-3025.

Sarosdy MF, Schelhammer PF, Johnson R, et al. Does prolonged combined androgen blockade have survival benefits over short-term combined androgen blockade therapy? *Urology.* 2000;55: 391-396.

Scheithauer W, McKendrick J, Begbie S, et al. Oral capecitabine as an alternative to IV 5-FU-based adjuvant therapy for colon cancer. Safety results of a randomized, phase III trial. *Ann Oncol.* 2003;14:1735-1743.

Schellhammer P, Sharifi R, Block N, et al. A controlled trial of bicalutamide versus flutamide, each in combination with luteinizing hormone-releasing hormone analogue therapy, in patients with advanced prostate cancer. *Urology.* 1995;45:745-752.

Schiller JH, Sudeshna A, Cella D, et al. Topotecan versus observation after cisplatin plus etoposide in extensive-stage small-cell lung cancer: E7593—A phase III trial of the Eastern Cooperative Oncology Group. *J Clin Oncol.* 2001;19:2114-2122.

Schmoll HJ. Development of treatment for advanced colorectal cancer: Infusional 5-FU and the role of new agents. *Eur J Cancer.* 1996;32A(suppl):S18-S22.

Seidman AD, Tiersten A, Hudis C, et al. Phase II trial of paclitaxel by 3-hour infusion as initial and salvage chemotherapy for metastatic breast cancer. *J Clin Oncol.* 1995;13:2575-2581.

Selker RG, Shapiro WR, Burger P, et al. A randomized comparison of surgery, external radiotherapy, and carmustine versus surgery, interstitial radiotherapy boost, external radiation therapy, and carmustine. The Brain Tumor Cooperative Group NIH Trial 87-01. *Neurosurgery.* 2002;51(2): 343-355.

Shingal S, Mehta J, Desikan R, et al. Antitumor activity of thalidomide in refractory multiple myeloma. *N Engl J Med.* 1999;341:1565-1571.

Shulman LN. Targeted therapy in metastatic breast cancer: A positive trial. Medscape. Available online at: http://www.medscape.com/viewarticle/506535.

Silverman LR, Demakos EP, Peterson BL, et al. Randomized controlled trial of azacitidine in patients with the myelodysplastic syndrome: A study of the Cancer and Leukemia Group B. *J Clin Oncol.* 2002;20:2429-2440.

Skarlos DV, Samantas E, Briassoulis E, et al. Randomized comparison of early versus late hyperfractionated thoracic irradiation concurrently with chemotherapy in limited disease small-cell lung cancer: A randomized phase II study of the Hellenic Cooperative Oncology Group (HeCOG). *Ann Oncol.* 2001;12(9):1231-1238.

Skubitz KM. Phase II trial of pegylated-liposomal doxorubicin (Doxil) in sarcoma. *Cancer Invest.* 2003;21(2):167-176.

Sledge GW. ECOG-E2100: Phase III randomized trial of paclitaxel with or without bevacizumab as first-line chemotherapy for metastatic disease. Breast Cancer Update. Available online at: http://www.breastcancerupdate.com/bcu2005/6/sledge.htm.

Smith RE, Brown AM, Mamounas EP, et al. Randomized trial of 3-hour versus 24-hour infusion of high-dose paclitaxel in patients with metastatic or locally advanced breast cancer. National Surgical Adjuvant Breast and Bowel Project Protocol B-26. *J Clin Oncol.* 1999;17(11):3403-3411.

Stewart DJ, Evans WK, Shepherd FA, et al. Cyclophosphamide and fluorouracil combined with mitoxantrone versus doxorubicin for breast cancer: Superiority of doxorubicin. *J Clin Oncol.* 1997;15:1897-1905.

Strauss GM, Herndon J, Maddaus MA, et al. Randomized clinical trial of adjuvant chemotherapy with paclitaxel and carboplatin following resection in Stage IB non-small-cell lung cancer. Report of Cancer and Leukemia Group B (CALGB) Protocol 9633. *J Clin Oncol.* 2004;22(suppl 14S): 621S. Abstract 7019.

Sundstrom S, Bremnes RM, Kaasa S, et al. Cisplatin and etoposide regimen is superior to cyclophosphamide, epirubicin, and vincristine regimen in small-cell lung cancer: Results from a randomized phase III trial with 5 years follow-up. *J Clin Oncol.* 2002;20(24):4665-4672.

Sutton GP, Blessing JA, Rosenshein N, et al. Phase II trial of ifosfamide and mesna in mixed mesodermal tumors of the uterus. A Gynecologic Oncology Group study. *Am J Obstet Gynecol.* 1989;161:309-312.

Sutton GP, Brunetto VL, Kilgore L, et al. A phase III trial of ifosfamide with or without cisplatin in carcinosarcoma of the uterus: A Gynecologic Oncology Group study. *Gynecol Oncol.* 2000;79(2): 147-153.

Swenerton K, Jeffrey J, Stuart G, et al. Cisplatin-cyclophosphamide versus carboplatin-cyclophosphamide in advanced ovarian cancer: A randomized phase III study of the National Cancer Institute of Canada Clinical Trials Group. *J Clin Oncol.* 1992;10:718-726.

Taïeb J, Artru P, Baujat B, et al. Optimisation of 5-fluorouracil (5-FU)/cisplatin combination chemotherapy with a new schedule of hydroxyurea, leucovorin, 5-FU and cisplatin (HLFP regimen) for metastatic oesophageal cancer. *Eur J Cancer.* 2002;38(5):661-666.

Takada T, Amano H, Yasuda H, et al. Is postoperative adjuvant chemotherapy useful for gallbladder carcinoma? A phase III multicenter prospective randomized controlled trial in patients with resected pancreaticobiliary carcinoma. *Cancer.* 2002;95(8):1685-1695.

Talpaz M, Siler RT, Druker BJ, et. al. Imatinib induces durable hematologic and cytogenetic responses in patients with accelerated phase chronic myelogenous leukemia: Results of a phase II study. *Blood.* 2002;99(6):1928-1937.

Tannock IF, de Wit R, Berry WR, et al. Docetaxel plus prednisone or mitoxantrone plus prednisone for advanced prostate cancer. *N Engl J Med.* 2004;351:1502-1512.

Tannock IF, Osoba D, Stockler MR, et al. Chemotherapy with mitoxantrone plus prednisone or prednisone alone for symptomatic hormone-resistant prostate cancer: A Canadian randomized trial with palliative endpoints. *J Clin Oncol.* 1996;14:1756-1764.

Tesch H, Diehl V, Lathan B, et al. Moderate dose escalation for advanced stage Hodgkin's disease using the bleomycin, etoposide, Adriamycin, cyclophosphamide, vincristine, procarbazine, and prednisone scheme and adjuvant radiotherapy: A study of the German Hodgkin's Lymphoma Study Group. *Blood.* 1998;92:4560-4567.

Thigpen JT, Brady MF, Homesley HD, et al. Phase III trial of doxorubicin with or without cisplatin in advanced endometrial carcinoma: A Gynecologic Oncology Group study. *J Clin Oncol.* 2004;22(19):3902-3908.

Tournigand C, Andre T, Achille E, et al. FOLFIRI followed by FOLFOX6 or the reverse sequence in advanced colorectal cancer: A randomized GERCOR study. *J Clin Oncol.* 2004;22:229-237.

Turrisi AT III, Kim K, Blum R, et al. Twice-daily compared with once-daily thoracic radiotherapy in limited small-cell lung cancer treated concurrently with cisplatin and etoposide. *N Engl J Med.* 1999;340(4):265-271.

Urba SG, Orringer MB, Ianettonni M, et al. Concurrent cisplatin, paclitaxel, and radiotherapy as preoperative treatment for patients with locoregional esophageal carcinoma. *Cancer.* 2003;98(10): 2177-2183.

Vachani C. Patient guide to tumor markers. OncoLink. Available online at: http://www.oncolink.org/custom_tags/print_article.cfm?Page=2&id=296&Section=Treatment_ Options. Accessed January 20, 2006.

Vallejo CT, Machiavelli MR, Perez JE, et al. Docetaxel as neoadjuvant chemotherapy in patients with advanced cervical carcinoma. *Am J Clin Oncol.* 2003;26(5):477-482.

Van Cutsem E, Findlay M, Osterwalder B, et al. Capecitabine, an oral fluoropyrimidine carbamate with substantial activity in advanced colorectal cancer: Results of a randomized phase II study. *J Clin Oncol.* 2000;18:1337-1345.

van der Burg MEL, de Wit R, van Putten WLJ, et al. Weekly cisplatin and daily oral etoposide is highly effective in platinum pretreated ovarian cancer. *Br J Cancer.* 2002;86(1):19-25.

Vanhoefer U, Rougier P, Wilke H, et al. Final results of a randomized phase III trial of sequential high-dose methotrexate, fluorouracil, and doxorubicin versus etoposide, leucovorin, and fluorouracil versus infusional fluorouracil and cisplatin in advanced gastric cancer: A trial of the European Organization for Research and Treatment of Cancer Gastrointestinal Tract Cancer Cooperative Group. *J Clin Oncol.* 2000;18:2648-2657.

Vasey PA, Jayson GC, Gordon A, et al. Phase III randomized trial of docetaxel-carboplatin versus paclitaxel-carboplatin as first-line chemotherapy for ovarian carcinoma. *J Natl Cancer Inst.* 2004; 96(22):1682-1691.

Verschraegen CF, Sittisomwong T, Kudelka AP, et al. Docetaxel for patients with paclitaxel-resistant Müllerian carcinoma. *J Clin Oncol.* 2000;18:2733-2739.

Verweij J, Casali PG, Zalcberg J, et al. Progression-free survival in gastrointestinal stromal tumours with high-dose imatinib: Randomised trial. *Lancet.* 2004;364(9440):1127-1134.

Viele C, Stern JM, Ippoliti C, et al. Symptom management of chemotherapy-induced diarrhea: A multidisciplinary approach. 27th Annual Congress of Oncology Nursing Society; 2002. Medical Association Communications. Available online at: http://www.cmecorner.com/macmcm/ons/ons2002_05.htm. Accessed January 20, 2006.

Vokes EE, Herndon JE II, Crawford J, et al. Randomized phase II study of cisplatin with gemcitabine or paclitaxel or vinorelbine as induction chemotherapy followed by concomitant chemoradiotherapy for stage IIIB non-small-cell lung cancer. Cancer and Leukemia Group B Study 9431. *J Clin Oncol.* 2002;20(20):4191-4198.

Volger WR, Velez-Garcia E, Weiner RS, et al. A phase III trial comparing idarubicin and daunoru-bicin in combination with cytarabine in acute myelogenous leukemia. A Southeastern Cancer Study Group study. *J Clin Oncol.* 1992;10(7):1103-1111.

von der Maase H. Gemcitabine in locally advanced and/or metastatic bladder cancer. *Crit Rev Oncol Hematol.* 2000;34(3):175-183.

von der Masse H, Hansen SW, Roberts JT, et. al. Gemcitabine and cisplatin versus methotrexate, vinblastine, doxorubicin, and cisplatin in advanced or metastatic bladder cancer: Results of a large, randomized, multinational, multicenter phase III study. *J Clin Oncol.* 2000;17(17):3068-3077.

Wadler S. Treatment guidelines for chemotherapy-induced diarrhea. *Oncology Special Edition.* 2005;8:105-110.

Walczak JR, Carducci MA. Phase III randomized trial evaluating second-line hormonal therapy versus docetaxel-estramustine combination chemotherapy on progression-free survival in asymp-tomatic patients with a rising prostate-specific antigen level after hormonal therapy for prostate cancer. An Eastern Cooperative Oncology Group (E1899), Intergroup/Clinical Trials Support Unit study. *Urology.* 2003;62(suppl 1):141-146.

Walsh TN, Noonan N, Hollywood D, et al. A comparison of multimodal therapy and surgery for esophageal adenocarcinoma. *N Engl J Med.* 1996;335(7):462-467.

Waltzman RJ, Capo G. Cancer-related anemia, fatigue, and quality of life. *Oncology Special Edition.* 2005;8:51-55.

Watanabe Y, Amikura T, Obata H, et al. Adjuvant chemotherapy as treatment of high-risk stage I and II endometrial cancer. *Gynecol Oncol.* 2004;94:333-339.

Waters JS, Norman A, Cunningham D, et al. Long-term survival after epirubicin, cisplatin and fluorouracil for gastric cancer: Results of a randomized trial. *Br J Cancer.* 1999;80(1-2):269-272.

Webb A, Cunningham D, Scarffe JH, et al. Randomized trial comparing epirubicin, cisplatin and fluorouracil versus fluorouracil, doxorubicin and methotrexate in advanced esophagogastric can-cer. *J Clin Oncol.* 1997;15:261-267.

Whittington R, Neuberg D, Tester WJ, et al. Protracted intravenous fluorouracil infusion with ra-diation therapy in the management of localized pancreaticobiliary carcinoma: A phase I Eastern Cooperative Oncology Group trial. *J Clin Oncol.* 1995;13(1):227-232

Wie CH, Hsieh RK, Chiou TJ, et al. Adjuvant methotrexate, vinblastine and cisplatin chemother-apy for invasive transitional cell carcinoma: Taiwan experience. *J Urol.* 1996;155:118-125.

Wijermans P, Lubbert M, Verhoef G, et al. Low-dose 5-aza-2'-deoxycytidine, a DNA hypomethy-lating agent, for the treatment of high-risk myelodysplastic syndrome: A multi-center phase II study in elderly patients. *J Clin Oncol.* 2000;18:956-962.

Wilke H, Preusser P, Fink U, et al. New developments in the treatment of gastric carcinoma. *Cancer Treat Res.* 1991;55:363-373.

Williams SD, Birch R, Einhorn LH, et al. Treatment of disseminated germ-cell tumors with cis-platin, bleomycin, and either vinblastine or etoposide. *N Engl J Med.* 1987;316:1435-1440.

Wils J, Bleiberg H, Dalesio O, et al. An EORTC Gastrointestinal Group evaluation of the combination of sequential methotrexate and 5-fluorouracil, combined with Adriamycin in advanced measurable gastric cancer. *J Clin Oncol.* 1986;4:1799-1803.

Witzig TE, Vukov AM, Habermann TM, et al. Rituximab therapy for patients with newly diagnosed, advanced-stage, follicular grade I non-Hodgkin's lymphoma: A phase II trial in the North Central Cancer Treatment Group. *J Clin Oncol.* 2005;23(6):1103-1108.

Wolff D, Culakova E, Poniewierski S, et al. Predictors of chemotherapy-induced neutropenia and its complications: Results from a prospective nationwide registry. *J Support Oncol.* 2005;3(suppl 4):24-25.

Wu LT, Averbuch SD, Ball DW, et al. Treatment of advanced medullary thyroid carcinoma with a combination of cyclophosphamide, vincristine, and dacarbazine. *Cancer.* 1994;73:432-436.

Yang JC, Sherry RM, Steinberg SM, et al. Randomized study of high-dose and low-dose interleukin-2 in patients with metastatic renal cancer. *J Clin Oncol.* 2003;21(16):3127-3132.

Yung WK, Prados MD, Yaya-Tur R, et al. Multicenter phase II trial of temozolomide in patients with anaplastic astrocytoma or anaplastic oligoastrocytoma at first relapse. Temodal Brain Tumor Group. *J Clin Oncol.* 1999;17(9):2762-2771.

Zangari M, Anaissie E, Barlogie B, et.al. Increased risk of deep-vein thrombosis in patients with multiple myeloma receiving thalidomide and chemotherapy. *Blood.* 2001;98:1614-1615.

Zinzani PL, Pulsoni A, Perrotti A, et al. Fludarabine plus mitoxantrone with and without rituximab versus CHOP with and without rituximab as front-line treatment for patients with follicular lymphoma. *J Clin Oncol.* 2004;22:2654-2661.

Index

A

abarelix, 25-26
Abbreviations, common oncology, 459-460
Abraxane, 288
Absolute neutrophil count, calculating, 468
ABVD regimen, 409
AC regimen, 377-378
Accutane, 210
ACE regimen, 417-418
acetaminophen and codeine phosphate, 26-28
acetaminophen and hydrocodone bitartrate, 28-30
acetaminophen and oxycodone hydrochloride, 31-32
Acquired autoimmune hemolytic anemia, methylprednisolone for, 255
ACT, 101-103
actinomycin D, 101-103
Actiq, 156
Acute lymphatic leukemia, mercaptopurine for, 243
Acute lymphoblastic leukemia
    clofarabine for, 90
    cyclophosphamide for, 93
    doxorubicin for, 128
    mercaptopurine for, 243
    methotrexate for, 249
    pegaspargase for, 291
    teniposide for, 331
Acute lymphocytic leukemia
    asparaginase for, 49
    cytarabine for, 96

Acute lymphocytic leukemia (continued)
    daunorubicin for, 107
    fludarabine for, 164
    idarubicin for, 189
    ifosfamide for, 191
    imatinib for, 193
    mercaptopurine for, 243
Acute monocytic leukemia, cyclophosphamide for, 93
Acute myeloblastic leukemia, doxorubicin for, 128
Acute myelocytic leukemia, etoposide for, 153
Acute myelogenous leukemia
    cyclophosphamide for, 93
    mercaptopurine for, 243
    sargramostim for, 316
Acute myeloid leukemia
    all-trans retinoic acid for, 370
    azacitidine for, 51
    cladribine for, 88
    clofarabine for, 90
    cytarabine for, 370, 371, 372
    daunorubicin for, 370
    drugs in development for, 489
    filgrastim for, 159
    gemtuzumab for, 174, 371
    idarubicin for, 189, 370, 371, 372
    regimens for, 370-372
Acute myelomonocytic leukemia, mercaptopurine for, 243
Acute nonlymphocytic leukemia
    cytarabine for, 96

Acute nonlymphocytic leukemia (*continued*)
   daunorubicin for, 107
   mitoxantrone for, 263
   thioguanine for, 337
Acute promyelocytic leukemia
   arsenic trioxide for, 46
   tretinoin for, 352
Adenocarcinoma
   epirubicin for, 139
   floxuridine for, 161
Admixture compatibilities, chemotherapy,
   462-465
AD regimen, 444
Adrenocortical carcinoma, mitotane for,
   262
Adrenocot, 112
Adriamycin, 128
Adriamycin PFS, 128
Adriamycin RDF, 128
Adrucil, 165
AIDA regimen, 370
AIM regimen, 445
AK-Dex, 112
Alanine aminotransferase, normal value for,
   467
Albumin, normal value for, 466
aldesleukin, 32-35, 441
alemtuzumab, 6, 36-38
Alimta, 294
alitretinoin, 7
Alkaline phosphatase, normal value for,
   467
Alkylating agents, 5
Alkylsulfonates, 5
all-*trans*-retinoic acid, 352-354, 370
Alopecia, 9
Aloxi, 290
altretamine, 38-39
Amen, 234
American Society for Testing and Materials,
   17
American Society of Health-System Phar-
   macists, 11
amifostine, 40-41

aminoglutethimide, 41-43
Amnesteem, 210
Amylase, normal value for, 467
Anal cancer, mitomycin for, 260
Anal cancer, regimens for, 389-394. *See also*
   Colorectal cancer.
anastrozole, 7, 43-44
Anemia
   azacitidine for, 51
   darbepoetin alfa for, 103, 104
   epoetin alfa for, 144
   lenalidomide for, 214
   managing, 8-9
   supportive therapy for, 474-476
Anergan, 310
Anexsia, 28
Anion gap, normal value for, 466
Anolor DH5, 28
Anorexia, megestrol for, 236
Anthracycline extravasation, dexrazoxane
   for, 116
Antiandrogens, nonsteroidal, 7
Antiangiogenic drugs, 9
Antibiotics, antitumor, 5
Antibodies, monoclonal, 6
Antimetabolites, 4
Antineoplastics. *See* Oncology drugs.
Antisense drugs, 9
Antitumor antibiotics, 5
Anxiety, lorazepam for, 228
Anzemet, 126
Apoptosis-inducing drugs, 6
Appetite stimulant, dronabinol for, 136
aprepitant, 45-46
Aranesp, 103
Arimidex, 43
Aromasin, 155
Aromatase inhibitors, 7
arsenic trioxide, 7, 46-48
asparaginase, 7, 48-51
Aspartate aminotransferase, normal value
   for, 467
Astrocytoma
   carmustine for, 74

Astrocytoma (*continued*)
  temozolomide for, 329
Astromorph PF, 267
Ativan, 228
ATRA, 352-354
Avastin, 55
Avinza, 267
azacitidine, 51-52, 425

B

Banaril, 119
Bancap HC, 28
Barrett's esophagus, porfimer for, 301
Basal cell carcinoma
  bleomycin for, 61
  5-fluorouracil for, 165
BEACOPP regimen, 409-410
BCG live, intravesical, 52-55
BCNU, 74-77
Benadryl, 119
Benzacot, 354
Benzocaine-Trimethobenzamide Adult, 354
Benzocaine-Trimethobenzamide Pediatric, 354
BEP regimen, 448
bevacizumab, 378
bevacizumab, 392
bevacizumab, 55-57
bexarotene, 57-59
Bexxar [131]I Dosimetric, 345
Bexxar [131]I Therapeutic, 345
Bexxar Dosimetric, 345
Bexxar Therapeutic, 345
bicalutamide, 7, 59-60, 440
BiCNU, 74
Biliary tract carcinomas, gemcitabine for, 172
Bilirubin, normal value for, 467
Biological response modifiers, 6
Bladder cancer
  BCG live, intravesical, for, 53
  carboplatin for, 71, 376

Bladder cancer (*continued*)
  cisplatin for, 85, 372, 373, 374, 375
  cyclophosphamide for, 94
  docetaxel for, 124, 372
  doxorubicin for, 128, 375
  drugs in development for, 489
  epirubicin for, 140
  gemcitabine for, 172, 373, 375
  ifosfamide for, 191, 374
  interferon alfa-n3 for, 202
  methotrexate for, 250, 372, 375
  mitomycin for, 260
  paclitaxel for, 374, 375, 376
  porfimer for, 301
  regimens for, 372-376
  thiotepa for, 340
  valrubicin for, 357
  vinblastine for, 359, 372, 375
Bladder outlet obstruction, abarelix for, 25
Blenoxane, 61
bleomycin sulfate, 61-63, 409, 410, 448, 449
Blood tests, standard, 466
Blood urea nitrogen, normal value for, 466
Body surface area, 8
Body surface area, calculating, 461
Bone cancer, doxorubicin for, 128
Bone lesions, strontium chloride Sr 89 for, 324
Bone marrow depression, amifostine for, 40
Bone marrow transplantation
  cisplatin for, 85
  etoposide for, 153
  melphalan for, 238
  sargramostim for, 316
  thiotepa for, 340
Bone pain
  abarelix for, 25
  strontium chloride Sr 89 for, 324
Bone sarcoma
  cyclophosphamide for, 376
  doxorubicin for, 376
  etoposide for, 376
  ifosfamide for, 376

Bone sarcoma (*continued*)
  leucovorin for, 377
  methotrexate for, 377
  regimens for, 376-377
  vincristine for, 376
bortezomib, 63-65, 422
Brain tumors
  carmustine for, 74
  dexamethasone for, 112, 113
  doxorubicin hydrochloride, liposomal,
      for, 132
  etoposide for, 153
  irinotecan for, 205
  lomustine for, 225
  thalidomide for, 335
  vincristine for, 362
Brainstem glioma, carmustine for, 74
Breast cancer
  aminoglutethimide for, 42
  anastrozole for, 43
  bevacizumab for, 55, 378
  capecitabine for, 69, 378
  cetuximab for, 78
  cyclophosphamide for, 93, 94, 377, 378,
      380, 381
  dexrazoxane for, 115
  docetaxel for, 123, 379
  doxorubicin for, 128, 377, 380, 382
  doxorubicin hydrochloride, liposomal,
      for, 132
  drugs in development for, 489
  epirubicin for, 139, 380, 381
  estrogens, conjugated, for, 149
  exemestane for, 155
  5-fluorouracil for, 165, 378, 380, 381
  fulvestrant for, 169
  gemcitabine for, 172, 381
  goserelin acetate for, 176
  idarubicin for, 189
  ifosfamide for, 191
  letrozole for, 217
  leuprolide for, 221
  lomustine for, 225
  medroxyprogesterone for, 234

Breast cancer (*continued*)
  megestrol for, 236
  methotrexate for, 250, 378
  mitoxantrone for, 263
  paclitaxel for, 285, 378, 381, 382
  paclitaxel protein-bound particles for,
      288
  raloxifene for, 312
  regimens for, 377-383
  tamoxifen for, 327
  testolactone for, 334
  thiotepa for, 340
  toremifene for, 344
  trastuzumab for, 350, 382
  vinblastine for, 359
  vinorelbine for, 364, 382
Bronchogenic carcinoma
  doxorubicin for, 128
  mechlorethamine for, 231
Burkitt's lymphoma
  cyclophosphamide for, 93
  methotrexate for, 250
busulfan, 65-68
Busulfex, 65
Butterfly clips, contaminated, disposal of, 19

C

Cachexia
  dronabinol for, 136
  megestrol for, 236
CAE regimen, 417-418
CAF regimen, 380-381
Calcium, normal value for, 466
Campath, 36
Camptosar, 203
Cancer risk, hazardous drug exposure and,
      14
capecitabine, 69-71
  as regimen component
    for breast cancer, 378
    for colon, rectal, anal cancers, 390,
        394

capecitabine, as regimen component
(continued)
for gastric cancer, 401
for pancreatic cancer, 436
Capital with Codeine Suspension, 26
CAP regimen, 452-453
Carac, 165
Carafate, 326
Carbon dioxide, normal value for, 466
carboplatin, 71-73
as regimen component
for bladder cancer, 376
for cervical cancer, 383, 386
for lung cancer, 412, 418
for ovarian cancer, 433, 434, 435
for skin cancer, 443
Carcinoid tumors
dacarbazine for, 99
doxorubicin for, 128
interferon alfa-2a, recombinant, for,
196
interferon alfa-n3 for, 202
ocreotide for, 273
Carcinoma
metastatic, mechlorethamine for, 231
of unknown primary site, etoposide for,
153
Cardiotoxicity, anthracycline-induced,
dexrazoxane for, 116
carmustine, 74-77, 388
Casodex, 59
CAV regimen, 376-377, 419
CAV with IE regimen, 376-377, 419-420
CeeNU, 224
Cell cycle, phases of, 3-4
Central nervous system tumors
carmustine for, 388
drugs in development for, 489
lomustine for, 388
procarbazine for, 388
regimens for, 388-389
temozolomide for, 389
vincristine for, 388
Cerebral edema, dexamethasone for, 112

Cerubidine, 107
Cervical cancer
carboplatin for, 383, 386
cisplatin for, 384, 385, 386
cyclophosphamide for, 94
docetaxel for, 385
doxorubicin for, 128
drugs in development for, 489
gemcitabine for, 386
ifosfamide for, 191, 386
irinotecan for, 205
mesna for, 386
paclitaxel for, 384, 387
regimens for, 383-387
topotecan for, 385
vinblastine for, 359
vinorelbine for, 364
Ceta Plus, 28
cetuximab, 77-79, 390
Chemistry studies, normal, 466
Chemo adjuncts, 16
Chemotherapy. See also Oncology drugs.
combination, 7. See also Regimens.
drug classifications in, 3-7
future of, 9-10
goal of, 3
managing, 8
origins of, 3
patient management during, 8-9
types of, 3
Chemotherapy protocols, 7. See also Regimens.
chlorambucil, 79-81, 427
Chloride, normal value for, 466
chlorpromazine hydrochloride, 81-84
Cholesterol, normal value for, 467
CHOP regimen, 427-428
Chorioadenoma destruens, methotrexate
for, 249
Choriocarcinoma
methotrexate for, 249
vinblastine for, 359
Chromosomal activity, effect of hazardous
drug exposure on, 14

Chronic granulocytic leukemia, cyclophosphamide for, 93
Chronic lymphocytic leukemia
  alemtuzumab for, 36
  chlorambucil for, 79
  cladribine for, 87
  cyclophosphamide for, 93
  drugs in development for, 489
  fludarabine for, 163
  mechlorethamine for, 231
  pentostatin for, 297
  prednisone for, 304
  rituximab for, 314
  sodium phosphate P 32 for, 319
Chronic lymphocytic lymphoma,
  denileukin diftitox for, 110
Chronic myelocytic leukemia
  cytarabine for, 96
  hydroxyurea for, 184
  interferon alfa-n3 for, 202
  mechlorethamine for, 231
  mitoxantrone for, 264
Chronic myelogenous leukemia
  busulfan for, 65, 66
  cytarabine for, 388
  daunorubicin for, 108
  imatinib for, 387
  interferon alfa-2a, recombinant, for, 196
  interferon alfa-2b for, 199
  interferon alfa-2b for, 388
  regimens for, 387-388
  thioguanine for, 338
Chronic myeloid leukemia
  arsenic trioxide for, 46
  imatinib for, 193
  sodium phosphate P 32 for, 319
Chronic myelomonocytic leukemia
  azacitidine for, 51
  topotecan for, 342
Chronic nonlymphocytic leukemia, mitoxantrone for, 264
cisplatin, 84-87
  as regimen component
    for bladder cancer, 372, 373, 374, 375

cisplatin, as regimen component (continued)
    for cervical cancer, 384, 385, 386
    for esophageal cancer, 395, 396, 397,
      398, 399
    for gastric cancer, 400, 401, 404,
      405, 406
    for head and neck cancer, 406, 407
    for lung cancer, 412, 413, 414, 419,
      420, 421
    for ovarian cancer, 433, 436
    for pancreatic cancer, 437
    for skin cancer, 443
    for testicular cancer, 448, 449, 450,
      451
    for uterine cancer, 452, 453, 455,
      456
Cisplatin-induced neurotoxicity, amifostine
  for, 40
13-cis-retinoic acid, 210-213
citrovorum factor, 218-220
cladribine, 87-89
Cladribine Novaplus, 87
Claravis, 210
Classifications, chemotherapy drug, 3-7
clofarabine, 89-91
Clolar, 89
CMF regimen, 378-379
CMV regimen, 372-373
Coagulation studies, normal, 466
Cockcroft-Gault method, for creatinine
  clearance calculation, 467
codeine phosphate, 91-93
codeine sulfate, 91-93
Codes, oncology drug, 484-488
CODOX-M regimen, 428-429
Co-Gesic, 28
Colon cancer. See Colorectal cancer.
Colorectal cancer
  bevacizumab for, 55, 392
  capecitabine for, 69, 390, 394
  cetuximab for, 77, 390
  daunorubicin citrate liposome for, 106
  drugs in development for, 489
  erlotinib for, 146

Colorectal cancer (continued)
 floxuridine for, 162
 5-fluorouracil for, 165, 389, 391, 392, 393
 irinotecan for, 204, 205, 390, 392, 393
 leucovorin for, 218, 389, 391, 392, 393
 lomustine for, 225
 oxaliplatin for, 278, 391, 394
 regimens for, 389-394
Compatibility, chemotherapy admixture, 462-465
Compazine Spansule, 308
Compazine, 308
Compro, 308
Contamination, packaging and, 15
Cortastat, 112
Cortastat LA, 112
Cortastat 10, 112
Cosmegen, 101
Cough, codeine for, 92
Coveralls, 17
CPT-11+CDDP regimen, 397
Creatinine, normal value for, 466
Creatinine clearance, calculating, 467
Curretab, 234
CVD regimen, 451-452
cyclophosphamide, 93-96
 as regimen component
 for bone sarcoma, 376
 for breast cancer, 377, 378, 380, 381
 for Hodgkin's disease, 409
 for lung cancer, 417, 419
 for non-Hodgkin's lymphoma, 427, 428, 429, 430, 431, 432
 for ovarian cancer, 433
 for thyroid cancer, 451
 for uterine cancer, 452
Cycrin, 234
Cytadren, 41
cytarabine, 96-99
 as regimen component
 for acute myeloid leukemia, 370, 371, 372

cytarabine, as regimen component (continued)
 for chronic myelogenous leukemia, 388
 for non-Hodgkin's lymphoma, 428, 429, 432
cytarabine liposome, 96-99
Cytosar-U, 96
Cytotoxic agents, diphenhydramine as premedication for, 119
Cytoxan, 93
Cytoxan Lyophilized, 93

D

dacarbazine, 99-101
 as regimen component
 for Hodgkin's disease, 409
 for skin cancer, 441
 for soft-tissue sarcoma, 444, 447
 for thyroid cancer, 451, 452
 for uterine cancer for, 455
dactinomycin, 101-103
Dalalone, 112
Dalalone D.P., 112
Dalalone L.A., 112
darbepoetin alfa, 103-105
daunorubicin citrate liposome, 105-107
daunorubicin hydrochloride, 107-110, 370
DaunoXome, 105
DCF regimen, 400-401
Decadron, 112
Decadron 5-12 Pak, 112
Decadron Phosphate, 112
Decaject, 112
decitabine, 425
de Gramont regimen, 389
Deltasone, 303
Demerol Hydrochloride, 240
denileukin diftitox, 6, 110-112
DepoCyt, 96
Depo-Medrol, 255
Depo-Provera, 234

Depression, lorazepam for, 228
Depression, modafinil for, 266
De-Sone LA, 112
Dexacen-4, 112
dexamethasone, 112-115
   as regimen component
      for multiple myeloma, 423, 424, 425
      for non-Hodgkin's lymphoma, 429,
        432
dexamethasone acetate, 112-115
Dexamethasone Intensol, 112
dexamethasone sodium phosphate, 112-
    115
Dexasone, 112
Dexasone LA, 112
Dexedrine, 117
Dexedrine Spansule, 117
Dexpak Taperpak, 112
dexrazoxane hydrochloride, 115-117
dextroamphetamine sulfate, 117-119
Dextrostat, 117
Diarrhea
   codeine for, 92
   diphenoxylate and atropine for, 121
   kaolin and pectin for, 213
   loperamide for, 227
   ocreotide for, 274
   supportive therapy for, 480-481
Dilaudid, 182
Dilaudid-5, 182
Dilaudid-HP, 182
Diphedryl, 119
diphenhydramine hydrochloride, 119-121
diphenoxylate hydrochloride and atropine
    sulfate, 121-123
docetaxel, 123-126
   as regimen component
      for bladder cancer, 372
      for breast cancer, 379
      for cervical cancer, 385
      for gastric cancer, 400, 401, 406
      for lung cancer, 412, 414, 415
      for ovarian cancer, 434
      for prostate cancer, 438, 439

docetaxel, as regimen component
   (continued)
      for soft-tissue sarcoma, 445
Docetaxel administration, dexamethasone
    as premedication for, 112
Dolacet, 28
dolasetron mesylate, 126-128
Dolophine, 247
Dosage calculation, 8
Douillard regimen, 393
Doxil, 131
doxorubicin hydrochloride, 128-131
   as regimen component
      for bladder cancer, 375
      for bone sarcoma, 376
      for breast cancer, 377, 380, 382
      for gastric cancer, 403
      for Hodgkin's disease, 409, 410
      for lung cancer, 417, 419
      for multiple myeloma, 422, 423, 425
      for non-Hodgkin's lymphoma, 427,
        428, 429, 430, 431, 432
      for soft-tissue sarcoma, 444, 445, 447
      for uterine cancer, 452, 453, 454,
        455, 456
doxorubicin hydrochloride, liposomal,
    131-135
dronabinol, 135-137
droperidol, 137-139
Droxia, 184
DTIC, 99-101
DTIC-Dome, 99
Duragesic, 156
Duramorph PF, 267
Dvd regimen, 422-423
Dvd-T regimen, 423
DXP regimen, 401
Dytan, 119

E

ECF regimen, 397-398, 401-402
ECOG performance status scale, 469

Efudex, 165
Ehrlich, Paul, 3
ELF regimen, 402
Eligard, 220
Ellence, 139
Eloxatin, 278
Elspar, 48
Emcyt, 148
Emend, 45
Emend 3-Day, 45
Emesis, risk levels for, 471-472. *See also* Nausea and vomiting.
Employee monitoring, hazardous drug safety program and, 22
Endocet, 31
Endocodone, 281
Endometrial cancer
   doxorubicin for, 128
   ifosfamide for, 191
   leuprolide for, 221
   medroxyprogesterone for, 234
   megestrol for, 236
Ependymoma, carmustine for, 74
Epidermal growth factor receptor over-expression, cetuximab for, 77, 78
epirubicin hydrochloride, 139-143
   as regimen component
      for breast cancer, 380, 381
      for esophageal cancer, 397
      for gastric cancer, 401
epoetin alfa, 143-146
Epogen, 143
EP regimen, 448-449
Equipment, personal protective, 17-19
Erbitux, 77
erlotinib, 146-147, 415
Erythroblastopenia, methylprednisolone for, 255
Erythropoietic therapy, for anemia, 475
Esophageal cancer
   cisplatin for, 395, 396, 397, 398, 399
   docetaxel for, 124
   drugs in development for, 489
   epirubicin for, 139, 397

Esophageal cancer (*continued*)
   5-fluorouracil for, 395, 397, 398, 399
   hydroxyurea for, 398
   irinotecan for, 397
   leucovorin for, 398
   mitomycin for, 398
   oxaliplatin for, 279
   paclitaxel for, 285, 395, 399
   porfimer for, 301
   regimens for, 395-400
   vinorelbine for, 396
Esophagogastric junction carcinoma, epirubicin for, 139
estramustine phosphate sodium, 148-149, 438, 439, 440
Estrogen/nitrogen mustard, 5
Estrogen receptors, cancers with, tamoxifen for, 327
estrogens, conjugated, 149-152
Ethylenimines, 5
Ethyol, 40
Etopophos, 152
etoposide, 152-155
   as regimen component
      for bone sarcoma, 376
      for gastric cancer, 402
      for Hodgkin's disease, 409, 410
      for lung cancer, 417, 418, 419, 420
      for non-Hodgkin's lymphoma, 428, 431
      for ovarian cancer, 433
      for skin cancer, 443
      for testicular cancer, 448, 451
etoposide phosphate, 152-155
Eulexin, 167
Evista, 312
Ewing's sarcoma
   cyclophosphamide for, 94
   dactinomycin for, 101
   doxorubicin for, 128
   etoposide for, 153
   ifosfamide for, 191
exemestane, 7, 155-156

Extravasation, anthracycline, dexrazoxane for, 116
Eye protection, 18
EZ III, 26

F

FAC regimen, 380-381
Face protection, 18
FAMTX regimen, 403
Fareston, 344
Faslodex, 169
Fatigue, dextroamphetamine for, 117
Febrile neutropenia, supportive therapy for, 477-479
FEC-100 regimen, 381
Femara, 216
fentanyl citrate, 156-159
fentanyl transdermal system, 156-159
fentanyl transmucosal, 156-159
Ferritin, normal value for, 466
Fever, dexamethasone for, 113
Fibrinogen, normal value for, 466
filgrastim, 159-161, 456
floxuridine, 161-163
Fludara, 163
fludarabine phosphate, 163-165, 429
Fluoroplex, 165
fluorouracil, 165-167
5-fluorouracil, 165-167
  as regimen component
    for breast cancer, 378, 380, 381
    for colon, rectal, anal cancers, 389, 391, 392, 393
    for esophageal cancer, 395, 397, 398, 399
    for gastric cancer, 400, 401, 402, 403, 404, 405
    for head and neck cancer, 407
    for hepatobiliary cancer, 407, 408
    for pancreatic cancer, 438
    for thyroid cancer, 452,
flutamide, 7, 167-169, 440

FOLFIRI regimen, 393
FOLFOX4 regimen, 391
FOLFOX6 regimen, 391, 403-404
Folic acid antagonists, 4
folinic acid, 218-220
5-FU, 165-167
FUDR, 161
fulvestrant, 7, 169-170
FUP regimen, 404

G

Gallbladder carcinomas, gemcitabine for, 172
Gastric cancer
  capecitabine for, 401
  cisplatin for, 400, 401, 404, 405, 406
  docetaxel for, 124, 400, 401, 406
  doxorubicin for, 128, 403
  drugs in development for, 490
  epirubicin for, 140, 401
  etoposide for, 402
  5-fluorouracil for, 165, 400, 401, 402, 403, 404, 405
  irinotecan for, 205, 404
  leucovorin for, 402, 403, 404, 405
  methotrexate for, 403
  mitomycin for, 260
  oxaliplatin for, 403
  paclitaxel for, 286, 405
  regimens for, 400-406
Gastroenteropancreatic tumors, ocreotide for, 274
Gastroesophageal junction carcinomas, docetaxel for, 124
Gastrointestinal neoplasia, floxuridine for, 161
Gastrointestinal stromal tumor, imatinib for, 193
gefitinib, 170-171
gemcitabine hydrochloride, 171-174
  as regimen component
    for bladder cancer, 373, 375

gemcitabine hydrochloride, as regimen
    component (*continued*)
    for breast cancer, 381
    for cervical cancer, 386
    for hepatobiliary cancer, 408
    for lung cancer, 413, 415, 416
    for pancreatic cancer, 437, 438
    for soft-tissue sarcoma, 445
gemtuzumab ozogamicin, 6, 174-175, 371
Gemzar, 171
Genasense, 6
Genotoxic activity, hazardous drug expo-
    sure and, 14
Germ-cell tumors
    doxorubicin for, 128
    vinblastine for, 359
Gestational trophoblastic neoplasia, dactin-
    omycin for, 101
Giant follicular lymphoma, chlorambucil
    for, 79
Gleevec, 193
Gliadel, 74
Glioblastoma
    carmustine for, 74
    doxorubicin hydrochloride, liposomal,
      for, 132
    procarbazine for, 306
Glioblastoma multiforme
    temozolomide for, 329
    thalidomide for, 335
Glioma
    erlotinib for, 146
    imatinib for, 193
    temozolomide for, 329
Gloves, 17
Glucose, normal value for, 466
GM-CSF, 316-318
Gonadal cancer, gemcitabine for, 172
goserelin acetate, 7, 176-177, 440
Gowns, 17
G_1 phase, of cell cycle, 3
G_2 phase, of cell cycle, 3
Graft-versus-host disease, denileukin difti-
    tox for, 110

granisetron hydrochloride, 177-179
Granulocytopenia, amifostine for, 40
GT regimen, 381-382
Gynecologic cancers
    doxorubicin hydrochloride, liposomal,
      for, 132
    megestrol for, 236

H

Hair coverings, 18
Hairy cell leukemia
    cladribine for, 87
    interferon alfa-2a, recombinant, for, 196
    interferon alfa-2b for, 199
    interferon alfa-n3 for, 202
    pentostatin for, 297
Hazardous drug exposure
    accidental, 21-22
    potential effects of, 12-15
    routes for, 14-15
Hazardous drugs, 11-22
    administration area for, 16
    compounding, 16
    defining, 12-14
    disposal of, 19
    guidelines for handling, 11
    labeling, packaging, and storing, 15-16
    list of, 13
    preparation environment for, 16
    preparing and administering, 20-22
    safe handling program for, 15-19
    transporting, 16
    waste management for, 19
Hazardous drug spills, 18-19
HDAC regimen, 371
Head and neck cancer
    amifostine for, 40
    cetuximab for, 77
    cisplatin for, 406, 407
    cyclophosphamide for, 94
    docetaxel for, 124
    doxorubicin for, 128

Head and neck cancer (continued)
  doxorubicin hydrochloride, liposomal,
    for, 132
  drugs in development for, 490
  5-fluorouracil for, 407
  hydroxyurea for, 184
  ifosfamide for, 191
  isotretinoin for, 210
  methotrexate for, 250
  oxaliplatin for, 279
  paclitaxel for, 285
  regimens for, 406-407
  vinblastine for, 359
Hematocrit, normal value for, 466
Hematology studies, normal, 466
Hemoglobin, normal value for, 466
Hemorrhagic cystitis
  estrogens, conjugated, for, 150
  mesna for, 245
Hepatobiliary cancer
  drugs in development for, 490
  5-fluorouracil for, 407, 408
  gemcitabine for, 408
  leucovorin for, 408
  regimens for, 407-409
Hepatocellular carcinoma
  doxorubicin for, 128
  epirubicin for, 140
  tamoxifen for, 327
Herceptin, 350
Hexadrol, 112
Hexadrol Phosphate, 112
Hexalen, 38
Hiccups, intractable
  chlorpromazine for, 82
  metoclopramide for, 258
Histiocytic lymphoma, cyclophosphamide
    for, 93
Histiocytosis, vinblastine for, 359
histrelin acetate implant, 179-180
HLFP regimen, 398
HN₂, 230
Hodgkin's disease
  bleomycin for, 61, 409, 410

Hodgkin's disease (continued)
  carmustine for, 74
  chlorambucil for, 79
  cyclophosphamide for, 93, 409
  cytarabine for, 97
  dacarbazine for, 99, 409
  doxorubicin for, 128, 409, 410
  epirubicin for, 140
  etoposide for, 153, 409, 410
  gemcitabine for, 172
  ifosfamide for, 191
  lomustine for, 225
  mechlorethamine for, 231, 410
  prednisone for, 303, 409, 410
  procarbazine for, 305, 409
  regimens for, 409-410
  thiotepa for, 340
  vinblastine for, 359, 409, 410
  vincristine for, 362, 409, 410
Hormonal antineoplastics, 6-7
Hycamtin, 342
Hydatidiform mole, methotrexate for, 249
Hydrea, 184
hydrocodone bitartrate and ibuprofen,
    180-182
hydromorphone hydrochloride, 182-184
Hydrostat IR, 182
hydroxyurea, 184-186, 398
Hypercalcemia
  methylprednisolone for, 255
  plicamycin for, 299
Hypercalciuria, plicamycin for, 299
Hyper CVAD regimen, 429-430
Hy-Phen, 28
Hyrexin, 119

I

ibritumomab tiuxetan, 6, 186-188
ICM regimen, 386-387
Idamycin PFS, 189
idarubicin hydrochloride, 189-191, 370
Ifex, 191

Ifex/Mesnex, 191
IFL/BV regimen, 392-393
IFLrA, 196-198
IFL regimen, 393
IFN-alfa 2, 198-202
IFN regimen, 442
ifosfamide, 191-193
  as regimen component
    for bladder cancer, 374
    for bone sarcoma, 376
    for cervical cancer, 386
    for non-Hodgkin's lymphoma, 428
    for soft-tissue sarcoma, 445, 447
    for testicular cancer, 449, 450, 451
    for uterine cancer for, 454, 455
I.M. administration, of hazardous drugs, 21
imatinib mesylate, 6, 193-196, 387, 446
Imodium, 227
Imodium A-D, 227
Inapsine, 137
Infection
  filgrastim for, 159
  pegfilgrastim for, 293
Infumorph, 267
In-111 Zevalin, 186
interferon alfa-2a, recombinant, 196-198, 411
interferon alfa-2b, recombinant, 198-202, 388, 442
interferon alfa-n3, 202-203
interleukin-2, 411, 441
International Normalized Ratio, normal value for, 466
Intracavitary effusion, thiotepa for, 340
Intracranial tumor, vincristine for, 362
Intron A, 198
Iressa, 170
irinotecan hydrochloride, 203-310
  as regimen component
    for colon, rectal, anal cancers, 390, 392, 393
    for esophageal cancer, 397
    for gastric cancer, 404
    for lung cancer, 421

Iron administration, for anemia, 475
Iron studies, normal, 466
Islet-cell carcinoma, dacarbazine for, 99
isotretinoin, 210-213
ITP regimen, 374-375
IVAC regimen, 428
I.V. administration, of hazardous drugs, 20
I.V. tubing, contaminated, disposal of, 19

J
Jelliffe method, for creatinine clearance calculation, 467

K
Kadian, 267
kaolin and pectin, 213-214
Kaopectate II, 227
Kapectolin, 213
Kaposi's sarcoma
  bleomycin for, 61
  daunorubicin citrate liposome for, 105
  doxorubicin hydrochloride, liposomal, for, 132
  interferon alfa-2b for, 199
  interferon alfa-n3 for, 202
  paclitaxel for, 285
  thalidomide for, 335
  vinblastine for, 359
  vincristine for, 362
Karnofsky performance index, 469
Kidney cancer
  drugs in development for, 490
  floxuridine for, 162
  interferon alfa-2a for, 411
  interferon alfa-n3 for, 202
  interleukin-2 for, 411
  lomustine for, 225
  medroxyprogesterone for, 234
  regimens for, 411-412
  vinblastine for, 411

K-P, 213
Kytril, 177

L

Labeling, for hazardous drugs, 15-16
Laboratory values, normal, 466-467
LED, 131-135
lenalidomide, 214-216
Lethargy, modafinil for, 266
letrozole, 7, 216-218
leucovorin calcium, 218-220
    as regimen component
        for bone sarcoma, 377
        for colon, rectal, anal cancers, 389,
            391, 392, 393
        for esophageal cancer, 398
        for gastric cancer, 402, 403, 404, 405
        for hepatobiliary cancer, 408
Leukemia. *See also specific type.*
    clofarabine for, 90
    daunorubicin citrate liposome for, 105
    dexamethasone for, 112
    methylprednisolone for, 255
    prednisone for, 303
    vincristine for, 362
Leukeran, 79
Leukine, 316
leuprolide acetate, 7, 220-222, 440
Leustatin, 87
Levo-Dromoran, 222
levorphanol tartrate, 222-224
Lipase, normal value for, 467
Lipid values, normal, 467
liposomal encapsulated doxorubicin, 131-
    135
Liquid Pred, 303
Liver cancer
    floxuridine for, 161
    vincristine for, 362
Liver function values, normal, 467
Logen, 121
Lomanate, 121

Lomotil, 121
lomustine, 224-227, 388
Lonox, 121
loperamide hydrochloride, 227-228
Lorazepam Intensol, 228
lorazepam, 228-230
L-PAM, 237
Lung cancer
    drugs in development for, 490
    non-small-cell
        amifostine for, 40
        bevacizumab for, 55
        carboplatin for, 71, 412, 418
        cisplatin for, 412, 413, 414
        docetaxel for, 123, 412, 414, 415
        epirubicin for, 140
        erlotinib for, 146, 415
        etoposide for, 153
        gefitinib for, 170
        gemcitabine for, 172, 413, 415, 416
        ifosfamide for, 191
        irinotecan for, 205
        lomustine for, 225
        oxaliplatin for, 279
        paclitaxel for, 285, 412, 414, 416
        pemetrexed for, 295
        porfimer for, 301
        procarbazine for, 306
        regimens for, 412-417
        topotecan for, 342
        vinblastine for, 359
        vinorelbine for, 364, 416, 417
    small-cell
        altretamine for, 38
        cisplatin for, 419, 420, 421
        cyclophosphamide for, 94, 417, 419
        docetaxel for, 123
        doxorubicin for, 417, 419
        epirubicin for, 140
        etoposide for, 417, 418, 419, 420
        etoposide for, 152
        imatinib for, 193
        irinotecan for, 421
        methotrexate for, 250

Lung cancer, small-cell *(continued)*
    paclitaxel for, 418
    procarbazine for, 306
    regimens for, 417-422
    teniposide for, 331
    topotecan for, 342, 421
    vincristine for, 362, 419
Lupron, 220
Lupron Depot, 220
Lymphocytic leukemia, vinblastine for, 359
Lymphocytic lymphoma, cyclophos-
    phamide for, 93
Lymphoid malignancies, isotretinoin for,
    210
Lymphomas. *See also specific type.*
  cisplatin for, 85
  dexamethasone for, 112
  doxorubicin for, 128
  methylprednisolone for, 255
  thiotepa for, 340
  vinblastine for, 359
Lymphomatous meningitis, cytarabine for,
    96
Lymphosarcoma
  chlorambucil for, 79
  mechlorethamine for, 231
  methotrexate for, 250
Lysodren, 261

M

Magnesium, normal value for, 466
MAID regimen, 447-448, 455-456
Malignant melanoma
  aldesleukin for, 33
  bleomycin for, 61
  carmustine for, 74
  dacarbazine for, 99
  interferon alfa-2b for, 199
  interferon alfa-n3 for, 202
Marinol, 135
Material Safety Data Sheet, 12, 15
Matulane, 305

Mayo regimen, 389
MCF regimen, 398-399
mechlorethamine hydrochloride, 230-234,
    410
Medical surveillance, hazardous drug safety
    program and, 22
Medrol Dosepak, 255
medroxyprogesterone acetate, 234-235
Medulloblastoma, carmustine for, 74
Megace, 235
Megace ES, 235
megestrol acetate, 7, 235-237
Melanoma
  cisplatin for, 85
  drugs in development for, 490
  lomustine for, 225
  temozolomide for, 329
  vinblastine for, 359
melphalan, 237-240, 423
Meningeal leukemia
  cytarabine for, 96
  methotrexate for, 249
Meningitis, carcinomatous, thiotepa for,
    340
meperidine hydrochloride, 240-242
mercaptopurine, 242-245
mesna for, 454, 455
mesna, 245-247
  as regimen component
    for cervical cancer, 386
    for soft-tissue sarcoma, 445, 447
    for testicular cancer, 449, 450, 451
Mesnex, 245
Mesothelioma
  cisplatin for, 85
  malignant pleural, pemetrexed for, 295
Metastatic carcinoid syndrome, ocreotide
    for, 274
Metastron, 324
methadone hydrochloride, 247-249
methotrexate sodium, 249-255
  as regimen component
    for bladder cancer, 372, 375
    for bone sarcoma, 377

methotrexate sodium, as regimen component (*continued*)
   for breast cancer, 378
   for gastric cancer, 403
   for non-Hodgkin's lymphoma, 428, 429, 432
Methotrexate overdose, leucovorin for, 218
Methylpred DP, 255
methylprednisolone, 255-257
methylprednisolone acetate, 255-257
methylprednisolone sodium succinate, 255-257
Meticorten, 303
metoclopramide hydrochloride, 257-259
mFOLFOX6 regimen, 392
Mithracin, 299
mithramycin, 299-301
mitomycin, 259-261, 398
mitotane, 261-263
mitoxantrone hydrochloride, 263-266, 440
Mixed-cell type lymphoma, cyclophosphamide for, 93
modafinil, 266-267
Monoclonal antibodies, 6
morphine sulfate, 267-271
Mostellar calculation, for body surface area, 461
M-Oxy, 281
M phase, of cell cycle, 3
MS Contin, 267
MSIR, 267
MS/S, 267
Mucositis
   amifostine for, 40
   kaolin and pectin for, 213
   sucralfate for, 326
   supportive therapy for, 482-483
Multiple myeloma
   arsenic trioxide for, 46
   bortezomib for, 63, 422
   carmustine for, 74
   cyclophosphamide for, 93

Multiple myeloma (*continued*)
   daunorubicin citrate liposome for, 106
   dexamethasone for, 112, 113, 423, 424, 425
   doxorubicin for, 128, 422, 423, 425
   doxorubicin hydrochloride, liposomal, for, 132
   drugs in development for, 490
   interferon alfa-n3 for, 202
   lomustine for, 225
   melphalan for, 237, 423
   prednisone for, 423
   regimens for, 422-425
   thalidomide for, 335, 423, 424
   vincristine for, 422, 423, 425
Mustargen, 230
Mutamycin, 259
MVAC regimen, 375
Mycosis fungoides
   cyclophosphamide for, 93
   interferon alfa-n3 for, 202
   lomustine for, 225
   mechlorethamine for, 231
   methotrexate for, 250
   pentostatin for, 297
   vinblastine for, 359
Myelodysplastic syndrome
   amifostine for, 40
   arsenic trioxide for, 47
   azacitidine for, 51, 425
   decitabine for, 425
   drugs in development for, 490
   filgrastim for, 160
   lenalidomide for, 214
   regimens for, 425-426
   topotecan for, 342
Myelosuppression, managing, 8-9
Myleran, 65
Mylocel, 184
Mylotarg, 174

N

National Institute for Occupational Safety
and Health, 11, 13
Nausea and vomiting, 9
 aprepitant for, 45
 chlorpromazine for, 82
 dexamethasone for, 113
 diphenhydramine for, 119
 dolasetron for, 126, 127
 dronabinol for, 136
 droperidol for, 138
 granisetron for, 178
 lorazepam for, 229
 methylprednisolone for, 255
 metoclopramide for, 257, 258
 ondansetron for, 276, 277
 palonosetron for, 290
 prochlorperazine for, 308
 promethazine for, 310
 supportive therapy for, 470-473
 trimethobenzamide for, 354
Navelbine, 364
Navogan, 354
Needles, contaminated, disposal of, 19
Neosar, 93
Nephroblastoma, vincristine for, 362
Neulasta, 293
Neupogen, 159
Neuroblastoma
 cyclophosphamide for, 93
 doxorubicin for, 128
 etoposide for, 153
 ifosfamide for, 191
 teniposide for, 331
Neuroendocrine tumors, regimens for, 426-
427
Neurotoxicity, drug-induced, amifostine
for, 40
Neutropenia
 degrees of, 468
 filgrastim for, 159, 160
 managing, 8
 pegfilgrastim for, 293

Neutropenia (continued)
 supportive therapy for, 477-479
Neutrophil recovery, sargramostim for, 316
Nexavar, 320
Nilandron, 271
nilutamide, 7, 271-273
nilutamide, 7
Nipent, 297
nitrogen mustard, 230
Nitrogen mustards, 5
Nitrosoureas, 5
Nolvadex, 327
Non-Hodgkin's lymphoma
 aldesleukin for, 33
 bleomycin for, 61
 bortezomib for, 64
 carmustine for, 74
 chlorambucil for, 427
 cladribine for, 87
 cyclophosphamide for, 427, 428, 429,
430, 431, 432
 cytarabine for, 97, 428, 429, 432
 denileukin diftitox for, 110
 dexamethasone for, 429, 432
 doxorubicin for, 427, 428, 429, 430,
431, 432
 drugs in development for, 490
 epirubicin for, 140
 etoposide for, 428, 431
 fludarabine for, 163, 429
 gemcitabine for, 172
 ibritumomab tiuxetan for, 186
 ifosfamide for, 191, 428
 interferon alfa-2a, recombinant, for, 196
 interferon alfa-2b for, 199
 interferon alfa-n3 for, 202
 lomustine for, 225
 melphalan for, 238
 methotrexate for, 428, 429, 432
 mitoxantrone for, 264
 prednisone for, 303, 427, 430
 procarbazine for, 306
 regimens for, 427-432
 rituximab for, 314, 429, 430, 431, 432

Non-Hodgkin's lymphoma (*continued*)
  teniposide for, 331
  tositumomab for, 346
  vincristine for, 362, 427, 428, 429, 430, 431, 432
Nonmyeloid cancers, filgrastim for, 159
Novantrone, 263

O

Occupational Safety & Health Administration, 11
ocreotide acetate, 273-276
Oncaspar, 291
Oncology drugs. *See also* Chemotherapy.
  classifying, 3-7
  developmental, 489-490
  hazardous. *See* Hazardous drugs.
  phase-nonspecific, 5
  phase-specific, 4-5
  unclassified, 5-7
Oncology Nursing Society, 11
Oncovin, 362
ondansetron hydrochloride, 276-278
Online resources, 492-494
Ontak, 110
Onxol, 285
Oral administration, of hazardous drugs, 21
Oramorph SR, 267
Orasone, 303
Osteosarcoma, 101
  cisplatin for, 85
  etoposide for, 153
  ifosfamide for, 191
  methotrexate for, 250
Ovarian cancer
  altretamine for, 38
  amifostine for, 40
  carboplatin for, 71, 433, 434, 435
  cisplatin for, 85, 433, 436
  cyclophosphamide for, 93, 94, 433
  docetaxel for, 123, 124, 434

Ovarian cancer (*continued*)
  doxorubicin for, 128
  doxorubicin hydrochloride, liposomal, for, 132
  drugs in development for, 491
  epirubicin for, 140
  etoposide for, 433
  floxuridine for, 162
  gemcitabine for, 172
  hydroxyurea for, 184
  ifosfamide for, 191
  interferon alfa-n3 for, 202
  irinotecan for, 205
  leuprolide for, 221
  megestrol for, 236
  melphalan for, 238
  oxaliplatin for, 279
  paclitaxel for, 285, 435, 436
  regimens for, 433-436
  sorafenib for, 320
  thiotepa for, 340
  topotecan for, 342
  vincristine for, 362
  vinorelbine for, 364
oxaliplatin, 278-281
  as regimen component
    for colon, rectal, anal cancers, 391, 394
    for gastric cancer, 403
    for prostate cancer, 438
oxycodone hydrochloride, 281-285
OxyContin, 281
Oxydose, 281
OxyFast, 281
OxyIR, 281

P

Packaging, for hazardous drugs, 15-16
paclitaxel, 285-288
  as regimen component
    for bladder cancer, 374, 375, 376
    for breast cancer, 378, 381, 382

paclitaxel, as regimen component
(continued)
for cervical cancer, 384, 387
for esophageal cancer, 395, 399
for gastric cancer, 405
for lung cancer, 412, 414, 416, 418
for ovarian cancer, 435, 436
for prostate cancer, 440
for testicular cancer, 449
for uterine cancer, 453, 456
paclitaxel protein-bound particles, 288-290
Paclitaxel-induced neurotoxicity, amifostine
for, 40
Pain
abarelix for, 25
acetaminophen and codeine for, 27
acetaminophen and hydrocodone for, 29
acetaminophen and oxycodone for, 31
codeine for, 92
fentanyl for, 157
hydrocodone and ibuprofen for, 180
hydromorphone for, 182
levorphanol for, 222
meperidine for, 240
methadone for, 247
mitoxantrone for, 263
morphine for, 268
oxycodone for, 281, 282
prednisone for, 304
strontium chloride Sr 89 for, 324
tramadol for, 348
palonosetron hydrochloride, 290-291
Pancreatic cancer
capecitabine for, 436
cisplatin for, 437
doxorubicin for, 128
drugs in development for, 491
erlotinib for, 146
5-fluorouracil for, 165, 438
gemcitabine for, 171, 437, 438
irinotecan for, 205
mitomycin for, 260
ocreotide for, 274
oxaliplatin for, 438

Pancreatic cancer (continued)
regimens for, 436-438
sorafenib for, 320
streptozocin for, 322
Pancreatic enzymes, normal values for, 467
Paraplatin, 71
Parathyroid hormone, intact, normal value
for, 467
Partial thromboplastin time, normal value
for, 466
Patient, managing, during chemotherapy,
8-9
Patient care resources, 494
PC regimen, 376
PCV regimen, 388-389
pegaspargase, 7, 291-293
pegfilgrastim, 293-294
pemetrexed, 294-296
Pentazine, 310
pentostatin, 297-299
Pepto Diarrhea Control, 227
Percocet-2.5/325, 31
Percocet-5/325, 31
Percocet-7.5/325, 31
Percocet-7.5/500, 31
Percocet-10/325, 31
Percocet-10/650, 31
Percolone, 281
PE regimen, 440-441
Performance scales, 469
Phenaphen with Codeine No. 2, 26
Phenaphen with Codeine No. 3, 26
Phenaphen with Codeine No. 4, 26
Phenergan, 310
Phenoject-50, 310
Pheochromocytoma
dacarbazine for, 99
vincristine for, 362
Phosphorus, normal value for, 466
Photodynamic therapy, 10
Photofrin, 301
Platelet count, normal value for, 466
Platinol-AQ, 84
Platinum agents, 5

Plenaxis, 25
Pleural effusion, malignant, bleomycin for, 61
plicamycin, 299-301
Polycythemia vera, mechlorethamine for, 231
porfimer sodium, 301-303
Potassium, normal value for, 466
prednisone, 303-305
    as regimen component
        for Hodgkin's disease, 409, 410
        for multiple myeloma, 423
        for non-Hodgkin's lymphoma, 427, 430
        for prostate cancer, 439, 440
Pregnancy, effect of hazardous drug exposure on, 12
Premarin, 149
Premarin Intravenous, 149
procarbazine hydrochloride, 305-308, 388, 409
prochlorperazine, 308-310
Procot, 308
Procrit, 143
Progenitor cell mobilization
    filgrastim for, 159
    sargramostim for, 316
Progenitor cell transplantation, busulfan for, 66
Proleukin, 32
promethazine hydrochloride, 310-312
Promethegan, 310
Prostate cancer
    abarelix for, 25
    aminoglutethimide for, 42
    bicalutamide for, 59, 440
    cyclophosphamide for, 94
    dexamethasone for, 112
    docetaxel for, 123, 438, 439
    doxorubicin for, 128
    doxorubicin hydrochloride, liposomal, for, 132
    drugs in development for, 491
    epirubicin for, 140

Prostate cancer (continued)
    estramustine for, 148, 438, 439, 440
    estrogens, conjugated, for, 150
    flutamide for, 167, 440
    goserelin for, 176, 440
    histrelin acetate implant for, 179
    imatinib for, 193
    leuprolide for, 221, 440
    megestrol for, 236
    mitoxantrone for, 263, 440
    nilutamide for, 271
    paclitaxel for, 286, 440
    prednisone for, 303, 304, 439, 440
    regimens for, 438-441
    thalidomide for, 335
    triptorelin for, 356, 440
    vinblastine for, 439,
Protective equipment, personal, 17-19
Protein, normal value for, 466
Prothrombin time, normal value for, 466
Protocols, chemotherapy, 7. See also Regimens.
Provera, 234
Provigil, 266
Purine analogues, 4
Purinethol, 242
PVB regimen, 449-450
Pyrimidine analogues, 4

Q

Q-Dryl, 119

R

raloxifene hydrochloride, 312-313
Rapi-Ject, 267
Reconstitution, of hazardous drugs, 20
Rectal cancer. See Colorectal cancer.
Red blood cell count, normal value for, 466
Red blood cell indices, normal value for, 466

Regimens
  for acute myeloid leukemia, 370-372
    AIDA, 370
    cytarabine, daunorubicin, 370-371
    gemtuzumab, 371
    HDAC, 371
    idarubicin, cytarabine, 371, 372
  for bladder cancer, 372-376
    cisplatin, docetaxel, 372
    CMV, 372-373
    gemcitabine, 373
    gemcitabine, cisplatin, 373-374
    ITP, 374-375
    MVAC, 375
    paclitaxel, 375
    paclitaxel, gemcitabine, 375-376
    PC, 376
  for bone sarcoma, 376-377
    CAV, 376-377
    CAV with IE, 376-377
    methotrexate, leucovorin, 377
  for breast cancer, 377-383
    AC, 377-378
    bevacizumab, paclitaxel, 378
    CAF, 380-381
    capecitabine, 378
    CMF, 378-379
    docetaxel, 379
    doxorubicin, 380
    epirubicin, 380
    FAC, 380-381
    FEC-100, 381
    GT, 381-382
    paclitaxel, 382
    pegylated liposomal doxorubicin, 382
    trastuzumab, vinorelbine, 382-383
  for cervical cancer, 383-387
    carboplatin, 383
    cisplatin, 384
    cisplatin, paclitaxel, 384
    cisplatin, topotecan, 384
    docetaxel, 384-385
    gemcitabine, cisplatin, 386
    ICM, 386-387

Regimens, for cervical cancer *(continued)*
    paclitaxel, 387
  for chronic myelogenous leukemia, 387-388
    imatinib, 387-388
    interferon alfa-2b, cytarabine, 388
  for CNS tumors, 388-389
    carmustine, 388
    PCV, 388-389
    temozolomide, 389
  for colon, rectal, and anal cancers, 389-394
    5-fluorouracil, 391
    5-fluorouracil, leucovorin, 389-390
    5-fluorouracil, leucovorin, oxaliplatin combinations, 391-392
    capecitabine, 390
    cetuximab, 390
    cetuximab, irinotecan, 390-391
    IFL/BV, 392-393
    irinotecan, 393
    irinotecan, leucovorin, 5-fluorouracil combinations, 393-394
    XELOX, 394
  de Gramont, 389
  Douillard, 393
  for esophageal cancer, 395-400
    cisplatin, 5-fluorouracil, 395
    cisplatin, paclitaxel, 395-396
    cisplatin, vinorelbine, 396-397
    CPT-11 + CDDP, 397
    ECF, 397-398
    HLFP, 398
    MCF, 398-399
    paclitaxel, 399
    paclitaxel, cisplatin, 5-fluorouracil, 399-400
  FOLFIRI, 393
  FOLFOX4, 391
  FOLFOX6, 391
  FOLFOX7, 392
  for gastric cancer, 400-406
    DCF, 400-401
    DXP, 401

Regimens, for gastric cancer (*continued*)
    ECF, 401-402
    ELF, 402
    FAMTX, 403
    FOLFOX6, 403-404
    FUP, 404
    irinotecan, 5-fluorouracil, leucovorin,
      404-405
    paclitaxel, cisplatin, 5-fluorouracil,
      leucovorin, 405-406
    TC, 406
    TCF, 400-401
  for head and neck cancer, 406-407
    cisplatin, 406-407
    cisplatin, 5-fluorouracil, 407
  for hepatobiliary cancer, 407-409
    5-fluorouracil, 407-408
    5-fluorouracil, leucovorin, 408
    gemcitabine, 408-409
  for Hodgkin's disease, 409-410
    ABVD, 409
    BEACOPP, 409-410
    Stanford V, 410
  IFL, 393
  for kidney cancer, 411-412
    interferon alfa-2a, interleukin-2, 411
    interleukin-2, 411
    vinblastine, interferon alfa-2a, 411-
      412
  for lung cancer, 412-422
    ACE, 417-418
    CAE, 417-418
    carboplatin, etoposide, 418
    carboplatin, paclitaxel, 412
    carboplatin, paclitaxel, etoposide,
      418-419
    CAV, 419
    CAV with EP, 419-420
    cisplatin, docetaxel, 412-413
    cisplatin, etoposide, 420-421
    cisplatin, gemcitabine, 413-414
    cisplatin, paclitaxel, 414
    docetaxel, 414-415
    erlotinib, 415

Regimens, for lung cancer (*continued*)
    gemcitabine, 415
    gemcitabine, docetaxel, 415-416
    gemcitabine, paclitaxel, 416
    gemcitabine, vinorelbine, 416-417
    irinotecan, cisplatin, 421
    topotecan, 421-422
    vinorelbine, 417
  Mayo, 389
  mFOLFOX6, 392
  for multiple myeloma, 422-425
    bortezomib, 422
    Dvd, 422-423
    Dvd-T, 423
    MP, 423-424
    thalidomide, 424
    thalidomide, dexamethasone, 424
    VAD, 425
  for myelodysplastic syndrome, 425-426
    azacitidine, 425
    decitabine, 425-426
  for neuroendocrine tumors, 426-427
    5-fluorouracilo, dacarbazine, epiru-
      bicin, 426-427
    doxorubicin, streptozocin, 426
  for non-Hodgkin's lymphoma, 427-432
    chlorambucil, 427
    CHOP, 427-428
    CODOX-M, 428-429
    fludarabine, rituximab, 429
    hyper CVAD, 429-430
    rituximab, 430
    rituximab/CHOP, 430-431
    rituximab/EPOCH, 431-432
    rituximab/hyper CVAD, 432
  for ovarian cancer, 433-436
    carboplatin, cyclophosphamide,
      433
    cisplatin, etoposide, 433-434
    docetaxel, 434
    docetaxel, carboplatin, 434
    paclitaxel, 435
    paclitaxel, carboplatin. 435-436
    paclitaxel, cisplatin, 436

Regimens (*continued*)
  for pancreatic cancer, 436-438
    5-fluorouracil, 438
    capecitabine, 436-437
    gemcitabine, 437
    gemcitabine, cisplatin, 437-438
    gemcitabine, oxaliplatin, 438
  for prostate cancer, 438-441
    docetaxel, estramustine, 438-439
    docetaxel, prednisone, 439
    estramustine, vinblastine, 439
    hormone therapy, 440
    mitoxantrone, prednisone, 440
    PE, 440-441
  Rosewell, 389
  Saltz, 393
  for skin cancer, 441-444
    aldesleukin, 441
    carboplatin, etoposide, 443
    cisplatin, etoposide, 443-444
    dacarbazine, 441-442
    IFN, 442
    temozolomide, 442
    topotecan, 444
  for soft-tissue sarcoma, 444-448
    AD, 444
    AIM, 445
    doxorubicin, 445
    gemcitabine, docetaxel, 445-446
    imatinib, 446
    liposomal doxorubicin, 447
    MAID, 447-448
  for testicular cancer, 448-451
    BEP, 448
    EP, 448-449
    paclitaxel, ifosfamide, cisplatin, mesna, 449
    PVB, 449-450
    VeIP, 450-451
    VIP, 451
  for thyroid cancer, 451-452
    CVD, 451-452
    dacarbazine, 5-fluorouracil, 452
  for uterine cancer, 452-456

Regimens, for uterine cancer (*continued*)
    CAP, 452-453
    cisplatin, doxorubicin, 453
    cisplatin, paclitaxel, 453-454
    doxorubicin, 454
    ifosfamide, 454-455
    ifosfamide, cisplatin, 455
    MAID, 455-456
    TAP, 456
Reglan, 257
Renal carcinoma. *See* Kidney cancer.
Renal cell carcinoma
  aldesleukin for, 33
  capecitabine for, 69
  erlotinib for, 146
  interferon alfa-2a, recombinant, for, 196
  interferon alfa-2b for, 199
  sorafenib for, 320
Renal toxicity, amifostine for, 40
Reproduction
  effect of chemotherapy on, 9
  effect of hazardous drug exposure on, 12
Resource Conservation and Recovery Act, 19
Resources, online, 492-494
Respiratory protection, 18
Retinoblastoma
  cyclophosphamide for, 93
  doxorubicin for, 129
Retinoids, 7
Revlimid, 214
Rhabdomyosarcoma
  dactinomycin for, 101
  etoposide for, 153
  vincristine for, 362
Rheumatrex Dose Pack, 249
rIFN-A, 196-198
Rituxan, 313
rituximab, 6, 313-315
  as regimen component, for non-Hodgkin's lymphoma, 429, 430, 431, 432
rituximab/CHOP regimen, 430-431
rituximab/EPOCH regimen, 431-432

rituximab/hyper CVAD regimen, 432
RMS, 267
Roferon-A, 196
Rosewell regimen, 389
Roxanol, 267
Roxanol-T, 267
Roxicet, 31
Roxicodone, 281
Roxilox, 31

S

Safe drug handling program, components
    of, 15-19
Salivary secretion disturbance, amifostine
    for, 40
Saltz regimen, 393
Sandostatin, 273
Sandostatin LAR Depot, 273
sargramostim, 316-318
Sézary syndrome, pentostatin for, 297
Sharps, contaminated, disposal of, 19
Shoe coverings, 18
Signal-transduction inhibitors, 6
Skeletal metastases, sodium phosphate P
    32 for, 319
Skin cancer
    aldesleukin for, 441
    carboplatin for, 443
    cisplatin for, 443
    dacarbazine for, 441
    etoposide for, 443
    interferon alfa-2b for, 442
    interleukin-2 for, 441
    regimens for, 441-444
    temozolomide for, 442
    topotecan for, 444
Small-molecule inhibitors, 6
Sodium, normal value for, 466
sodium phosphate P 32, 318-320
Soft-tissue sarcoma
    cisplatin for, 85
    dacarbazine for, 99, 444, 447

Soft-tissue sarcoma (continued)
    docetaxel for, 445
    doxorubicin for, 128, 444, 445, 447
    epirubicin for, 140
    etoposide for, 153
    gemcitabine for, 445
    ifosfamide for, 191, 445, 447
    imatinib for, 193, 446
    mesna for, 445, 447
    regimens for, 444-448
Solid cancers
    dactinomycin for, 101
    doxorubicin hydrochloride, liposomal,
      for, 132
    floxuridine for, 162
    fludarabine for, 164
Solu-Medrol, 255
Solurex, 112
Solurex LA, 112
Solutions, for drug and fluid administra-
    tion, codes for, 487
sorafenib, 320-322
Sotret, 210
S phase, of cell cycle, 3
Spill kit, 18
Spills, hazardous drug, 18-19
Squamous-cell carcinoma, bleomycin for, 61
Stagesic, 28
Stagesic-10, 28
Sterapred, 303
Stomatitis, sucralfate for, 326
Storage, of hazardous drugs, 15-16
streptozocin, 322-324
strontium chloride Sr 89, 324-325
Subcutaneous administration, of hazardous
    drugs, 21
sucralfate, 326-327
Supportive therapies, 470-483
    for anemia, 474-476
    for diarrhea, 480-481
    for febrile neutropenia, 477-479
    for mucositis, 482-483
    for nausea and vomiting, 470-473
Syringes, contaminated, disposal of, 19

T

Tabloid, 337
tamoxifen citrate, 7, 327-329
TAP regimen, 456
Tarceva, 146
Targeted cancer therapies, 6
Targretin, 57
Taxanes, 5
Taxol, 285
Taxotere, 123
TC regimen, 406
T-cell lymphoma, cutaneous
    bexarotene for, 57
    cladribine for, 87
    denileukin diftitox for, 110
    interferon alfa-2a, recombinant, for, 196
    isotretinoin for, 210
    mechlorethamine for, 231
    methotrexate for, 250
    pentostatin for, 297
TCF regimen, 400-401
Tebamide, 354
Tebamide Pediatric, 354
Temodar, 329
temozolomide, 329-330, 389, 442
teniposide, 331-333
Teslac, 333
Testicular cancer
    bleomycin for, 61, 448, 449
    cisplatin for, 85, 448, 449, 450, 451
    dactinomycin for, 101
    doxorubicin for, 128
    etoposide for, 152, 448, 451
    gemcitabine for, 172
    ifosfamide for, 191, 449, 450, 451
    mesna for, 449, 450, 451
    paclitaxel for, 449
    plicamycin for, 299
    regimens for, 448-451
    vinblastine for, 359, 449, 450
    vincristine for, 362
testolactone, 7, 333-334
T-Gesic, 28

thalidomide, 334-337, 423, 424
Thalomid, 334
TheraCys, 52
thioguanine, 337-339
thiotepa, 339-341
Thorazine, 81
Thorazine Spansule, 81
Thrombocytopenia
    amifostine for, 40
    managing, 9
    methylprednisolone for, 255
Thymic carcinoma, ifosfamide for, 191
Thymoma, ifosfamide for, 191
Thyroid cancer
    cyclophosphamide for, 451
    dacarbazine for, 451, 452
    doxorubicin for, 128
    5-fluorouracil for, 452
    regimens for, 451-452
    vincristine for, 451
Thyroid-stimulating hormone, normal val-
        ue for, 467
Thyroid studies, normal, 467
Thyrotropin-secreting tumors, ocreotide
        for, 274
Thyroxine, normal value for, 467
Tice BCG, 52
Tigan, 354
Tigan Adult, 354
Tigan Pediatric, 354
Topoisomerase inhibitors, type I, 5
Toposar, 152
topotecan hydrochloride, 342-343
    as regimen component
        for cervical cancer, 385
        for lung cancer, 421
        for skin cancer, 444
toremifene citrate, 7, 344-345
tositumomab, 345-348
tositumomab and iodine ^{131}I, 345-348
tramadol hydrochloride, 348-350
Transfer devices, drug, 16
Transferrin, normal value for, 467
trastuzumab, 350-352, 382

Trelstar Depot, 356
Trelstar LA, 356
tretinoin, 7, 352-354
Trexall, 249
Triazenes, 5
Triglycerides, normal values for, 467
Triiodothyronine, normal value for, 467
trimethobenzamide hydrochloride, 354-356
triptorelin pamoate, 7, 356-357, 440
Trisenox, 46
Trux-Adryl, 119
Tylenol with Codeine, 26
Tylenol with Codeine #2, 26
Tylenol with Codeine #3, 26
Tylenol with Codeine #4, 26
Tylox, 31

U

"U" list, of commercial chemicals, 19
Ultram, 348
Ureteral outlet obstruction, abarelix for, 25
Uric acid, normal value for, 466
Uterine cancer
  cisplatin for, 452, 453, 455, 456
  cyclophosphamide for, 452
  dacarbazine for, 455
  doxorubicin for, 452, 453, 454, 455, 456
  filgrastim for, 456
  ifosfamide for, 454, 455
  mesna for, 454, 455
  paclitaxel for, 453, 456
  regimens for, 452-456

V

VAD regimen, 425
valrubicin, 357-359
Valstar, 357
Value-Dryl, 119
Vanacet, 28

Vantas, 179
Vasoactive intestinal polypeptide tumors,
  ocreotide for, 273
VeIP regimen, 450-451
Velcade, 6, 63
Ventilation, for hazardous drug preparation, 16
VePesid, 152
Vesanoid, 352
Viadur, 220
Vicodin, 28
Vicodin ES, 28
Vicodin HP, 28
Vicoprofen, 180
Vidaza, 51
vinblastine sulfate, 359-361
  as regimen component
    for bladder cancer, 372, 375
    for Hodgkin's disease, 409, 410
    for kidney cancer, 411
    for prostate cancer, 439
    for testicular cancer, 449, 450
Vinca alkaloids, 4
Vincasar PFS, 362
vincristine sulfate, 362-364
  as regimen component
    for bone sarcoma, 376
    for CNS tumors, 388
    for Hodgkin's disease, 409, 410
    for lung cancer, 419
    for multople myeloma, 422, 423, 425
    for non-Hodgkin's lymphoma, 427,
      428, 429, 430, 431, 432
    for thyroid cancer, 451
vinorelbine tartrate, 364-366
  as regimen component
    for breast cancer, 382
    for esophageal cancer, 396
    for lung cancer, 416, 417
VIPomas, ocreotide for, 273
VIP regimen, 451
Vomiting. *See* Nausea and vomiting.
VP-16, 152-155
Vumon, 331

W

Waste, hazardous drug, managing, 19
White blood cell count, normal value for,
    466
White blood cell differential, normal value
    for, 466
Wilms' tumor
    dactinomycin for, 101
    doxorubicin for, 128
Winpred, 303

XYZ

Xeloda, 69
XELOX regimen, 394
Xerostomia, amifostine for, 40
Y-90 Zevalin, 186
Zanosar, 322
Zinecard, 115
Zofran, 276
Zofran ODT, 276
Zoladex, 176
Zydone, 28

The ELSEVIER Guide to ONC DRUGS

WWW.ONCOLOGYDRUGGUIDE.COM

New oncology drug approvals
New drugs in the pipeline

Calculating dosages
Monitoring laboratory values
Supportive therapy guidelines
  Managing CINV
  Managing Anemia
  Managing Neutropenia
  Managing Diarrhea
  Managing Stomatitis

Oncology drug codes
Links to best oncology websites

The companion website
The Elsevier Guide t

The all-purpose oncolog

Whether you're an oncologist
other professional working in
a wide range of your professi
formation required to prescrib
drugs safely and effectively.

  This website will keep you
help you stay up to date on th
pies used to treat cancer pati

Turn to oncologydrugguide

- accurate, up-to-date monog
- selected combination chemo
- information on newly approv
- HCPCS codes
- guidelines on managing che
- crucial laboratory values
- calculations to use for body
  absolute neutrophil count
- supportive therapies—incluc
  induced nausea and vomitin
  and mucositis
- patient teaching aids you ca

Your online source for reliable,
supportive care drugs